Thieme

The Craniotomy Atlas

Editor
Andreas Raabe, MD
Professor, Chairman, and Director
Department of Neurosurgery
Inselspital, Bern University Hospital
Bern, Switzerland

Associate Editors
Bernhard Meyer, MD
Professor, Chairman, and Director
Department of Neurosurgery
University Hospital rechts der Isar
Technical University of Munich
Munich, Germany

Karl Schaller, MD
Professor, Chairman, and Director
Division of Neurosurgery
Department of Clinical Neurosciences
University Hospital of Geneva
Geneva, Switzerland

Peter Vajkoczy, MD
Professor, Chairman, and Director
Department of Neurosurgery
Charité - Universitätsmedizin Berlin
Berlin, Germany

Peter A. Winkler, MD
Professor, Chairman, and Director
Department of Neurosurgery
University Hospital – Salzburg University
Salzburg, Austria

926 illustrations

Thieme
Stuttgart • New York • Delhi • Rio de Janeiro

Library of Congress Cataloging-in-Publication Data is available from the publisher

Important note: Medicine is an ever-changing science undergoing continual development. Research and clinical experience are continually expanding ourknowledge, in particular ourknowledge of proper treatment and drug therapy. Insofar as this book mentions any dosage or application, readers may rest assured that the authors, editors, and publishers have made every effort to ensure that such references are in accordance with **the state of knowledge at the time of production of the book.**

Nevertheless, this does not involve, imply, or express any guarantee or responsibility on the part of the publishers in respect to any dosage instructions and forms of applications stated in the book. **Every user is requested to examine carefully** the manufacturers' leaflets accompanying each drug and to check, if necessary in consultation with a physician or specialist, whether the dosage schedules mentioned therein or the contraindications stated by the manufacturers differ from the statements made in the present book. Such examination is particularly important with drugs that are either rarely used or have been newly released on the market. Every dosage schedule or every form of application used is entirely at the user's own risk and responsibility. The authors and publishers request every user to report to the publishers any discrepancies or inaccuracies noticed. If errors in thiswork are foundafter publication, errata will be posted atwww. thieme.com on the product description page.

Some of the product names, patents, and registered designs referred to in this book are in fact registered trademarks or proprietary names even though specific reference to this fact is not always made in the text. Therefore, the appearance of a name without designation as proprietary is not to be construed as a representation by the publisher that it is in the public domain.

Thieme Publishers Stuttgart
Rüdigerstrasse 14, 70469 Stuttgart, Germany
+49 [0]711 8931 421, customerservice@thieme.de

Thieme Publishers New York
333 Seventh Avenue, New York, NY 10001 USA
+1 800 782 3488, customerservice@thieme.com

Thieme Publishers Delhi
A-12, Second Floor, Sector-2, Noida-201301
Uttar Pradesh, India
+91 120 45 566 00, customerservice@thieme.in

Thieme Publishers Rio de Janeiro,
Thieme Publicações Ltda.
Edifício Rodolpho de Paoli, 25° andar
Av. Nilo Peçanha, 50 – Sala 2508
Rio de Janeiro 20020-906 Brasil
+55 21 3172 2297

MIX
Papier aus verantwortungsvollen Quellen
FSC www.fsc.org FSC® C089473

Cover design: Thieme Publishing Group
Typesetting by DiTech Process Solutions, India

Printed in Germany by Beltz Grafische Betriebe

5 4 3 2

ISBN 978-3-13-205791-3

Also available as an e-book:
eISBN 978-3-13-205801-9

To my wonderful wife, Katrin; my children, Tanja, Max, and Clemens; my parents; my family, who are my life.
To my residents, who always inspire me.
To my colleagues, who are mentors, teachers, and friends.
To those who help to take care of my patients, making me feel grateful for their efforts.
To my patients, who trusted me and who were my reason to strive for excellence.

Andreas Raabe

Contents

Foreword

The Craniotomy Atlas, edited by Professor Raabe, is intended to be a resource for residents and new neurosurgeons with the goal of providing precise instructions for performing common neurosurgical exposures. Professor Raabe and his coauthors have used high-quality operative photographs accompanied by excellent illustrations to compile an atlas that far exceeds expectations. The beautiful step-by-step compilation for each approach will make this volume an essential companion for every neurosurgical resident and a useful reference for the new neurosurgeon. The precision and attention to detail that we have come to expect from Raabe has reached a new high in this book. With the introduction of intraoperative indocyanine green angiography to the neurosurgical community, Andreas Raabe had already cemented his place as a foremost contributor to our specialty—with this book, he will have created the neurosurgical primer that every resident will own and study.

As with any neurosurgical procedure, there are differences among neurosurgeons based on experience and training. For example, with the exception of the sigmoid sinus, I routinely cross all other sinuses by just using the footplate of the drill rather than multiple burr holes. After washing out the bone dust with irrigation, one can look right down the bone cut and verify that the footplate is extradural, and the dura can be separated from the bone by placing sufficient pressure on the underside of the bone while crossing the sinus as readily as with multiple burr holes and any other instrument. Although many roads lead to Rome, I find that this volume, except for a few inconsequential differences, provides the best highway to get there. I congratulate the authors for this detailed, beautifully illustrated, step-by-step guide to performing the routine craniotomies that all residents and neurosurgeons need to master.

Robert F. Spetzler, MD
Phoenix, Arizona
United States

Foreword

There is no doubt among neurosurgeons that a correct and tailored craniotomy, apart from the detailed preoperative planning, represents the decisive first step toward a successful intracranial operation. *The Craniotomy Atlas,* edited by Professor Andreas Raabe and compiled with contributions of a large number of experienced neurosurgeons, is primarily aimed at the neurosurgical resident and younger neurosurgeon. However, as a seasoned and experienced neurosurgeon, who has selected over the years his own armamentarium of favorite craniotomies and surgical variations, I have found it highly interesting to wander through the abundance of beautiful and detailed illustrations as well as the exact and informative step-by-step descriptions of the various craniotomies presented in this atlas. Although there exists a large number of neurosurgical textbooks with detailed descriptions of surgical approaches, these are mostly presented within the context of the underlying intracranial target, mainly a tumorous or vascular lesion.

I am not aware of a comparable and up-to-date compilation of craniotomies, covering all aspects—basic considerations such as positioning and attention to surgical landmarks, routine craniotomies, and elaborate skull base craniotomies and its extensions. The outstanding attention to details presented in this atlas reflects the meticulous way of preparation and performance of every craniotomy by Professor Raabe, as I have seen over the many years during which we have both worked together. Within this context, it is a pleasure and an honor to applaud the editor and his co-authors for this excellent contribution to the art of craniotomy, which will surely stand as a surgical reference for many years to come.

Volker Seifert, MD, PhD
Frankfurt
Germany

Preface

Craniotomies are an essential part of brain surgery. They are regarded as important but rather basic procedures that are the prelude to the intradural neurosurgical operation proper. An optimally placed craniotomy provides the basis for a simple or sophisticated intradural approach and a straightforward case. Wrongly placed, it completely changes the operation, making access to the neurosurgical target traumatic or impossible.

Neurosurgeons start with simple craniotomies early on in their training. Junior residents learn how to perform a specific craniotomy from senior residents or attendings. Many textbooks and journal articles describe the various craniotomies in detail and serve as excellent reference sources.

Despite being "mainstream" knowledge, for the first "Frankfurt craniotomy course" that Bernhard Meyer, Peter Vajkoczy, Peter Winkler, and I organized in 2004, there was an overwhelming number of applications for only 20 course seats. The applicants were searching for a systematic collection and teaching of information related to craniotomies. We learned from the course participants that craniotomies are far from being standardized, with numerous variations even within the same department. Since then, yearly courses have been held in Frankfurt and, since 2008, also in Bern and Geneva with an equally high number of applicants for the restricted number of available course seats.

This book is a logical effort to continue this teaching and extend the systematic collection of knowledge about standard and some extended craniotomies and related aspects. I hope that it contributes to a better understanding of the underlying concept and anatomy, greater standardization of the operations, and an improved technique when performing the planned craniotomy.

Andreas Raabe, MD

Acknowledgments

I would like to express my deep gratitude to Anja Giger and Alain Blank, who provided the superb illustrations for this book. Over a period of 3 years, it was always a pleasure to sit together and discuss the details of the authors' photographs and how these should be depicted in the illustrations. Without their artistic skills and their invaluable contribution, this book would not have been possible.

I am specifically grateful to Luisa Tonarelli, who accompanied the development of this book from the very first chapter to the final printed version. Her help, advice, expertise, and hard work were indispensable in bringing this volume to publication.

Finally, I would like to thank Susan Kaplan, Irena Zubak, Janine Abu-Isa, Katharina Lutz, Michael Murek, David Bervini, Johannes Goldberg, Levin Häni, and Jonathan Rychen for their time and advice during the review of the chapters of this book.

Andreas Raabe

Call for Submissions

The techniques and knowledge described in this book reflect the personal views, teaching, and experience of its authors. We know that the content of this book is far from comprehensive. We are also aware that skilled surgeons around the world have their own tricks and modifications of craniotomies, usually derived from personal experience and for good reasons.

Therefore, we invite authors to submit their modification, nuance, or technique in the form of a step-by-step series of photographs with a text description, like the chapters in this book. The topic may range from a craniotomy not yet included in this book to a technical note or a nuance of an already described craniotomy; however, it should be recognized as useful, reproducible, and potentially suitable for routine use. These submissions will undergo peer review by experienced neurosurgeons as well as young residents. If accepted, illustrations will be produced to complement the photographs, and a corresponding chapter will be added to the book.

We are aware that only a limited number of carefully selected additional chapters on a craniotomy or a nuance can be included in this collection. But, despite having arrived in the digital age, we still believe in the educational value of a book, in which a compilation of the most important craniotomies and the related knowledge can be found. All contributions have been peer-reviewed and selected as pearls of wisdom for neurosurgical residents.

Before submitting a manuscript, authors should contact the Editorial Office to request for the technical specifications and to have the topic checked for potential duplication and suitability.

Inquiries and submissions should be sent to:

Editorial Office Craniotomy Book
Department of Neurosurgery
Inselspital, University of Bern
3010 Bern
Switzerland
Email: craniotomyatlas@insel.ch

Contributors

Janine Abu-Isa, MD
Department of Neurosurgery
Inselspital, Bern University Hospital
Bern, Switzerland

Hugo Andrade-Barazarte, PhD
Juha Hernesniemi International Center for Neurosurgery
Henan People's Provincial Hospital
Zhengzhou, China

Jörg Baldauf, MD, PD
Department of Neurosurgery
University Medicine Greifswald
Greifswald, Germany

Jürgen Beck, MD
Professor and Medical Director
Department of Neurosurgery
Neurocenter
University of Freiburg
Freiburg, Germany

David Bervini, MD
Department of Neurosurgery
Inselspital, Bern University Hospital
Bern, Switzerland

Marco Caversaccio, MD
Professor, Chairman, and Director
Department of ENT, Head and Neck Surgery
Inselspital, Bern University Hospital
Bern, Switzerland

Mihai A. Constantinescu, MD
Professor, Chairman, and Director
Department of Plastic and Hand Surgery
Inselspital, Bern University Hospital
Bern, Switzerland

Philipp Dammann, MD
Department of Neurosurgery
University Hospital of Essen
Essen, Germany

Florian H. Ebner, MD
Professor
Department of Neurosurgery
University of Tübingen
Tübingen, Germany

Jens Fichtner, MD
Department of Neurosurgery
Inselspital, Bern University Hospital
Bern, Switzerland

Christian F. Freyschlag, MD
Department of Neurosurgery
University Hospital Innsbruck
Medical University of Innsbruck
Innsbruck, Austria

Christian Fung, MD
Department of Neurosurgery
Neurocenter
University of Freiburg
Freiburg, Germany

Johannes Goldberg, MD
Department of Neurosurgery
Inselspital, Bern University Hospital
Bern, Switzerland

Daniel Hänggi, MD
Professor, Chairman, and Director
Department of Neurosurgery
University Hospital Mannheim
University of Heidelberg
Mannheim, Germany

Levin Häni, MD
Department of Neurosurgery
Inselspital, Bern University Hospital
Bern, Switzerland

Juha Hernesniemi
Professor Emeritus, Former Chairman, and Director
Department of Neurosurgery
Helsinki University Hospital
University of Helsinki
Helsinki, Finland

Nikolai Hopf, MD
Professor and Director
NeuroChirurgicum
Center for Endoscopic and Minimally Invasive Neurosurgery
Stuttgart, Germany

Marton König
Department of Neurosurgery
Oslo University Hospital
University of Oslo
Oslo, Norway

Andreas Kramer, MD
Department of Neurosurgery
University of Mainz
Mainz, Germany

Sandro Krieg, MD, PD
Department of Neurosurgery
and TUM-Neuroimaging Center
University Hospital rechts der Isar
Technical University of Munich
Munich, Germany

Torstein R. Meling, MD
Professor
Division of Neurosurgery
Department of Clinical Neurosciences
University Hospital of Geneva
Geneva, Switzerland

Michael Murek, MD
Department of Neurosurgery
Inselspital, Bern University Hospital
Bern, Switzerland

Georgios Naros, MD
Department of Neurosurgery
University of Tübingen
Tübingen, Germany

Robert Reisch, MD
Professor
Endomin Center for Endoscopic and Minimally Invasive Neurosurgery
Hirslanden Clinic
Zurich, Switzerland

Florian Ringel, MD
Professor, Chairman, and Director
Department of Neurosurgery
University of Mainz
Mainz, Germany

Henry Schroeder, MD
Professor, Chairman, and Director
Department of Neurosurgery
University Medicine Greifswald
Greifswald, Germany

Philippe Schucht, MD
Department of Neurosurgery
Inselspital, Bern University Hospital
Bern, Switzerland

Ulrich Sure, MD
Professor, Chairman, and Director
Department of Neurosurgery
University Hospital of Essen
Essen, Germany

Marcos Tatagiba, MD
Professor, Chairman, and Director
Department of Neurosurgery
University of Tübingen
Tübingen, Germany

Claudius Thomé, MD
Professor, Chairman, and Director
Department of Neurosurgery
Medical University of Innsbruck
Innsbruck, Austria

Irena Zubak, MD
Department of Neurosurgery
Inselspital, Bern University Hospital
Bern, Switzerland

1 Basics

1.1 Craniotomies Overview

Andreas Raabe and Peter A. Winkler

There are four basic categories of supratentorial and infratentorial craniotomy:

1. Convexity craniotomies may be performed anywhere according to the surgical target and goal of the operation. They range from burr holes and mini-craniotomy to decompressive hemicraniectomy, which is the most extensive variant.
2. Midline craniotomies are used for midline approaches that take advantage of subdural anatomical corridors to reach superficial, deep, or contralateral targets. The supratentorial suboccipital craniotomy with an intradural approach along the falx and the tentorium or an infratentorial suboccipital craniotomy with a supracerebellar approach are possible variants.
3. Skull base craniotomies range from the frontal midline to the foramen magnum, covering the entire skull base. ▶Fig. 1.1 and ▶Fig. 1.2 demonstrate the continuum of approaches which are often overlapping and are named according to their location at the skull base.
4. Skull base extensions are added to standard skull base craniotomies. They allow access with angles of approach or to structures that cannot be easily reached with standard skull base craniotomies. Typical skull base extensions are anterior clinoidectomy, removal of the orbital rim or zygoma (orbitozygomatic), transpetrosal approaches, the suprameatal extension after retrosigmoid craniotomy or the far- (enough) lateral extension to the foramen magnum (see Chapter 6, Skull Base Extensions).

Supratentorial skull base craniotomies can be divided according to their location, their frontal and temporal extension (size), and their relation to the sylvian fissure. There is no uniform classification, but the following general rules may serve as a guide to the terminology (see ▶Table 1.1).

Table 1.1 Systematics of skull base craniotomies—supratentorial

Location	Description
Median frontobasal	Mostly bilateral. Target: medial frontal base, anterior midline.
Frontolateral	Extends 1–3 cm lateral to the midline to approximately the sphenoid wing, but does not cross it. The proximal sylvian fissure is exposed intradurally, and targets within the sylvian fissure, the anterior skull base, and the temporal lobe can be reached. There are mini- and standard sizes. "Frontolateral" is the term that was historically first used for this approach.
Supraorbital	Usually a smaller variant of the frontolateral approach; typically by eyebrow (transciliary) incision, which limits the size of the craniotomy. Extends 2.5–3 cm lateral to the midline to approximately the sphenoid wing, but does not cross it. The proximal sylvian fissure is exposed intradurally, and targets in the sylvian fissure, skull base, and temporal lobe can be reached. Some surgeons use the term supraorbital as synonymous with frontolateral.
Pterional	Extends 1–3 cm lateral to the midline to the anterior temporal region: centered around the "H" of the sutures that form the pterion (see Chapter 2.2, Craniocerebral Topography). The sphenoid wing is always crossed. Typically defined as two-thirds of the craniotomy frontal and one-third temporal exposure of variable sizes (2:1). There is also a mini-pterional variant.
Frontotemporal	Usually a large exposure (1:1 to 2:1 frontal:temporal) centered above the sphenoid wing = sylvian fissure.
Anterior temporal	Sphenoid wing is crossed.
Temporobasal	The exact position varies according to the surgical target: does not cross the sphenoid wing. Typically used for subtemporal intradural approaches. There may be a more anterior and a more posterior variant.

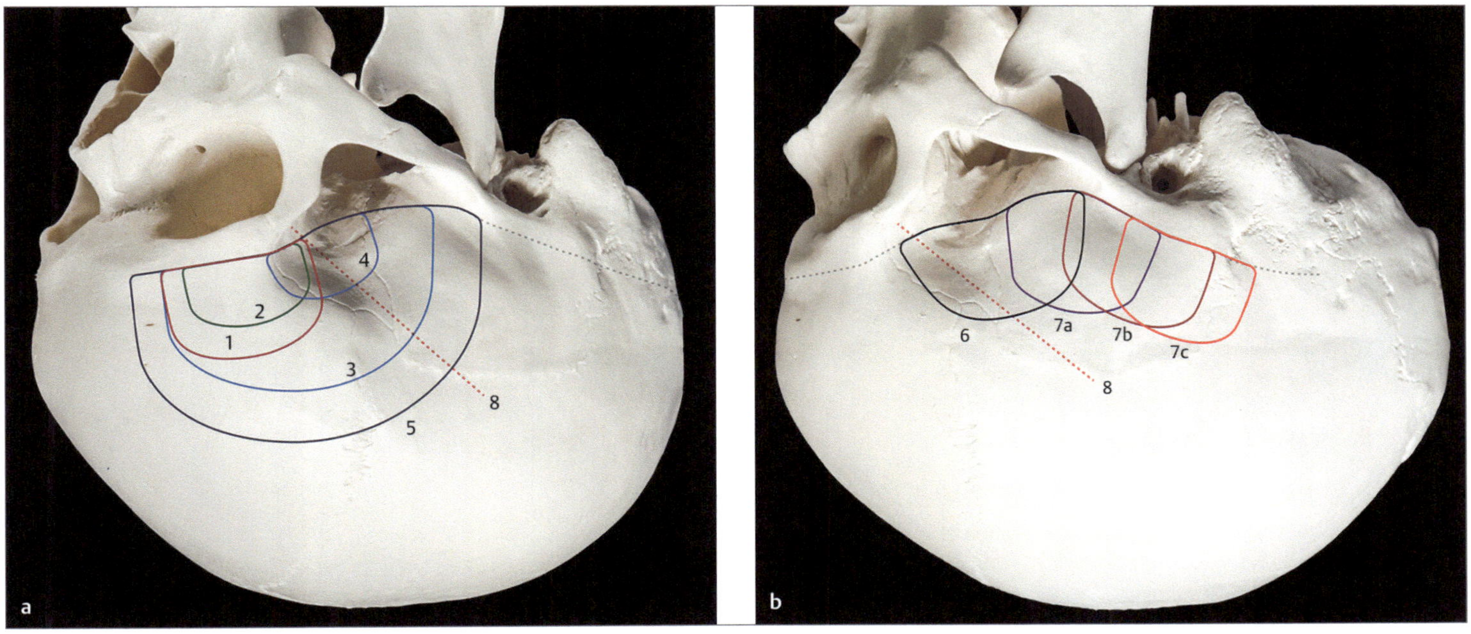

Fig. 1.1 Systematics of skull base craniotomies—supratentorial. Supratentorial frontotemporal skull base craniotomies, 45° view **(a)** and lateral view **(b)**. 1, frontolateral; 2, supraorbital; 3, standard pterional; 4, mini-pterional; 5, frontotemporal; 6, anterior temporal; 7a–c anterior, middle, posterior temporobasal; 8, sylvian fissure/sphenoid wing.

Infratentorial skull base craniotomies are performed along the sigmoid sinus or the foramen magnum (see ▶ Table 1.2 for further details).

Table 1.2 Systematics of skull base craniotomies—infratentorial

Location	Description
Suboccipital median infra-transverse-sinus	Midline craniotomy for supracerebellar median or paramedian approaches, e.g., for access to the pineal region or tentorial dural fistulas.
Suboccipital lateral infra-transverse-sinus	These are craniotomies based on the same principle as the midline craniotomies for an intradural approach along the subdural space parallel to the tentorium. Typically, they are used for supracerebellar lateral approaches to the midbrain or other regions. They are horizontally oriented compared to the retrosigmoid craniotomy, with more exposure along the transverse sinus and less along the sigmoid sinus. A modification is the suboccipital far-lateral infra-transverse-sinus craniotomy.
Retrosigmoid	Typically ranges from the transverse sinus to the base of the posterior fossa along the sigmoid sinus to gain access to the cerebellopontine angle. May vary in size and be centered more superiorly or inferiorly: vertically oriented.
Suboccipital median peri-foraminal craniotomy with opening of the foramen magnum	Typically bilateral, there is a mini-version, for example, in Chiari-decompression surgery.
Suboccipital lateral perifo-raminal craniotomy with opening of the foramen magnum	The lateral suboccipital craniotomy with opening of the foramen magnum is the basic craniotomy for the far lateral approach which can be regarded as a skull base extension of the basal suboccipital craniotomy.

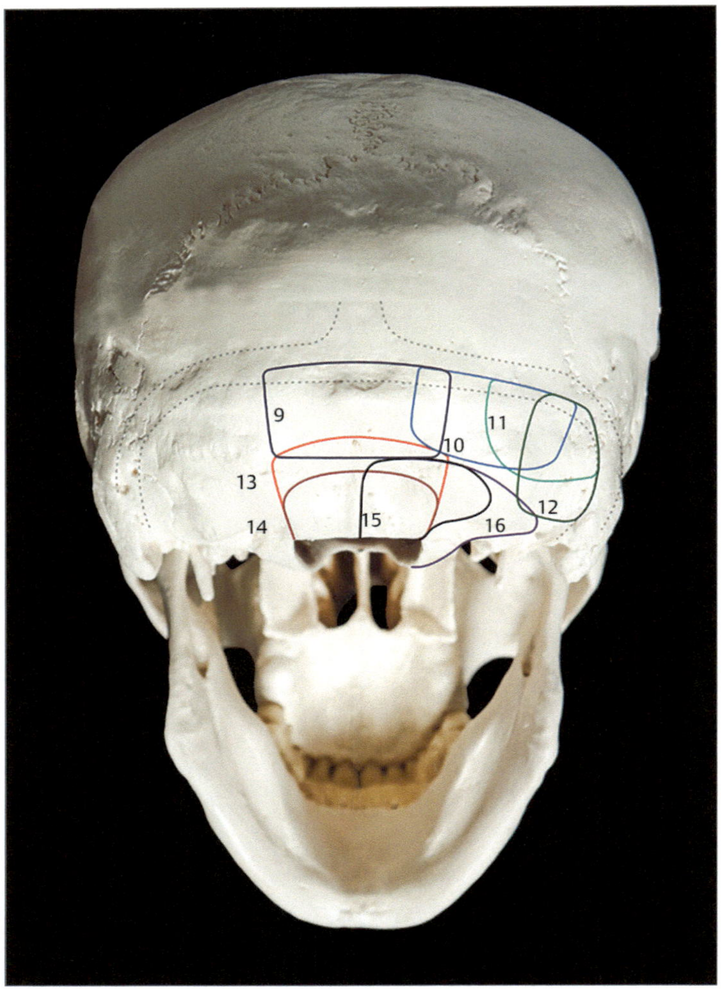

Fig. 1.2 Systematics of skull base craniotomies—infratentorial. Craniotomies of the posterior fossa. 9, suboccipital median infra-transverse-sinus; 10, suboccipital lateral infra-transverse-sinus; 11, suboccipital far-lateral infra-transverse-sinus; 12, retrosigmoid; 13, suboccipital median periforaminal (with opening of the foramen magnum); 14, mini-suboccipital median periforaminal (with opening of the foramen magnum); 15, suboccipital lateral periforaminal (with opening of the foramen magnum); 16, far-lateral extension.

1.2 Difference between Approach and Craniotomy

Andreas Raabe

Although often used synonymously, there is a difference between a craniotomy and an approach. Approach is the broader term and is often used for craniotomy and intradural preparation. In this book, we discuss only the steps of the craniotomy, i.e., to reach bony exposure. With a few exceptions, we stay outside the dura. We will therefore mostly use the term craniotomy instead of approach, and generally reserve the latter to describe the dissection and exposure after opening the dura mater. Craniotomy and approach may be different as in the examples given below. However, as already mentioned, the term "approach" often overlaps with craniotomy and intradural preparation.

Examples:

- Supraorbital craniotomy and subfrontal approach.
- Pterional craniotomy and transsylvian approach.
- Temporobasal craniotomy and subtemporal approach.
- Suboccipital lateral craniotomy and supracerebellar lateral approach.
- Median suboccipital craniotomy and telovelar approach.

1.3 Craniotomies We Have Omitted from This Book and Why

Andreas Raabe, Bernhard Meyer, Peter Vajkoczy, and Karl Schaller

This book is intended primarily for young residents, to serve as a guide to understanding the various craniotomies. It describes the most often used craniotomies, but we decided not to include those that are used only very rarely. Therefore, it does not cover highly specialized skull base craniotomies and their extension, such as posterior transpetrosal, translabyrinthine, transcochlear, or combined approaches, nor is it our aim to provide a complete atlas of approaches and extensions.

We acknowledge that these specialized skull base approaches had their place in the heyday of skull base surgery. However, nowadays they are often replaced by a staged procedure or a combination of simpler craniotomies that provide a less invasive strategy with lower morbidity than a technically demanding and more invasive approach. Moreover, radiosurgery and endovascular treatment often complete a less invasive treatment for many patients.

We are also aware that the nomenclature for the craniotomies varies around the world and that experienced surgeons use their own tricks and modifications when performing craniotomies.

1.4 Positioning

1.4.1 Basic Rules

Andreas Raabe and Janine Abu-Isa

Time spent on careful positioning is time well spent. Mistakes in positioning may render any surgical plan, even if it is conceptually perfectly elaborated, impossible. Positioning is the first strategic step for the operation; it is the first digit of the code number to unlock the door to the target of brain surgery. Correct positioning can open the surgical field, achieve gravity retraction, reduce bleeding, and provide the most relaxing position for the surgeon.

Positioning should be highly standardized in each department to improve communication, to save time, and to achieve the goal of the surgery. Use of photographs, step-by-step instructions, and a checklist is recommended.

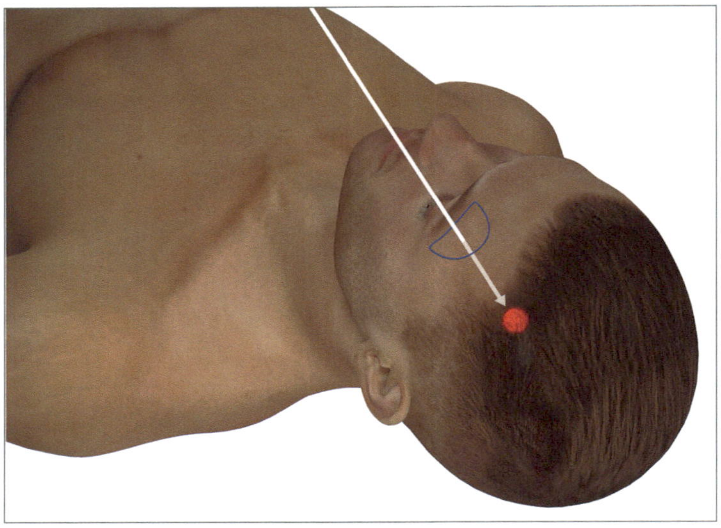

Fig. 1.3 Craniotomy-to-lesion trajectory. This is the first and most important factor determining the position of the head.

The position of the head depends on the following factors (also see ▶ Fig. 1.3, ▶ Fig. 1.4, ▶ Fig. 1.5, and ▶ Fig. 1.6):

1. Planned Surgical Trajectory

The surgical trajectory is the line between the craniotomy and the surgical target, i.e., the midline craniotomy and the tumor in the third ventricle, or the subtemporal craniotomy and the midbrain cavernoma, or the convexity craniotomy and the underlying meningioma (▶ Fig. 1.3).

2. Position of the Surgeon

The same surgical trajectory can vary according to the preferred position of the surgeon (see below).

3. Gravity Retraction or Drainage

When gravity retraction is a major part of the surgery, it may become the dominant principle, for instance, in contralateral or midline approaches via the dependent hemisphere or when the semisitting position is preferred in some cases for posterior fossa surgery for pineal or cerebellopontine targets.

4. Measures for Avoiding Potential Position-Related Complications

Such measures include positioning to minimize intracranial pressure, venous congestion, and air embolism, as well as improved orientation if only standardized head positions are allowed.

Every head position can be achieved by combining head rotation (▶ Fig. 1.4a) with patient's body positioning (▶ Fig. 1.4b):

- Rotation of the head from 0° to 60° (this can be tested in the awake patient before surgery: in younger patients a rotation up to 90° may be possible, whereas in elderly patients head rotation may be limited to 30°), with the desired degree of head flexion and tilting.
- Selection of one of five supplemental positions of the patient's body to achieve the final desired head position. These five body positions should be standardized.

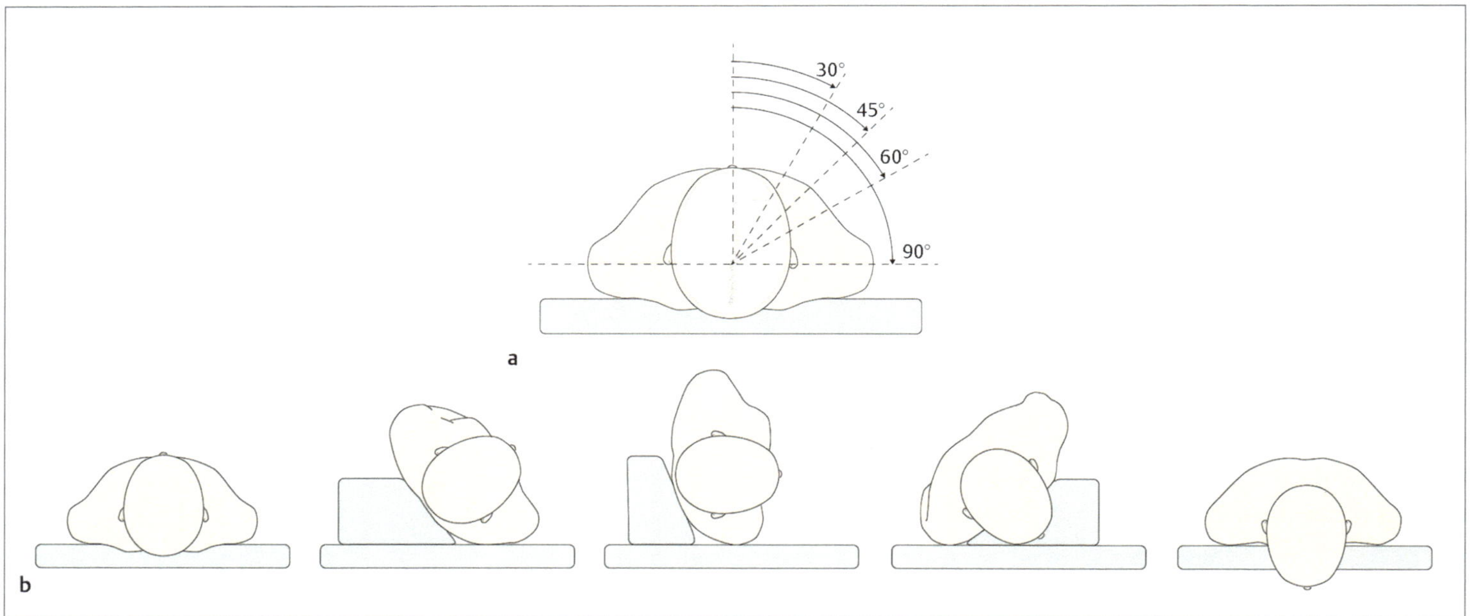

Fig. 1.4 Combining positioning of the head and the body of the patient. Head rotation **(a)** combined with five body positions **(b)** allows the surgeon to gain access to every trajectory. Special positions are also possible (e.g., semisitting).

Except for special positions (e.g., semisitting), one of the following five basic positions are applied (▶Fig. 1.4b):

- Supine: quick and easy.
- Supine oblique (45°) upper body rotation with the pelvis and legs supine: still quick.
- Lateral recumbent: more complicated, takes more time.
- Lateral oblique or park bench (135°): more complicated, takes more time.
- Prone: more complicated, takes more time and should be avoided if possible because of increased venous congestion.

For instance, a horizontal head position can be achieved by combining:

- 90° head rotation and supine body position or
- 45° head rotation and 45° upper body rotation or
- 0° head rotation and lateral recumbent position.

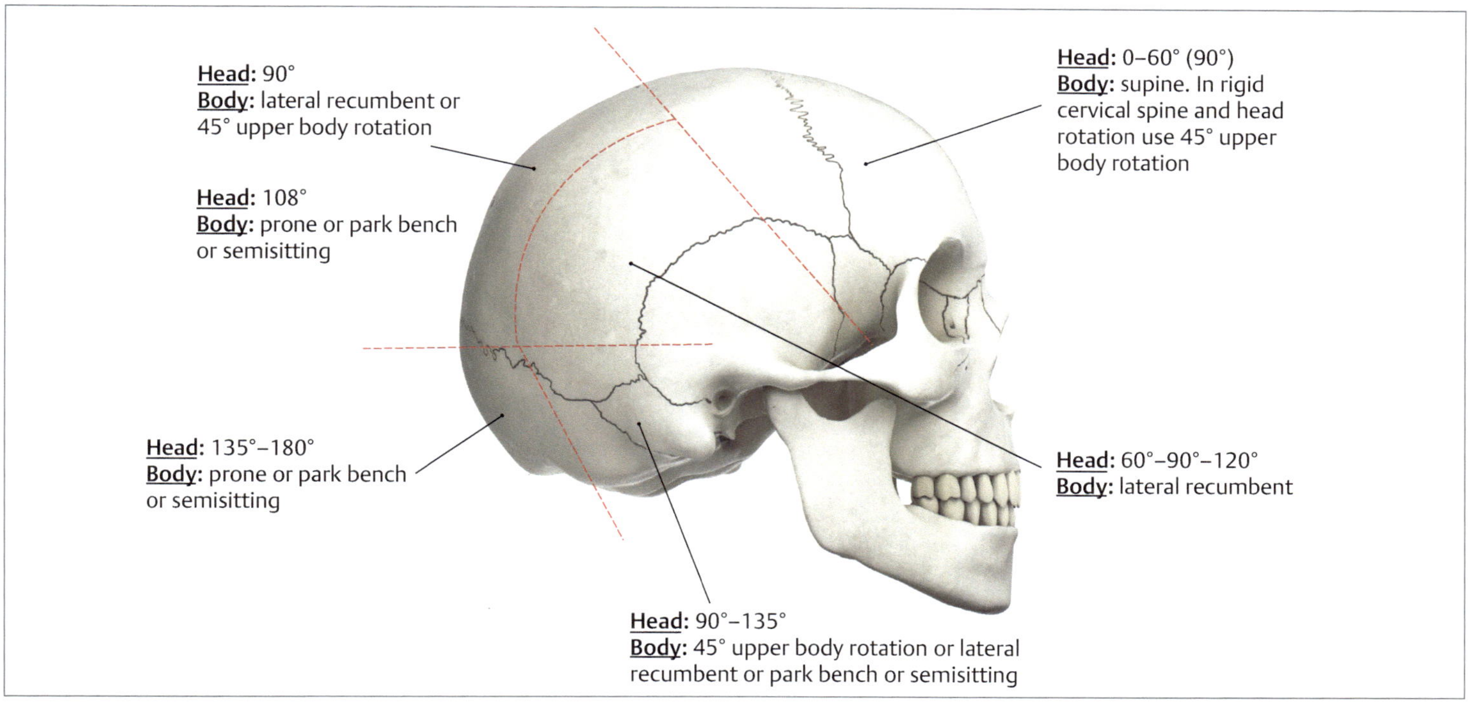

Fig. 1.5 Positioning of the patient's body. Typical positioning for different locations of craniotomies.

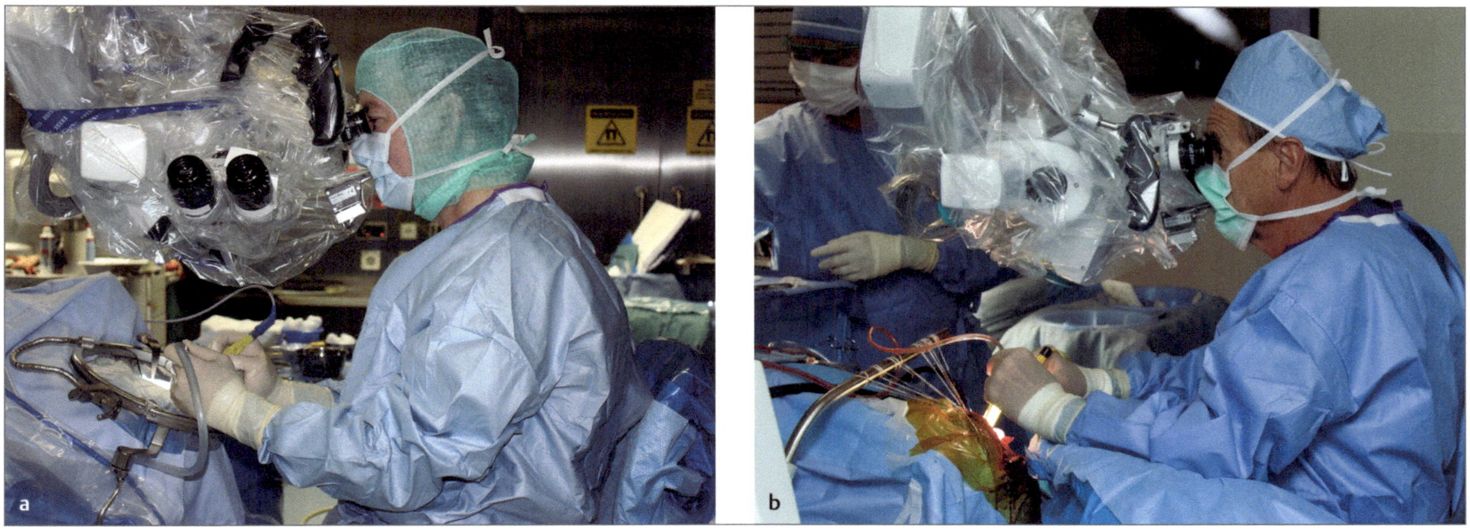

Fig. 1.6 Position of the surgeon. There are two basic positions for the surgeon: the first is more upright, closer to the surgical field and short instruments, and the hands or fingers are supported **(a)**. The second is a somewhat more oblique position with slightly longer instruments, and forearms or elbows supported **(b)**. Both can achieve the goals of a relaxed surgeon, excellent stability, minimized trembling, and soft instrument movements with maximum haptic feedback about resistance of structures and tactile information. Normally, the positioning of the microscope and the patient's head follows the position of the surgeon. Make yourself comfortable and then adjust the microscope and the patient, unless otherwise required by the planned surgical trajectory and the specific goals. (▶Fig. 1.6a is reproduced courtesy of Volker Seifert and ▶Fig. 1.6b courtesy of Robert F. Spetzler.)

1.4.2 Supine

Philippe Schucht

See ▸ Fig. 1.7 and ▸ Fig. 1.8.

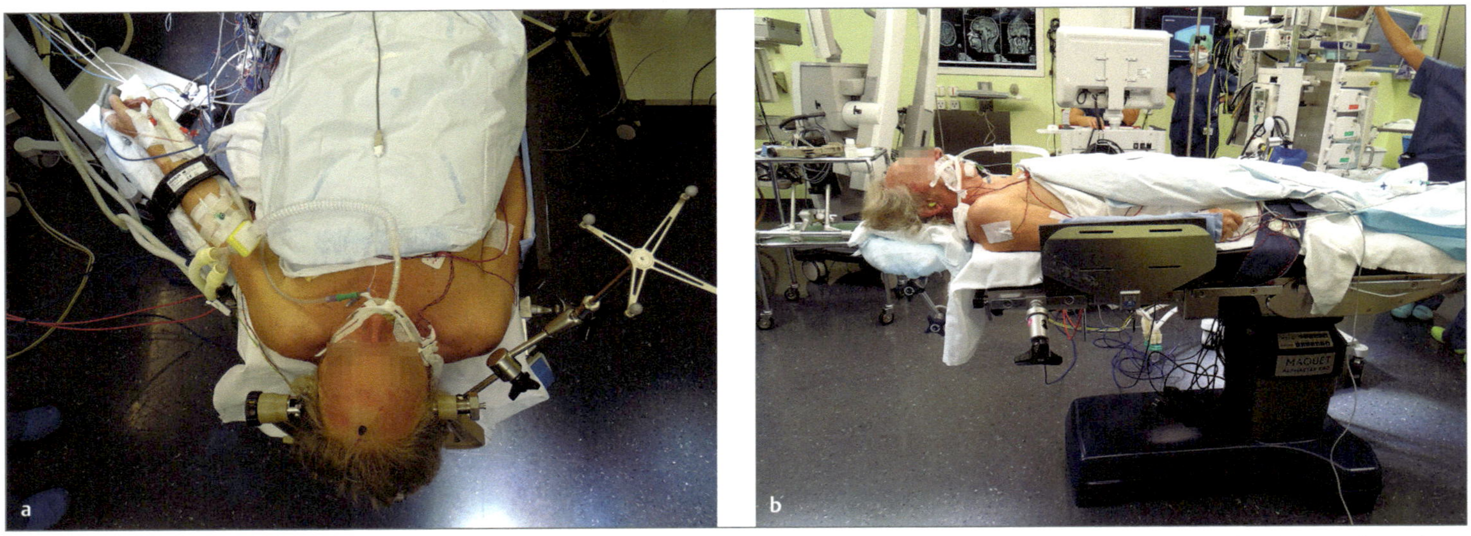

Fig. 1.7 Body position. View from the top **(a)** and the side **(b)**. The supine position is the simplest position. The body and the legs lie straight and the right arm lies parallel to the body. The left arm lies at an angle on a separate armrest to allow insertion of arterial and venous lines and should be loosely fixed.

Attention should be paid to making sure that the body is well cushioned and that the sheets beneath the patient have no wrinkles. In particular in long procedures, incorrect patient positioning may result in decubiti.

Rotating the patient during surgery may give you a better angle of view. For rotating during surgery, prop the patient with additional side pads.

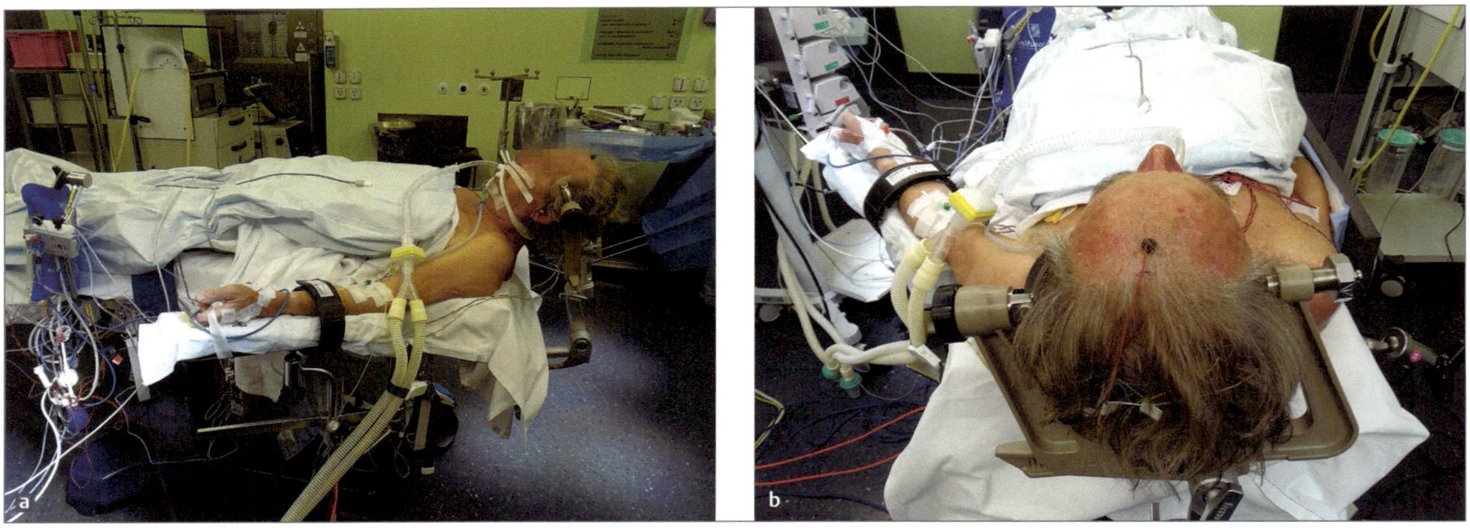

Fig. 1.8 (a, b) Head position. The shoulders should reach the edge of the table. The head is elevated by approximately 5–10 cm in order to facilitate venous drainage

Checklist

- Use side pads to prop the patient if you consider rotating the patient during surgery.
- Cushion the patient well and avoid wrinkles in the sheets to prevent decubiti.
- Elevate the head by approximately 5 to 10 cm to facilitate venous drainage.

1.4.3 Supine Lateral

Christian F. Freyschlag and Claudius Thomé

Supine lateral positioning (45°) of the patient's upper body is used to enable access to the posterior fossa and the cerebellopontine angle, but may also be used for other approaches where the head is placed with the midline horizontally. In our experience, a sitting or semisitting position offers no advantage over lateral positioning. Although this has long been debated, we do not consider that gravitation-facilitated dissection outweighs disadvantages such as the complexity of positioning, need for exclusion of a persistent foramen ovale, and the risk of venous air embolism.[1,2] Furthermore, operating on a patient in the sitting or semisitting position is less ergonomic and more exhausting for most surgeons. Refer to ▶Fig. 1.9, ▶Fig. 1.10, ▶Fig. 1.11, and ▶Fig. 1.12.

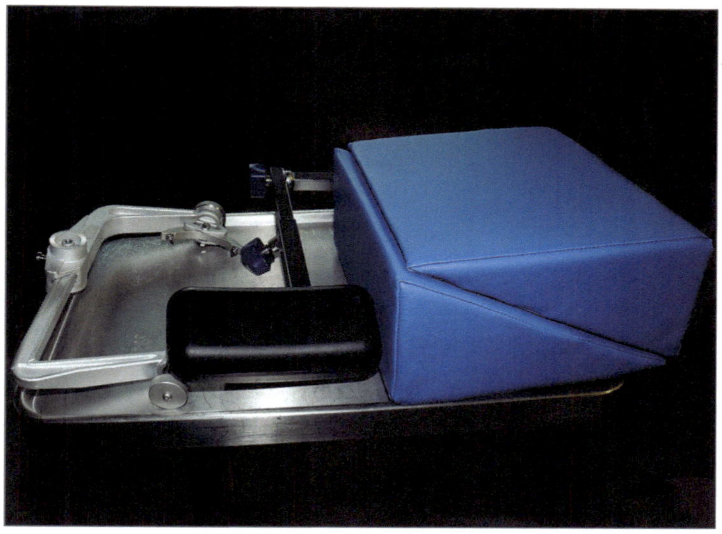

Fig. 1.9 Equipment. The devices needed for supine lateral positioning are found in the basic neurosurgical OR: a three-pin Mayfield clamp, two wedge-shaped cushions, and a support for the pelvis that can be attached to the table.

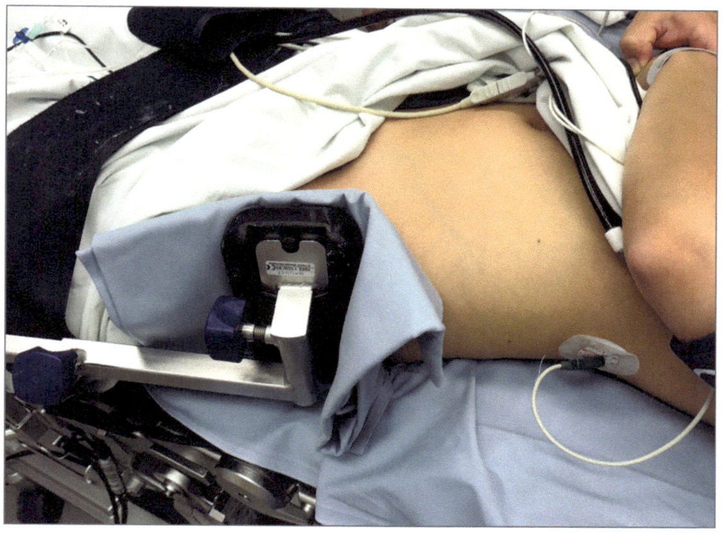

Fig. 1.10 Positioning of the patient. Supporting the pelvis helps maintain the position during rotation of the table.

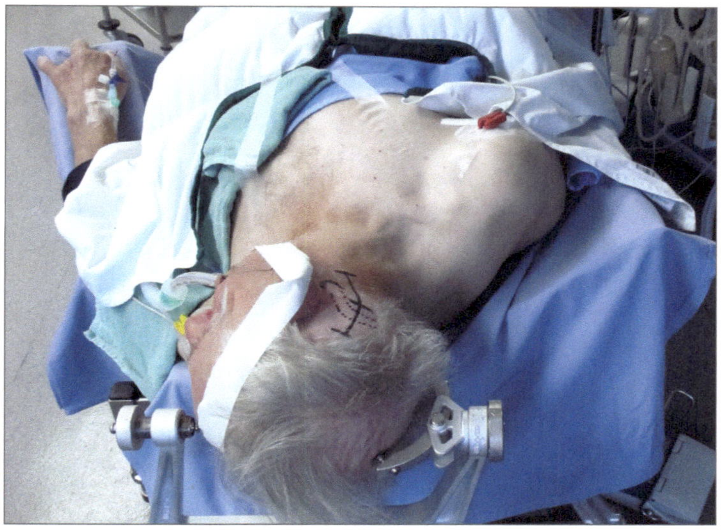

Fig. 1.11 Body positioning. It is possible to place the patient flat on the operating table.[3] However, the positioning is easier and rotation of the cervical spine and vascular structures is minimized if the shoulder is elevated by a wedge-shaped cushion. In older patients, this support is mandatory due to the patients' limited neck movement.

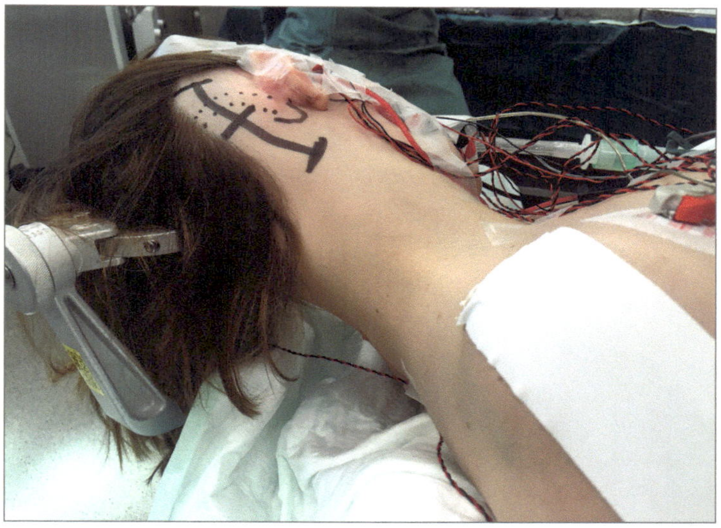

Fig. 1.12 Positioning. To obtain optimal conditions and exposure for a retrosigmoid approach, it is necessary to rotate the head (without creating excessive tension on the neck) away from the surgical site. The head is moved in three directions[4]: (1) contralateral rotation toward a position parallel to the floor, (2) bending of the vertex toward the floor (retroflexion), and (3) inclination of the head to open the cervical-suboccipital angle. This maneuver raises the mastoid process so that it becomes the highest point, while creating space between shoulder and head, which can be increased by retracting the upper shoulder caudally and securing it with adhesive tape.

If the patient has limited neck mobility, the table can be easily rotated to compensate for this limitation. The use of a support prevents the patient from sliding.

Finally, pressure points of the upper and lower extremities are meticulously padded to avoid any injury during surgery.

Checklist

- Make sure the patient's body is moved sufficiently toward the top end of the operating table (when operating on a patient in a supine lateral position, you tend to sit at 90° to the patient's longitudinal axis).
- Always support the patient's position—you might want to rotate the table for better exposure.
- Positioning needs three crucial head movements: rotation, inclination, and lateral flexion.

References

[1] Nozaki K. Selection of semisitting position in neurosurgery: essential or preference? World Neurosurg 2014;81(1):62–63
[2] Feigl GC, Decker K, Wurms M, et al. Neurosurgical procedures in the semisitting position: evaluation of the risk of paradoxical venous air embolism in patients with a patent foramen ovale. World Neurosurg 2014;81(1):159–164
[3] Wait SD, Gazzeri R, Galarza M, Teo C. Simple, effective, supine positioning for the retrosigmoid approach. Minim Invasive Neurosurg 2011;54(4):196–198
[4] Elhammady MS, Telischi FF, Morcos JJ. Retrosigmoid approach: indications, techniques, and results. Otolaryngol Clin North Am 2012;45(2):375–397, ix

1.4.4 Lateral

Philippe Schucht

See ▶ Fig. 1.13, ▶ Fig. 1.14, ▶ Fig. 1.15, ▶ Fig. 1.16, and ▶ Fig. 1.17 for reference on lateral positioning.

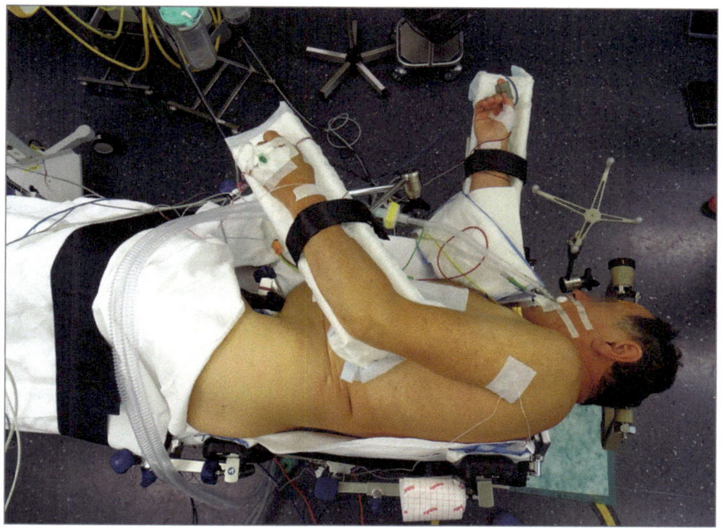

Fig. 1.13 View of the lateral position from above. Both arms lie secured and tension-free on separate armrests. The legs are slightly flexed and fixed. The position of the arms and legs, as well as the side pad just below the abdomen, increases the body's stability and allows rotation of the patient to the surgeon's right side if necessary during surgery.

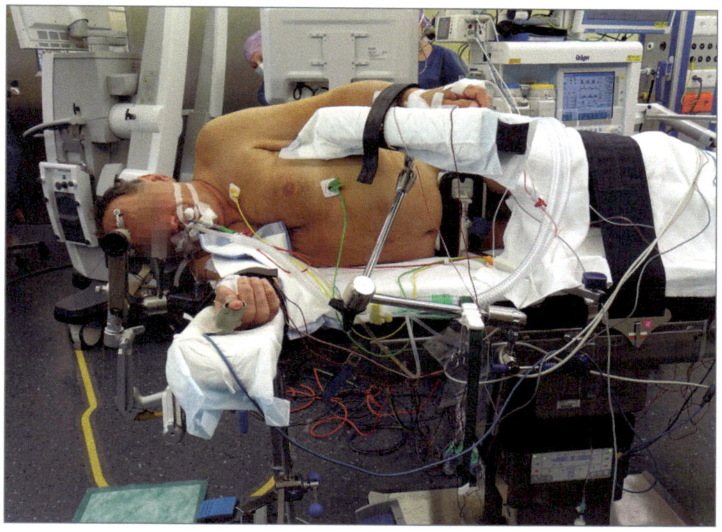

Fig. 1.14 Side view of the lateral position. The head lies aligned with the body's axis and can be tilted and flexed as required. The ventral supporting side pad is positioned below the abdomen to avoid an increase of the abdominal pressure. The lower arm lies aligned with the top edge of the table at a 90° angle to the body. A cushion is placed between the legs to prevent pressure sores on the knees and ankles. Both arms and legs are secured by belts.

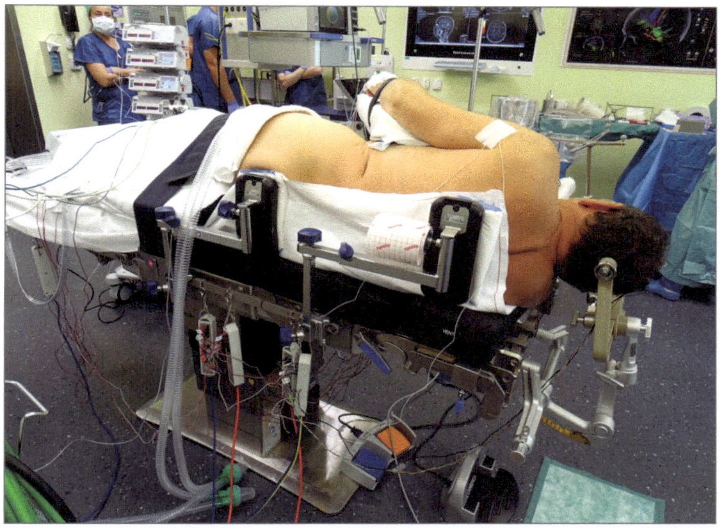

Fig. 1.15 Lateral position from posterior. Two posteriorly supporting side pads, positioned just beneath the scapulae and over the buttocks, provide lateral stability and allow the patient to be rotated to the left if necessary during surgery. The patient's back is aligned with the left edge of the table at an angle of 90°.

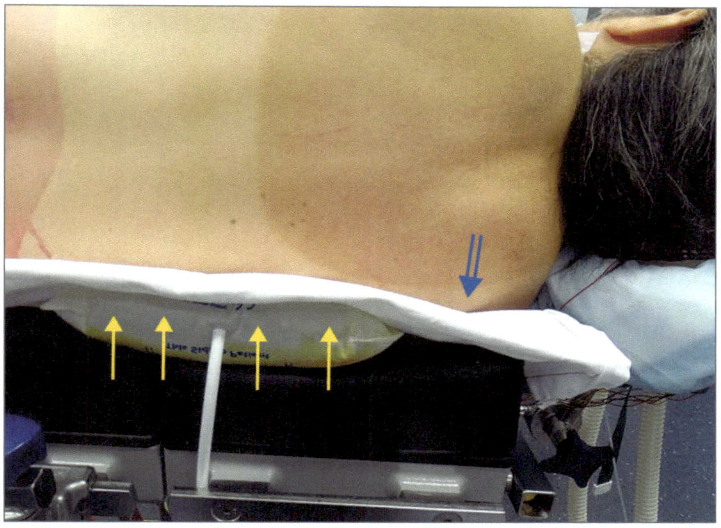

Fig. 1.16 Relieving pressure from the shoulder by a supporting cushion below the axilla. It is important to prevent putting pressure on the lower shoulder. The arm and shoulder are both positioned exactly in line with the upper edge of the table, but still on the table. To relieve pressure on the shoulder, a special supporting cushion should be placed beneath the thorax and immediately below the lower arm. We use a pneumatic cushion (*yellow arrows*), which lifts the thorax slightly while relieving the pressure from the shoulder (*blue double arrow*).

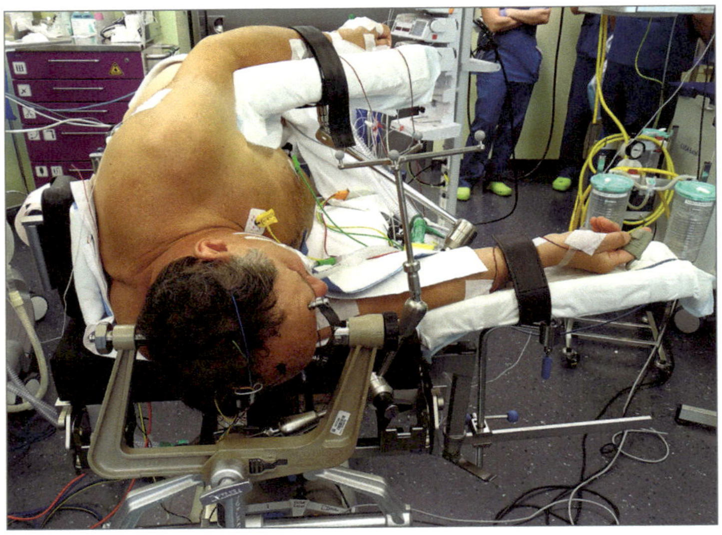

Fig. 1.17 **Lateral position from above.** The shoulder should reach the edge of the table but still entirely lie on it. Special care should be taken to cushion the shoulder and the hips well in order to avoid decubiti. The head can now be adjusted to the surgical position. Maximal flexion of the head should be limited to a chin–manubrium distance of two fingers.

Checklist

- Use separate armrests for both arms; use a cushion between the legs.
- Flexing the legs, correct positioning of the arms, and using a subabdominal side pad stabilize the patient ventrally.
- Propping with pads on the patient's buttock and scapulae stabilizes the patient dorsally.
- Cushion the shoulder and the hips well to avoid decubiti.

1.4.5 Lateral Oblique or Park Bench

Daniel Hänggi

The lateral oblique (135°) or park bench position with the arm on the table is suitable for posterior fossa or occipital midline and lateral craniotomies as well as for subtemporal and temporal approaches. It allows rapid positioning of the patient and is less often associated with serious complications—including venous air embolism, hypotension, pneumocephalus, and laryngeal trauma—than the sitting position. In addition, in comparison to the prone position, it offers considerable advantages to the neurosurgeon in terms of gravity-assisted drainage and reduced cerebellar retraction.

The patient should be positioned on the left or right side to achieve a surgical corridor without using a spatula-assisted retraction. See ▶Fig. 1.18, ▶Fig. 1.19, ▶Fig. 1.20, ▶Fig. 1.21, ▶Fig. 1.22, and ▶Fig. 1.23.

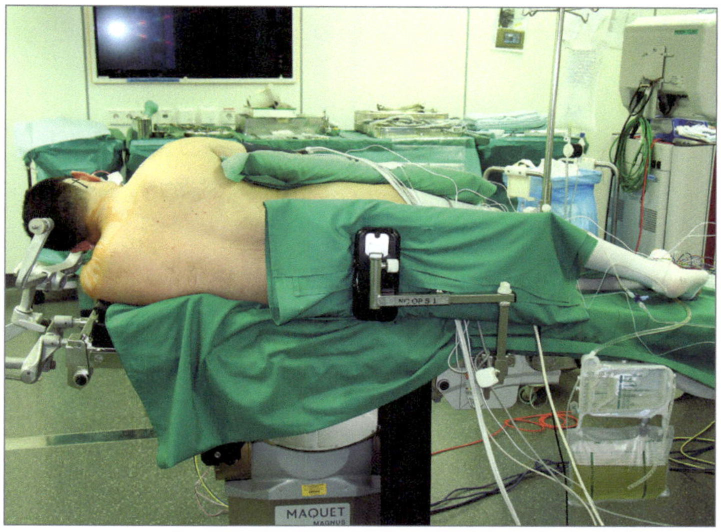

Fig. 1.18 Body positioning and support. The patient is placed in a lateral recumbent position with the contralateral (lower) arm stretched out on top of the table. A support is mounted at the lumbar spine and opposite at the pelvis to make sure that the patient can be rotated up to 30° during surgery. Cushions or soft padding of the lower arm, below and between the knees, and below and between the ankles is important to avoid pressure marks and neural or vascular complications.

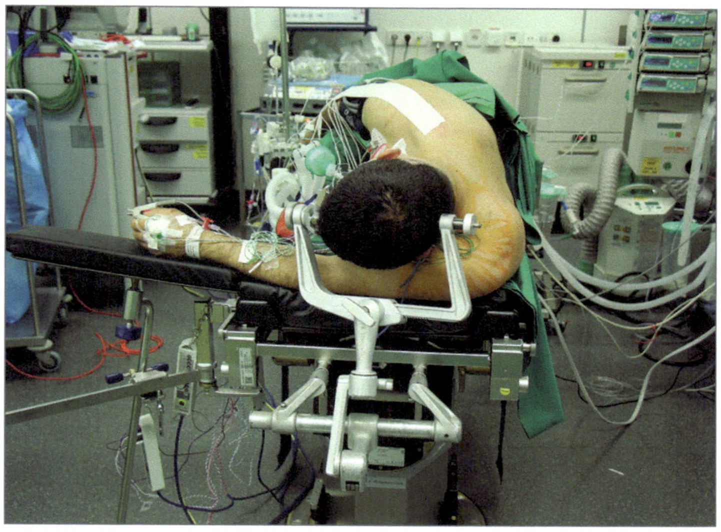

Fig. 1.19 Ipsilateral shoulder and arm. The shoulders should be rotated about 45° away from the surgeon so that they are out of the line of access. An additional option is to tape the ipsilateral shoulder inferiorly to provide more room for the surgeon to work. Traction during taping should be applied carefully to avoid neural injury. The ipsilateral (upper arm) is positioned and fixed on a cushion positioned anteriorly at the level of the patient's abdomen.

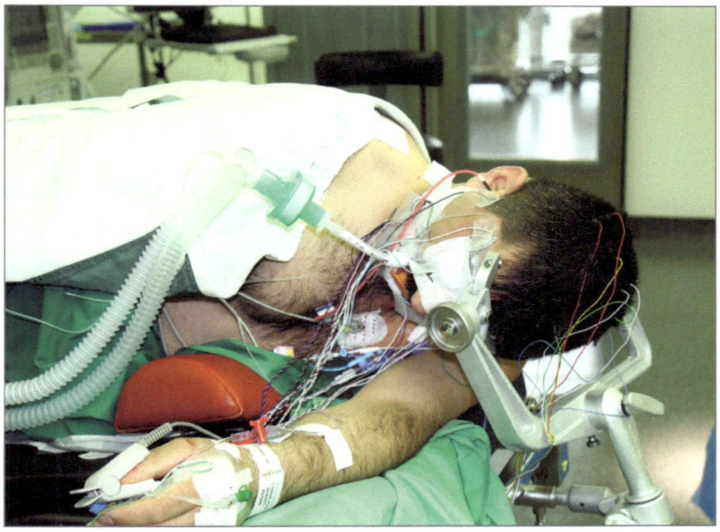

Fig. 1.20 Head flexion. The head should be inclined as much as possible, but two fingers' distance should be left between the chin and the jugulum.

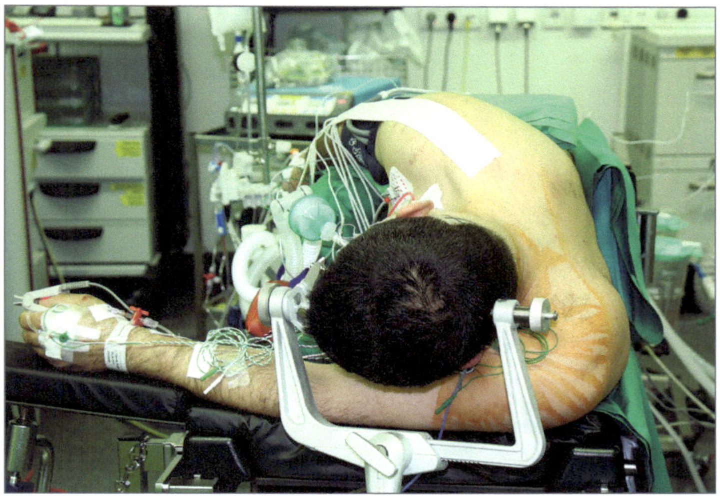

Fig. 1.21 Head rotation. Head rotation varies depending on the point of access required for posterior fossa midline or lateral craniotomies as well as for subtemporal and temporal approaches. The Mayfield pins must be placed in a plane perpendicular to the planned line of access, and the paired pins should be placed on the underside of the head. This is important for later positioning of the retraction system.

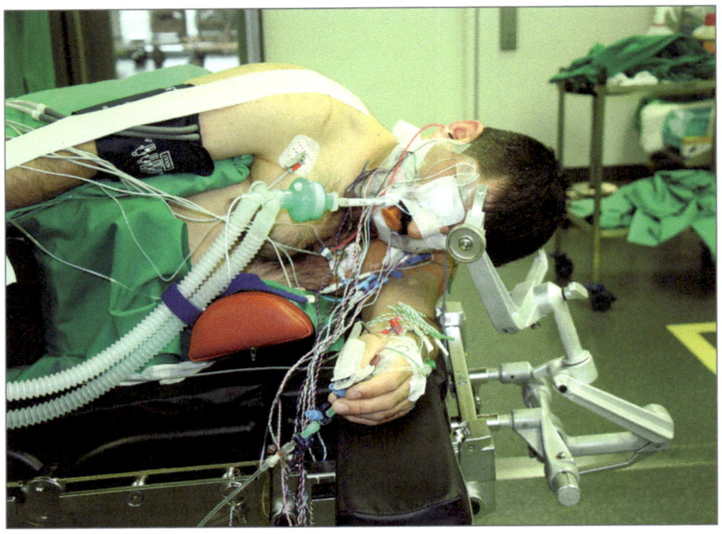

Fig. 1.22 Body tilt. Finally, the operating table is turned into reverse Trendelenburg position to achieve maximal gravity-assisted drainage and to minimize venous congestion.

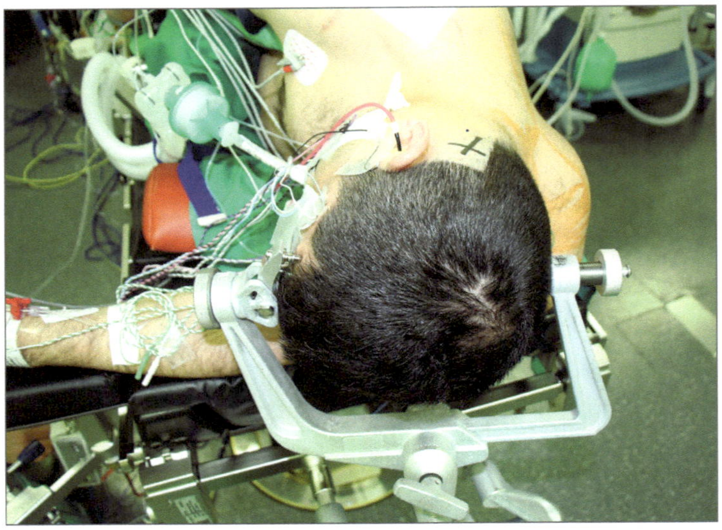

Fig. 1.23 Final head position. The craniotomy site is at or near the highest point. In summary, this position with the shoulder rotated anteriorly and the head flexed and tilted toward the floor provides an excellent position for the surgeon with ample space for both hands.

Checklist

- The patient is placed in a lateral recumbent position with the contralateral (lower) arm stretched out on top of the table.
- The shoulders should be rotated about 45° away from the surgeon.
- The head should be inclined as much as possible.
- Head rotation depending on the point of access required for posterior fossa midline or lateral craniotomies.
- Finally, the operating table is turned into reverse Trendelenburg position.

1.4.6 Park Bench

David Bervini and Janine Abu-Isa

The park bench position is suitable for approaches to the posterior fossa, including retrosigmoid and occipital midline, and for lateral infratentorial craniotomies in general. Unlike in the lateral recumbent position, the patient's shoulder and lower arm hang over the edge of the table. This may allow greater contralateral head flexion and tilt, and hence a wider opening of the lateral craniocervical corridor. See ▶ Fig. 1.24, ▶ Fig. 1.25, ▶ Fig. 1.26, ▶ Fig. 1.27, ▶ Fig. 1.28, ▶ Fig. 1.29, and ▶ Fig. 1.30.

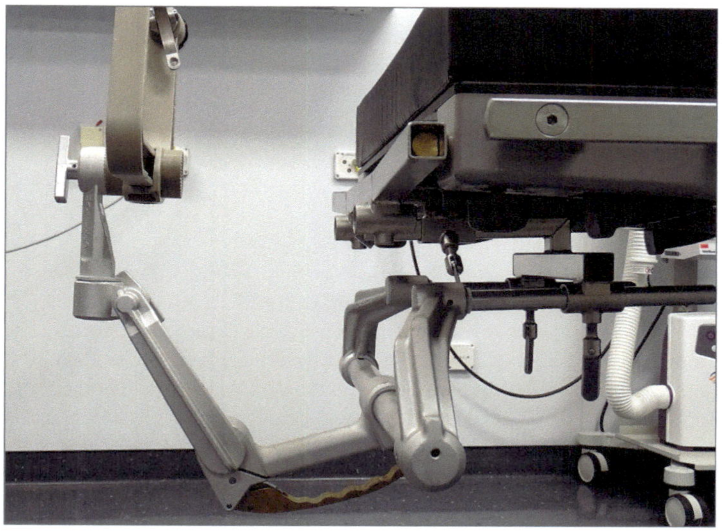

Fig. 1.24 Attachment of the Mayfield clamp. Ideally, the base of the Mayfield clamp is attached to the operating table with a special connection piece, which moves the vertical main base of the clamp underneath the edge of the table and away from the down-hanging arm.

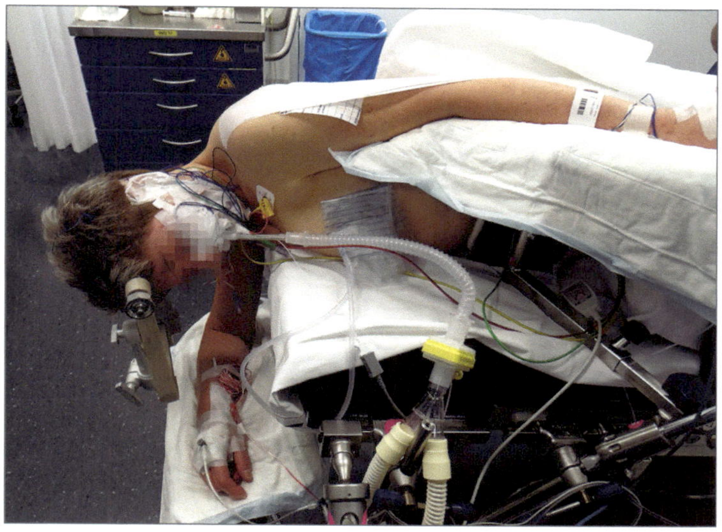

Fig. 1.25 Positioning of the patient's body. The intubated patient is turned into a lateral recumbent position to rest on his/her lateral chest. The axilla is positioned 5 cm beyond the edge of the table. The axilla and the upper arm are carefully padded.

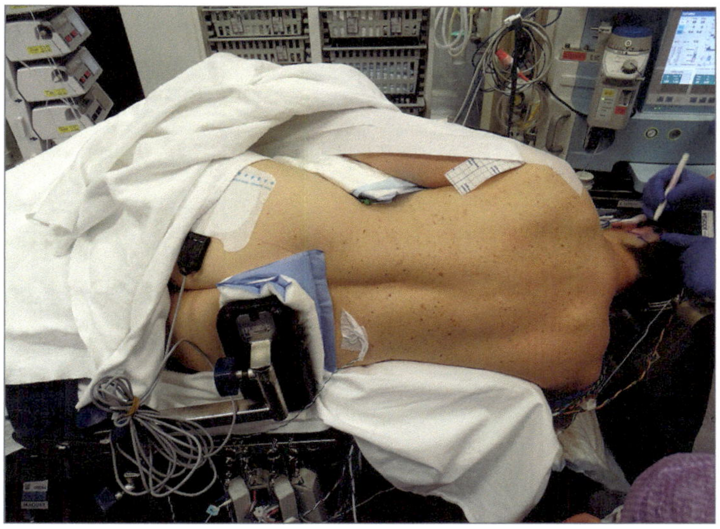

Fig. 1.26 Support of the lower body. The patient's lower body is secured by a support at the level of the lumbosacral spine and pelvis (see also ▶ Fig. 1.25).

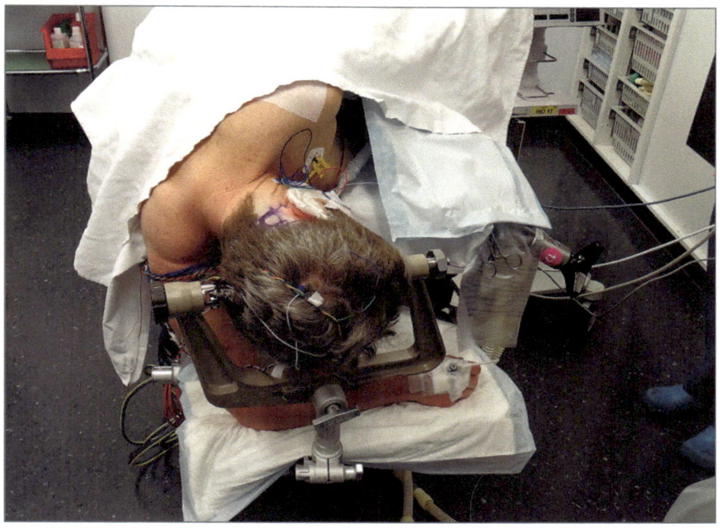

Fig. 1.27 Positioning of the patient's head. The head is secured in the Mayfield pin holder, one pin anteriorly and two pins posteriorly. Alternatively, the Mayfield clamp can be placed vertically with two pins pointing down and one pin up. The head is rotated as far as needed, depending on the laterality of the surgical approach. After rotation, the head is flexed and slightly tilted downward, making sure to preserve a distance of two finger widths between the chin and the manubrium. This helps to prevent venous congestion and/or kinking of the tracheal tube. The craniotomy site should be at or near the highest point. Finally, the operating table is tilted in the reverse Trendelenburg position to minimize venous congestion. If needed, additional lateral tilting can be performed after verifying that the body is properly supported.

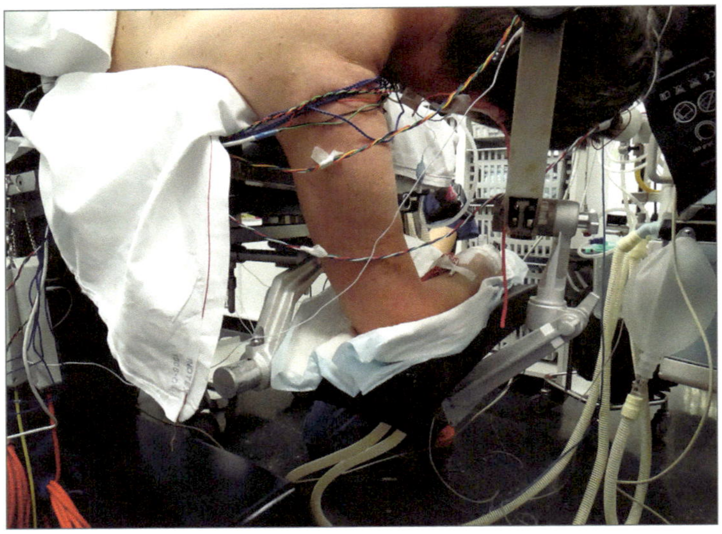

Fig. 1.28 Positioning of the lower arm. The lower arm rests on a soft arm board or a sling inserted above the flexible attachment arm of the Mayfield clamp, between the operating table and the clamp itself. Special care should be taken to avoid compression of the ulnar nerve, the axilla, and elbow.

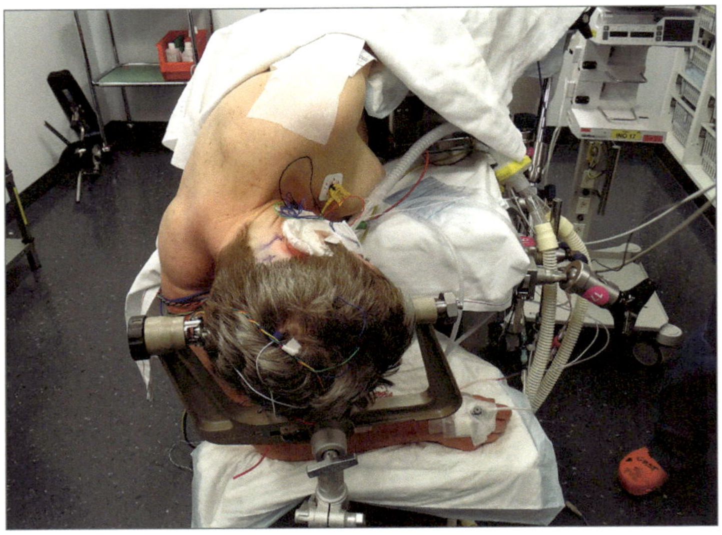

Fig. 1.29 Fixation of the upper arm and shoulder. The superior shoulder falls at an angle of 30–45° anteriorly, away from the surgical approach and from the line of sight of the surgeon. If the surgeon needs more room, the shoulder can be taped and pulls inferiorly toward the feet. Traction during taping has to be applied carefully to avoid neural injury. The superior arm rests on a jelly board, slightly elevated to avoid venous congestion.

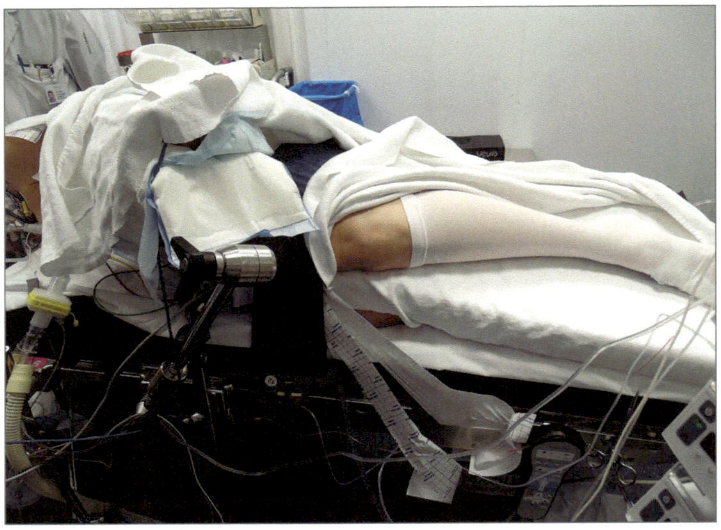

Fig. 1.30 Padding the knee and ankles. Jelly cushions between and under the knees and the ankles are important to reduce the risk of pressure sores and neural compression.

Potential Complications of Park Bench Position

Potential complications of the park bench position include pressure palsies of the shoulder or arm, brachial plexus injuries, and stretch injuries. Excessive head flexion can cause jugular vein compression and venous outflow congestion.

Checklist

- Lateral position, upper body tilted 15 to 30° in anti-Trendelenburg position to minimize venous pressure in the head.
- Body secured at the level of the lumbosacral spine and pelvis with two supports.
- Pay special attention to possible pressure points (elbow, axilla, knee, ankle).
- Lower arm on arm board between the table and the Mayfield clamp; support the arm so that it does not hang from the shoulder.
- Upper shoulder rotated by gravity about 30 to 45° away from the surgeon.
- Further gentle downward draping of the shoulder may be needed; avoid excessive traction.
- Head is rotated and tilted as far as needed.
- Maximum head flexion limited to two finger widths between the chin and clavicle/sternum.
- Final adjustment of the table position is made to suit the surgeon.

Further Reading

Rozet I, Vavilala MS. Risks and benefits of patient positioning during neurosurgical care. Anesthesiol Clin 2007;25(3):631–653

1.4.7 Prone/Concorde

Christian Fung

The prone position is used to access lesions in the occipital or superior parietal lobe and the posterior cervical spine. Putting the patient into the prone position increases abdominal pressure and decreases venous reflux. Special tables or frames (e.g., Wilson frame, Jackson table) enable free movement of the abdominal wall and increase venous backflow, therefore decreasing surgical bleeding due to venous congestion. Higher head positions improve venous reflux but increase the risk of air embolism.

The Concorde position is a modification of the prone position and enables access to the suboccipital region. It is a position often used for craniotomies of the posterior fossa for cerebellar approaches, approaches to the infratentorial supracerebellar region, and the foramen magnum. See ▶Fig. 1.31, ▶Fig. 1.32, ▶Fig. 1.33, and ▶Fig. 1.34.

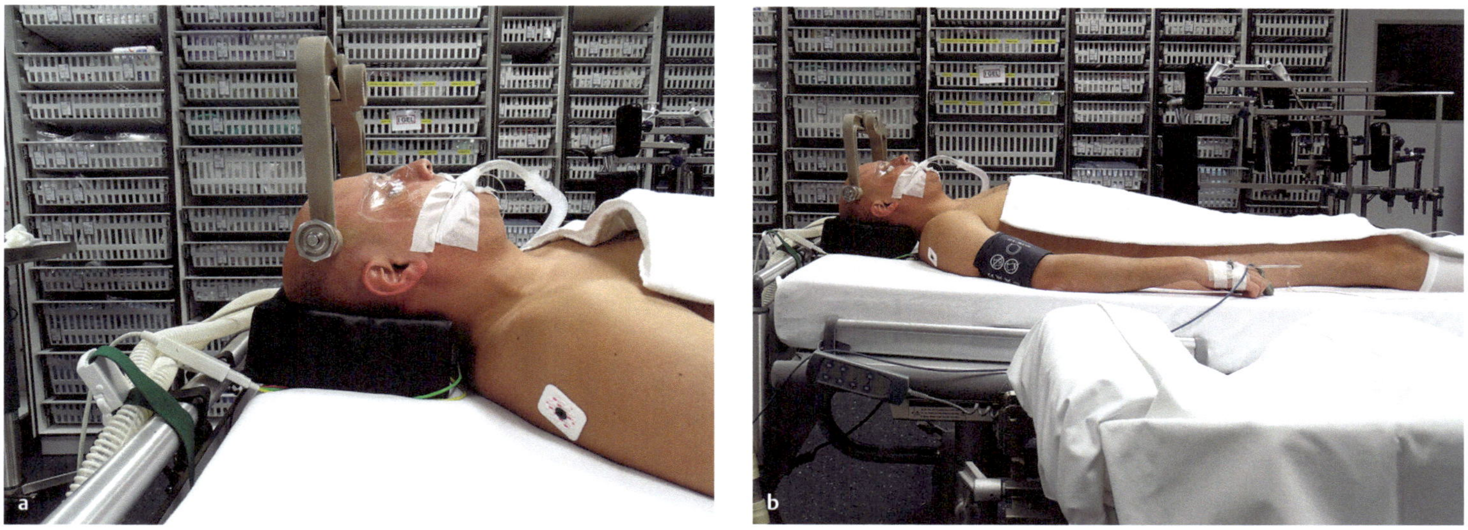

Fig. 1.31 (a, b) Supine position. It is easier for the surgeon to place the Mayfield clamp when the patient is still in the supine position. Care has to be taken to place the pins of the Mayfield clamp anteriorly (about 2–3 cm above the helix of the auricular), to achieve secure head fixation after the patient is turned into the prone position. For a patient in the prone position, a horseshoe headrest can be used instead, depending on the surgical target and the preferences of the surgeon. All lines and tubes need to be fixed securely, since after turning and draping, access to the patient is very limited. Especially for the Concorde position, the patient needs to overhang the cranial end of the operating table. Therefore, the operating table should be put in the right position before the patient is turned **(b)**.

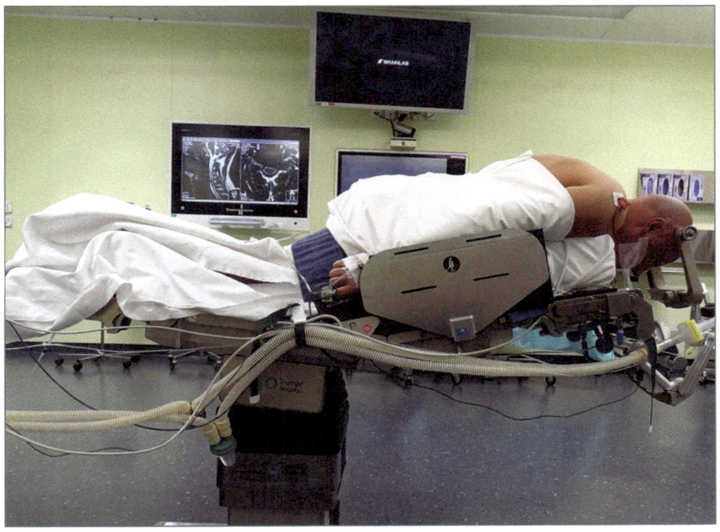

Fig. 1.32 Prone position. For a simple prone position, the Mayfield clamp can be fixed in the required position. This depends on the planned surgical target and the preference of the surgeon. Depending on the flexion of the head, also in prone position the operating table can be positioned in a slight reversed Trendelenburg position to increase venous reflux and align the operating field horizontally (e.g., cervical spine). If necessary, the shoulders can be taped caudally to provide better exposure of the surgical field. For patients in prone position, female breasts and nipples should be mobilized medially and male genitalia should hang freely. For a simple prone position, the patient requires less cranial overlap. Some surgeons use a head support system or specific cushions for positioning of the head instead of a Mayfield clamp or a horseshoe headrest. When such devices are used, the patient does not overhang the operating table.

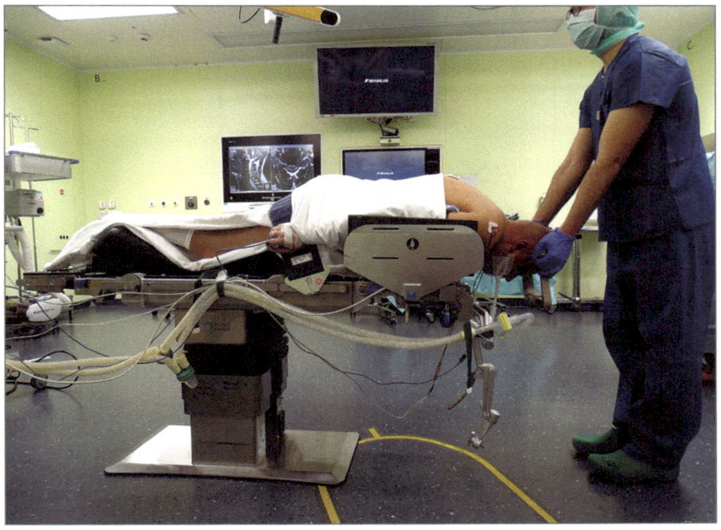

Fig. 1.33 Progress to Concorde position. When progressing to a Concorde position, further steps have to be taken before bringing the head into its final position. Note that the patient overhangs the cranial end of the operating table. This is necessary to enable sufficient flexion of the head in the Concorde position. For the Concorde position, the patient has to be placed in a reversed Trendelenburg position. The knees are properly cushioned and the lower legs are supported with padding in a slightly flexed position. Flexion of the knees and securing the patient with a strap around the buttocks or thighs will prevent the patient from slipping downward while in the reversed Trendelenburg position. This position can be achieved gently by alternately flexing the knees and increasing the reversed Trendelenburg position.

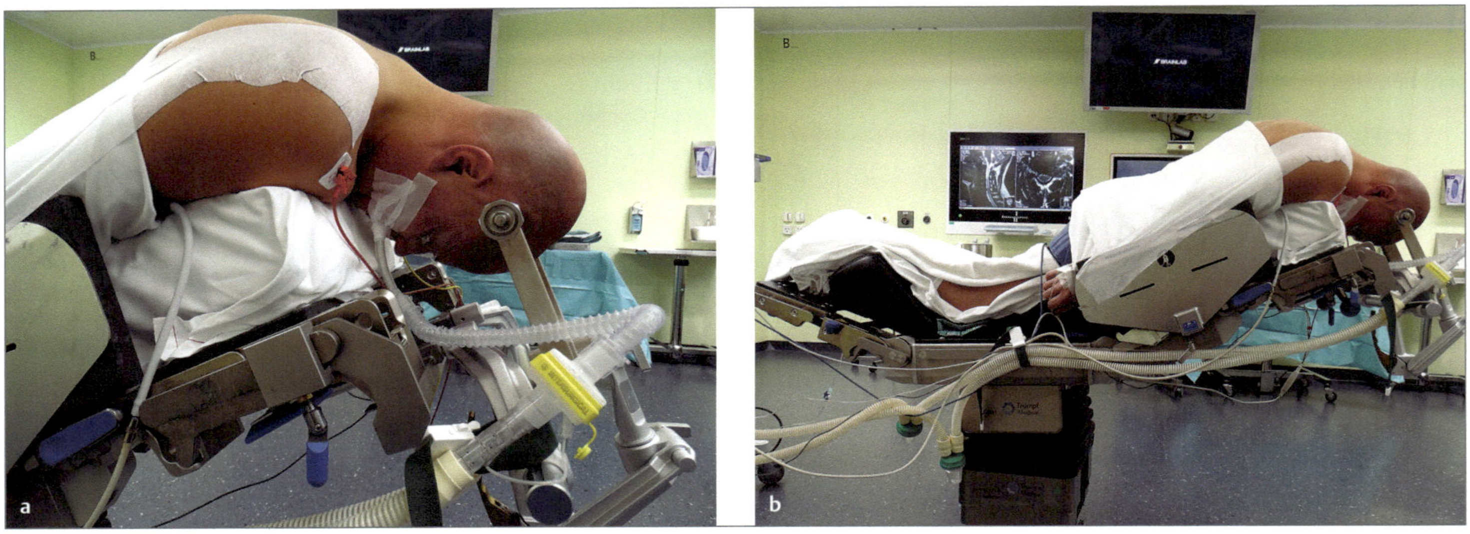

Fig. 1.34 (a, b) **Head position.** The Mayfield clamp should be screwed to the base unit after the patient has been put into the right position. To achieve sufficient exposure of the posterior fossa, the head has to be maximally flexed with just two fingers of space between the chin and the manubrium. The head should be positioned at the level of the heart to achieve a sufficient venous reflux while not increasing the risk of air embolism. To achieve better exposure of the cervical spine and suboccipital region, it is advisable to tape the shoulders toward the feet. The surgeon has to check that the whole face, eyes and especially the chin, is free of any compression by either the Mayfield clamp or the table. The arms are padded and wrapped to the sides of the patient.

Potential Complications of Prone/Concorde Position

Potential complications of the prone/Concorde position include cervical strains with postoperative pain. Patients can develop skin necrosis due to compression and insufficient padding. Excessive downward taping of the shoulders can lead to brachial plexus injury. If the patient is in the prone or Concorde position, the risk of air embolism is lower than in a sitting position but may still occur. In addition, an obstruction of the cerebral lymphatic and venous outflow can cause swelling of the face, tongue, and neck, leading to macroglossia and airway obstruction. The same mechanism can also cause intraoperative brain swelling with increased intracranial pressure. Occasionally, blindness or corneal abrasion after a patient has been in the prone position has been described.

Checklist

- Place Mayfield clamp before turning the patient.
- For Concorde position, remember the cranial overhang to enable sufficient head flexion.
- Maximal head flexion with two fingers of space between chin and manubrium.
- Avoid pressure sores.
- Head at the level of the heart.

Further Readings

Nadar R, Gragnaniello C, Berta SC, et al. Neurosurgery Tricks of the Trade: Cranial. Thieme; 2015

Ellenbogen RG, Abdulrauf SI, Sekhar LN. Principles of Neurological Surgery. 3rd ed. Elsevier; 2012

1.4.8 Semisitting

Andreas Raabe

Introduction

Arguments in favor of the semisitting position for surgery of lesions in the posterior fossa, in occipital or occipitoparietal locations, include: (1) better access to the lesion, (2) improved cerebral venous drainage and less swelling or pressure, (3) less retraction, and (4) promotion of gravity drainage of blood and cerebrospinal fluid. There are also beneficial effects of this position on the cardiovascular and respiratory system, especially in obese patients. Disadvantages include: (1) less comfortable position for the surgeon, (2) potential venous air embolism (VAE) and paradoxical air embolism, (3) tension pneumocephalus, and (4) positioning-related injuries such as spinal cord injury or compressive peripheral neuropathy. The reported incidence of these complications ranges from 0.5 to 30%; however, this number largely depends on correct or incorrect positioning, monitoring, and surgical principles. A dedicated protocol for semisitting positioning and monitoring can reduce clinically relevant VAE to less than 1%.[1]

Intraoperative Anesthesiological Preparation

The patient is prepared with a central line in the right atrium inserted by using a syringe with ECG-monitoring capability and a peripheral catheter in the radial or femoral artery for invasive continuous arterial pressure measurement. Before and during the procedure, the patient is monitored using a transesophageal echocardiography (TEE) device. Preoperative TEE studies are performed to rule out a patent foramen ovale. Routine monitoring should include ECG, pulse oximetry, electrophysiology, invasive arterial pressure, right atrial pressure, and urine output. Continuous monitoring of end tidal CO_2 is used throughout the operation to detect clinically significant VAEs. End tidal CO_2 in combination with TEE is used as the most sensitive parameter.

Positioning

See ▶Fig. 1.35, ▶Fig. 1.36, ▶Fig. 1.37, ▶Fig. 1.38, ▶Fig. 1.39, ▶Fig. 1.40, ▶Fig. 1.41, and ▶Fig. 1.42.

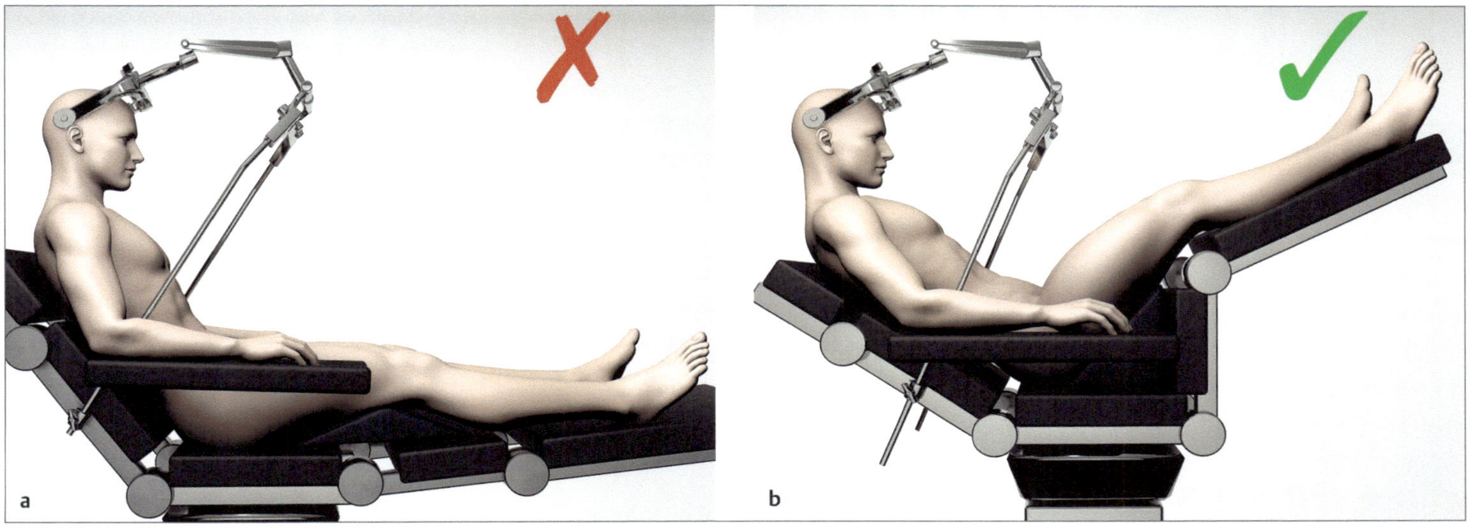

Fig. 1.35 Sitting (wrong) or semisitting position. The illustration on the left **(a)** demonstrates the major error in positioning and the cause of significant complications. The pressure in the transverse and sigmoid sinus determines the risk of air embolism. Using the position shown on the left, pressure in the venous sinus will likely be negative and a venous vessel will not bleed to the outside but suck air in and cause air embolism. The correct position, shown on the right **(b)**, increases the pressure of the right atrium of the heart to eventually achieve a positive pressure in the transverse and sigmoid sinus during the entire expiration cycle of artificial ventilation. The head is much further down in relation to the legs and the body and venous return and pressure is maximized in this position.

Before surgery, the patient should be placed in his or her bed in exactly the same position as that planned for the intraoperative procedure, to ensure that the movements and positioning correspond to the patient's physiological range. This position and the movements are then tested, and the patient is asked to pay attention to report any clinical sign of paresthesia, numbness, Lhermitte's sign, etc.

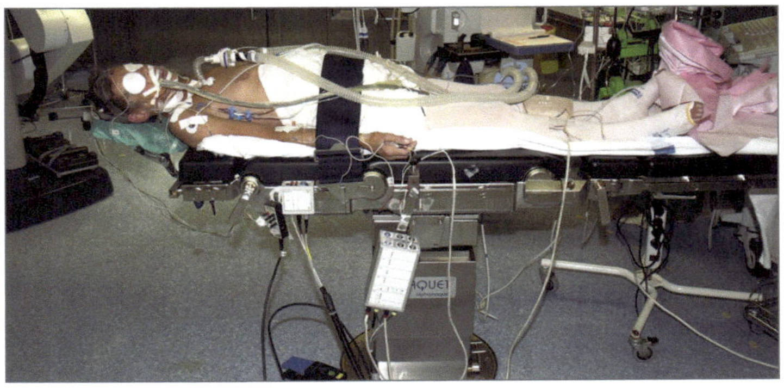

Fig. 1.36 Starting position. Positioning is best achieved with a combination of adjustments of the different parts of the operating table and special cushions. There should be two people working together during positioning.

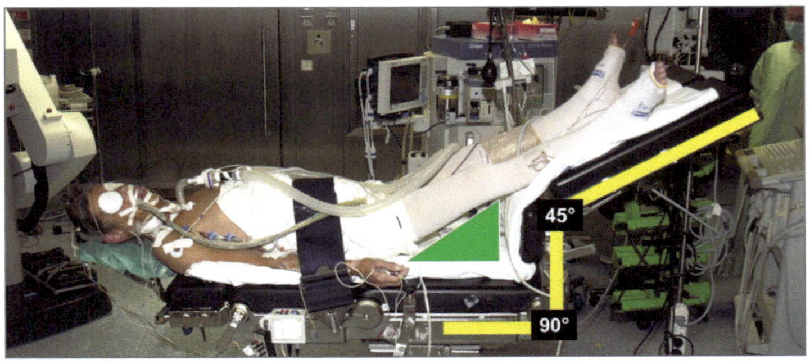

Fig. 1.37 Adjusting leg rise and knee flexion. First, the table is brought into a 30°–45° position to elevate the legs. A triangular cushion is used to bolster the backs of the upper legs. With this step, the hips are flexed to a 30°–45° position. The patient's shoulders should protrude 2–5 cm beyond the upper edge of the table to provide access to the operative field (e.g., retrosigmoid or suboccipital approach).

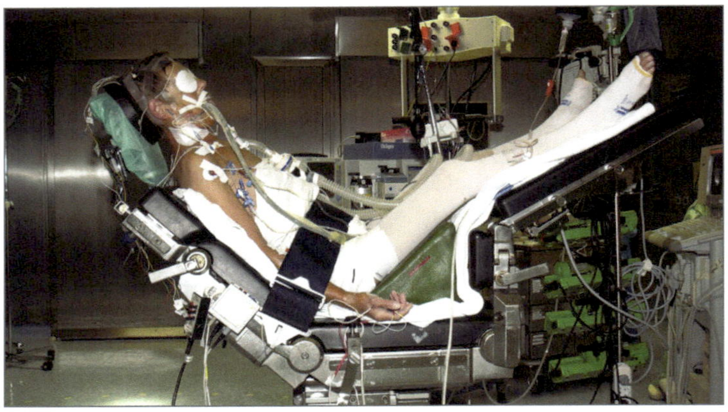

Fig. 1.38 Elevating upper body. Now the patient's upper body is elevated 45° to achieve hip flexion of a maximum of 80°–90°. Then another triangular cushion is used to flex the knees to a 20°–30° angle to avoid overstretching of the tendons and nerves of the legs. We use intraoperative electrophysiological monitoring of somatosensory evoked potential and motor evoked potential when performing this type of positioning and surgery. This monitoring provides an additional safety measure for the patient.

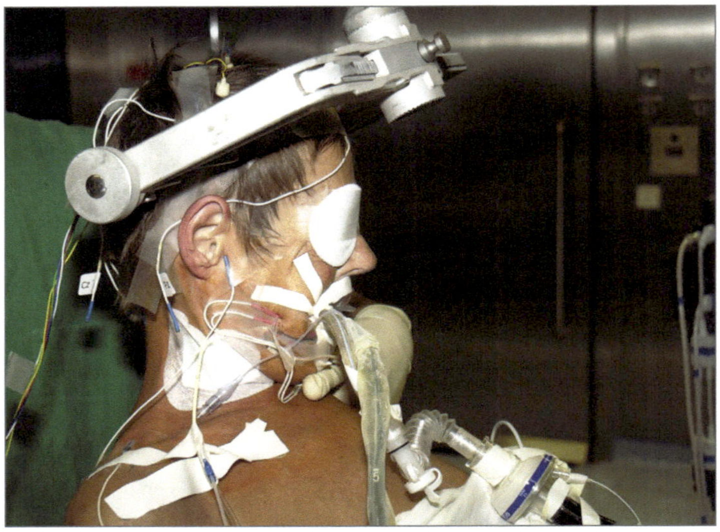

Fig. 1.39 Head flexion. Next, the patient's head is flexed anteriorly in a slow and cautious manner. A two-finger space should be maintained between the jugulum and the patient's chin to avoid venous outflow and airway obstruction. If an increase in resistance occurs during anteflexion of the patient's head, further flexion should be avoided and the head should be fixed in that position. As mentioned earlier, the physiological range of head flexion should be tested in the awake patient before surgery. If preferred, the head may be turned to the side of surgery up to about 45° and tilted laterally to open the space between the shoulder and the mastoid.

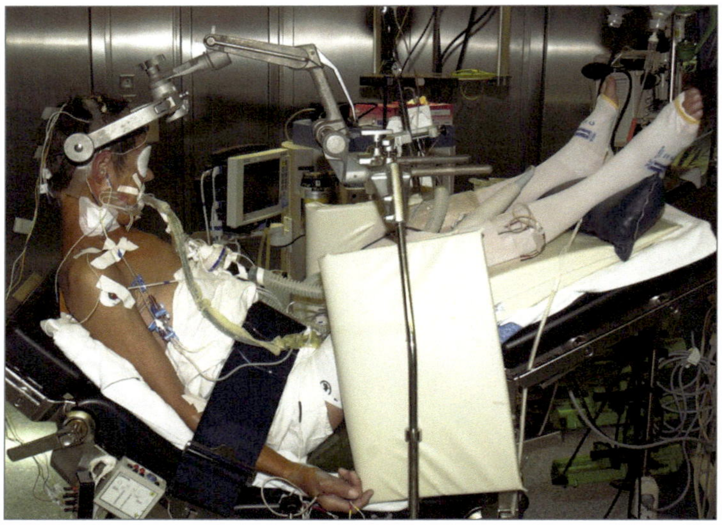

Fig. 1.40 Checking, padding, and locking the table. After securing the patient in that position, the anesthesiologist should ensure that the central line is working and measurements of central venous pressure can be obtained. The Mayfield clamp holder should be fixed as high as possible to provide a maximum amount of working space for the anesthesiologist. The legs, arms, and especially the heels are padded. Now the different platforms of the operating table should be locked to avoid separate movements caused by accidentally pressing the wrong buttons of the remote control during surgery, which can have disastrous consequences. It should only be allowed to move the entire table into a Trendelenburg or reverse Trendelenburg position.

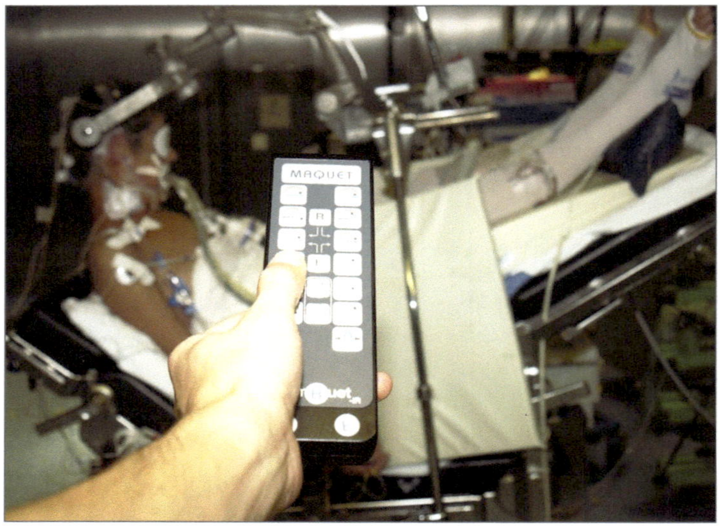

Fig. 1.41 Adjusting final head to heels position. The inclination of the whole operating table is now changed to a lower head and higher legs position, where the feet of the patient are as high as the vertex. This maneuver is performed to increase venous pressure and ultimately achieving a continuous positive venous pressure at the operation site, together with other measures such as fluid input and positive end-expiratory pressure (PEEP) ventilation.

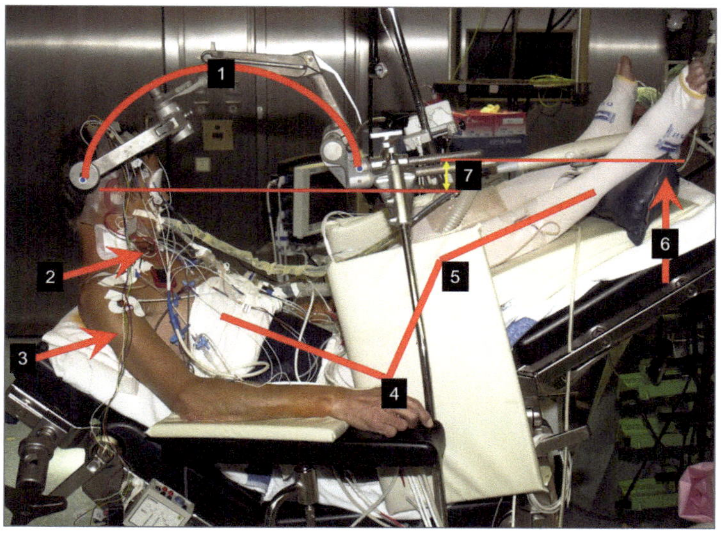

Fig. 1.42 Final position. The patient's arms may be positioned along the body or in special arm holders, but they have to be supported to avoid traction of the shoulder. Once this has been done, the final position is achieved. It can still be adjusted by tilting the table to suit the surgeon's and the anesthesiologist's needs. After the semisitting position has been achieved, TEE position is checked with an intravenous 0.25-mL air injection. Fluid input and urine output is monitored, aiming at a 5–12 cm H_2O pressure in the right atrium. Mechanical ventilation is adjusted to achieve a PEEP of 5–10 mm Hg, which is to be maintained throughout the surgical procedure. A 20-mL syringe is prepared to aspirate air from the right atrium if VAE occurs.

During Surgery: How to Avoid Air Embolism

Air embolism occurs when the pressure in injured and noncollapsed venous vessels is permanently or temporarily decreased to a level where air can enter and be transported to the heart by the bloodstream. Depending on the pressure in the sinus or vein, there are three pressure scenarios.

- If the pressure proximal and distal to the injured vessel is constantly positive, continuous bleeding occurs. The risk of air embolism is low, and the site of bleeding is easily identified.
- If the pressure is constantly negative, bleeding of the injured vessel is absent. In this situation, air is sucked into the vessel and the source of the embolism is difficult for the surgeon to identify. Therefore, intermittent moderate jugular compression performed by the anesthesiologist in a repeated and regular manner is an important safety maneuver. Often, these cases are only identified by jugular compression or, when missed, by the anesthesiologist monitoring for air embolism.
- The third scenario is also very common, with positive pressure in the injured sinus or vein during the inspiration phase of artificial ventilation and negative pressure during the expiration phase of ventilation. In this situation, air may enter the vessel in the expiration phase. The site of the potential air embolism can be found by identifying intermittent venous bleeding that occurs during the inspiration phase of ventilation. Again, jugular compression helps to identify the locations.

The most critical situation in which an air embolism can occur is during craniotomy. Injured venous structures are not visible, and access to sources of air embolism is limited while the craniotomy is being performed. Therefore, critical steps such as moving the craniotome close to the upper part of the sigmoid sinus should be performed as the final step of craniotomy to allow quick removal of the flap and covering of the injured sinus using, for example, gelatin foam. Special care should be taken not to push any material into the sinus but only to cover the site of the bleeding. The ultimate goal should be to avoid injury to the sinus. There are several techniques, such as using navigation or drilling the bone over the sinus instead of using the craniotome, which can be helpful. Which pressure scenario applies to the patient may be recognized even before the craniotomy by watching typical venous bleeding sites, such as the emissary vein at the mastoid, and appropriate measures can be taken to increase the venous pressure before beginning the craniotomy. After the craniotomy, the dura is immediately inspected for injuries and the bone is waxed. Injuries to the sinus are best closed with sutures or by gluing gelatin foam, muscle, or fascia, or both techniques together. Close communication between the surgeon and the anesthesiologist is required. The surgeon can pass the information about the pressure in the transverse and sigmoid sinus to the anesthesiologist—i.e., whether the sinus is inflated or collapsed, or intermittently inflated and collapsed during the respiration cycle. Often the team can create a scenario less likely to favor air embolism, when PEEP is increased, fluid is administered, and the patient is put in a more head-down and feet-up position. As mentioned earlier, we recommend repeated moderate jugular compression, e.g., after creating the skin flap and detaching the skin/muscle/fascia layer from the occipital bone, after craniotomy, and after dural incision before starting the intradural part of the procedure, which may last many hours in some cases.

Checklist

- Use TEE to check for patent foramen ovale before considering a semisitting position.
- Test the positioning with head anteflexion, head turning, and leg positioning with the patient awake the day before surgery.
- The Mayfield clamp holder should be placed with the metal arm upward to increase space for the anesthesiologist to work.
- The chin should be at two fingers distance from the jugulum.
- Traction on the shoulder should be avoided by placing the arms on armrests.
- The hip is flexed not more than 90°.
- The knee is extended not more than 20–30°. More flexion avoids nerve tension.
- The heels should be kept in the air by bolstering the lower leg.
- Finally, the table should be tilted so that the heels are higher than the transverse sinus.
- Remote control of the tables positioning system should be locked.

Reference

[1] Jadik S, Wissing H, Friedrich K, Beck J, Seifert V, Raabe A. A standardized protocol for the prevention of clinically relevant venous air embolism during neurosurgical interventions in the semisitting position. Neurosurgery 2009;64(3):533–538, discussion 538–539

1.5 Rigid Head Fixation

Christian Fung

See ▶ Fig. 1.43, ▶ Fig. 1.44, ▶ Fig. 1.45, and ▶ Fig. 1.46.

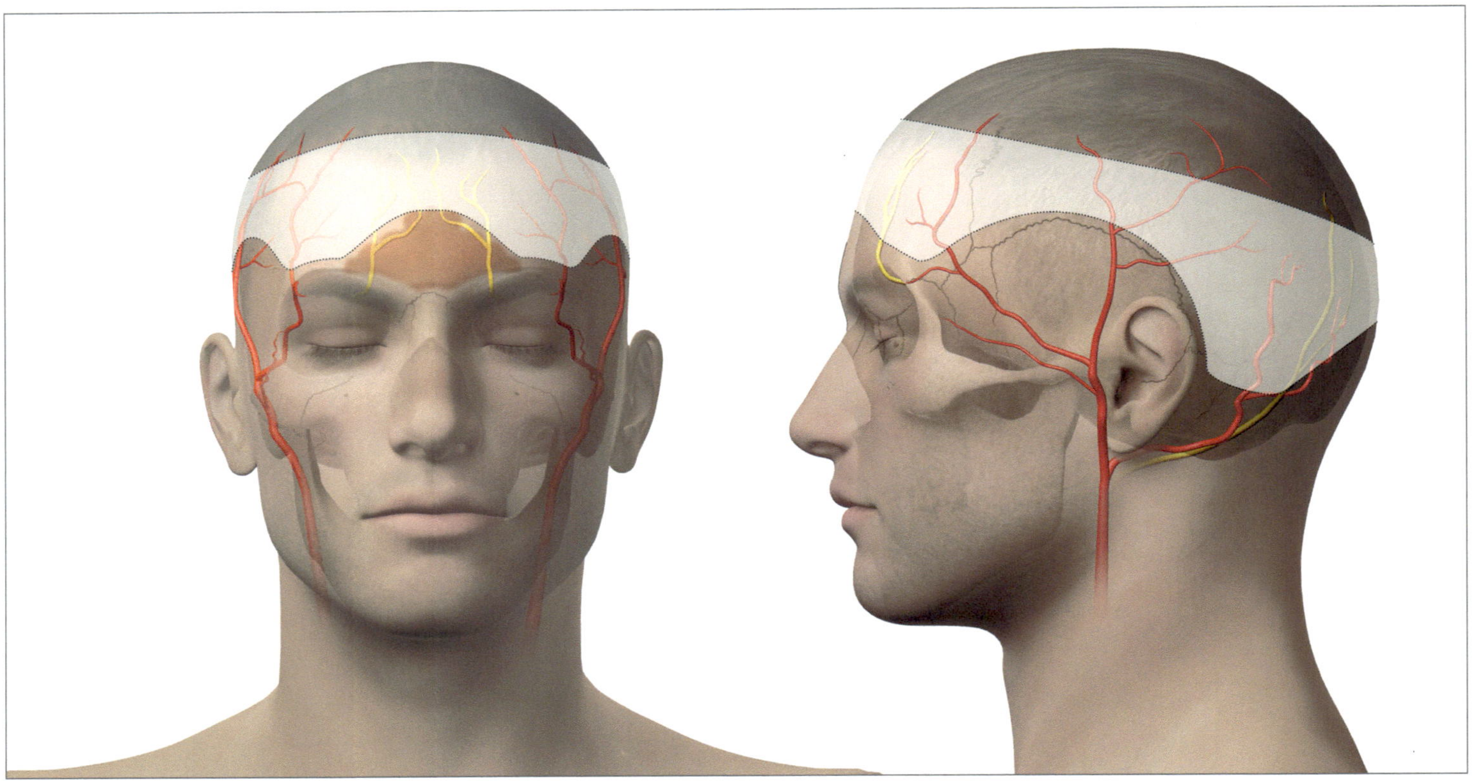

Fig. 1.43 Anatomy of the head and danger zones for rigid fixation. The purpose of rigid head fixation is safe immobilization of the head during neurosurgical procedures (cranial and cervical). It prevents unwanted movements of the head during surgery and enables us to use neuronavigation. Care has to be taken to avoid vascular (superficial temporal artery, occipital artery) and neuronal (supraorbital, occipital nerve) structures, and areas where the bone is thin and fragile to prevent a fracture or penetrating with a pin. Attention should also be paid to avoiding structures like the orbit and the pinna, prior craniotomy defects, or foreign material (shunts, electrodes running subcutaneously).

The safe zone for the placement of the rigid head fixation is often depicted as a circumferential headband. This is not entirely correct, because the width of this area changes from anterior to posterior. It does not extend:

- Frontally at the area of the frontal sinus.
- Temporally below the superior temporal line, because of the thin bone and the temporalis muscle.
- Occipitally, in the area of the nuchal muscles.
- Above the "headband," where the curvature of the bone may prevent correct fixation because the pins can slip off when minimal movements occur.

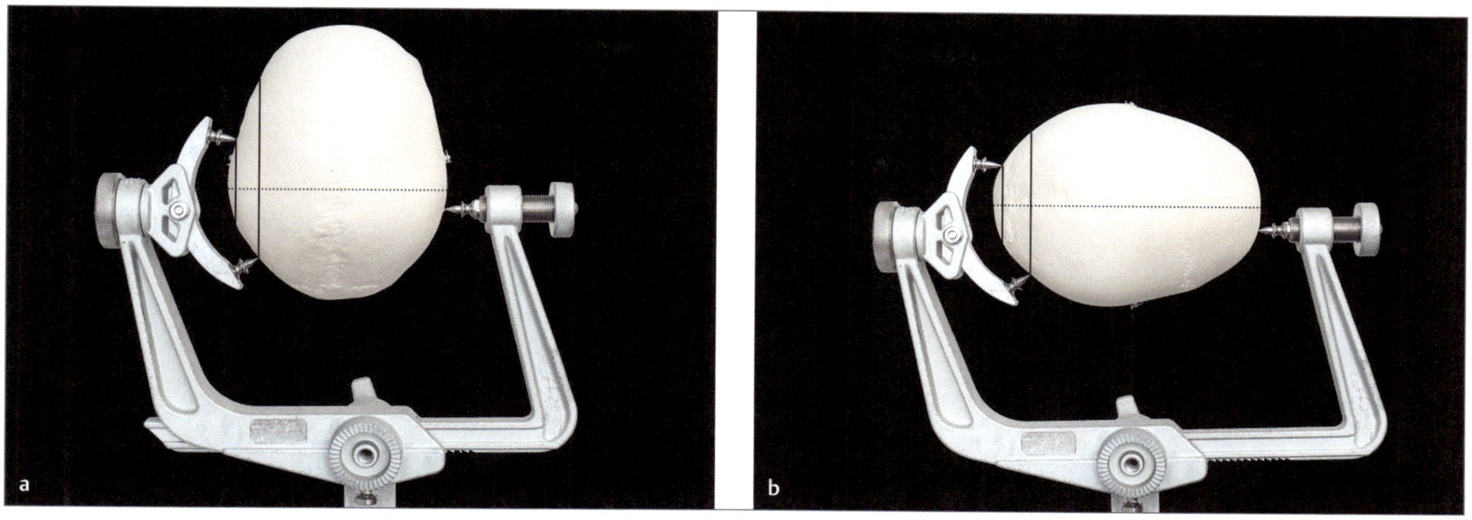

Fig. 1.44 (a, b) Pin placement to avoid dislocation. The pins fix the head at the level of the cortical bone but do not penetrate it. Thus, the head may move when excessive pressure or traction is applied to the head, e.g., due to too much pressure during trephination, a forceful craniotomy or insufficient mobilization of the skin, muscular structures, or a scar (traction by fish hooks). Also, if pins are placed near a convexity curve of the skull, they may lose bone contact within few millimeters of displacement.

The two-pin swivel should be placed first, followed by the single pin. Two of the three pins should be positioned below the largest diameter (equator) of the skull. This prevents downward displacement even when extensive pressure is applied from above. One pin should be above the equator to prevent dislocation by upward traction or rotational forces (e.g., by fish hooks).

In addition, the two-point swivel should be positioned so that the lower pin is located further "inward" (see vertical lines) than the upper pin. This placement of the pins ensures strong and safe positioning because the head is "pushed into" the pins. In adults, the usual pin pressure is 60 lbs (each line on the torque knob corresponds to 20 lbs).

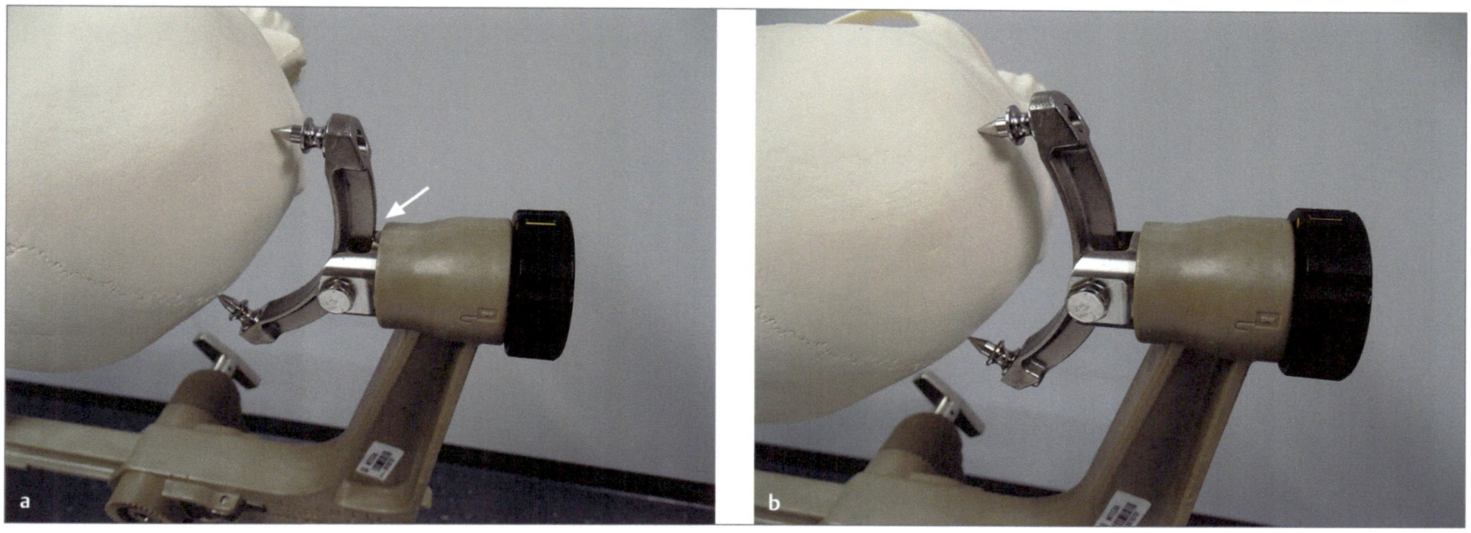

Fig. 1.45 Avoidance of a blocked two-pin swivel. The head clamp should not hinder the movements of the hands during surgery. Thus, both sides should usually be placed below the surgical field except in special positions (semisitting or lateral or oblique surgical fields). The two-pin swivel should have the necessary range of movement and not be blocked on one side. This ensures an even distribution of the applied force between the two pins of the two-point swivel. Image **(a)** shows a blocked two-point swivel at its superior aspect (*arrow*) which may cause the lower pin to have less or no bone contact, in contrast to a swivel with a preserved range of motion **(b)**.

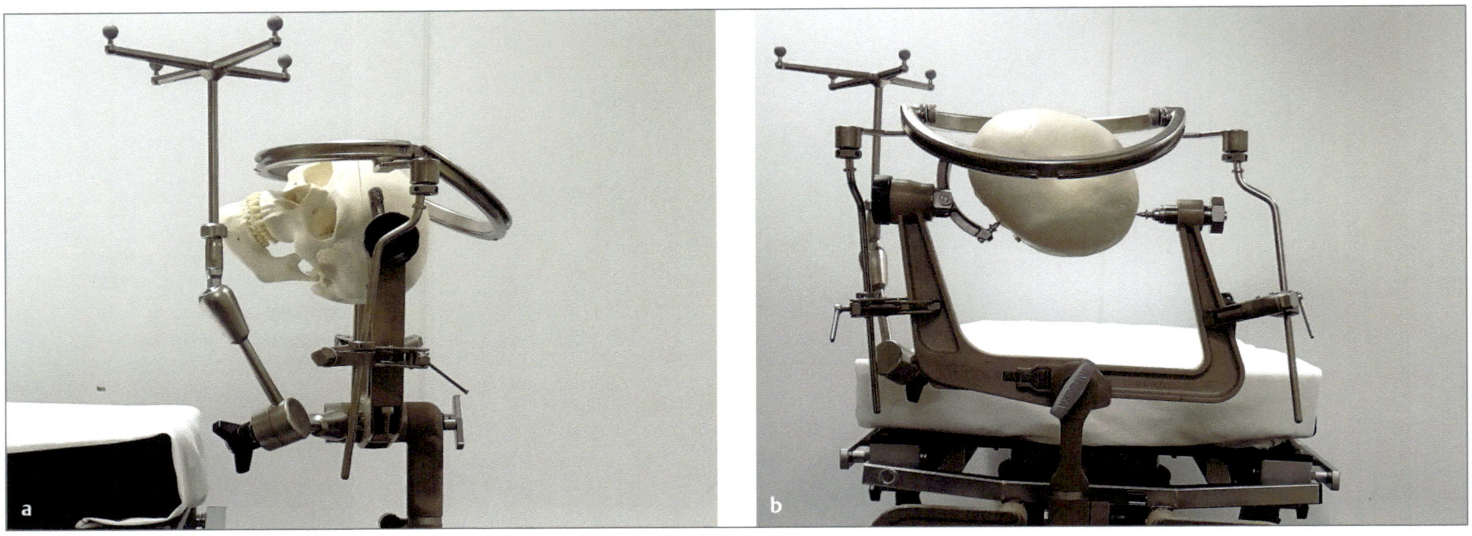

Fig. 1.46 (a, b) Mayfield clamp as base for attachment of other equipment. The position of the Mayfield clamp should allow the addition of equipment such as a Halo retractor horizontally without forcing it into an oblique position. Some textbooks show an obliquely applied Mayfield clamp. This is necessary when the patient's position and the surgical target require this position, but the general rule is that the more horizontally the Mayfield clamp is situated, the more easily the Halo retractor can be added and the more room there is for the surgeon's hands.

During awake craniotomies, a free airway and free deglutition must also be assured, for the comfort of the patient.

The fixation of the head and tightening of the pins may cause tachycardia and hypertension; therefore, the application of the rigid head fixation should be done in agreement with the anesthetist after administration of an additional analgesic bolus and waiting for 1 minute (▶ Fig. 1.47, ▶ Fig. 1.48, and ▶ Fig. 1.49).

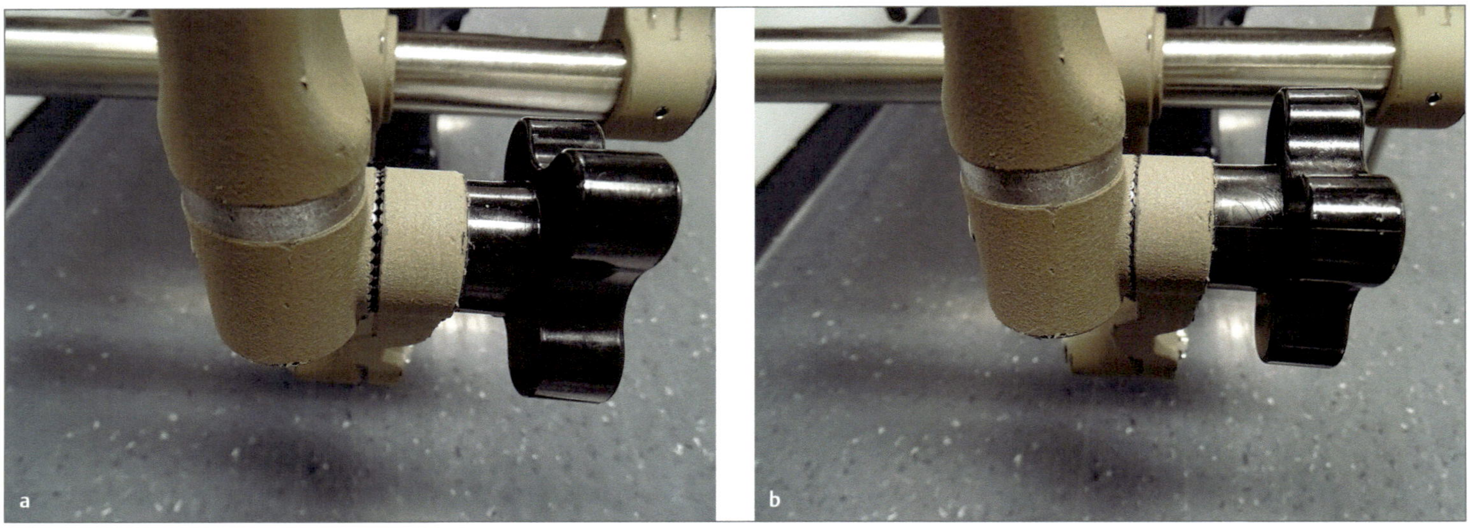

Fig. 1.47 (a, b) Correct clamp fixation. Before placing the pins, some surgeons apply antibiotic ointment to decrease the risk of infection and to seal the skin in order to protect against air embolism. This may be considered, especially when the head is positioned higher than the heart, such as in a patient in the semisitting position or supine position and when the head is extensively flexed. The fixation of the head clamp is screwed to the table and the clamp arm should be checked to make sure that all the joints are tightly fixed and in the correct position **(a)**. As final check, some pressure should be put on the fixed head in an upward and downward direction imitating the pressure of trepanation and the pulling force of the fish hooks to make sure that the head does not dislocate. By using this maneuver, a loose joint below the clamp can also be detected.

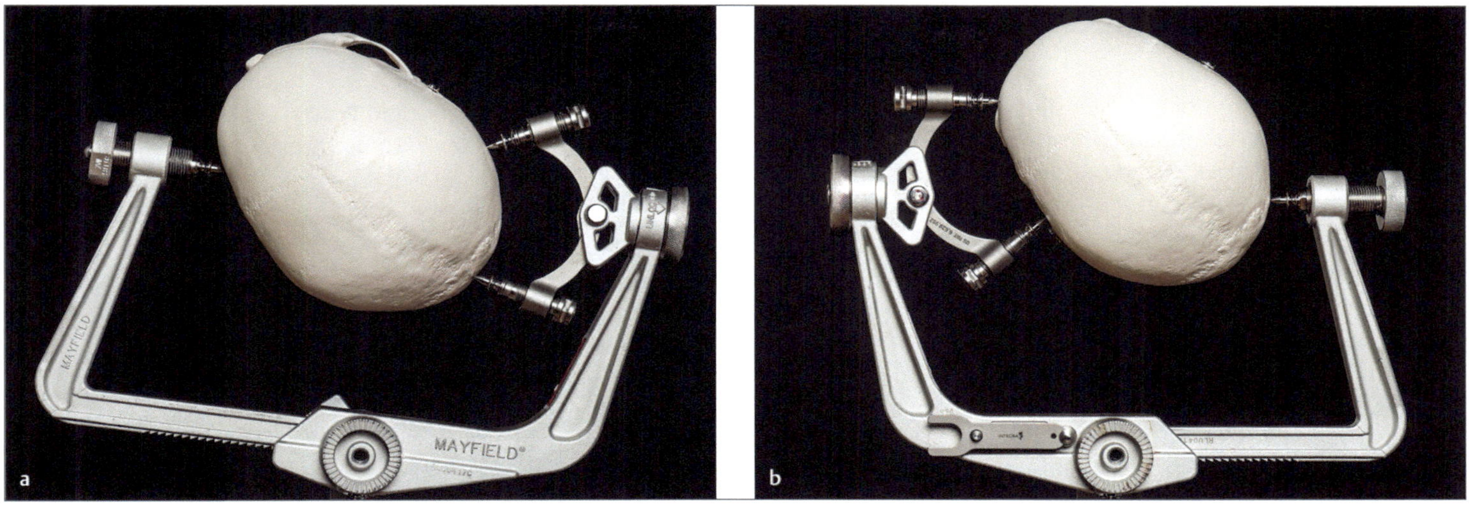

Fig. 1.48 (a, b) Two pins anterior or posterior. The position of the pins must be adapted according to the desired head position and the skin incision. Whether the two-point swivel is placed anteriorly or posteriorly depends on the surgeon's preference. Both provide a rigid fixation. Our preference is to position the two pins frontally because this gives a right-handed surgeon more room for manual maneuvering during surgery.

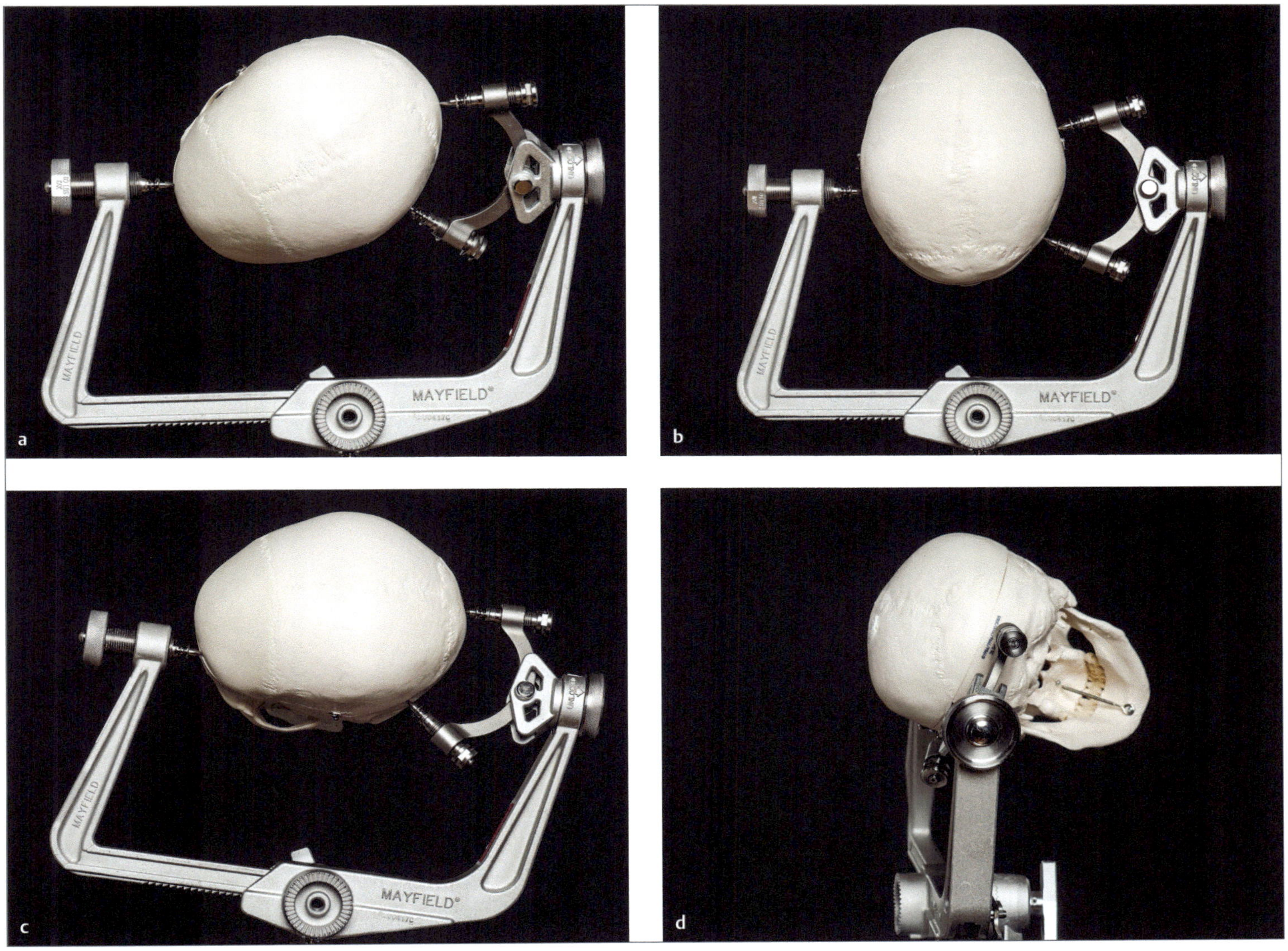

Fig. 1.49 More examples of different positions. These are examples of positions for retrosigmoid craniotomy **(a)**, frontal craniotomy **(b)**, and hemicraniectomy **(c, d)**.

Rigid Head Fixation in Children

The variable thickness of a developing cranium poses an increased risk during application of the rigid head fixation. The surgeon has to pay special attention to the thickness of the cranial vault, patency of the fontanelle, status of fusion of the bony sutures, and factors that might cause a thinning of the cranial vault (e.g., chronic hydrocephalus).

In children under the age of 3 years, rigid head fixation should be avoided. A padded horseshoe headrest can be used instead. The fixation of the head can be supported using adhesive tape.

For children between 3 and 10 to 12 years of age, smaller pins should be used and the pin pressure should not exceed 20 to 40 lbs. The lower pin carries the higher risk of slippage; therefore, excessive force during trephination, craniotomy, and retraction should be avoided. The pressure and size of the pin should be adapted according to the individual head and scalp of the child. For example, the shoulder of the pediatric pin may sometimes cause pressure lacerations in children with a thick scalp. To avoid skin necrosis, surgeons sometimes prefer to use pins designed for use in adults when operating on children, but with reduced pin pressure. Finally, there are no standardized recommendations for rigid head fixation in children. The surgeon has to choose according to his experience and needs, taking the individual child's anatomy into account.

Potential Complications of Rigid Head Fixation

Potential complications of rigid head fixation include skin lacerations due to movement of the pins or skin necrosis (especially in pediatric patients) and bleeding from the sites of pin location. Occasionally, patients develop infections at the site of the pins. Fractures (ping pong fractures in infants) with or without accompanying epidural hematoma may result from incorrect location or a pin pressure that is too high. Rare cases of air embolism or a cerebrospinal fluid leak have been described, mainly in patients in sitting positions and pediatric patients, respectively.

Further Readings

Cohen AR. Pediatric Neurosurgery: Tricks of the Trade. Thieme; 2015

Ellenbogen RG, Abdulrauf SI, Sekhar LN. Principles of Neurological Surgery. 3rd ed. Elsevier; 2012

Winn H. Youmans Neurological Surgery. 6th ed. Elsevier; 2011

Greenberg MS. Handbook of Neurosurgery. 7th ed. Thieme; 2010

1.6 Esthetic Considerations in Neurosurgical Procedures

Mihai A. Constantinescu, Irena Zubak, and Andreas Raabe

Although everybody agrees that esthetic considerations have always been a part of the neurosurgical procedure, both patients and surgeons nowadays have higher expectations of optimal result. Patient dissatisfaction can result from unesthetic sequelae, for example, burr holes that can be seen or felt, asymmetric appearance of the head, or an avoidable visible scar.

1.6.1 Skin Incision

Basic Considerations

The skin incision is planned in the area covered by the patient's hair, while allowing good exposure of the operation field. A minimum distance of 1 to 2 cm to the hairline should be respected to reduce visibility. The superficial temporal artery should be spared as it can be useful for later reconstructive microsurgical procedures.

Particular considerations apply to bald patients where the classical curved frontotemporal skin incision extending from the tragus to the midline behind the forehead makes less sense. Here, either a bicoronal, or transciliary, or supraciliary, or forehead (=frontal wrinkle) incision can be used (▸Fig. 1.50). Many maxillofacial surgeons prefer the bicoronal incision to an incision in a visible wrinkle of the forehead. If the latter is used, it must be made in a frontal wrinkle at least 3 to 4 cm above the eyebrow to avoid the motor branches of the facial nerve.

An eyebrow incision usually also gives an esthetically pleasing result with an almost invisible scar. Some authors prefer a supraciliary incision to spare the hair follicle immediately above and following the eyebrow, starting lateral to the supraorbital foramen and nerve, and extending 4 to 5 cm laterally. Plastic surgeons also use infraciliary incision, but this often further limits the space for a supraorbital craniotomy. For safety zones of the facial nerve, see Chapter 5.2.1, Facial Nerve Anatomy and Protection by Raabe and Winkler.

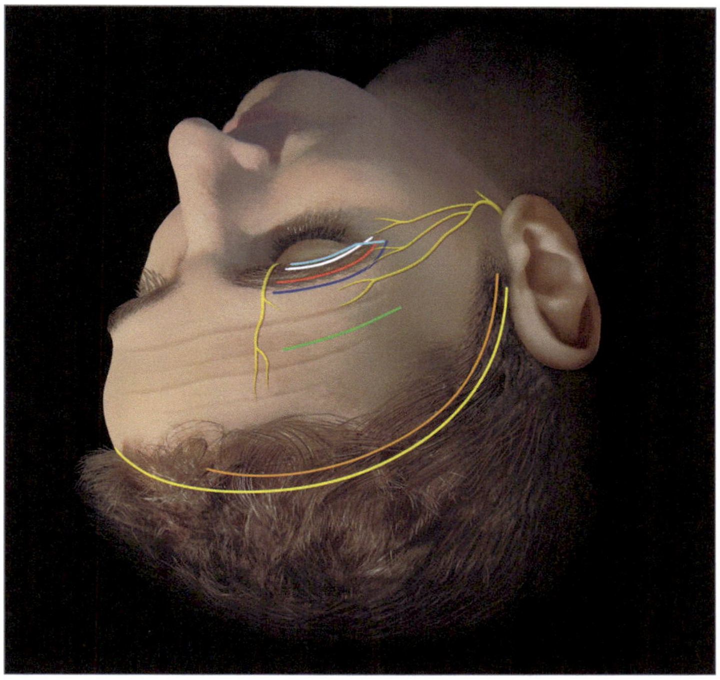

Fig. 1.50 Skin incision. Transpalpebral (*light blue*), infraciliary (*white*), transciliary (*red*), supraciliary (*dark blue*), transfrontal skin wrinkle (*green*), frontotemporal curved (*orange*), and bicoronal (*yellow*) skin incision.

Reducing Scar Formation and Visibility

Monopolar and bipolar cautery should be minimized because of the thermal damage to the hair follicles. Infiltration with vasoconstrictors like adrenaline (epinephrine) 1:100,000 (1 mg epinephrine added to 100 mL of Ringer's solution or local anesthetics) 5 to 10 minutes before incision may markedly reduce bleeding and thus the need for coagulation. Preserve hair follicles by incising slightly oblique, holding the blade parallel to the direction of hair growth.

Coagulation should also be minimized at closure because the galeal and superficial sutures or staples will provide reliable hemostasis. The subcutaneous sutures can be either running or interrupted using 2–0 or 3–0 resorbable sutures. Make sure the knots are deep beneath the galea and threads do not stick out of the skin incision. Otherwise, they may serve as entry points for bacteria and will result in small local ulcerations that may persist for weeks. Underlying implants (Palacos, mesh, etc.) have a higher risk of infection in such cases. After tension of the skin has been reduced by a deep suture, closure of the superficial wound layer should be performed tension-free using either nonresorbable single stitches (usually 3–0, to be removed after 7–14 days) or with staples (which are both authors' preference and are believed to interfere least with the hair follicle perfusion).

In non-hair bearing areas, incision should be along the tension lines and not crossing cosmetic units. ▸Fig. 1.51 depicts the typical tension lines of the skin as described by Langer, a Viennese anatomist of the 19th century, who found out that skin folds usually run perpendicular to the underlying musculature and thus the scars produced in these folds tend to become less visible since they are subject to weaker transverse tension forces. If in doubt about the exact course of these lines, ask the patient to give you a big smile or to frown while you mark the folds.

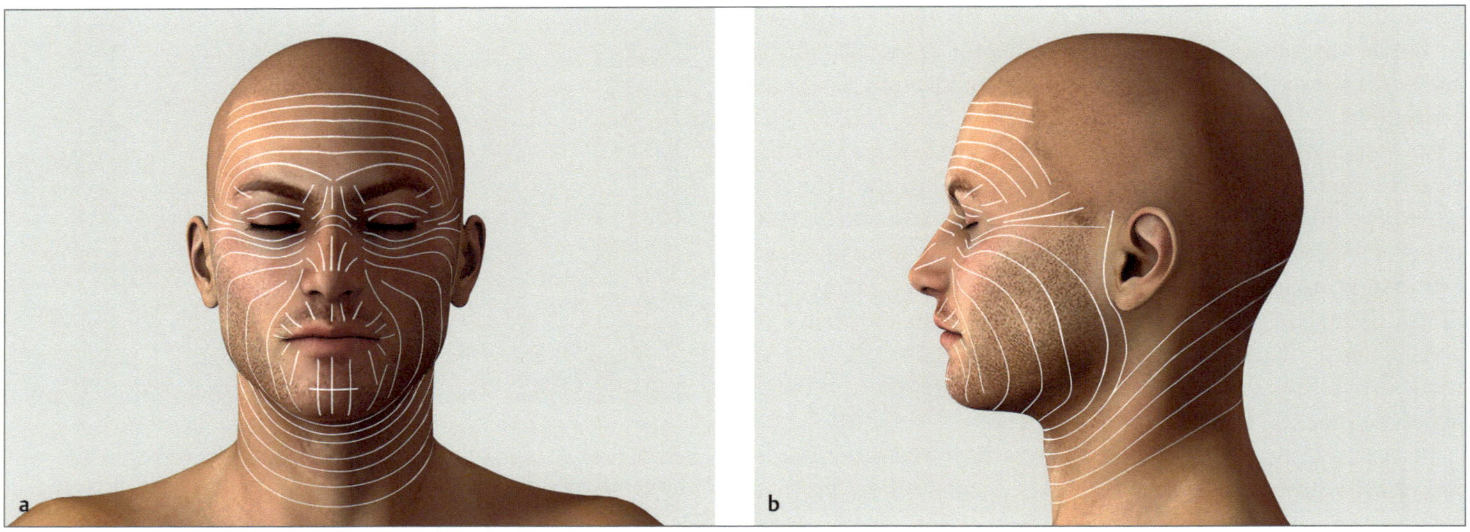

Fig. 1.51 Typical tension lines of the skin. (a) Anteroposterior view. **(b)** Lateral view.

Optimizing Soft Tissue Perfusion and Wound Healing

At the convexity, we prefer straight incisions because they have bilateral 180° vascular supply, are easy to readapt, well covered by the hair of the patient, and do not usually need scalp clips for hemostasis when a wound retractor spreads the skin with slight pressure.

For some regions, for instance, above the ear, or for some approaches such as the far-lateral approach, it makes sense to use a horseshoe incision to allow sufficient exposure or to preserve the integrity of underlying muscular layers.

Another important factor for optimal wound healing is the intraoperative pressure on the edges of the wound and its duration. Excessive pressure by a retractor or by fish hooks can cause small necroses of the skin resulting in wound crusts, loss of hair follicles, and visible scars. This also applies to the frontotemporal flap where kinking and excessive tension should be avoided as it may result in skin necrosis. A compress folded below the turned skin flap can help avoid the kinking of the skin.

We recommend that after having performed the craniotomy, the tension on the skin edges is checked and reduced to the amount required to keep the surgical field optimally open. In most cases, tension of the retractors or fish hooks on the skin can be reduced considerably.

Revision Surgery

If you need to expand your surgical approach and extending the preexisting scar is not enough, the golden rule is that the new incision should not cross the existing scar. If this is unavoidable, then a T-design with the scars at right angles to one another will heal better than a V-shape (with acute angles) or a "cross" design with four corners joined together. Each of these designs limits tissue perfusion which has a direct bearing on how well the incision will heal.

Wound Dressing

The wound dressing of a dry freshly performed suture or staple line should provide dryness and stability while allowing the wound to "breathe." There is no particular evidence in favor of any specific brand or dressing technique. The stapling or suturing of gauze onto the closed wound is our preferred technique for places covered by hair, but the dressing has to be removed after a maximum of 3 to 5 days, or earlier if the dressing is continuously wet, because otherwise skin maceration will occur. If the wound closure line appears repeatedly damp, the application of iodine solution twice daily and leaving the area to dry in the air can be helpful. Our personal opinion is that a surgically well-adapted and closed wound will heal in spite of the dressing chosen rather than because of it (▶ Fig. 1.52).

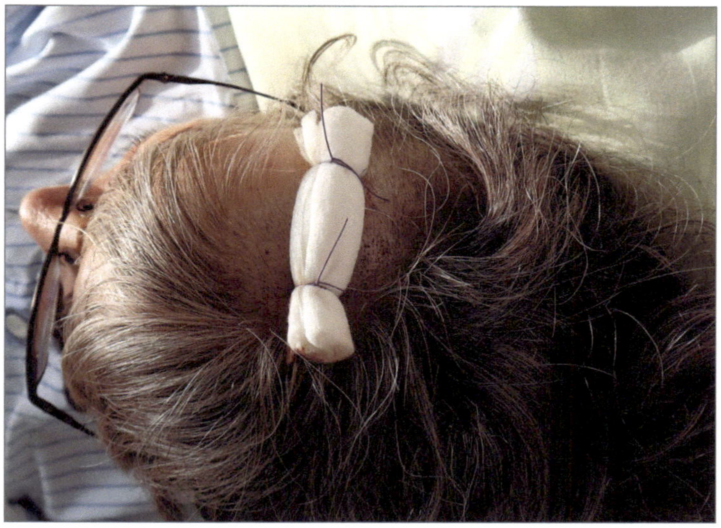

Fig. 1.52 Sutured wound dressing. The compress is sutured on to the wound with two to three stitches. It is removed on the third day.

Wound Crusts

Despite the best surgical planning and tissue handling, crusts and poor wound healing can still occur. In former times, the crusts were left in place in the hope that the tissue would heal underneath until they fell off on their own. It is, however, important to ask two questions when deciding how to handle a crust:

- Is the crust due to dried blood or due to necrotic skin?
- What is most likely to be underneath this crust (implant, Palacos, perfused bone)?

Crusts resulting from dried blood can be washed or picked away as soon as possible, resulting in a clean and dry wound that will continue to heal. A crust formed from dead skin harbors bacteria and will be detrimental to the local wound bed; therefore, they can also be removed. Particular caution is recommended when the crusts are located over an implant or unperfused calvarial bone. In this case, the removal should be performed in the operating theater under sterile conditions followed by an immediate secondary closure or soft tissue reconstruction. Unfortunately, necrotic skin does not present a barrier to bacteria, which will quickly contaminate and colonize any underlying foreign material, to the point where it will frequently require replacement.

1.6.2 Burr Holes

Burr holes may result in a visible disfigurement if not handled correctly. Immediately after surgery, the skin covers the burr hole and the esthetic appearance seems to be preserved. However, over time, the scar within the hole retracts the skin and a visible and palpable skin depression develops. This also affects burr holes covered by hair, because the patient will still feel them when combing the hair or touching the skin.

The degree of deformity depends on the size of the burr hole and its location. The following rules help to achieve good results.

The burr hole(s) should be:

- As small as is safe for the procedure; most craniotomies can be performed using a small or medium-sized cutter.
- Covered by the temporalis muscle.
- Avoided or minimized in frontal visible areas.
- Covered by a cap or plate or mesh (may still be palpable, when not drilled flash with the bone) or with bone cement.
- Avoided in the cosmetically sensitive frontotemporal area where the temporalis muscle is prone to atrophy or asymmetry.

Therefore, our teaching is to avoid the classical MacCarty "keyhole-burr-hole," especially when no orbitotomy is planned. The MacCarty burr hole is usually placed 5 mm posterior and 7 mm superior the frontozygomatic suture[1] to expose the dura and the periorbita with only one burr hole, allowing a craniotome to be used for orbitotomy, but this is not required for a typical frontolateral, supraorbital, or pterional craniotomy.

1.6.3 Mini-plates or Craniotomy Fixation Caps

Bone fixation is usually performed with mini-plates or fixation clamps. These help to reestablish the correct contour, but some special considerations apply to their use. Although they are advertised as being "low profile," they can still be felt beneath the skin or, in some cases, may even disturb the esthetic appearance when placed prominently in a frontal visible region. To achieve the best esthetic results, the mini-plates can be drilled into the bone so that they are absolutely flush with the surface (▶Fig. 1.53).

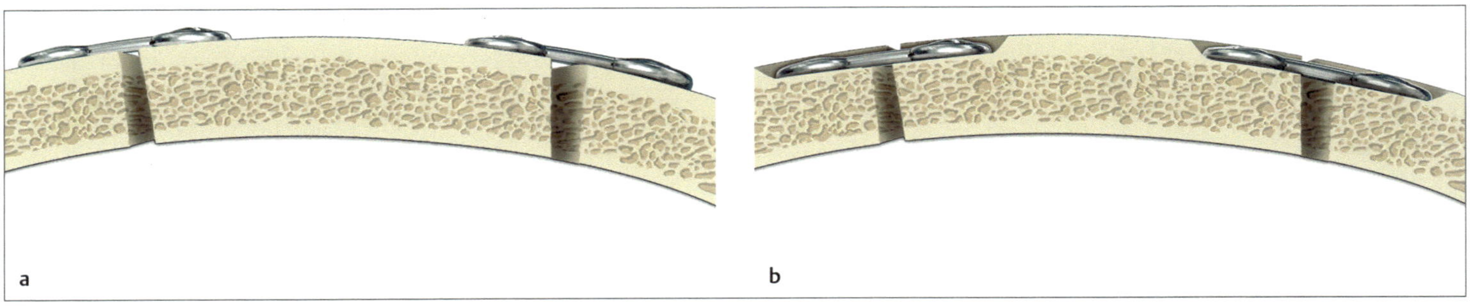

Fig. 1.53 Mini-plates milled into the bone. Although "low profile," many mini-plates may still be palpated or even seen in cosmetically sensitive areas **(a)**. Drilling a groove and placing them with the upper surface of the plate flush with the bone surface may optimize patient satisfaction **(b)**.

1.6.4 Craniotomy Caps

The standard craniotomy blade removes about 2 mm of bone at the craniotomy line. The classical, but not uniformly accepted teaching is that the bone flap should be in contact with the intact bone at least on one side to reduce resorption (▶Fig. 1.54a). This may result in a larger gap on the other two sides, which can easily be tolerated in the deep temporal or occipital region when covered by a thick muscle. However, in esthetically sensitive regions, such as the frontal and frontolateral areas, a large gap should be filled using bone cement or by placing the bone flap centrally and using bone chips saved during placement of the burr hole (▶Fig. 1.54b). We recommend keeping the bone dust or chips in just a few milliliters of a 240 mg/1,000 mL gentamycin solution, and covering the container to prevent any bacterial contamination, until completion of the surgery and the refixing of the bone flap.

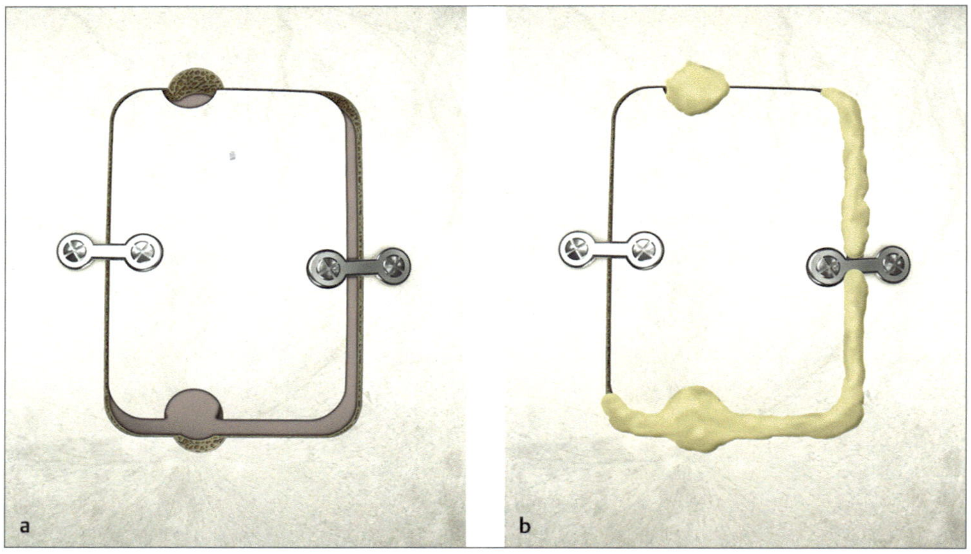

Fig. 1.54 Closing the bone gap for best cosmesis. The craniotomy blade may create a considerable bone gap in some cases, especially when the bone is fixed with two sides in direct contact with the skull **(a)**. In these cases, the gap and the burr holes should be filled with Palacos cement or hydroxylapatite or similar material to ensure good esthetic contouring **(b)**.

1.6.5 The Temporalis Muscle

This muscle is an important soft tissue filler for the underlying bony temporal fossa and its atrophy or retraction can lead to visible and disturbing contour deformities that cannot always be sufficiently hidden by hair. During surgery, this muscle should thus be handled with care and excessive use of monopolar or bipolar coagulation should be avoided. The retraction force of fish hooks that may be required to expose the craniotomy site should be checked and minimized before starting the surgical procedure because excessive pressure can cause muscle damage and necrosis. The best cosmetic results can be achieved with the combined musculocutaneous flap and by avoiding a MacCarty burr hole at the spheno-fronto-zygomatic region.

Some surgeons use a technique that involves leaving a muscle cuff at the superior temporal line to resuture the muscle, but this is rarely required for pterional craniotomy when using the musculocutaneous flap because the cosmetic results are usually excellent. Dissecting the temporal muscle subfascially or interfascially, dissecting it from the orbit and zygoma and folding it posteroinferiorly, may be more likely to lead to atrophy. In these cases, suturing the temporalis muscle and its fascia back to a cuff may be helpful.

1.6.6 Secondary Procedures for Restoration of Contour after Temporal Muscle Atrophy

As previously mentioned, the bony fossa temporalis is a concave area normally filled by the temporalis muscle. If the muscle retracts from its origins or atrophies, a noticeable contour deformity disturbs the esthetic appearance.

The lack of local volume can be successfully treated by autologous fat transfer, also known as lipofilling (▶ Fig. 1.55). In this procedure, liposuction is performed in an area of abundant fat (usually the abdomen or thighs) and the harvested fat cells are separated from the other tissues and fluids using different techniques (i.e., centrifugation, sieving, etc.). The fat and stem cells obtained are then injected with special cannulas into the previously marked area aiming at overinjecting about 30% of the necessary volume, since a certain amount of the cells will be resorbed. The procedure is usually repeated twice more with a delay of at least 3 to 6 months between treatments, depending on the individual`s resorption, and will usually achieve a steady lifelong contour correction with the patients' own perfused tissues.

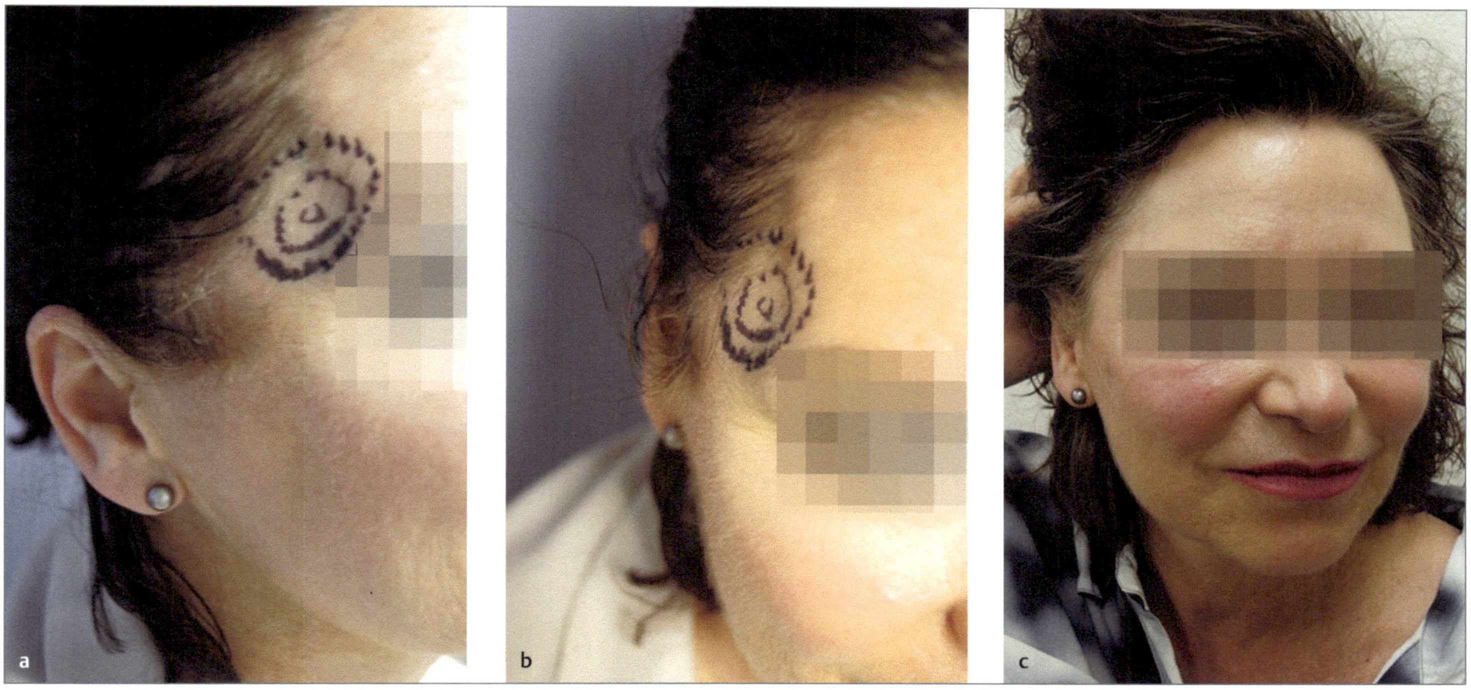

Fig. 1.55 Lipofilling for restoring cosmesis in patients with temporal muscle atrophy. After a frontolateral approach, this patient developed a visible and aesthetically disturbing volume loss caused by temporal muscle atrophy between the anterior edge of the superior temporal line and the lateral orbital rim **(a, b)**. Complete restoration of the temporal contour is achieved after two sessions of autologous fat graft transfer (lipofilling) **(c)**.

Reference

[1] Tubbs RS, Loukas M, Shoja MM, Cohen-Gadol AA. Refined and simplified surgical landmarks for the MacCarty keyhole and orbitozygomatic craniotomy. Neurosurgery 2010;66(6, Suppl Operative):230–233

1.7 Protection of the Dura Mater

Andreas Raabe and David Bervini

1.7.1 Potential Problems Arising from a Laceration of the Dura Mater

Ideally, the dura mater should remain intact during craniotomy. However, inadvertent tearing of the dura is quite common. The following problems may arise from this injury:

- Dura laceration at the rim of the craniotomy where suturing or patching the dura is difficult or impossible. This may increase the likelihood of a cerebrospinal fluid leak, depending on the location.
- Penetrating the dura may lead to injury of a sinus or a cortical vein, a cortical contusion with or without cortical subarachnoid hemorrhage, or intracerebral hemorrhage.

1.7.2 Measures to Protect the Integrity of the Dura Mater

Burr Hole

When drilling a burr hole, the pressure applied with the trephine perpendicular to the skull should be gentle. When the trephine does not advance into the bone, it is more likely to be because of a blunt cutting edge than insufficient pressure. Excessive pressure can dislocate the skull from the Mayfield clamp. With some craniotomes, excessive pressure can even perforate the dura or a venous sinus. Neurosurgeons need a high sensitivity to haptic or tactile feedback during the procedures they perform. Training can start at the burr hole with being able to feel that immediately before perforating the inner tabula of the skull, the trephine starts to "eat" deeper into the burr hole, getting slightly slower because of the greater resistance from the inner tabula, but also advancing almost by itself. This can and should be felt by the surgeon. During this moment, pressure should further be eased.

Detaching the Outer Dura Leaf from the Tabula Interna

Using a small hook or dissector, or a punch, the thin bone shell that often covers the dura within a burr hole should be removed. The first detachment of the dura from the inner tabula should include the outer (periosteal) leaf of the dura mater. Taking one's time and assuring proper detachment is important, because this is the entry and starting point for the craniotomy.

Additional Dural Detachment during Craniotomy

This can be performed using instruments via:

- Burr hole: a curved instrument can be used to detach the dura. The correct amount of bending is such that the instrument does not cause a contusion at the cortex. It is easier to use in larger burr holes than in smaller ones (▶Fig. 1.56).
- Craniotomy line or smaller burr holes: special instruments equipped with a 90° blade can detach and separate the dura from the bone (▶Fig. 1.57). Again, tactile feedback is essential, to avoid perforating the dura during this maneuver.

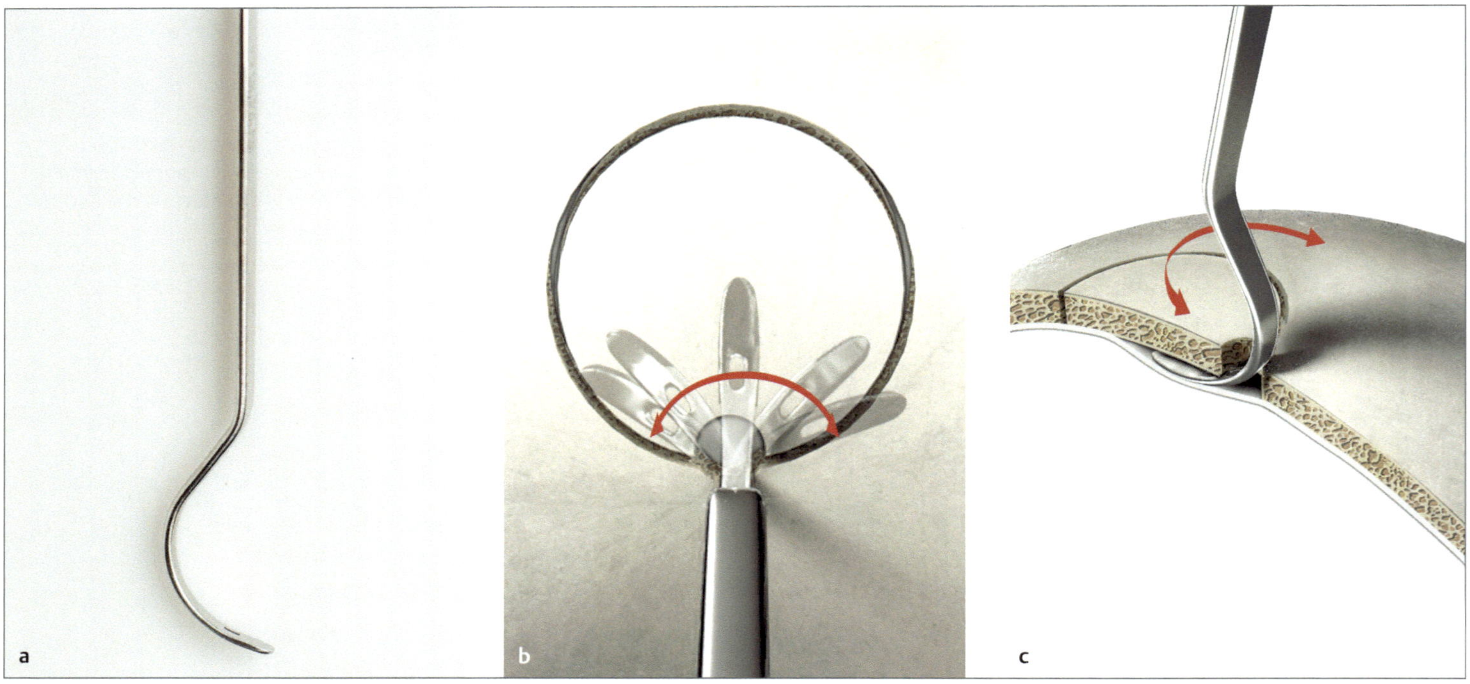

Fig. 1.56 (a–c) Detaching the dura. A set of curved instruments with different radiuses can be used to detach the dura along the craniotomy line and beyond. It requires one or more burr holes to be used.

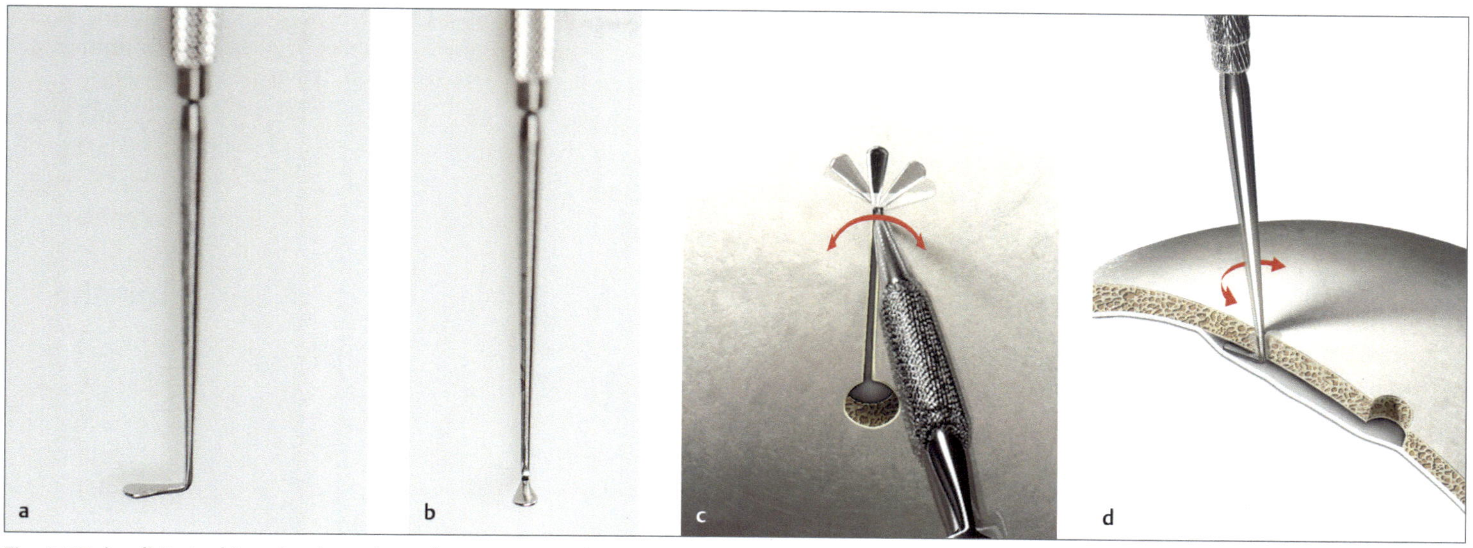

Fig. 1.57 (a–d) Detaching the dura along the craniotomy line. A 90° angled instrument with a thin base that allows the surgeon to introduce it into the craniotomy line where it can be used to detach the dura mater, especially at points where the craniotomy turns or to check whether the craniotomy is basal enough. It allows palpation beyond the point of the craniotomy line.

The Correct Use of the Craniotome

First, the geometry of the craniotome should be checked. The metal leg that protects the dura should be in a correct 90° position below the rotating blade (▸Fig. 1.58). The tip of the rotating blade should be covered by the bent anterior edge of the protecting leg. If bent out of shape, it will not work correctly. The craniotome should be held gently with two fingers like a pencil (▸Fig. 1.59a) or with four fingers for better haptic feedback (▸Fig. 1.59b), but not in a closed fist like a hand ax (▸Fig. 1.59c). It should be advanced in a strictly perpendicular (90°) or very slightly backward-tilted position that keeps the anterior edge of the protecting leg separating the dura from the bone. Leaning the craniotome forward will open the space between the dural attachment and the craniotome and often causes dural laceration (▸Fig. 1.60).

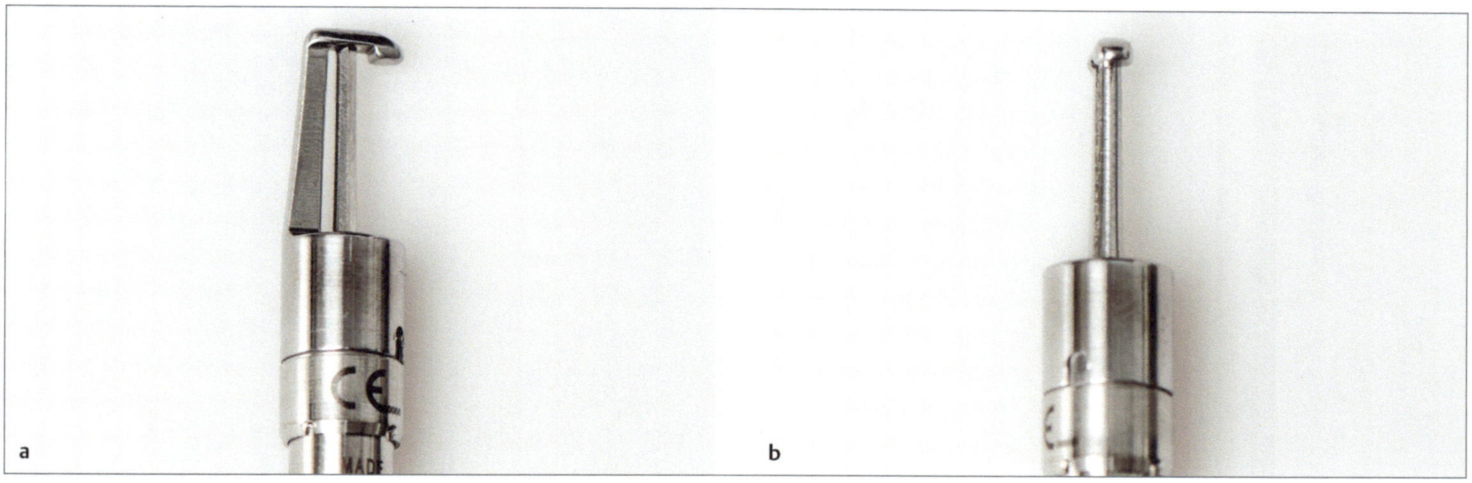

Fig. 1.58 (a, b) Check footplate position. If the footplate is bent, the craniotome may injure the dura.

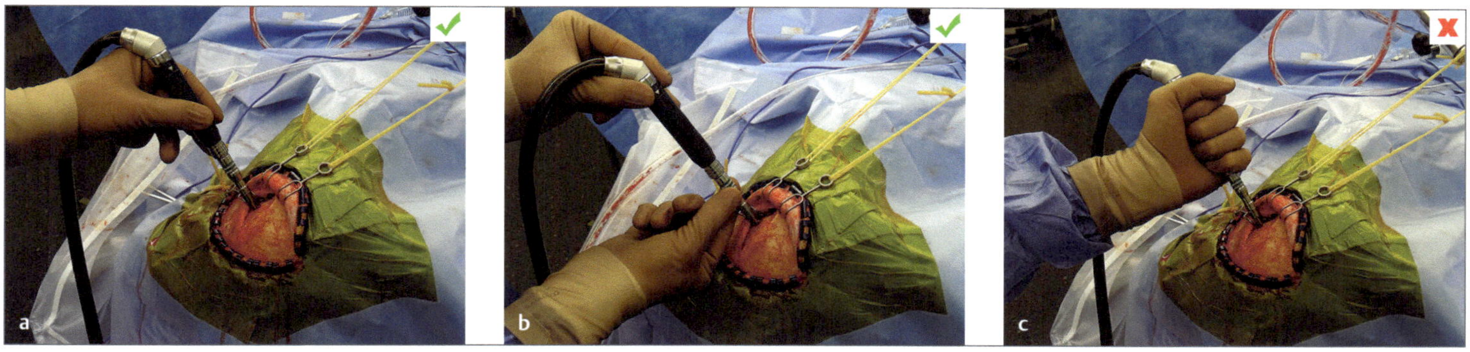

Fig. 1.59 Correct (a, b) and wrong (c) handling of the craniotome. The craniotome should be held with the fingers to obtain tactile feedback. Normally not much force is needed and holding it in a fist results in excessive pressure, less haptic feedback, and an increased likelihood of dural laceration.

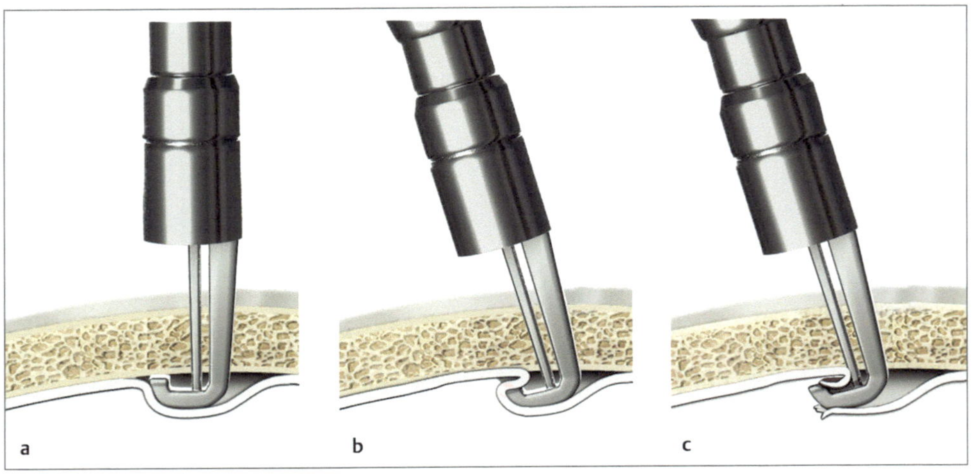

Fig. 1.60 (a–c) Angulation of the craniotome. The craniotome should be moved maintaining a 90° position. Tilting the craniotome anteriorly pushes the footplate into the dura.

The craniotome should be used at the full RPM speed of the motor, which helps to minimize the moving pressure, but with gentle forward pressure and advancing slowly to prevent heat generation. Ideally, it should be easy to advance. Copious irrigation should be used to prevent heat transmission to the cortex and heat necrosis of the bone. The craniotome should stop every 2 to 4 cm and be moved backward, washing the craniotomy dust out of the craniotomy line, and the integrity of the dura mater should be checked (suction-irrigation-assisted visual inspection).

The craniotome should be moved parallel to the surface of the skull and neither be pulled upward nor pushed downward. When the internal tabula of the skull is not parallel to the outer surface, such as where there are bony irregularities and when nearing the skull base, it may be necessary to give a millimeter more depth to the craniotome to pass it further. This may be critical when coming, for example, to the anterior skull base. The transition to the skull base is not a 90° angle but rather a curve. Stopping at the first sign of resistance will result in a craniotomy that is too high to gain access that is flush with the skull base. At this transition, the craniotome should be slightly moved toward the depth (▸ Fig. 1.61).

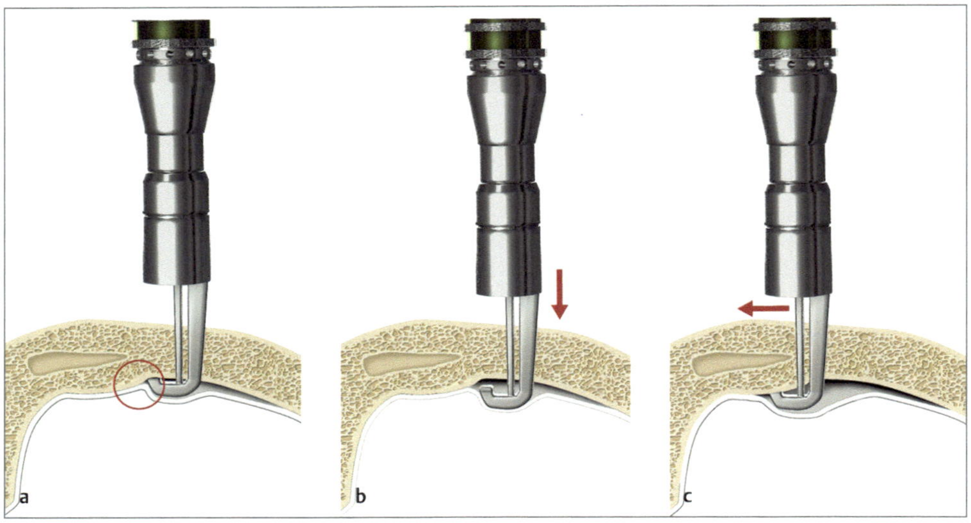

Fig. 1.61 Bony bumps. They may block the craniotome especially when it is pulled upward. Increasing the depth of the craniotome by 1–2 mm facilitates the continuation of the craniotomy.

Suction-Irrigation-Assisted Visual Inspection

The craniotome should be regularly moved back every 2 to 4 cm or whenever any resistance is encountered or the surgeon is not sure whether the dura is still intact. The light is directed perpendicularly into the craniotomy slit. At one end of the slit, a suction tube is placed, and at the other end (of the 2–4 cm segment) the slit is flushed with irrigation water. Usually, it is easy to see, at the bottom of the craniotomy line, whether the dura is still intact or not (▶ Fig. 1.62).

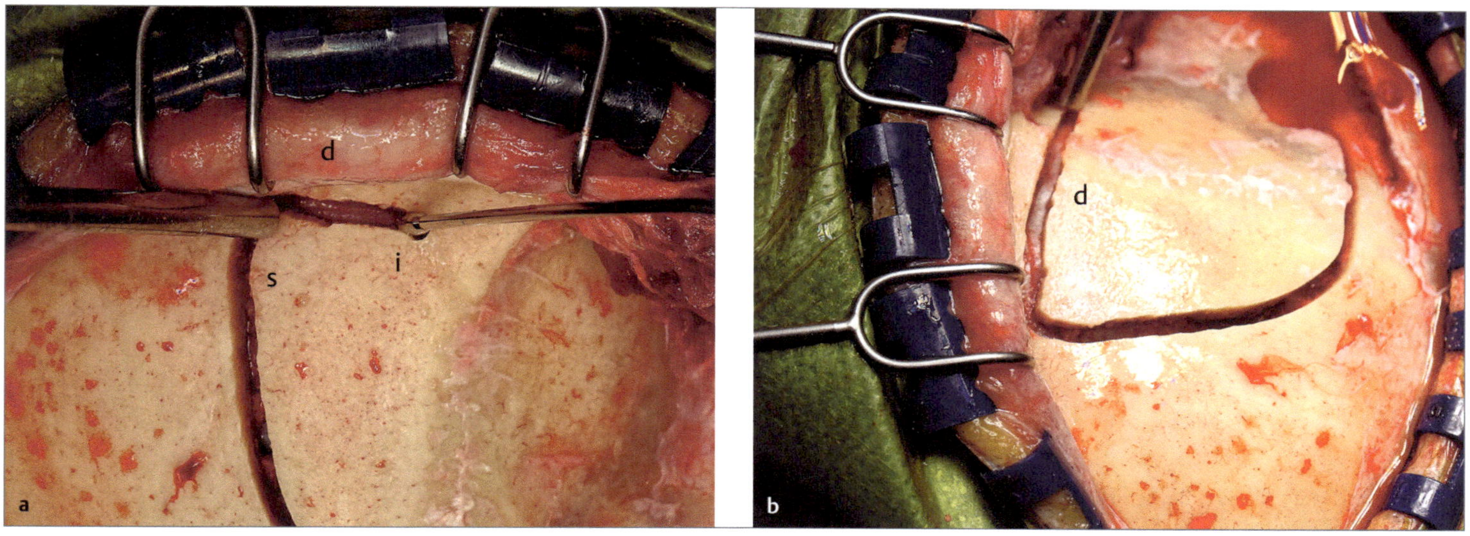

Fig. 1.62 Visualizing the dura beneath the craniotomy line. (a) Using suction (s) at one end of a 1–2 cm portion of the craniotomy line and irrigation (i) at the other end, the intact dura (d) can be seen at the bottom of the craniotomy line (or the cortex in the case of a dural laceration). **(b)** A perpendicular straight or oblique light illumination and view helps to visualize the dura mater (d).

Haptic Control and Tactile Feedback

Haptic feedback on whether the blade is gliding smoothly or whether the craniotome is pushing against a resistance is an important learning objective. Moving the craniotome back and forth further improves this haptic feeling, as does guiding the craniotome with two hands and 2 × 2 fingers (▶ Fig. 1.59b). When resistance is noticed, additional detachment of the dura or an additional burr hole can be performed.

Additional Burr Holes at Sites of Dural Adhesion

In case of further resistance or when a dural perforation is detected, additional burr holes on the adhesion or the next intact part of the craniotomy line should be made. From the intact dura in the burr hole, the craniotome can first be moved backward to connect to the craniotomy line and then forward with a new chance to keep the dura intact.

Away-from-Sinus Direction of Craniotomy

A craniotomy close to, above, or crossing a venous sinus is often performed but requires additional safety measures. Usually the Pacchioni granulations are weak spots for entering below the dura with the craniotome. This may not only injure the dura but cause a larger laceration of the sinus. Therefore, burr holes should be situated on the sinus (except for the sigmoid sinus) and the craniotomy should be performed away from the sinus. The craniotomy toward the sinus should stop at a distance of 1.5 cm from the sinus (see also Chapter 4.1, Sinus Crossing, by Sure and Dammann and Chapter 1.8, Sinus Laceration, by Krieg and Meyer).

1.8 Sinus Laceration

Sandro Krieg and Bernhard Meyer

1.8.1 Introduction

The walls of the venous sinuses consist of a double dural layer lined with endothelium. In contrast to normal venous blood vessels, they lack valves and a full set of tissue layers, such as a tunica media. Moreover, due to anatomical variations, including varying diameter between individuals and also between sides in the same individual, diagnosis of sinus pathologies, such as sinus thrombosis can be difficult.

Sinus lacerations usually happen during craniotomy but may also occur during tumor removal. This chapter will give a brief overview of the relevant sinus anatomy, technical steps for sinus wall reconstruction, and strategies to prevent sinus laceration.

1.8.2 Prevention Strategies

Burr holes are placed directly above the sinus (superior sagittal sinus, transverse sinus), except for the sigmoid sinus (see below). The most fragile part is at the level of the lacunae laterales and their connection with the sinus paramedian of the sinus. When performing a craniotomy over the sagittal or transverse sinus, the surgeon works above the sinus from both sides, or burr holes for the craniotomy are made directly over the sinus. Particularly at the bregma, dura and sinus walls can be firmly attached to the bone, increasing the risk of injury. Working from the burr holes toward the middle of the sinus provide initial visualization that the craniotome is in the epidural space.

When making the bone cuts laterally, the safer direction is away from the sinus, because the epidural position of the craniotome can be confirmed at the burr hole. Using the craniotome in the opposite direction, i.e., toward the sinus, carries a higher risk that the craniotome could run into the lateral lacunae and then into the wall of the sinus (see ▸ Fig. 1.63).

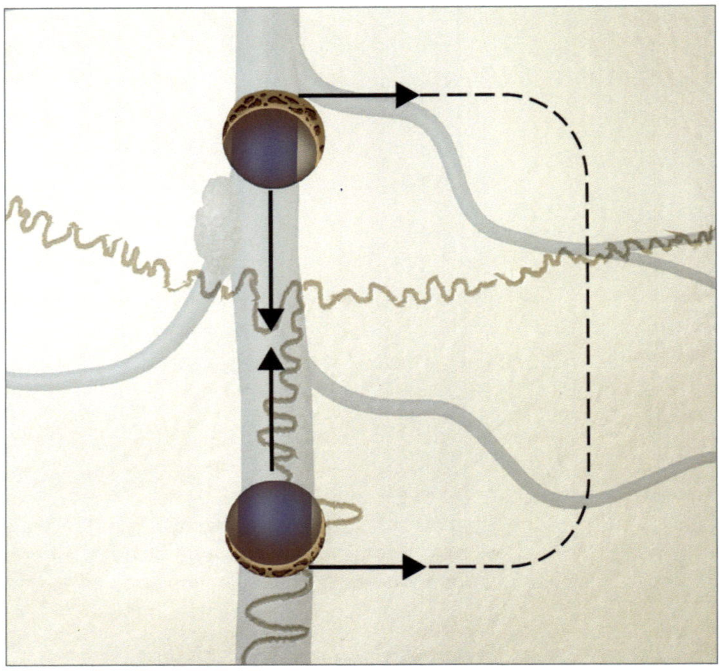

Fig. 1.63 Craniotomy. Recommended directions when performed above the superior sagittal sinus and for connecting the rest of the bone flap. The wall of the sinus is usually tighter and more resistant to injury in the midline compared to paramedian.

1.8.3 Management of Sinus Laceration

Initial Management

At the moment a severe injury to a sinus occurs, the bleeding should be stopped immediately by gentle pressure (finger, compress) and the head should be slightly elevated. Once bleeding is under control, think about further steps and notify the anesthesiologist to prepare for major blood loss. Fortunately, the majority of bleeding from the sinus are minor and can be managed initially by placing one or more wet pads on the site of the hemorrhage.

Onlay Patch

Following a sinus laceration, adhesive sealant patches (e.g., Tachosil, Hemopatch) or Gelfoam combined with a few minutes of gentle pressure usually lead to immediate closure of the laceration.[1,2] A compress can help to distribute the pressure evenly.

If the bleeding continues and constant pressure is required to keep the patch on the sinus wall, oblique burr holes at the bony rim of the craniotomy can be made every 2 mm, and the dura lateral of the sinus can be flipped over and sutured to the bone. Some Gelfoam is placed in between the dural leaves for constant compression (▶ Fig. 1.64**a**).

The use of hemostatics as sealants, however, carries the risk of promoting the coagulation cascade, causing sinus thrombosis.

The same is true for fibrin sealants, which, additionally, are much more likely to be washed away.[1] Fibrin glue requires a dry surface for application to enable it to polymerize, and does not stick properly to wet or bloody tissue. Moreover, the time needed for preparation of fibrin glue further limits its sefulness for sinus lacerations when significant hemorrhage occurs.

Temporary Hemostasis for Suturing

In order to achieve temporary hemostasis for direct suture or patch application, small pieces of hemostatic material, such as Surgicel or Gelfoam or even bone wax can be put into the lumen of the sinus and the openings of draining veins.[3] Balloons are not recommended since they can injure the sinus' endothelium.

Bridging veins, including their ostia into the sinus, need to be preserved, especially those draining the central region. If the bleeding cannot be stopped by intraluminal measures, clips can be used (▶ Fig. 1.64**b**). However, due to the risk of sinus wall injury, their use should be limited.[3]

Direct Suture

If the sinus injury is a sharp and clear cut, a direct suture using 5–0 or 6–0 monofilament (e.g., Prolene) is the first choice. However, the sinus walls are typically thin and fragile. Careful attention should be paid to the preservation of sufficient lumen of the sutured sinus (▶ Fig. 1.64**c, d**).

Suturing a Patch

As an alternative to the use of adhesive sealant patches to cover the sinus wall defect, some authors prefer autologous dural or venous patches to avoid the thrombogenic potential of any synthetic material as mentioned above. Moreover, some sinus injuries are too extensive for direct suture or adhesive sealant patches to be successful. Reconstruction of the venous sinuses is performed using autologous patches. Local tissue, such as temporal fascia, dura mater, and pericranium are suitably rigid. Note that the graft should not be compressed, e.g., by swollen brain parenchyma.[3] Patches can be applied in an onlay fashion (▶ Fig. 1.64**e**), as a free patch from temporal fascia or pericranium (▶ Fig. 1.64**f**) or as an inverted dural patch (▶ Fig. 1.64**g**). An inverted patch harvested from the falx cerebri can also be used (▶ Fig. 1.64**h**).

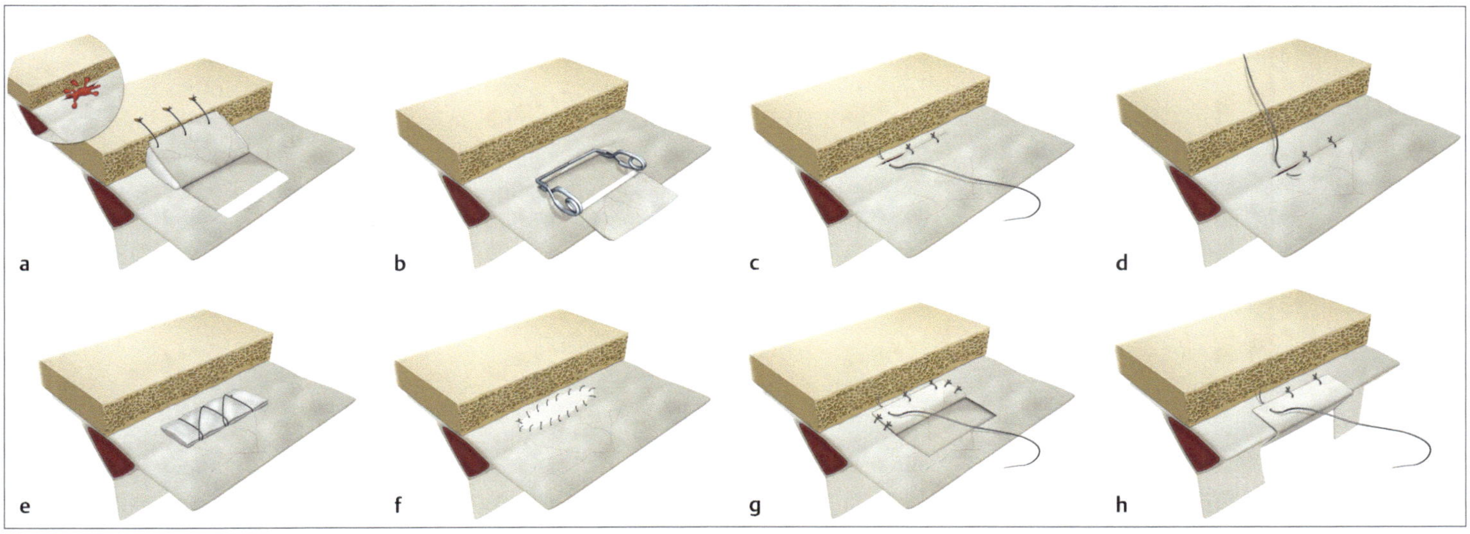

Fig. 1.64 Variants of managing sinus lacerations. Compression with flipped dura **(a)**, clip **(b)**, direct sutures **(c, d)**, patch sutures **(e, f)**, and sutures with flipped dura **(g, h)**.

Besides local tissue, tissue from the saphenous vein can also be used. However, its preparation from the thigh is time-consuming.[4] Since the likelihood of graft thrombosis is high if Goretex is used, autologous materials are preferred.[3]

After suturing is complete, patency is confirmed by a Doppler probe or by indocyanine green fluorescence angiography. Some authorities recommend antiplatelet therapy for 3 months after surgery if a patch was used.[5]

Sinus Thrombosis

Treatment for sinus laceration needs to avoid the introduction of any thrombogenic material inside the lumen of the sinus and any reduction of the sinus width, particularly of the superior sagittal sinus. It is of paramount importance not to push Gelfoam or other material inside the sinus during the initial attempt to control bleeding. Postoperative heparin has to be evaluated carefully on a case-by-case basis. For prophylaxis against sinus thrombosis, intravenous heparin is applied during the repair. If there is any concern about blood flow or thrombogenesis, heparinization should be considered for 5 to 7 days. In these cases, heparin is initiated during the sinus repair and continued after surgery to maintain a partial thromboplastin time of 40 to 60 s.[5]

1.8.4 Special Considerations

Sinus Occlusion

The only venous sinuses that can undergo complete iatrogenic occlusion in most cases are the superior petrosal sinus, the cavernous sinus, the nondominant collateralized transverse, and sigmoid sinus.[4]

Bleeding from Arachnoid Granulations and Venous Lacunae

Bleeding from arachnoid granulations and venous lacunae can be severe and stopping it can be complicated. While bleeding from small arachnoid granulations can be controlled with bipolar coagulation, bleeding from larger arachnoid granulations will normally only stop after continuous compression with or without adhesive sealant patches and is handled similarly to sinus laceration. Where feasible, very large arachnoid granulations and venous lacunae should be avoided by the craniotomy.

Superior Sagittal Sinus

The superior sagittal sinus drains diploic veins, veins from the pericranium and the dura as well as large parts of both hemispheres by collecting blood from the superior cerebral veins. These cortical veins run in a slightly anterior instead of 90° or a posterior direction immediately before entering the sinus. Many superior cerebral veins drain into venous lacunae before draining into the superior sagittal sinus.

While the closure of the anterior third of the superior sagittal sinus (ventral to the bregma) or of the complete occipital sinus is generally well tolerated (easiest by suture/ligation), closure of the superior sagittal sinus behind the bregma should only be done if sufficient (mainly tumor-induced) collaterals are present. This requires careful assessment of preoperative MRI or angiography.

Sigmoid Sinus

While all other sinus walls are composed of a double dural layer, the sigmoid sinus only consists of one tissue layer between the skull and the endothelium of the sinus. This makes the sigmoid sinus significantly more vulnerable. Due to the different blood volume provided by the Labbé veins, the sigmoid sinuses can differ significantly in size from their corresponding transverse sinus and vice versa, due to extensive draining by mastoid, occipital, or condylar emissary veins.

Depending on the asymmetry of the transverse sinus and the results of preoperative evaluation, closure of the sigmoid sinus of one side might also be well tolerated. This is usually done with Surgicel, Gelfoam, or suture. But it is important to bear in mind that injury to the dominant (i.e., major draining) sigmoid sinus is a life-threatening complication and preservation of venous outflow is absolutely mandatory. Here, the sinus has to be unroofed by drilling away the covering bone before repair is done with adhesive sealant patches, direct suture, or a dural patch.

Cavernous Sinus

The cavernous sinus consists of multiple compartments and only plays a minor role in the drainage of the brain. Lacerations of the cavernous sinus can usually be stopped by injecting fibrin glue, Gelfoam, or Flowseal.

Occipital Sinus

The occipital sinus is the smallest of the cranial sinuses. It is located in the attached margin of the falx cerebelli. It originates around the foramen magnum and drains into the confluence of the sinuses. It is more common in young children and is rarer and also smaller in adults. Surgically, it can be important for posterior fossa approaches since it can cause significant bleeding during incision of the dura. When this occurs, the occipital sinus should be completely closed by suture, ligation, or by using titanium clips.

References

[1] Gazzeri R, Galarza M. In reply: advanced hemostatics in the management of cerebral dural sinus lacerations. Neurosurgery 2015;77(4):E673–E674

[2] Kim YS, Jung SH, Lim DH, Kim TS, Kim JH, Lee JK. Traumatic dural venous sinus injury. Korean J Neurotrauma 2015;11(2):118–123

[3] Sindou M. Meningiomas invading the sagittal or transverse sinuses, resection with venous reconstruction. J Clin Neurosci 2001;8(Suppl 1):8–11

[4] Sekhar LN, Chanda A, Morita A. The preservation and reconstruction of cerebral veins and sinuses. J Clin Neurosci 2002;9(4):391–399

[5] Mantovani A, Di Maio S, Ferreira MJ, Sekhar LN. Management of meningiomas invading the major dural venous sinuses: operative technique, results, and potential benefit for higher grade tumors. World Neurosurg 2014;82(3–4):455–467

1.9 Frontal Sinus Breach and Repair

Andreas Raabe and Marco Caversaccio

In typical frontobasal and frontotemporal craniotomies, for example, bifrontal, frontolateral, supraorbital, and pterional craniotomies, the goal is to gain intradural subfrontal access without retracting the brain. Besides measures to relax, release, and gravity retract the brain, a craniotomy flush to the frontal base is required. This inevitably causes frontal sinus breach in some patients; however, the flush access to the base remains a higher priority than avoiding a potential breach of the frontal sinus.

Injury of the frontal sinus and the mucosa leads to contamination of the sterile intra- and extradural space. There is controversy in the literature as to whether this may cause more surgical site infections. Repairing the breach of the sinus and mucosa remains the mainstay of preventing infections and mucocele.

The procedure for repairing smaller breaches that occur during routine craniotomy is different from the procedure used in trauma patients that have more complex and extensive injuries. Note that in patients with chronic sinusitis, mucocele, and other diseases of the frontal sinus, more extensive procedures up to cranialization of the sinus have to be used, although the latter has become rare in the era of modern rhinology.

The literature still describes exenteration of the frontal sinus and plugging the frontonasal duct with abdominal fat or split calvarial bone as the standard procedure for treating a breach in the mucosa. We have abandoned these more invasive procedures; instead, we recommend a minimal procedure to maintain or reestablish the frontal sinus.

1.9.1 Landmarks for the Frontal Sinus

The frontal sinus is symmetric in only 50% of cases and asymmetric with considerable differences between the sides in the other 50%. Knowledge of the frontal sinus extension is not only helpful for craniotomies but also for placement of the Mayfield head pins. The following distances can be used as a rule of thumb (▸Table 1.3, ▸Fig. 1.65):

Table 1.3 Extensions of the frontal sinus

Distances	Maximum	Most commonly
Nasion to superior border of frontal sinus	4 cm	< 3 cm
Midline to lateral border of frontal sinus	4 cm	< 3 cm
Extension of the frontal sinus laterally to the midpupillary line	1 cm	at the midpupillary line

Source: Modified from Tubbs et al.[1]

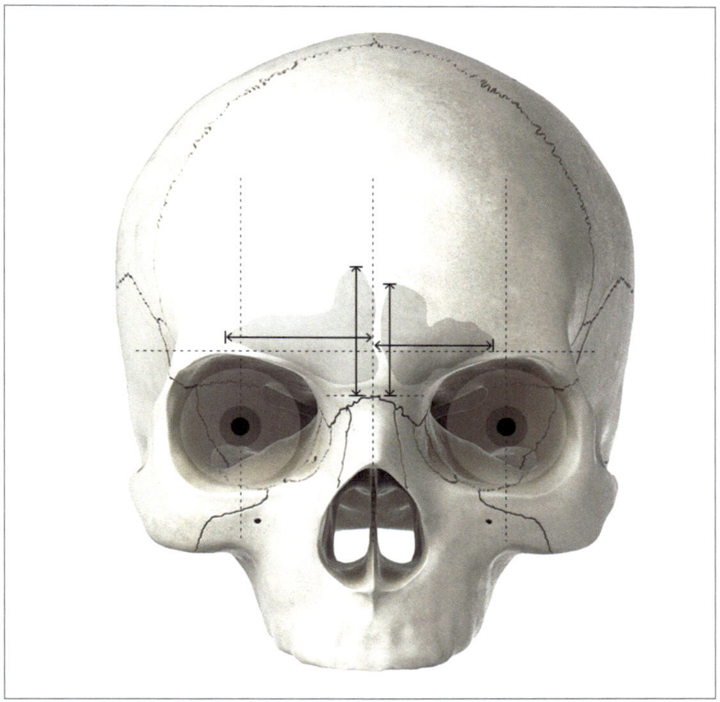

Fig. 1.65 Landmarks for the frontal sinus. In most patients, the frontal sinus does not extend superiorly more than 3 cm (maximum 4 cm) from the nasion and laterally not more than 3 cm (maximum 4 cm) from the midline (not crossing the midpupillary line). These distances vary considerably between patients and, therefore, individual measurements should be taken from the images of each patient undergoing surgery. (Reproduced with permission from Tubbs et al.[1])

1.9.2 Principles of Repair

After a craniotomy that breaches the sinus, there are two parts of the sinus to consider (▶ Fig. 1.66): (A) the frontal sinus main cavity, which is at the frontal base, and (B) the part of the wall involved in the craniotomy, which is situated in the bone flap.

For the main (skull base) part of the sinus (A), the rules are:

- Keep the mucosa.
- Keep the ostium to the nasal cavity open, i.e., remove craniotomy debris from the sinus and do not plug it.
- Reestablish the missing part of the sinus wall (the part involved in the craniotomy) without spreading mucosa and bacteria to the intra- or extracranial compartment.

For the part of the sinus wall that has been removed with the craniotomy (B), the rules are:

- Remove the mucosa to the very last cell.
- Keep this part clean and separate from the remaining part of the sinus (i.e., A).
- Use it to permanently fix and close the upper wall of the main sinus, i.e., use B to seal and close A (see ▶ Fig. 1.66).

1.9.3 Surgical Technique for Repairing in the Case of a Frontal Sinus Breach

1. Lifting the Bone Flap

Because of the presence of bacteria that constitute the natural flora of the frontal sinus, care should be taken not to touch the open sinus and not to spread any of the mucosa at the moment when the flap is lifted. The bone must be carefully inspected.

2. Preventing Bacterial Contamination

When a breach of the sinus is observed, the nurse should place the bone flap in a separate bowl of betadine or other disinfectant solution. The visible sinus at the skull should be covered with patties soaked in disinfectant. The surrounding intra- and extradural surface is covered with a layer of patties. Then the cavity of the frontal sinus is irrigated and cleaned using water irrigation. The mucosa in the main sinus is left intact. If any part of the mucosa overlaps the rim of the craniotomy, it should be pushed back into the frontal sinus. Then, a freshly prepared patty soaked in disinfectant is placed on top of the sinus, and covered by another layer of patties. They remain there until closure.

3. Preparation of the Bone Flap

The bone flap is taken out of the bowl containing the disinfectant, and the mucosa of the frontal sinus is removed using a diamond drill. Drilling should remove every part of the mucosa in every hidden recess because this part of the former sinus will be trapped and will no longer communicate with the remaining frontal sinus.

4. Completion of the Intracranial Surgery

The surgery is performed as planned. Care should be taken not to inadvertently remove the compress covering the frontal sinus.

5. Preparation of a Galea-Periosteal Flap

A galea-periosteal flap—ideally with a vascularized pedicle—is prepared. It should be long enough not only to place it as one layer on the sinus, but to be able to fold it into two layers covering the frontal sinus and obliterating the upper part.

6. Fixation of the Galea-Periosteal Flap with the Bone Flap

The bone flap is now reinserted. It should hold the galea-periosteal flap in place (▶ Fig. 1.66). The position of the galea-periosteal flap should be checked to rule out dislocation during closing. The area is disinfected again. Then, closure of the skin flap is completed. As previously described, more extensive and invasive procedures are available to manage frontal sinus breach, but there is no proof that they reduce infection at the surgical site, or have any other advantage.

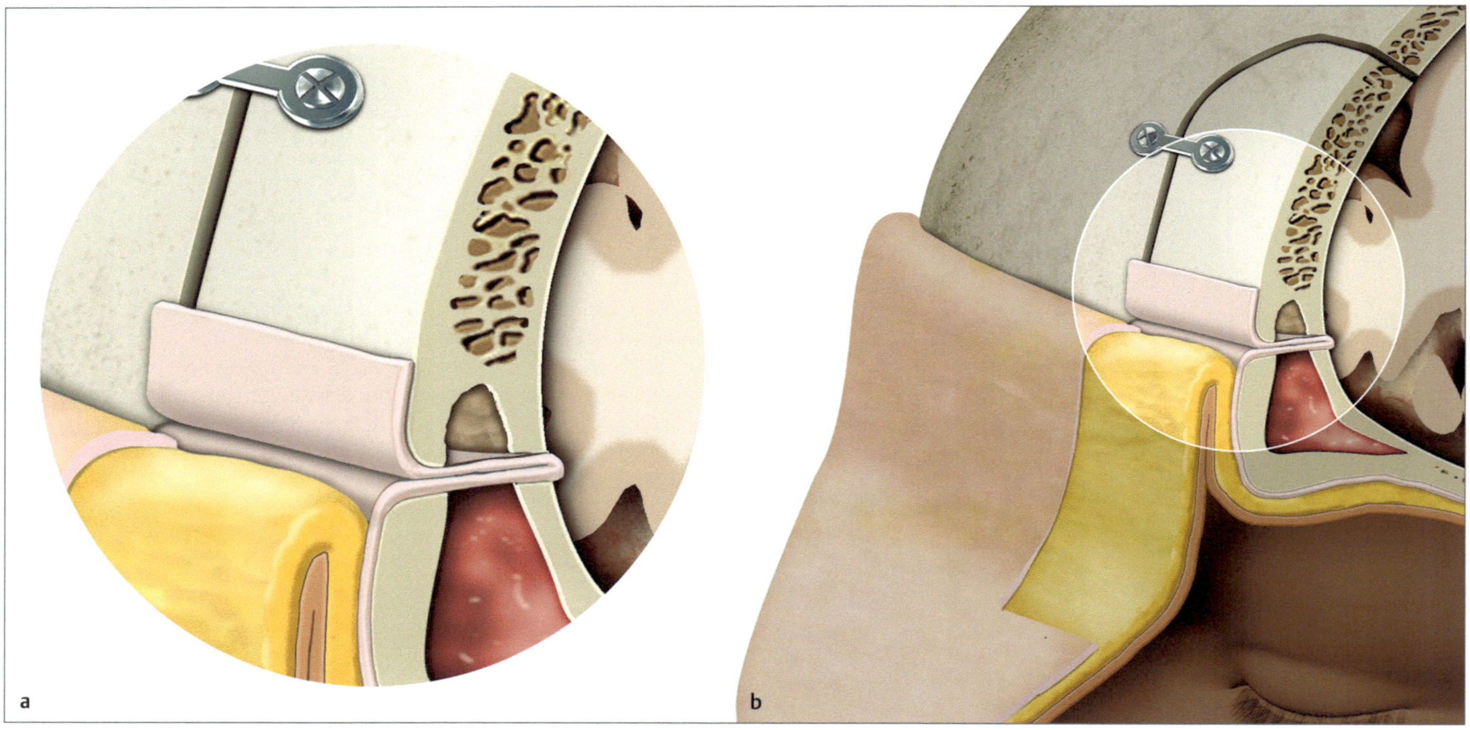

Fig. 1.66 Surgical technique for repairing in the case of a frontal sinus breach. Surgical closure of a small frontal sinus breach. The mucosa is removed completely from the craniotomy part **(a)**, which will be trapped by the closing procedure. The mucosa is left intact in the basal main part of the sinus **(b)**. The (galea)-periosteal flap is folded in and used to close the sinus.

Reference

[1] Tubbs RS, Elton S, Salter G, Blount JP, Grabb PA, Oakes WJ. Superficial surgical landmarks for the frontal sinus. J Neurosurg 2002;96(2):320–322

2 Landmarks

2.1 Schematic Cortical Anatomy

Andreas Raabe and Peter A. Winkler

Lateral Surface

The anatomy of the surface of the brain is complex, highly variable, and difficult to identify intraoperatively. Neurosurgeons often expose only a limited part of the cortex, which, in addition, is covered by the arachnoidal membrane and cortical vessels that cross gyri and small sulci. Thus, reliably recognizing the gyri and sulci of the brain surface is often not possible. Image guidance and brain mapping help with intraoperative orientation.

Preoperatively, we rely on knowledge of brain anatomy from MRI and CT scans. On the one hand, these images give more information than the classical surface anatomy view because we can scroll beneath the surface and visualize "true" deep sulci. On the other hand, we only have the three classical planes of axial, coronal, and sagittal view and miss the surface view.

In this chapter, we use a mixture of surface and neuroimaging features to provide a simplified cortical anatomy of the brain for neurosurgeons based on two landmark publications.[1,2]

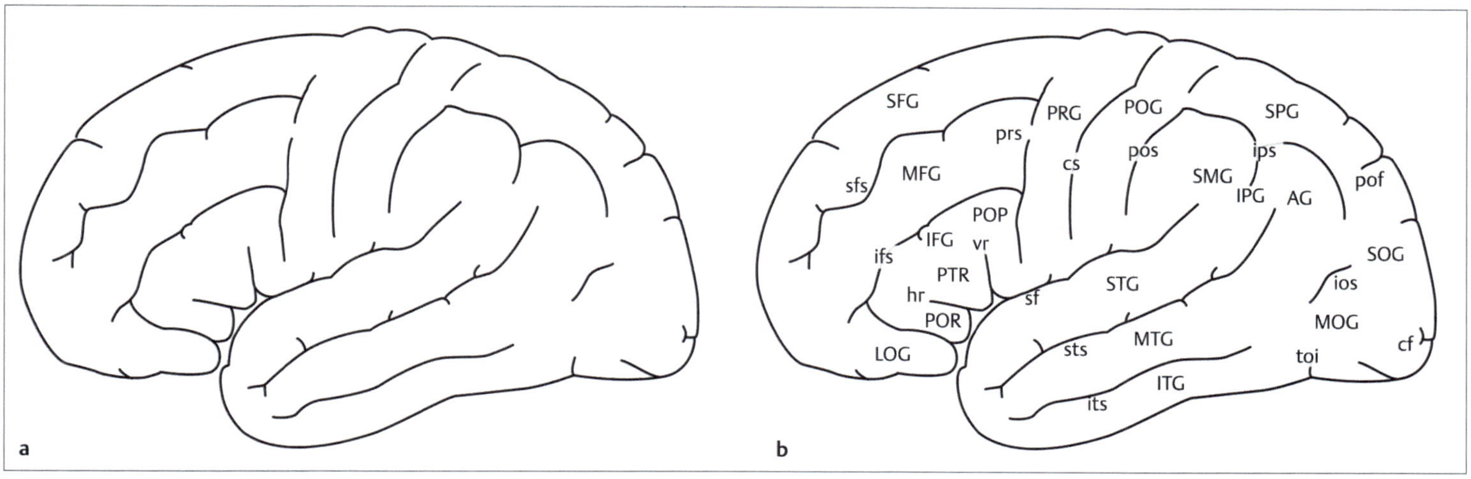

Fig. 2.1 (a, b) Lateral surface. Schematic cortical anatomy—lateral view. Gyri are denoted with large letters, sulci with small letters.

cf: calcarine fissure
cs: central sulcus
hr: horizontal ramus of the sylvian fissure
ifs: inferior frontal sulcus
ios: intraoccipital sulcus
ips: intraparietal sulcus
its: inferior temporal sulcus
pof: parieto-occipital fissure
pos: postcentral sulcus
prs: precentral sulcus
sf: sylvian fissure
sfs: superior frontal sulcus
sts: superior temporal sulcus
toi: temporo-occipital incisura
vr: vertical ramus of the sylvian fissure

AG: angular gyrus
IFG: inferior frontal gyrus (F3)
IPG: inferior parietal gyrus (P2)
ITG: inferior temporal gyrus (T3)
LOG: lateral orbital gyrus
MFG: middle frontal gyrus (F2)
MOG: middle occipital gyrus (O2)
MTG: middle temporal gyrus (T2)
POG: postcentral gyrus
POP: pars opercularis
POR: pars orbitalis
PRG: precentral gyrus
PTR: pars triangularis
SFG: superior frontal gyrus (F1)
SMG: supramarginal gyrus
SOG: superior occipital gyrus (O1)
SPG: superior parietal gyrus (P1)
STG: superior temporal gyrus (T1)

Frontally, the superior and inferior frontal sulci separate the superior, middle, and inferior frontal gyrus. The inferior frontal gyrus often has a characteristic appearance. A horizontal ramus and a vertical ramus arising from the sylvian fissure divide it into three parts: the pars orbitalis anteriorly, the pars triangularis in the middle, and the pars opercularis posteriorly, abutting the precentral gyrus. Following the typical "M" configuration of the inferior frontal gyrus from anterior to posterior, the pars opercularis gyrus runs down and connects posteriorly and inferiorly to the precentral gyrus. Thus, it is used to localize the precentral gyrus and the central sulcus on lateral images. The inferior frontal sulcus connects to the precentral sulcus, also locating the precentral gyrus. The classical Brodmann area 44 (pars opercularis) and 45 (posterior half of pars triangularis) are traditionally assigned to Broca's expressive language center, but the modern theory is much more complex.

Parietally, the intraparietal sulcus divides the superior and inferior parietal lobes. The inferior lobe consists of the supramarginal gyrus and the angular gyrus. Both are involved in higher neuropsychological or receptive language functions on the dominant side or bilaterally.

Temporally, the classical Wernicke area is localized starting anteriorly below the postcentral gyrus—the Heschl gyrus is larger and "kisses" the postcentral gyrus at the sylvian fissure—and extends to the posterior limit of the superior temporal gyrus (▶ Fig. 2.1 and ▶ Fig. 2.2).

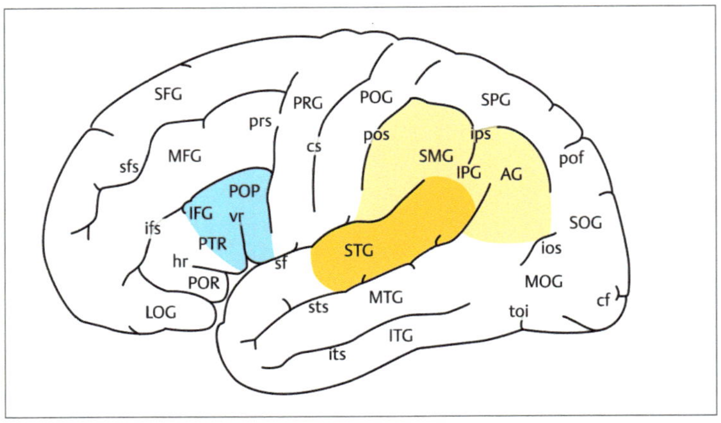

Fig. 2.2 Lateral surface. Lateral cortical surface with simplified language and higher neuropsychological function areas for expressive (*blue*) and receptive language functions (*orange*).

Superior Surface

The superior surface is divided by the central sulcus. Frontally both the superior and the inferior frontal sulcus connect to the precentral sulcus, thus localizing the precentral gyrus. However, the precentral sulcus does not connect to the midline, creating the typical "L" sign where the superior frontal gyrus connects to the precentral gyrus (this "L" also exists for the sulcus). The central sulcus resembles an obliquely flying bird and does not entirely connect to the midline. Its mid part—the body of the bird—represents the larger and typical omega- or epsilon-like hand knob.

Parietally, the ramus supramarginalis of the cingulate sulcus cuts into the superior parietal lobe and is a consistent sign—the bracket sign—that is used to localize the central sulcus, which is one sulcus anteriorly to it. The intraparietal sulcus divides the superior and inferior parietal lobes (▶ Fig. 2.3).

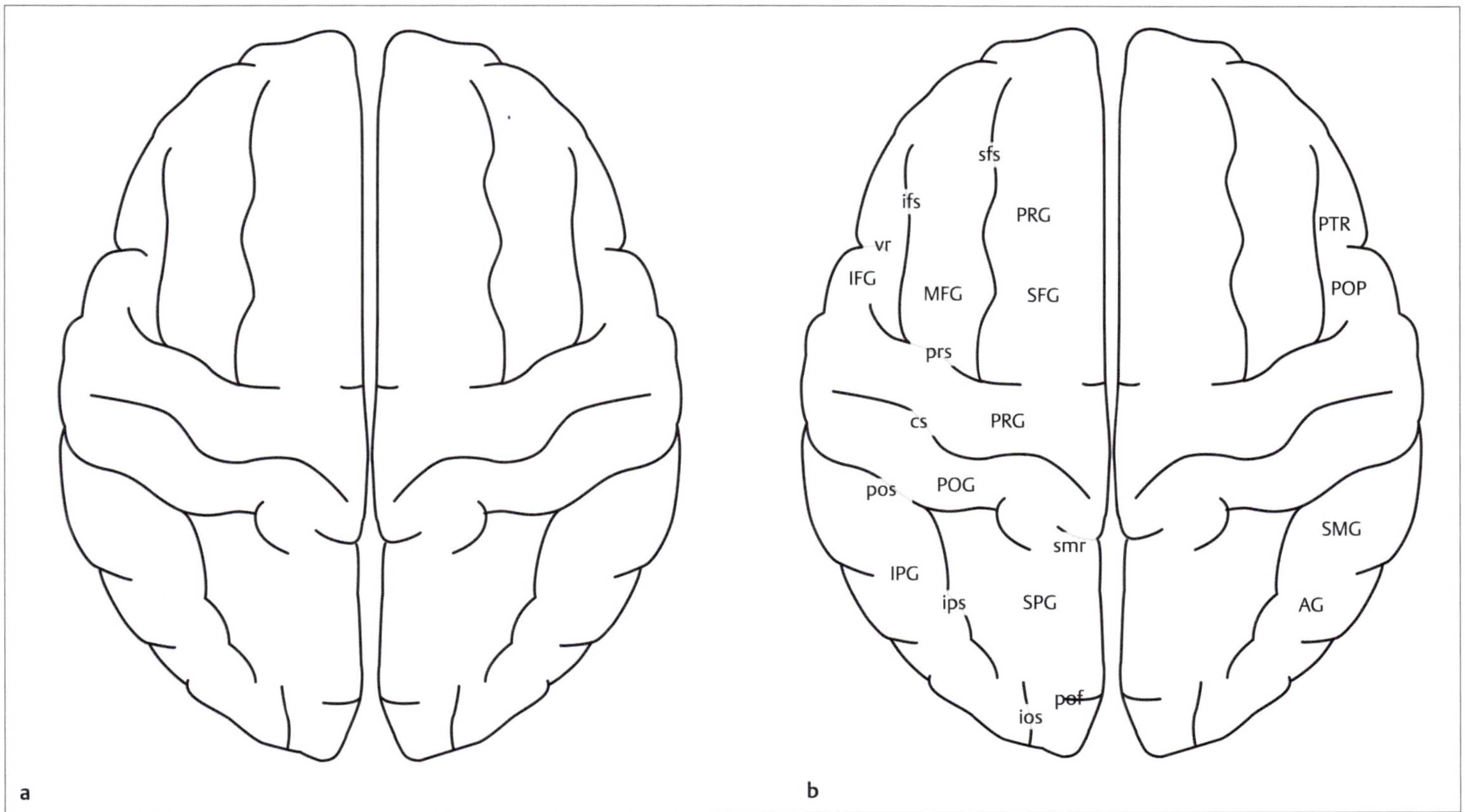

Fig. 2.3 (a, b) Superior surface. Schematic cortical anatomy—superior view.

cs: central sulcus
ifs: inferior frontal sulcus
ios: intraoccipital sulcus
ips: intraparietal sulcus
pof: parieto-occipital fissure
pos: postcentral sulcus
prs: precentral sulcus
sfs: superior frontal sulcus
smr: supramarginal ramus of cingulate sulcus
vr: vertical ramus

AG: angular gyrus
IFG: inferior frontal gyrus (F3)
IPG: inferior parietal gyrus (P2)
MFG: middle frontal gyrus (F2)
POG: postcentral gyrus
POP: pars opercularis
PRG: precentral gyrus
PTR: pars triangularis
SFG: superior frontal gyrus (F1)
SMG: supramarginal gyrus
SPG: superior parietal gyrus (P1)

Inferior Surface

The inferior surface is structured frontally by the typical "H" configuration of the intraorbital sulci. At the temporal and occipital surface, there are four gyri and three fissures. From lateral to medial, the inferior temporal gyrus (T3) is separated from the lateral occipitotemporal gyrus (T4 + O4) by the occipitotemporal sulcus. In the literature, the fusiform gyrus is most often taken as being synonymous for the lateral occipitotemporal gyrus; however, some restrict the fusiform gyrus to the major central part, but not the entire occipitotemporal gyrus. The collateral sulcus separates the lateral occipitotemporal gyrus (T4 + O4) from the medial occipitotemporal gyrus (T5 + O5), which is synonymous with the parahippocampal (T5) and the lingual gyrus (O5). The lingual gyrus is an additional gyrus that runs from posteriorly into the space between the parahippocampal (T5) and the posterior part (O4) of the lateral occipitotemporal gyrus (▶ Fig. 2.4).

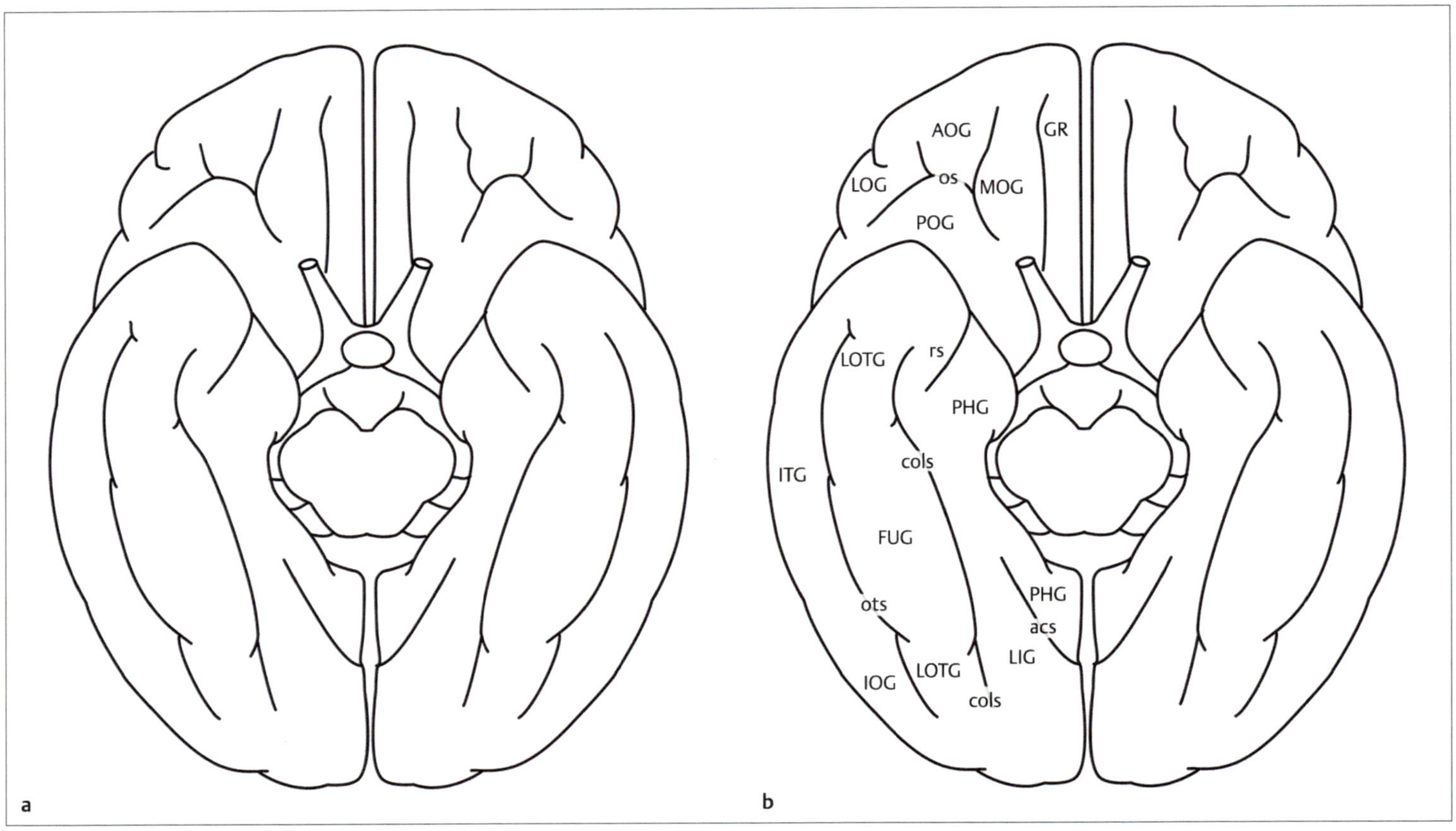

Fig. 2.4 (a, b) Inferior surface. Schematic cortical anatomy— inferior view.

acs: anterior calcarine sulcus
cols: collateral sulcus
os: orbital sulci
ots: occipitotemporal sulcus
rs: rhinal sulcus

AOG: anterior orbital gyrus
FUG: fusiform gyrus (=LOTG)
GR: gyrus rectus
IOG: inferior occipital gyrus (O3)
ITG: inferior temporal gyrus (T3)
LIG: lingual gyrus (O5)
LOG: lateral orbital gyrus
LOTG: occipitotemporal gyrus (=FUG)
MOG: medial orbital gyrus
PHG: parahippocampal gyrus (T5)
POG: posterior orbital gyrus

Medial Surface

At the medial cortical surface, the sulcus cinguli runs posteriorly and superiorly, finishing as the ramus marginalis sulcus cinguli within the medial cortex, creating the typical "bracket" sign on axial images. The parieto-occipital fissure separates the parietal lobe (the precuneus) from the occipital lobe (the cuneus). The calcarine fissure and the parieto-occipital fissure form a characteristic "Y"-shaped sign which ends behind the splenium of the corpus callosum where the parahippocampal gyrus connects with the cingulate gyrus (▶ Fig. 2.5).

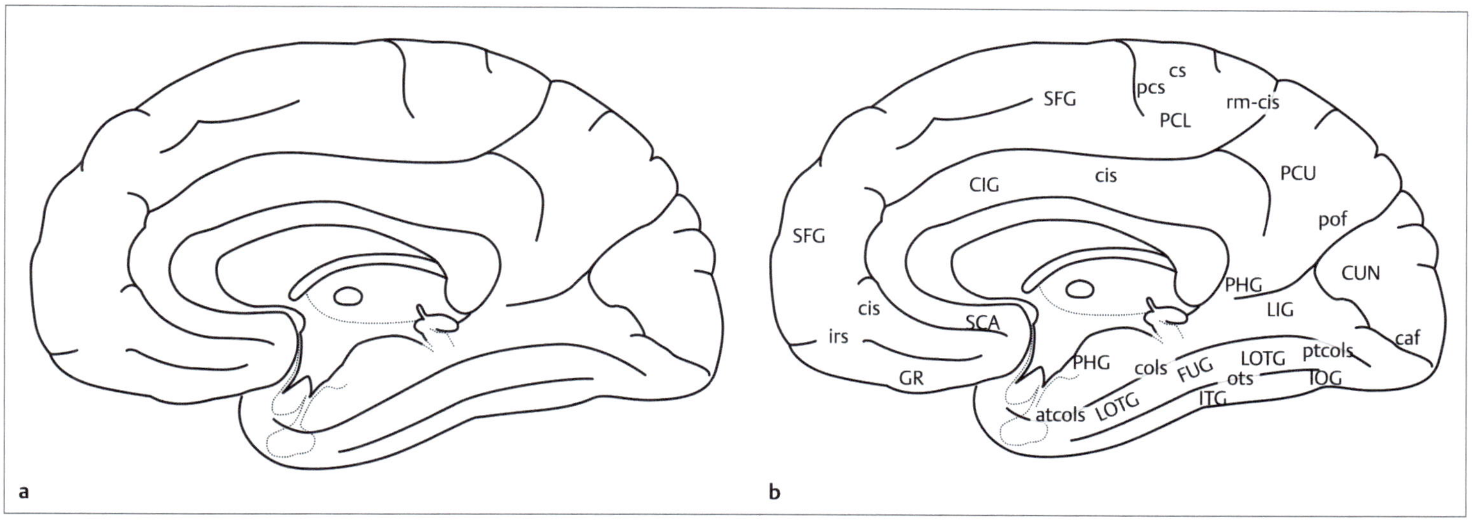

Fig. 2.5 (a, b) Medial surface. Schematic cortical anatomy—medial view. atcols:

atcols: anterior temporal collateral sulcus
caf: calcarine fissure
cis: cingulate sulcus
cols: collateral sulcus
cs: central sulcus
irs: inferior rostral sulcus
ots: occipitotemporal sulcus
pcs: precentral sulcus
pof: parieto-occipital fissure
ptcols: posterior temporal collateral sulcus
rm-cis: ramus marginalis cingulate sulcus
CIG: cingulate gyrus
CUN: cuneus
FUG: fusiform gyrus (=LOTG)
GR: gyrus rectus
IOG: inferior occipital gyrus (O3)
ITG: inferior temporal gyrus (F3)
LIG: lingual gyrus (O5)
LOTG: lateral occipitotemporal gyrus (=FUG)
PCL: paracentral lobule
PCU: precuneus
PHG: parahippocampal gyrus
SCA: subcallosal area
SFG: superior frontal gyrus (F1)

References

[1] Tamraz JC, Comair YG. Atlas of Regional Anatomy of the Brain Using MRI. Berlin: Springer; 2006
[2] Naidich P, Tang CY, Ng JC, Delman BN. Surface anatomy of the cerebrum. In: Naidich T, Castillo M, Cha S, Smirniotopoulos JG, eds. Imaging of the Brain. Philadelphia, PA: Saunders Elsevier; 2013

2.2 Craniocerebral Topography

Irena Zubak, Andreas Raabe, and Karl Schaller

2.2.1 Introduction

The human skull contains anthropological bony surface landmarks that are present in almost all human beings. These bony prominences or particular sutures are not only interesting anatomical features, but also helpful in terms of how they overlay or relate to cortical structures. Thus, a thorough knowledge of these topographical points can be crucial to neurosurgeons performing surgery in situations where no neuronavigation is available.

Some of these landmarks can easily be palpated through the scalp, whereas others can only be reliably identified after the scalp has been opened. Sutures are best visualized after removal of the periosteum with a rather sharp raspatorium, and even better by rubbing a compress soaked in hydrogen peroxide over the area of interest to enhance the contrast with the surrounding bone. Do not hesitate to use sterile pens during surgery to mark the skin and bone and to visualize and confirm these landmarks. This can facilitate the planning of surgical procedures and improve the accuracy of the approach.

Note that some of these landmarks are less reliable than others. In general, cortical key points may vary in the range of 1 to 2 cm. Although this may sound negligible, these variations may add up to considerable differences between patients (▶Fig. 2.6).

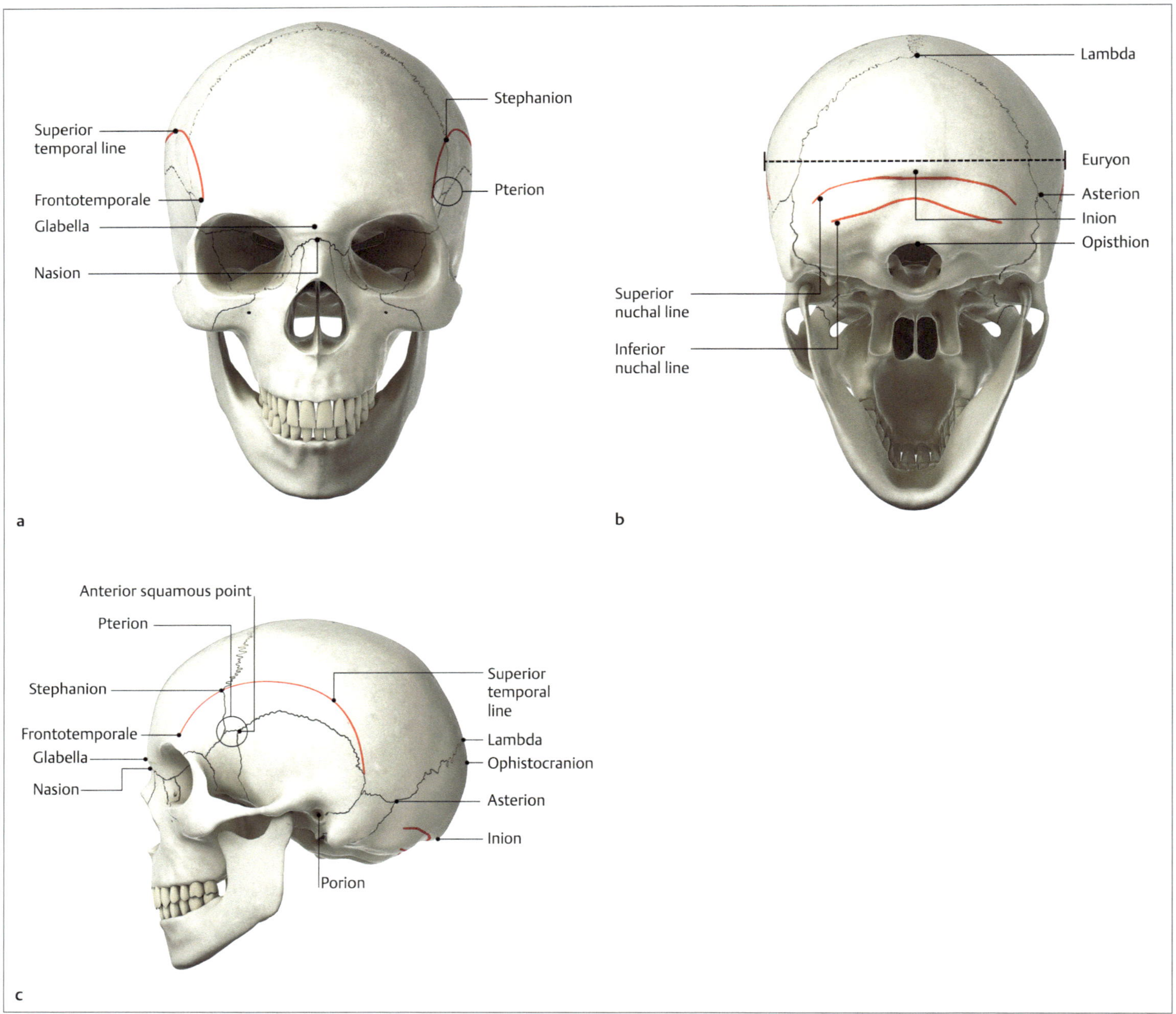

Fig. 2.6 Bony surface landmarks. **(a)** Anterior-to-posterior view; **(b)** posteroinferior-to-anterosuperior view; **(c)** lateral view.

2.2.2 Craniometric Points and Lines and Their Reference to Intracranial Structures

Most Important Cranial Landmarks

Anterior Squamous Point[1]

The connection of the squamous suture to the horizontal line of the "H" of the pterion.

- Corresponds to the base of the pars triangularis of the inferior frontal gyrus at the level of the sylvian fissure, i.e., the anterior sylvian point. It is usually a retraction in the middle of the typical "M" configuration of the inferior frontal gyrus and small widening of the fissure (see ▸Fig. 2.7).

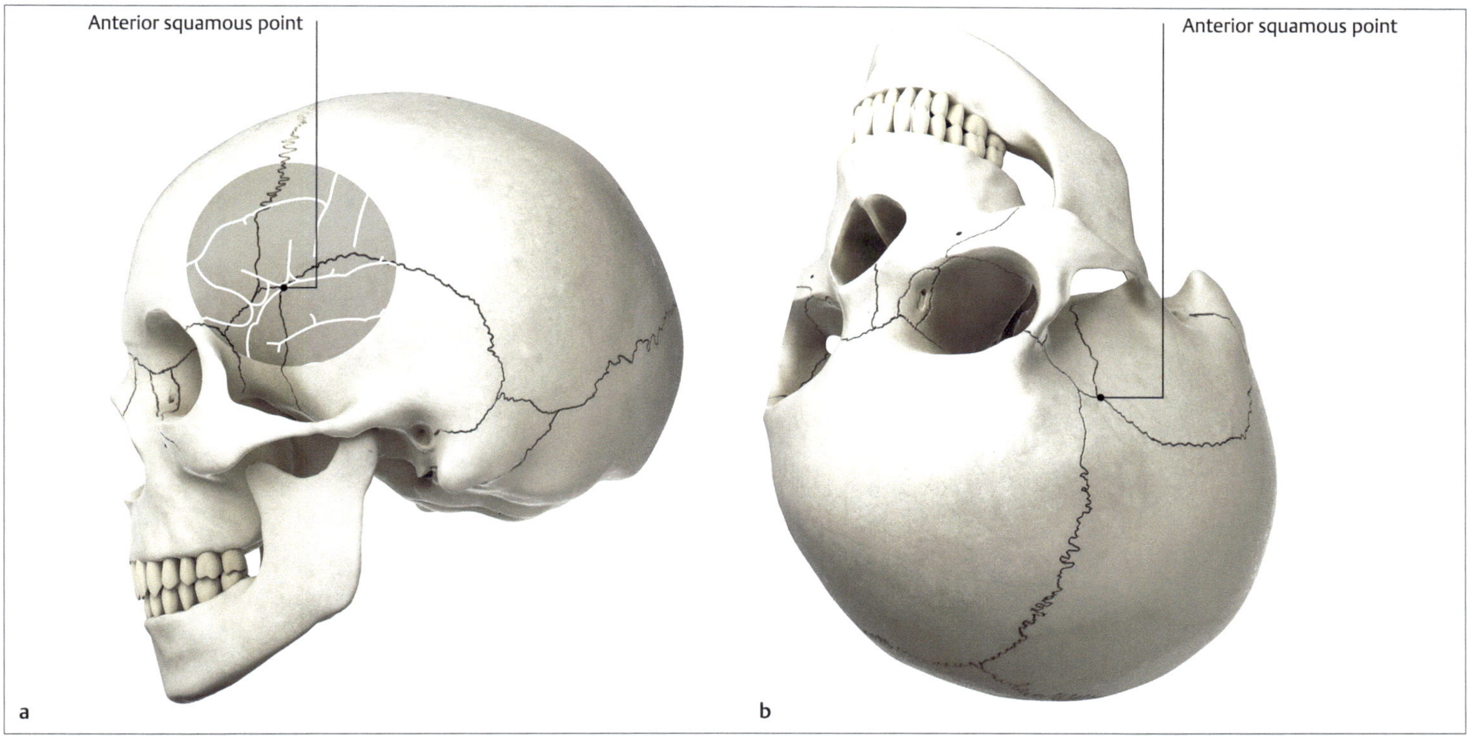

Fig. 2.7 Anterior squamous point. (a) Lateral view with transparent cortical structures. **(b)** Surgeon's view during a pterional approach.

Asterion[2,3]

Connection of the lambdoid, occipitomastoid, and parietomastoid sutures.

Important for localization of the transition from the transverse to the sigmoid sinus (sinus "knee"). Mostly on the distal transverse sinus (two-thirds); sometimes below the sinus (one-third); only rarely above (see ▸Fig. 2.8).

Around 5 to 10 mm proximal = posterior to the beginning of the sigmoid sinus, and never on the sigmoid sinus. Unlike the transverse sinus, the sigmoid sinus has a thin and fragile wall. Placement of burr holes and movement of the craniotome over the sigmoid sinus must be avoided to prevent laceration.

- Should be visualized in retrosigmoid and lateral suboccipital approaches. The transverse sinus has a resistant wall and direct exposure helps to complete the craniotomy.
- Cave: Can be variable, and thus tricky to identify due to additional confounding sutural components or even ossa suturarum (bony islands between sutural convolutions). Rub a compress soaked in hydrogen peroxide over the sutures concerned to allow better visualization.

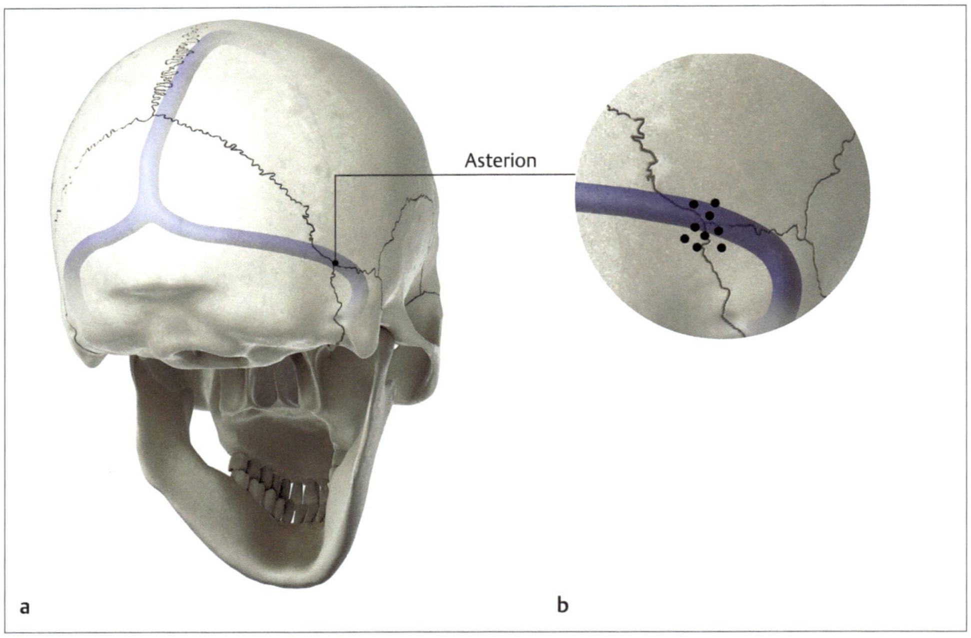

Fig. 2.8 Relationship of asterion to sinus. **(a)** Posterolateral view. **(b)** The center of the asterion burr hole is usually situated on the inferior third of the transverse sinus, but there is considerable variability.

Bregma

The connection between the sagittal suture and the coronal suture (see ▸Fig. 2.9). Located 12 to 13 cm posterior to the nasion. On palpation of the scalp, it can usually, but not always, be felt as a midline protuberance. It is a classical landmark, for example, for planning the placement of an external ventricular drain. For measurements lateral to the midline, the coronal suture is often used as a reference instead of the bregma.

- The upper end of the central sulcus is located on average 5 to 5.5 cm behind the bregma at the midline; however, some sources quote distances ranging from 4 to 6 cm.[1,4–6]
- The precentral sulcus is located on average 3 to 3.5 cm behind the bregma in the midline,[4,7] but also varies considerably.

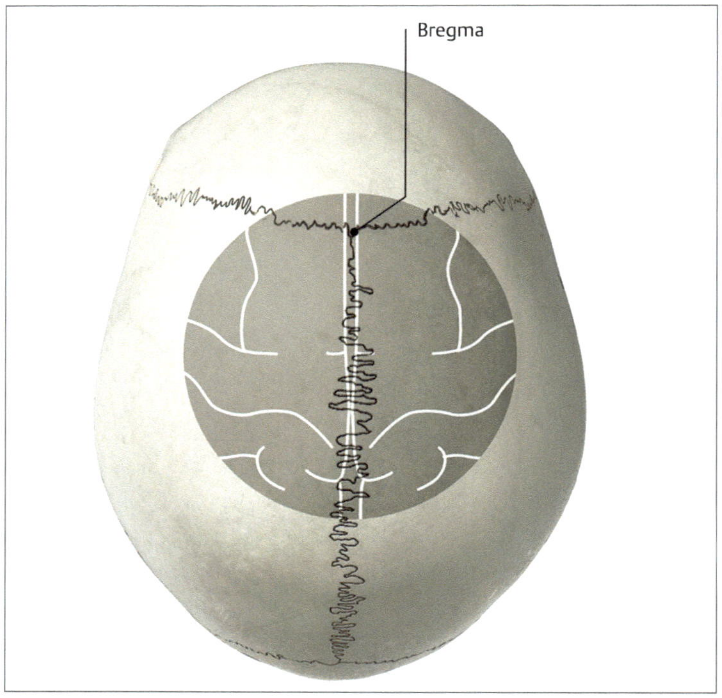

Fig. 2.9 Bregma and related cortical anatomy in the midline. For coronal suture and related anatomy of the precentral gyrus, see ▸Fig. 2.21.

Coronal Suture

For measurements lateral to the midline, instead of the bregma, the coronal suture is used as a reference. The more lateral we get, the more anterior the coronal suture runs in relation to the bregma (see ▶Fig. 2.10).

The coronal suture is located:

- 0.5 cm anterior to the bregma at a point 3 cm lateral to the midline.
- 1 cm anterior to the bregma at a point 5 cm lateral to the midline.
- 2 cm anterior to the bregma at a point 7 to 8 cm lateral to the midline (stephanion):
  - Compared to the coronal suture, the precentral and the central sulcus run even more anteriorly. Thus, the anterior border of the precentral gyrus may approach the coronal suture at the lateral part coming as close as 0.5 cm (on average 1.5–2 cm) at the level of the superior temporal line = stephanion[5] (see ▶Fig. 2.21).

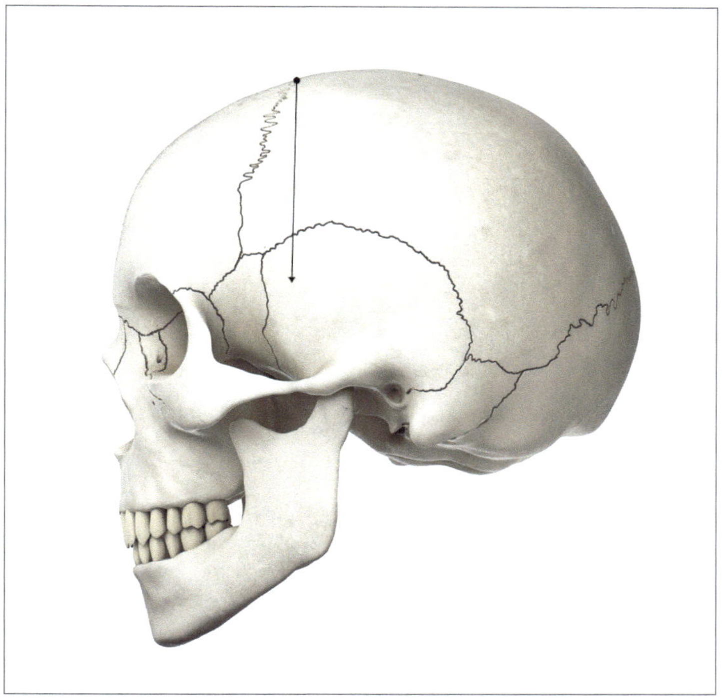

Fig. 2.10 Plumb line. Relationship between the coronal suture and the bregma.

Frontotemporale

The name "frontotemporale" is a classical term for this point, but almost not used in neurosurgery. It corresponds to the palpable bony prominence of the base of the zygomatic process of the frontal bone and forms the starting point of the superior temporal line. It is the innermost part of this line, usually immediately behind the orbital rim. In textbooks on craniometrics, it is defined as the narrowest bilateral point of the frontal bone (see ▶Fig. 2.11).

- It is a frequently used landmark for the floor of the lateral anterior cranial fossa, but usually described rather than named with one term. When lifting the scalp flap during a pterional or frontolateral approach, this is the landmark that indicates sufficient basal exposure to reach the floor of the anterior fossa flush with the craniotomy, i.e., it is the anterolateral skull base point.

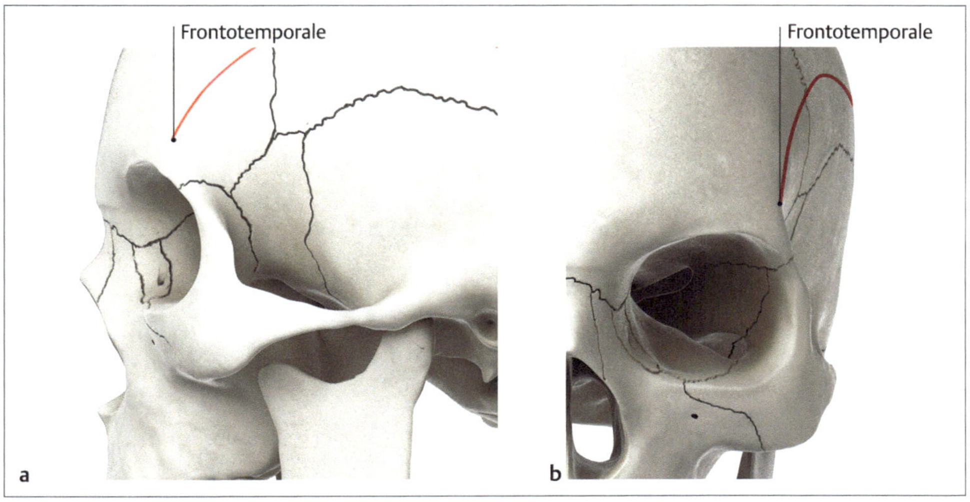

Fig. 2.11 Frontotemporale (anterior skull base point). (a) Lateral view. **(b)** Anterior view.

Inion

Most prominent part of the occipital bone, also referred to as the protuberantia occipitalis externa. It is formed by the midline junction of the bilateral superior nuchal lines (attachment of occipital and sternocleidomastoid muscles). Usually 7 cm inferior to the origin of the lambdoid suture (see ▶ Fig. 2.12).

- Serves as a demarcation line for supratentorial versus infratentorial (or combined supra-/infratentorial) approaches. Normally overlying torcular herophili (confluens sinuum), but varies widely (see ▶ Fig. 2.13). It marks the origin of trapezius muscle.
- Cave: Can deviate considerably to one side. May form a spoiler-like bony spur, rendering placement of burr holes hazardous. Only to be used as landmark in combination with information from CT or MRI due to high variability.

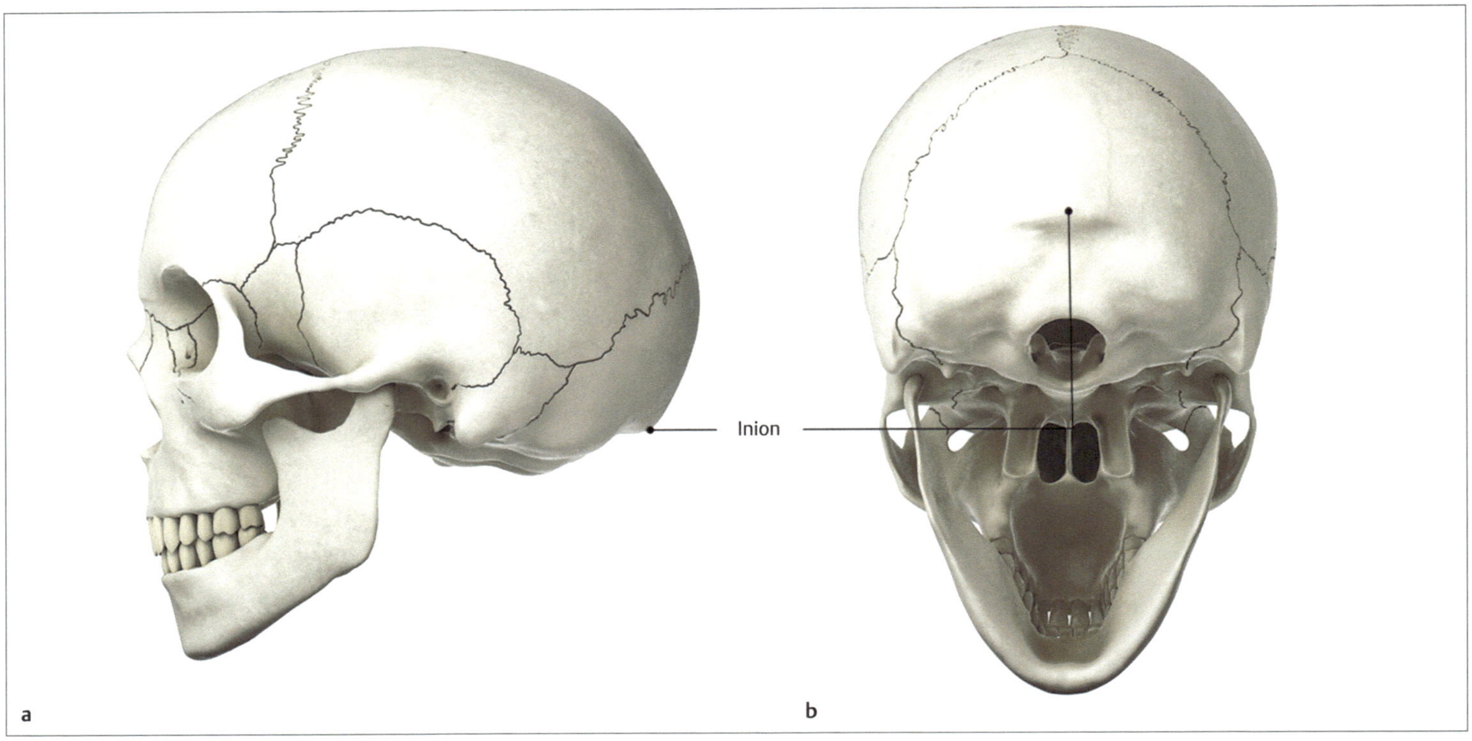

Fig. 2.12 Inion. (a) Lateral view. **(b)** Posterior view.

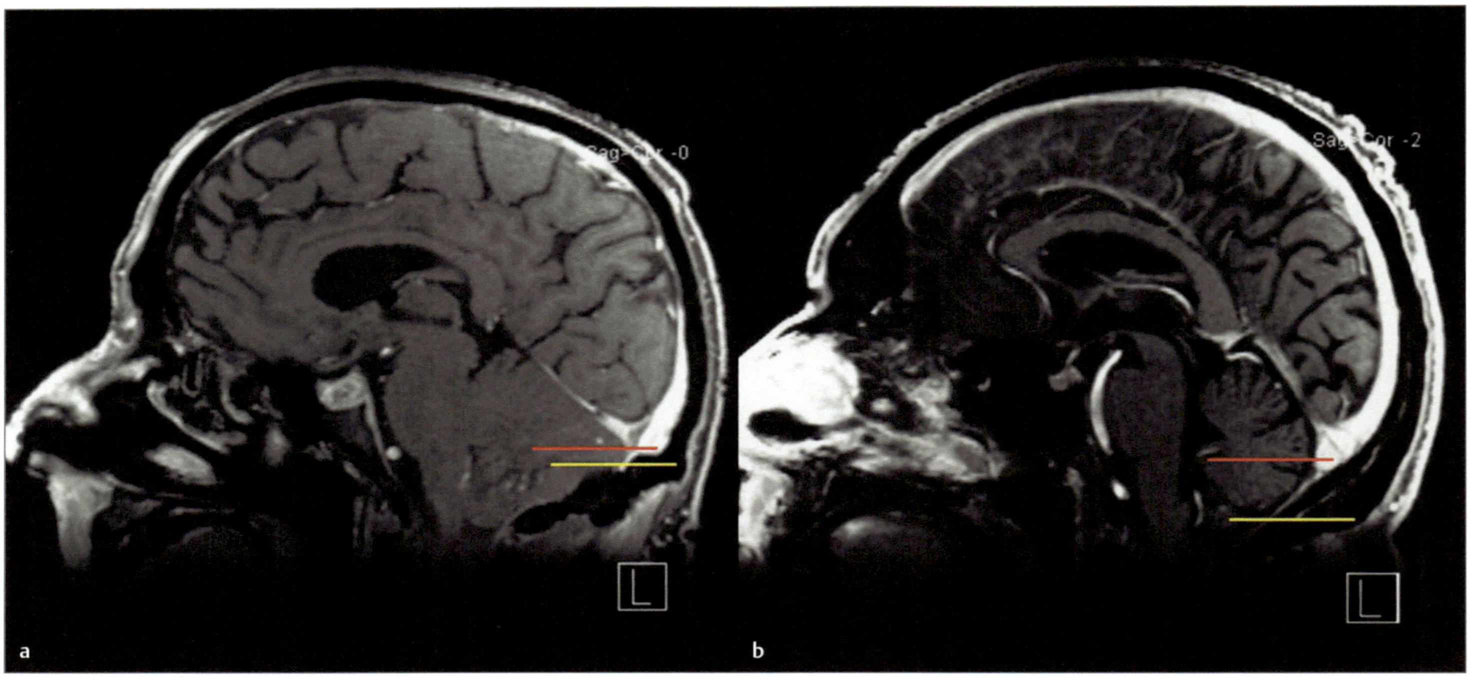

Fig. 2.13 (a, b) Sagittal MRI of two patients. The images show the high variability of the association between the inion and confluens sinuum.

Opisthion

The midline point of the posterior rim of the foramen magnum (see ▶ Fig. 2.14).

- Useful during midline posterior fossa approaches and for approaches to the craniocervical junction, which necessitate opening of the foramen magnum, e.g., during decompression procedures for Arnold–Chiari malformations.
- Care must be taken when palpating the opisthion to avoid forceful penetration of the atlanto-occipital membrane. The membrane can be very thick and firmly attached to this part of the occipital bone.
- Part of many radiographic lines that help in diagnosing atlanto-occipital dislocation, basilar invagination, and platybasia, such as the McRae line, Chamberlain line, Powers ratio, etc.

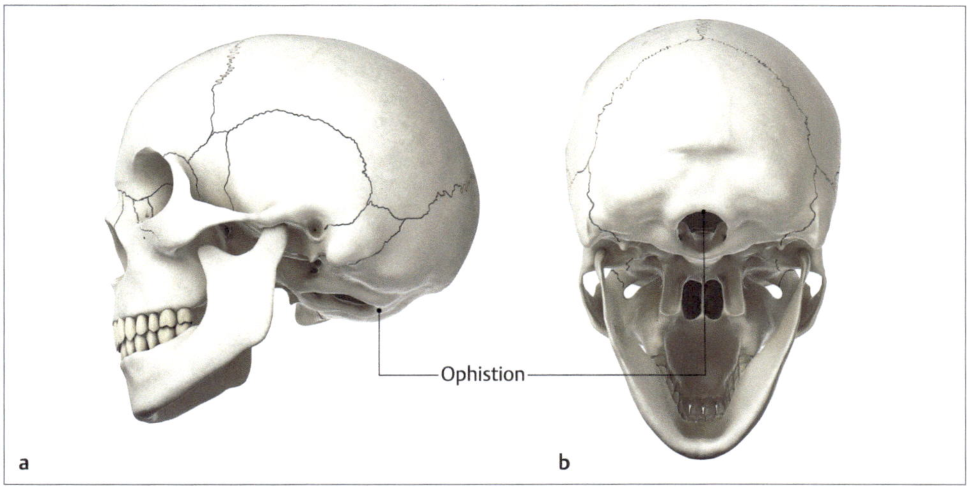

Fig. 2.14 Opisthion. Lateral **(a)** and posterior view **(b)**.

Pterion

This is not a single *point*. It is a small region, where four bones meet, namely ala major of sphenoid bone, squama temporalis, frontal bone, and parietal bone. Thus, in this region, the coronal, sphenofrontal, sphenosquamous, squamous, and sphenoparietal sutures unite in a typical H-like configuration (see ▶ Fig. 2.15).

Situated 2 to 2.5 finger's breadth above the zygomatic arch and 1 to 1.5 finger's breadth behind the lateral orbital rim.

- Virtual central point for important standard craniotomies, to provide (transsylvian) access to, e.g., the anterior part of the circle of Willis and the (para- and supra-) sellar region, orbital roof and apex, insula, and temporomesial region.
- Indicates the lower border of the inferior frontal gyrus close to the sylvian fissure at the level of the lateral orbital gyrus.
- The base center of the “M” of the inferior frontal gyrus is just posterior to the pterion at the anterior squamous point (see ▶ Fig. 2.7).

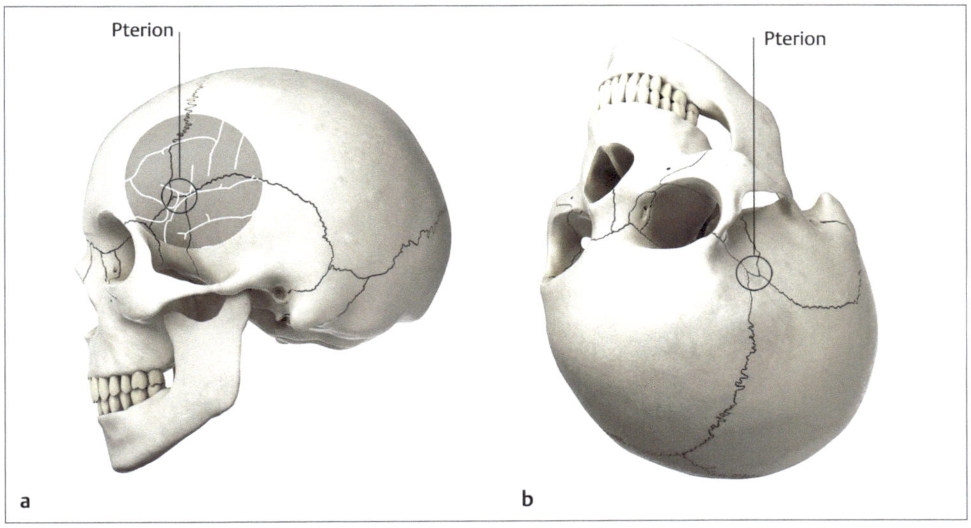

Fig. 2.15 Pterion. **(a)** Lateral view with underlying cortical anatomy. **(b)** Surgeon's view.

Stephanion

Intersection of coronal suture with the superior temporal line (STL).

- Indicates the level of the inferior frontal sulcus.
- On average, the precentral sulcus is 1.5 to 2 cm posterior to the stephanion, but it may come as close as 0.5 cm to it.[5]
- Can be used to localize the motor speech area by drawing a rectangle as follows:
  - Start at the stephanion.
  - Draw a line to the anterior squamous point (▸ Fig. 2.16a).
  - The potential "wider motor speech area" is situated 1 cm immediately anterior to this line (includes the pars triangularis) and 3 cm posterior to this line (includes the pars opercularis and inferior precentral gyrus) (▸ Fig. 2.16b).

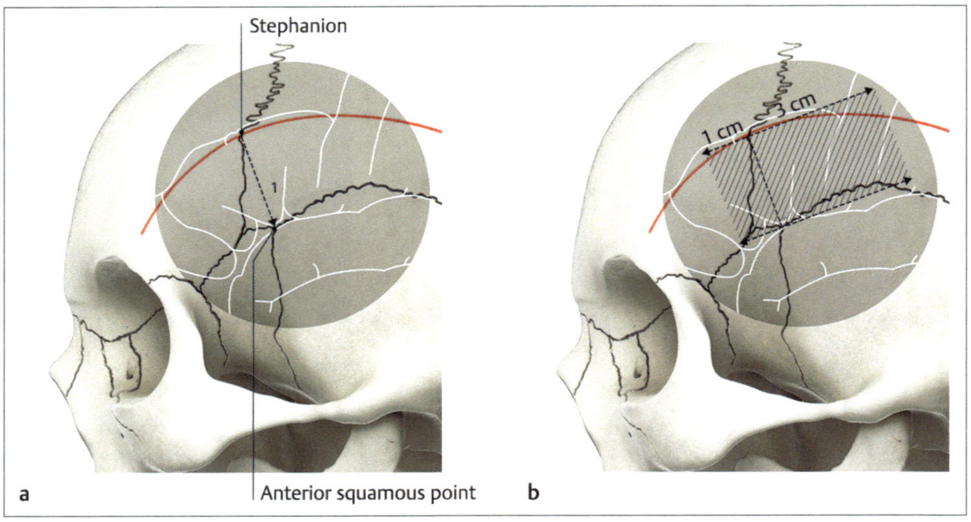

Fig. 2.16 Wider motor speech area. **(a, b)** Using the stephanion and the anterior squamous point, a "wider motor speech area" can be delineated; this is where the expressive language area is most often localized, but it is highly variable.

2.2.3 Skull Base Points

These landmarks are helpful to localize the floor of the various cranial fossae. They are important during skin incision, lifting of the skin flap, and in providing the appropriate bony exposure for making the burr holes and craniotomy.

Nasion	Bony floor of the medial anterior cranial fossa
Frontotemporale	Bony floor of the lateral anterior cranial fossa
Zygomatic arch	Bony floor of the middle cranial fossa

2.2.4 Other Cranial Landmarks (see ▶ Fig. 2.6a–c)

Landmark	Relevance
Euryon	
Not exactly a defined point, but is instrumentally determined as the most lateral and prominent point of the parietal skull bone. It is located at or just above the superior temporal line and at the level of a vertical line passing through the incisura mastoidea (▶ Fig. 2.6**b**)	Poorly defined landmark of little clinical relevance. Some sources assume that it projects to the supramarginal gyrus[1]
Glabella	
Most prominent anterior projecting point at the supraorbital level (▶ Fig. 2.6**a**, **c**)	Of merely historical relevance
Lambda	
Junction of posterior end of sagittal suture and origin of both lambdoid sutures. Its shape resembles the Greek letter lambda (▶ Fig. 2.6**b**,**c**)	On average 12–13 cm posterior to the bregma and 7 cm above the inion. Approximately 3 cm below the obelion. Nicely visible, yet unreliable landmark. Distances to the bregma and the inion may vary considerably. In addition, ossa interparietalia may be present
Nasion	
The point where the frontal bone connects through the nasofrontal suture with the right and left nasal bones. Easily visible and palpable as it forms a clear depression underneath the glabella, in the midline (see ▶ Fig. 2.6**a**, **c**)	• Determines the position of the bregma • Determines the exact midline • Used to check the accuracy of neuronavigation • Landmark for the trajectory of ventriculostomy in the coronal plane Note that the nasofrontal suture marks the lowest point for frontal approaches and must be visualized, e.g., for bifronto-orbital advancement procedures, and for certain techniques of frontal sinus and frontobasal revisions
Obelion	
A midline point, where the sagittal suture is at level with both foramina of the parietal emissary veins	No particular relevance, except as a landmark 3 cm above the lambda
Ophistocranion	
Not a real point, but is instrumentally determined as the posterior end of the maximum skull diameter Usually between the upper one-third to one-half of the lambda–inion line in the midline (see ▶ Fig. 2.6**c**) Described as the most posterior point of the distal cortical end of the calcarine fissure and the base of the cuneus	Of merely historical relevance May not even be recognizable in people with a flat occiput such as one of the authors
Porion	
Upper (bony) part of the external acoustic meatus. Easily visible and palpable (see ▶ Fig. 2.6**c**)	Relevant, e.g., when putting a (gloved) finger inside for the determination of the sagittal trajectory before placement of a ventricular catheter The porion is visible on lateral X-rays of the skull and on CT and MRI scans. Therefore, it is part of many measurements for craniotomy planning Used for checking the accuracy of neuronavigation It is part of the Frankfurt horizontal plane

There are many other craniometric points that are for connoisseurs only: Alare, Ectoconchion, Gnation, Prosthion, Rhinion, Ophryon, Gonion, Vajkonion, Meyrion, etc., but apart from the Schallerion they have no importance for craniotomies.

When the Schallerion was first discovered, it did not mean anything. Then, after much research had been done, it continued not to mean anything. Therefore, it is regarded as the 42 of craniometry.[8]

Most Important Craniocerebral Topography Lines

Craniocerebral topography lines	Relevance
Anterior commissure–posterior commissure (AC–PC) line (= bicommissural line)	
• Introduced by Talairach in 1952 as the line connecting the upper anterior commissure with the lower posterior commissure • Slightly more angled (0–10°) than the canthomeatal line (= orbitomeatal line) used in CT scanning (▶ Fig. 2.17)	• Not a craniometric line, but the standard plane for axial MR imaging
Canthomeatal line	
Also orbitomeatal line, from the center of the canthus to the center of the porion	• Traditional line for tilting the CT gantry, because it is easy to identify on the CT scout • A CT with this tilt is associated with a relatively high dose to the cornea • Increasingly, the AC–PC line is used instead, as it is routine in MR imaging; the AC–PC line is slightly more angled (0–10°)

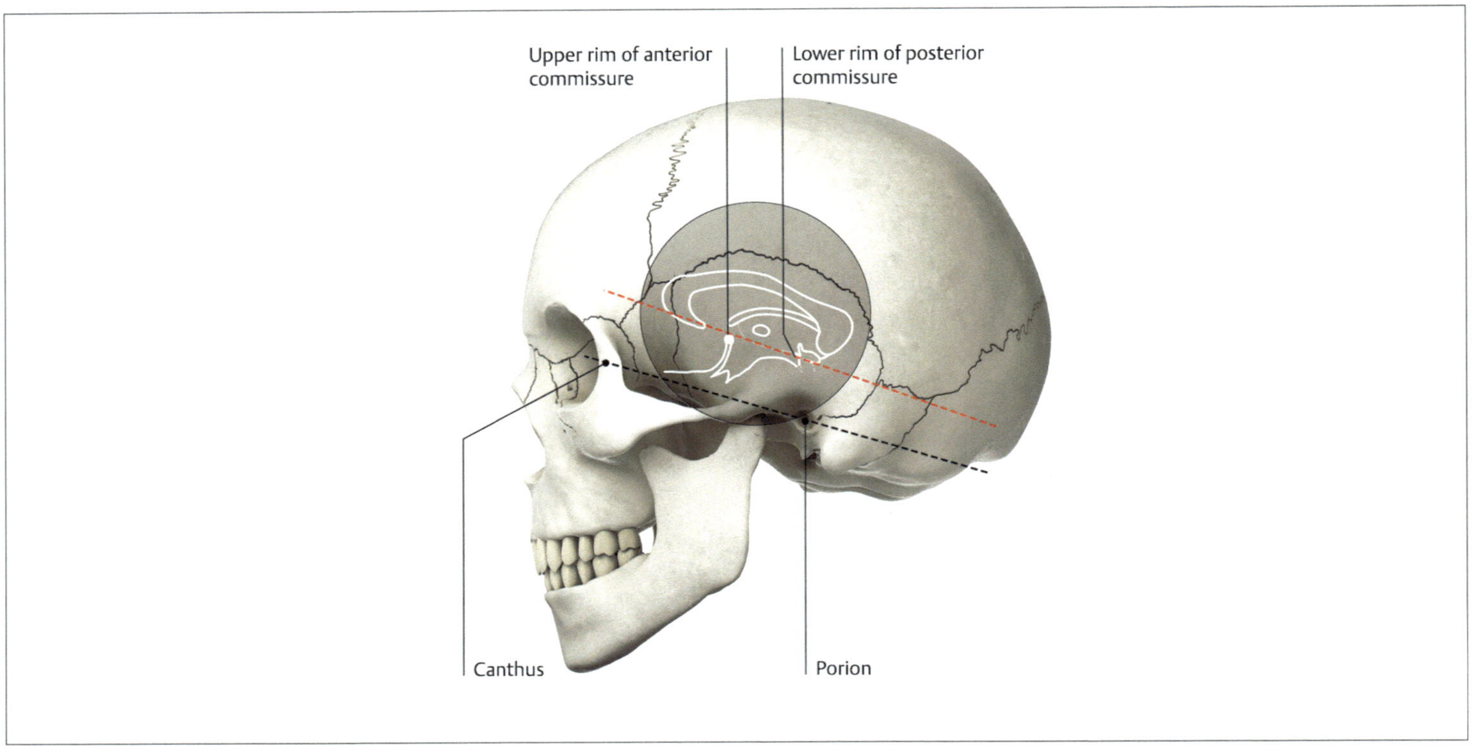

Fig. 2.17 Craniocerebral topography lines for radiologic imaging. AC–PC line (*red*) connecting the superior edge of the anterior commissure with the inferior edge of the posterior commissure. The similar, but not identical, canthomeatal line (*black*), which connects the lateral canthus with the porion, courses with slightly less angulation than the AC–PC line.

Craniocerebral topography lines	Relevance
Frankfurt horizontal plane and associated lines	
A line connecting the lower rim of the orbit with the upper rim of the porion	• Indicates the deepest point of the middle fossa (±7 mm) • When planning a craniotomy without image guidance, this line may help to transfer distances and angles from the CT or MRI image to the patient • By drawing a perpendicular line to the Frankfurt horizontal plane through the tip of the mastoid, the position of the apical part of the central sulcus can be estimated (▶ Fig. 2.18). Note that this measurement can result in considerable error in estimation
Taylor–Haughton lines	

Using these lines, the position of the central sulcus and the sylvian fissure can be estimated. There are lines, connecting:
• Nasion, bregma, and inion in the midsagittal line
• Frankfurt horizontal plane with two perpendicular planes:
  • Condylar
  • Mastoid
	Measuring the distance from the nasion to the inion gives approximations of the following structures:
	• Half of the distance plus 2 cm locates the most posterior point of the central sulcus in the midline (very accurate)[9]
	• A line connecting a point three-fourths of the distance to the canthus combined with the condylar and mastoid lines locates the central sulcus and the sylvian fissure (not very accurate)

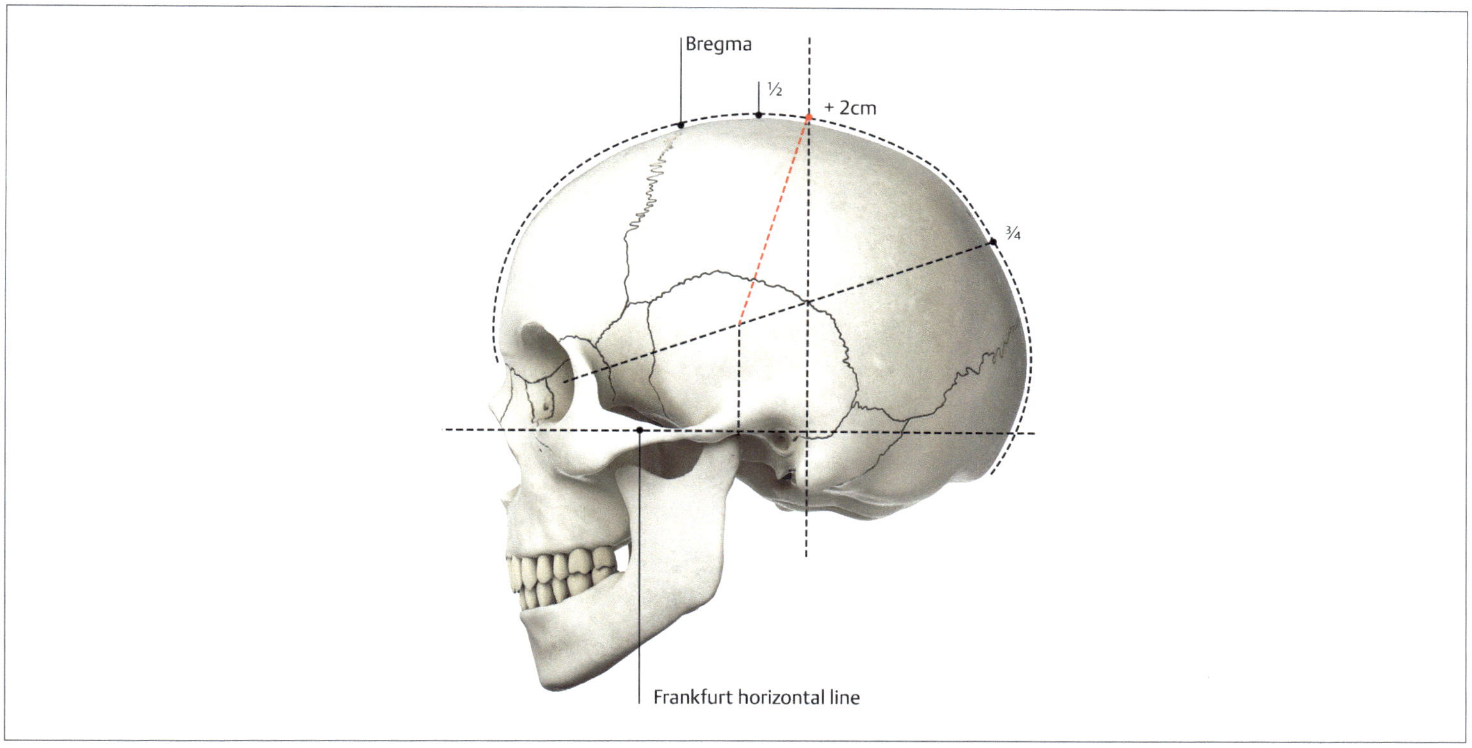

Fig. 2.18 Taylor–Haughton lines. Estimating the position of the central sulcus (*red line*).

Most Important Cerebral Landmarks

Cerebral landmark	Location in relation to cranial landmarks
Anterior sylvian point	
Enlargement of the sylvian fissure by the retraction (2–7 mm) of the base of the triangular part of the inferior frontal gyrus from the sylvian fissure Indicates the center of the base of the **M**-shaped inferior frontal gyrus Often used to start opening the sylvian fissure	Beneath the anterior squamous point, i.e., the most anterior segment of the squamous suture, before it connects to the pterion (see ▶Fig. 2.7 **and** ▶Fig. 2.19)

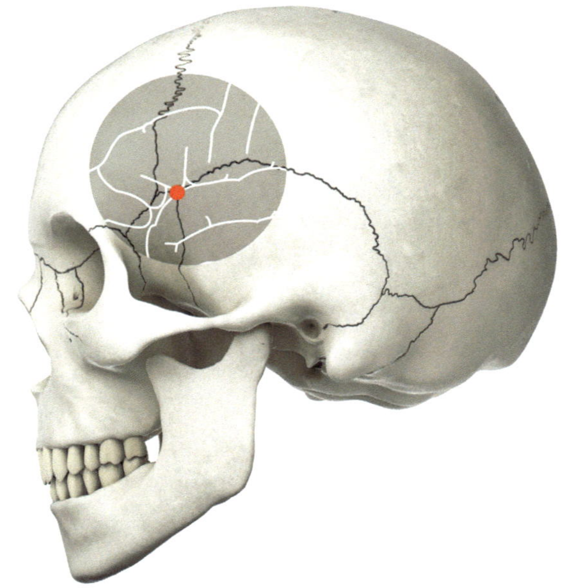

Fig. 2.19 Anterior sylvian and anterior squamous point. Cortical and cranial relationship between the anterior sylvian point and the anterior squamous point, which are basically identical.

Cerebral landmark	Location in relation to cranial landmarks
Broca or motor speech area	
Although this term is mainly of historical significance, it covers the most frequent sites of the "expressive" or motor language area. It comprises the dorsal part of the pars triangularis and the pars opercularis of the inferior frontal gyrus (see Chapter 2.1, Schematic Cortical Anatomy, ▶Fig. 2.2). During language mapping, we find that the positive sites are most often in this area. However, sites outside this area may also be positive for speech arrest or anomia and/or the "Broca area" may be negative and thus safe for approach and resection.	The following points and lines can be used to define a "wider motor speech area" window, which includes the pars triangularis, pars opercularis of the inferior frontal gyrus, and the relevant area of the precentral gyrus: A rectangle is drawn as follows (see ▶Fig. 2.16b and ▶Fig. 2.20): Start at the stephanion Draw a line to the anterior squamous point The potential "wider motor speech area" is situated 1 cm immediately anterior (includes pars triangularis) to this line and extending 3 cm posteriorly (includes pars opercularis and lower precentral gyrus) Note that all these measures are rough estimates and only serve for basic anatomical orientation.

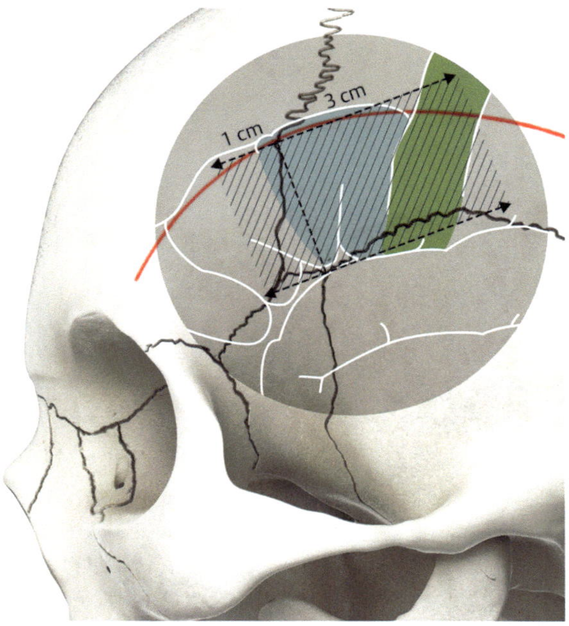

Fig. 2.20 Wider motor speech area. Definition of a "risk zone" where the motor speech area can be expected. The classical Brodmann area 44 and 45 ("Broca," *blue shading*) and the primary motor cortex (*green shading*) are shown.

Cerebral landmark	Location in relation to cranial landmarks
Precentral sulcus	
• The position in relation to the coronal suture depends on the distance to the midline (see ▶Fig. 2.21).	• 3–3.5 cm posterior to the coronal suture at the midline[4,7] • At the level of the stephanion, it may come as close as 0.5 cm (on average 1.5–2 cm) to the coronal suture[5]
Central sulcus	

• The central sulcus runs from the midline downward in an anterolateral direction
• It almost never intersects completely with the midline because the precentral and postcentral gyri fuse medially forming the paracentral lobulus
• For axial landmark based measurements, it is important to visualize the central sulcus as an obliquely flying bird. It has two anteriorly convex wings connected by the concave "body," which is the hand knob
Taking these two features into account, the distance of the central sulcus behind the coronal suture depends on the distance from the midline
	• It is located behind the bregma[1]:
	  • At the midline: 5–5.5 cm (range 4–6 cm)[4,5,6]
	  • At the level of the hand knob: 4–5 cm
	• The upper end at the midline can more accurately be estimated as half of the distance between the nasion and the inion, plus 2 cm more posteriorly[9] (see ▶Fig. 2.18)

Precentral gyrus	
Although often mentioned in the literature, it does not make sense to discuss the location of the central sulcus alone and whether it is situated 4 or 6 cm behind the bregma. Ultimately, these measurements should define a risk zone for injury of the precentral gyrus. To take the potential variability into account, the maximum (= range) data should be used, still indicating a likelihood of 5% of being outside our model shown in ▶Fig. 2.21 The wide variability seen in ▶Fig. 2.21 demonstrates the low accuracy of using landmarks	In ▶Fig. 2.21, we have transferred the "average" and "range" measurements of 20 cadaveric hemispheres as published by Frigeri et al[5] on to a 3D model, also taking into account the location and slope of the coronal suture Naturally, neurosurgeons should take into account the "range" to make sure that the precentral gyrus is not injured during emergency craniotomies or making of burr holes, for example, burr hole trepanations in patients with chronic subdural hematomas. For planned procedures, image guidance and electrophysiology should be used

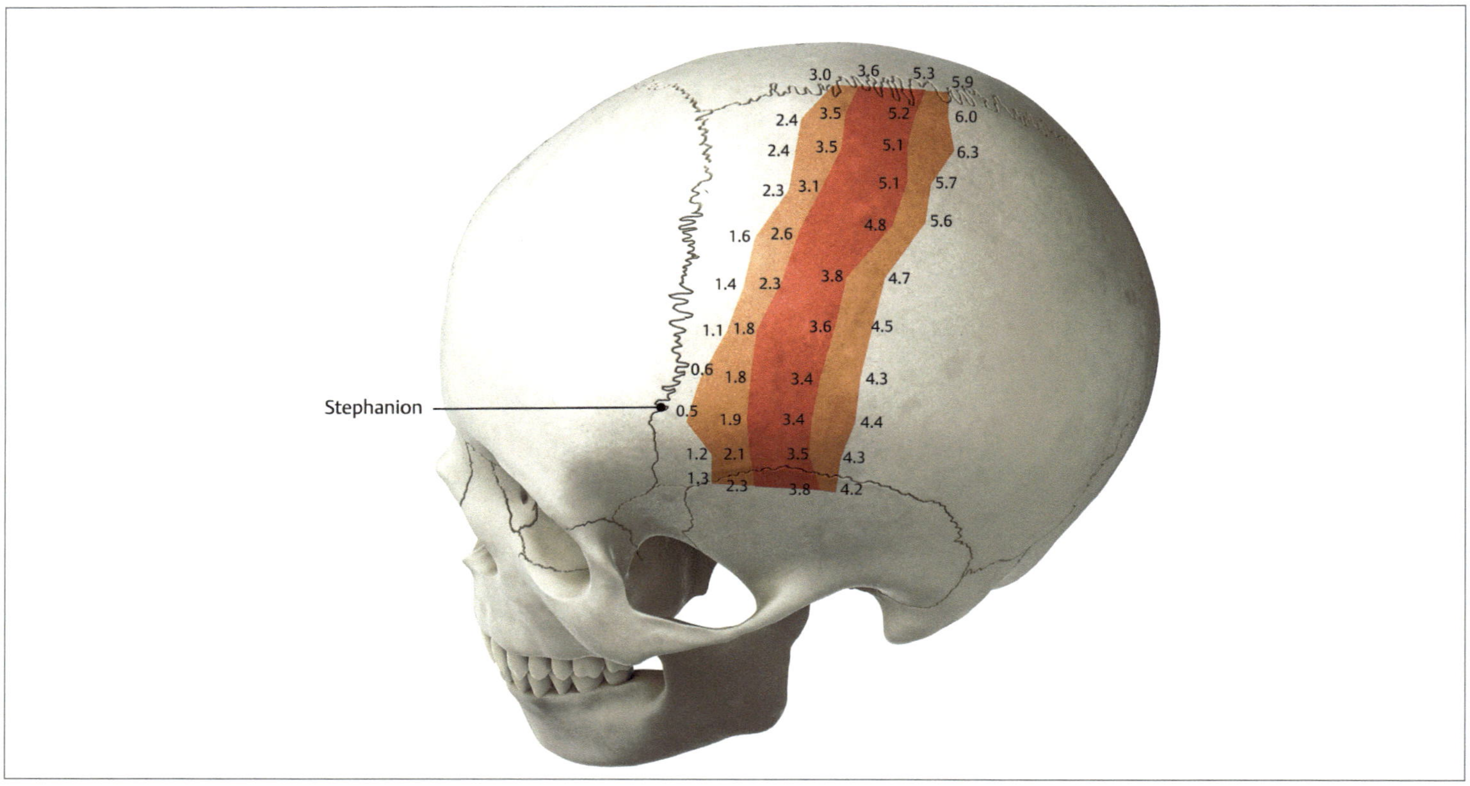

Fig. 2.21 Precentral gyrus. The precentral gyrus, precentral sulcus, and postcentral sulcus run from the midline downward in an anterolateral direction. The position in relation to the coronal suture depends on the distance to the midline. Even more oblique than the coronal suture, the precentral gyrus may approach it as close as 0.5 cm (average 1.5–2 cm) at the level of the stephanion. Each number represents the distance from the coronal suture in centimeters, as measured in 20 cadaveric hemispheres.[5] The *red-shaded zone* represents the mean values and the *orange zone* the maximal range of the position of the anterior and posterior limits of the precentral gyrus in relation to the coronal suture.

Cerebral landmark	Location in relation to cranial landmarks
Hand knob	
Omega- or epsilon-like anatomic structure. The thumb is located laterally and the fifth finger medially.	The center of the hand knob is located 4 cm behind the coronal suture and 3–4 cm lateral to the midline (see ▶Fig. 2.22). The anteroposterior width of the hand knob is 1.5–2 cm.[10]

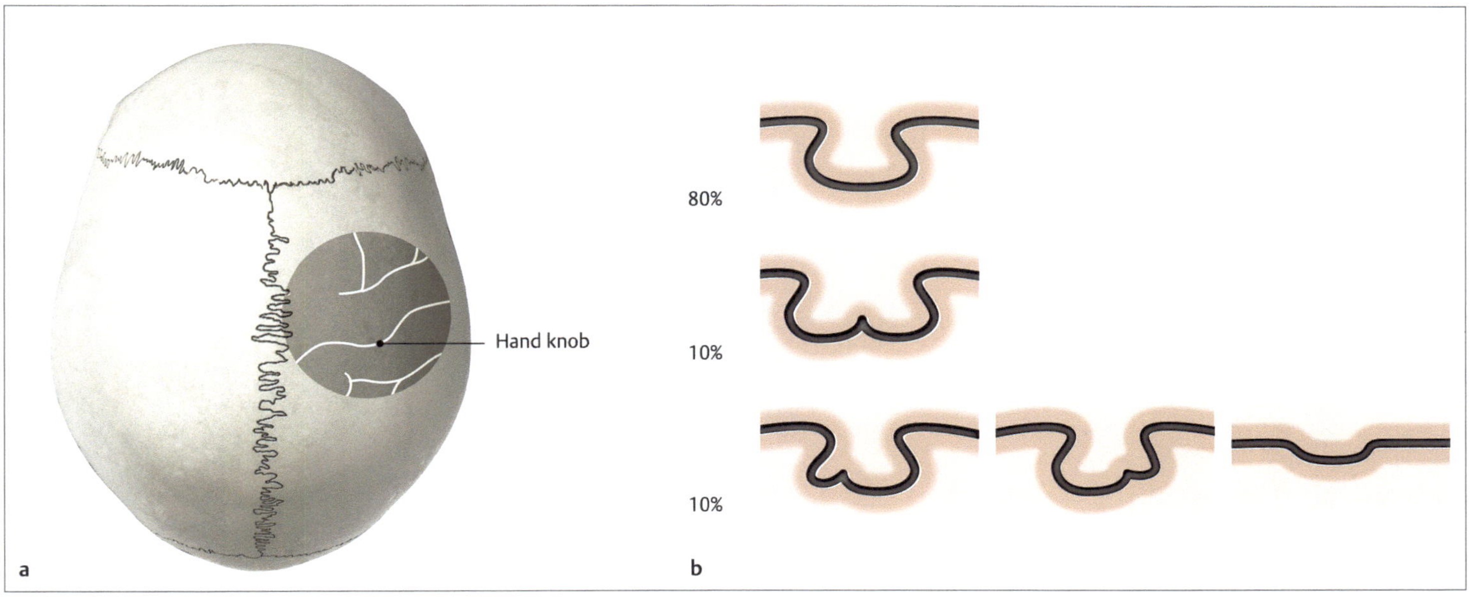

Fig. 2.22 (a, b) Hand knob. Schematic drawings of the so-called hand knob of the precentral gyrus. In most cases, it has an "omega" or an "epsilon"-like appearance.

Cerebral landmark	Location in relation to cranial landmarks
Inferior frontal and precentral sulcus meeting point (IFS/preCS)	
Intersection of the inferior frontal and the precentral sulcus. It delineates: • The posterior and superior limits of the opercular part of the inferior frontal gyrus. • The anterior border of the precentral sulcus at the level of the motor face area.	It is located on average: • 1.5–2 cm posterior to the stephanion at the superior temporal line; however, in some patients, it may come as close as 0.5 cm to the coronal suture.[5] • 3 cm above the sylvian fissure (see ▶Fig. 2.23).[1]

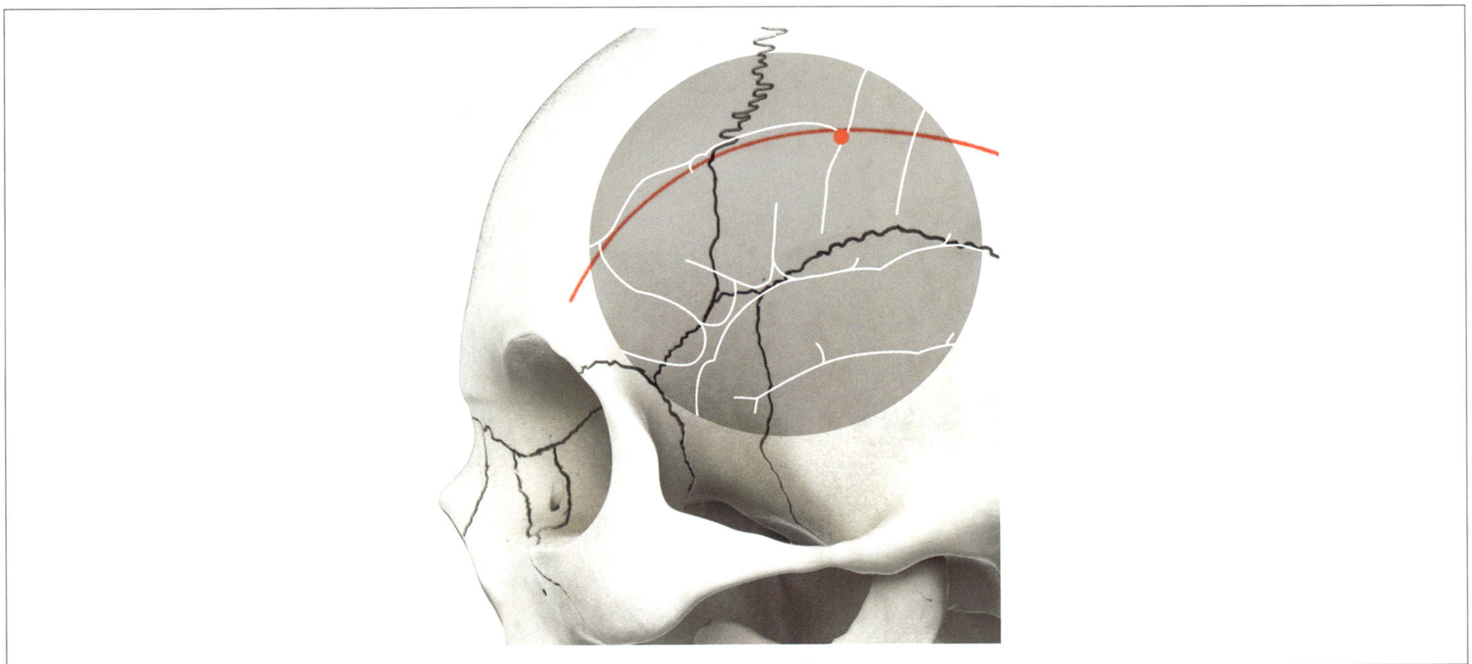

Fig. 2.23 IFS/preCS meeting point. Lateral view showing the relationship between the IFS/preCS meeting point which localizes the most superior and posterior edge of the pars opercularis of the inferior frontal gyrus.

Cerebral landmark	Location in relation to cranial landmarks
Inferior rolandic point (iRo)[1]	
Real or virtual intersection of the central sulcus with the sylvian fissure It indicates the motor cortex superiorly, but also the Wernicke area posterior to it. It is the anterior limit of the transverse gyrus of Heschl, which kisses the postcentral gyrus, and part of the Wernicke area.	• 2.5 cm behind the anterior squamous point (= 2.5 cm behind the anterior sylvian point) and 4–5 cm above the zygomatic arch. • Using the orbitomeatal line as reference: approximately 2–3 cm anterior to the porion and perpendicular to this line 4–5 cm up (see below: localizing sylvian fissure) (see ▶Fig. 2.24).

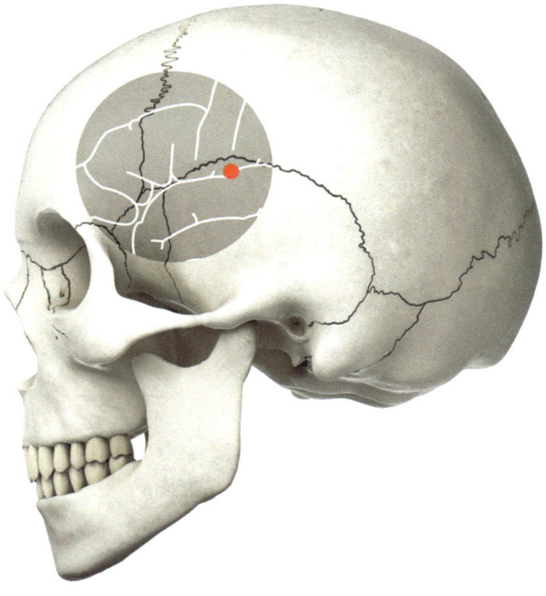

Fig. 2.24 Inferior rolandic point. Intersection of the sylvian fissure with the projected inferior end of the central sulcus.

Cerebral landmark	Location in relation to cranial landmarks
Intraparietal and postcentral sulci meeting point (IPS/postCS)[1]	
• Intersection of the intraparietal and postcentral sulcus. • The intraparietal sulcus runs almost parallel to the interhemispheric fissure, and starts at the postcentral sulcus. • Indicates the supramarginal gyrus below.	It is located: • 4 cm lateral to the midline.[1] • 6–7 cm posterior to the bregma (see ▶Fig. 2.25).

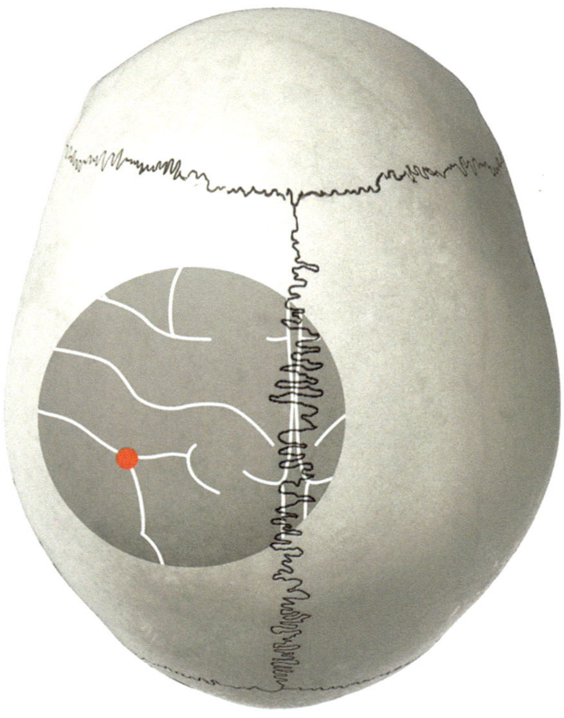

Fig. 2.25 IPS/postCS meeting point. Superior view.

Cerebral landmark	Location in relation to cranial landmarks
Sylvian fissure.	Use orbitomeatal = canthomeatal line. Lines perpendicular to the orbitomeatal line help to localize the sylvian fissure as shown in ▸Fig. 2.26.[11] The squamous suture is identical to the sylvian fissure from the anterior squamous point to 2 cm posterior to it. The Taylor–Haughton line is less accurate.

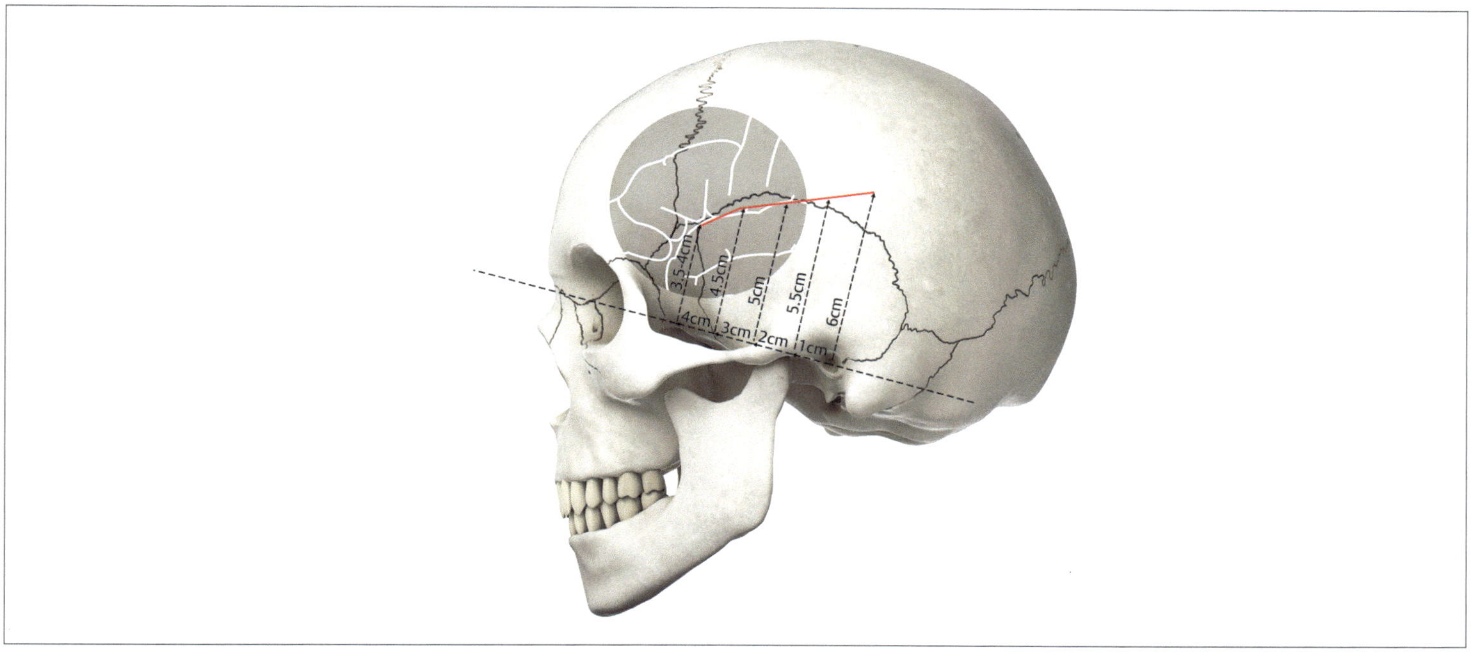

Fig. 2.26 Sylvian fissure. Localizing the sylvian fissure using the orbitomeatal line and squamous suture.

References

[1] Ribas GC, Yasuda A, Ribas EC, Nishikuni K, Rodrigues AJ Jr. Surgical anatomy of microneurosurgical sulcal key points. Neurosurgery 2006;59(4, Suppl 2):ONS177–ONS210, discussion ONS210–ONS211

[2] Ribas GC, Rhoton AL Jr, Cruz OR, Peace D. Suboccipital burr holes and craniectomies. Neurosurg Focus 2005;19(2):E1

[3] Seeger W. Planning Strategies of Intracranial Microsurgery. Vienna: Springer; 1986

[4] Sarmento SA, Jácome DC, de Andrade EM, Melo AV, de Oliveira OR, Tedeschi H. Relationship between the coronal suture and the central lobe: how important is it and how can we use it in surgical planning? Arq Neuropsiquiatr 2008;66(4):868–871

[5] Frigeri T, Paglioli E, de Oliveira E, Rhoton AL Jr. Microsurgical anatomy of the central lobe. J Neurosurg 2015;122(3):483–498

[6] Rhoton AL. Cranial anatomy and surgical approaches. Neurosurgery 2003;53:1–746

[7] Seeger W. Atlas of Topographical Anatomy of the Brain and Surrounding Structures. Vienna: Springer; 1978

[8] Adams D. The Hitchhiker's Guide to the Galaxy. New York, NY: Harmony Books; 1980

[9] Rhoton ALJ Jr. The cerebrum. Neurosurgery 2002;51(4, Suppl):S1–S51

[10] Caulo M, Briganti C, Mattei PA, et al. New morphologic variants of the hand motor cortex as seen with MR imaging in a large study population. AJNR Am J Neuroradiol 2007;28(8):1480–1485

[11] Rahmah NN, Murata T, Yako T, Horiuchi T, Hongo K. Correlation between squamous suture and sylvian fissure: OSIRIX DICOM viewer study. PLoS One 2011;6(3):e18199

2.3 Identifying Cortical Landmarks and Fiber Tracts in MRI

Johannes Goldberg, Michael Murek, Levin Häni, Karl Schaller, and Andreas Raabe

Introduction

Neurosurgeons should be able to identify the most important sulci, gyri, and tracts on MR images to appropriately plan their operations and to decide whether monitoring and mapping should be used. This chapter presents some useful guidance. For further reading, please refer to the seminal work of Naidich et al.[1]

Keep in mind that any mass lesion will shift the cortical area or subcortical tract and identification will therefore be much more difficult than in normal anatomy. In these situations, it helps to start by identifying the landmarks on the contralateral side first. They can then be translated to the side of the mass lesion taking into consideration the lesion's location and the direction of the shift.

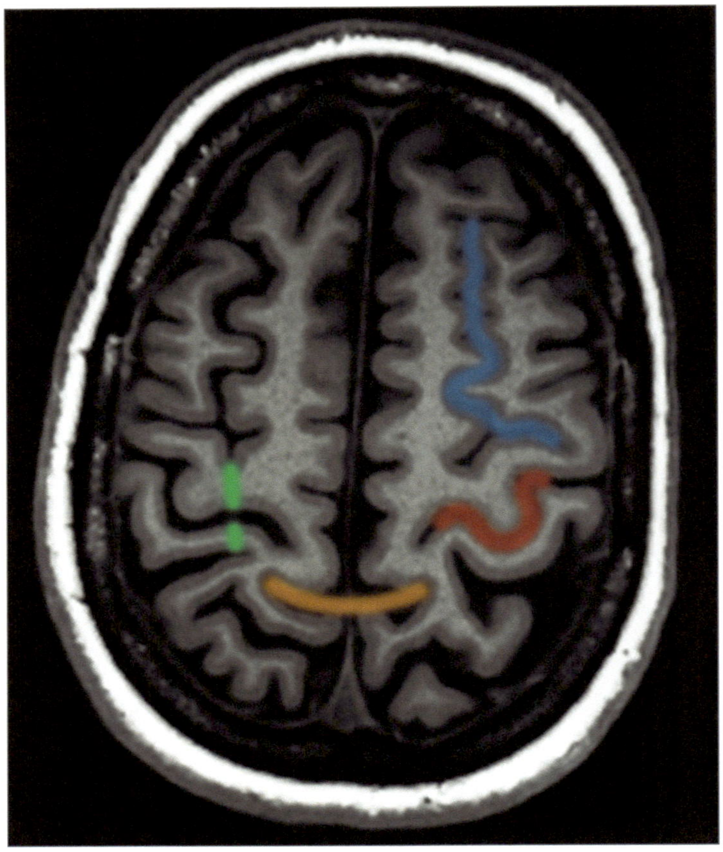

Fig. 2.27 Identification of the central sulcus on axial MRI. There are usually four signs that help to localize the central sulcus and the precentral gyrus: L-sign (*blue*), omega sign (*red*), bracket sign (*orange*), and thickness sign (*green*).

Cortical Landmarks—Primary Motor and Sensory Cortex

Axial MRI Signs

See ▶Fig. 2.27.

L-Sign

The superior frontal sulcus meets the precentral sulcus at an angle of almost 90° resembling the capital letter "L" (L-sign). This sign can be used for the gyri too: the connection between the superior frontal gyrus and the precentral gyrus also resembles a capital letter L. The central sulcus is the next sulcus posterior to the precentral sulcus.

"Hand Knob" Omega-sign

The motor hand area corresponds to a knob-like posteriorly pointing convolution of the precentral gyrus—the "hand knob"—where the central sulcus is shaped into an inverted omega or (more rarely) an epsilon. The hand knob contains the primary motor neurons of the hand, with a somatotopic organization where the fifth finger is most medial and the thumb lateral. The hand knob identifies the precentral gyrus.

Thickness Sign

The anteroposterior diameter of the precentral gyrus is larger than that of the postcentral gyrus.

Bracket Sign

On midline sagittal MRI sections (see also ▶Fig. 2.30), the pars marginalis of the distal cingulate sulcus ascends to the surface of the parietal lobe. It separates the paracentral lobule from the precuneus. In axial MRI, it forms a characteristic anteriorly opened bracket at the medial surface. It marks the posteromedial border of the postcentral gyrus. The next sulcus anterior to it is the central sulcus. Sometimes the splitting of the postcentral gyrus by the bracket sign is described as the "bifid postcentral sulcus sign."

Sagittal MRI Signs

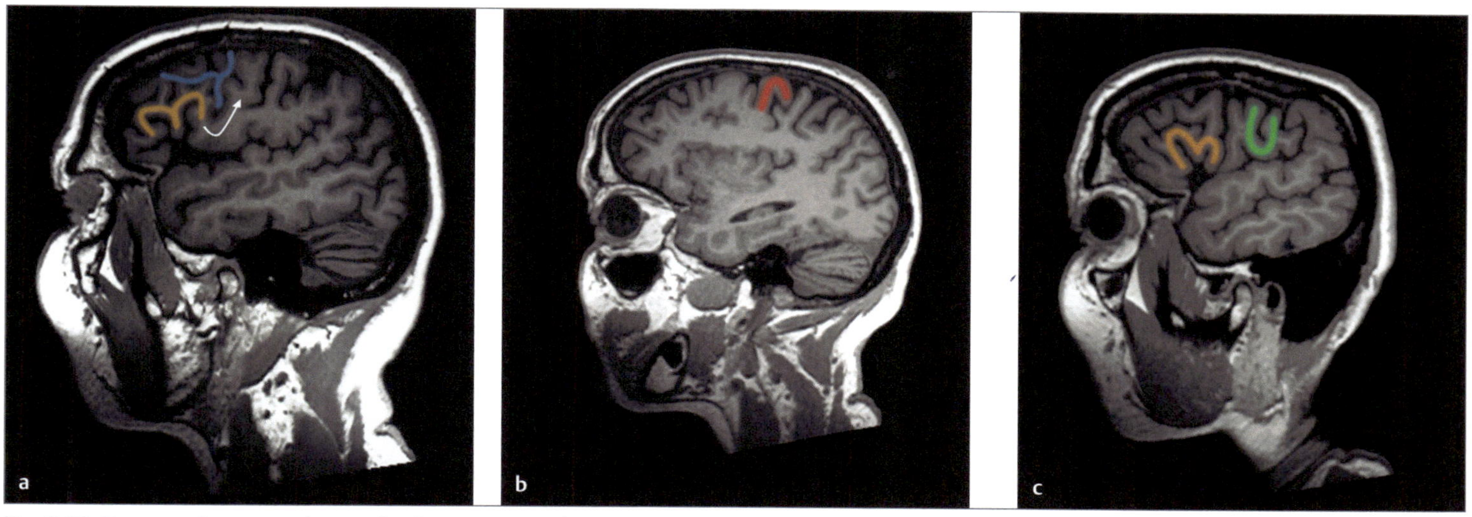

Fig. 2.28 Precentral gyrus and central sulcus on sagittal MRI. There are four signs in sagittal MRI that help to localize the central sulcus and the precentral gyrus. M-around sign (*orange*), T-sign (*blue*), U-sign (*green*), and hook sign (*red*). The first three are visible on more lateral slices **(a,b)**, the last is visible on more medial slices at the level of the hand knob **(c)**.

M-around Sign

The horizontal and the ascending ramus of the sylvian fissure give the inferior frontal gyrus its typical M-like configuration. The posterior border of the M is the precentral sulcus. Writing the M from anterior to posterior and then joining to an imaginary next letter around the caudal precentral sulcus leads up into the precentral gyrus (*arrow* in ▸Fig. 2.28a).

T-sign

The inferior frontal sulcus and the precentral sulcus form a capital T tilted 90° clockwise (T-sign). The top of the T marks the precentral sulcus and the precentral sulcus identifies the precentral gyrus. The central sulcus is located immediately parallel and posterior to it ▸Fig. 2.28a).

U-sign

The central sulcus does not extend to the sylvian fissure. There is a gyrus connecting the precentral with the postcentral gyrus, which is called the subcentral gyrus. The U-sign is the horizontal subcentral gyrus connecting both lower ends of the vertical precentral and postcentral gyrus (▸Fig. 2.28c).

Hook Sign

The fourth sign in the sagittal plane is the hand knob, but here it shows a less typical configuration than seen in axial MRI. In more median MRI sections, the hand knob rises out of the parenchyma like a backward-oriented hook or, as some see it, the head of an animal looking back toward the postcentral gyrus (▸Fig. 2.28b).

2.3.3 Cortical Landmarks—Language Areas

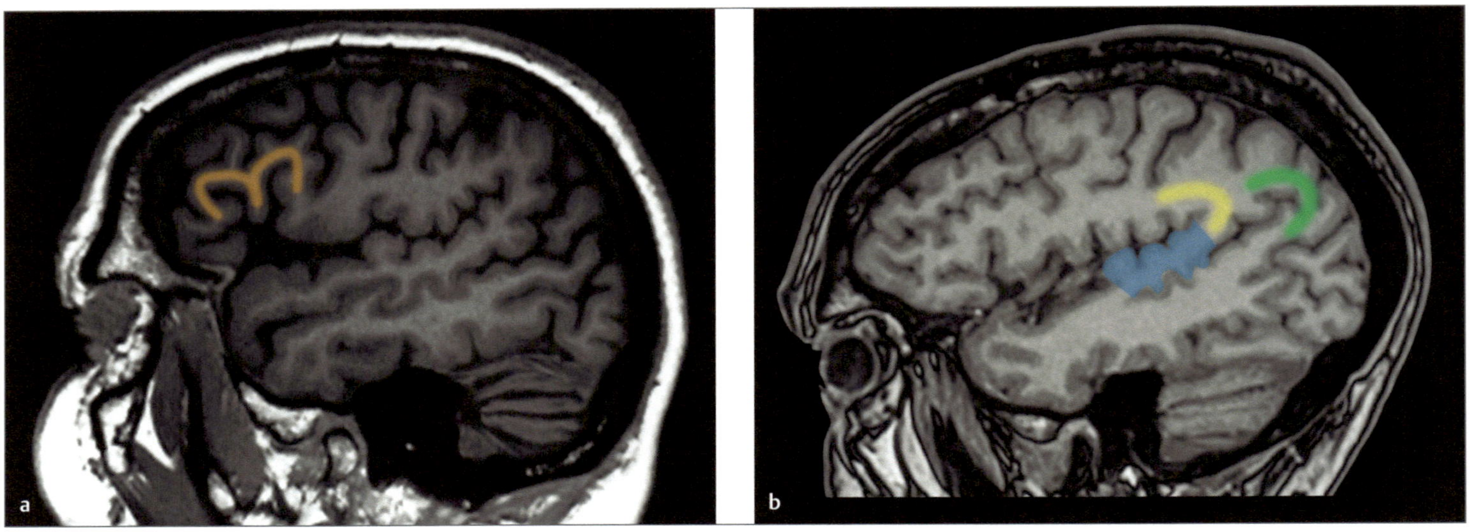

Fig. 2.29 Sagittal MRI showing frontal (a) and parietotemporal (b) cortical language areas. The M-sign (*orange*) identifies the pars orbitalis (anterior leg of the M), the pars triangularis (middle leg), and the pars opercularis (posterior leg). The other two signs are the horseshoe-like shapes of the supramarginal (*yellow*) and angular gyrus (*green*). The traditional Wernicke area is located in the dorsal superior temporal gyrus (*blue*) behind the more prominent Heschl gyrus, which is opposite the projection of the central sulcus on the other side of the sylvian fissure.

M-sign

In the sagittal plane, the inferior frontal gyrus is subdivided by the horizontal ramus and ascending ramus of the sylvian fissure. They form the pars orbitalis, pars triangularis, and pars opercularis, giving the inferior frontal sulcus a typical heart-like or upper case M shape on sagittal MRI sections. The dorsal triangular and opercular parts of the dominant hemisphere are supposedly involved in semantic and word generation tasks and are traditionally known as Broca's area. Sometimes, accessory sulci may be present within the M-shape, making identification more difficult (▶ Fig. 2.29a, *orange*).

Dorsal Superior Temporal Gyrus

The traditional Wernicke area is located in the dorsal half of the superior temporal gyrus. It can be easily recognized in the sagittal plane by the sylvian fissure and the parallel and inferior running superior temporal sulcus. Its anterior border connects to the auditory cortex (Heschl)—which kisses the subcentral to postcentral gyrus—and its posterior border connects to the supramarginal gyrus (▶ Fig. 2.29b, *blue*).

Supramarginal Gyrus

The posterior ramus of the sylvian fissure ascends into the anterior part of the inferior parietal lobule. There it is embraced in a semicircular fashion by the supramarginal gyrus, which resembles a horseshoe. On the dominant side, this part is involved in phonological word choices and visual word recognition (▶ Fig. 2.29b, *yellow*).

Angular Gyrus

Inferior and parallel to the sylvian fissure run the superior temporal gyrus and the superior temporal sulcus. The posterior ramus of the latter is called the angular sulcus. Like the shape of the supramarginal gyrus, the angular gyrus equally forms a horseshoe—by embracing the angular sulcus. The angular gyrus plays a role in language processing, arithmetic (on the dominant side), and spatial cognition (on the nondominant side). Damage to the dominant angular gyrus can manifest as Gerstmann's syndrome (▶ Fig. 2.29b, *green*).

2.3.4 Cortical Landmarks—Primary Visual Cortex

See ▶ Fig. 2.30.

Parieto-occipital Sulcus and Calcarine Sulcus—Lazy-Y-Sign

The occipital and parietal lobes are separated by the parieto-occipital sulcus (separates precuneus and cuneus). The anatomy can best be identified in paramedian sagittal MRI sections. The parieto-occipital sulcus separates the parietal (precuneus) from the occipital lobe (cuneus) and ascends in an oblique fashion from anteroinferiorly to superoposteriorly, where it reaches the hemispherical surface. The calcarine sulcus forms the lower limb of the oblique lazy-Y travelling toward the occipital pole in a posteroinferior direction. The parieto-occipital sulcus and the calcarine fissure unite anteriorly to form the anterior calcarine sulcus, the lower limb of an oblique Y immediately below and posterior to the splenium of the corpus callosum at the inferomedial side of the brain. The gyri on the superior and on the inferior side of the calcarine sulcus contain the primary visual cortex.

2.3.5 Determining the Position of Important Fiber Tracts on MRI—Corticospinal Tract (CST)

Preoperative diffusion tensor imaging (DTI) combined with functional information from navigated transcranial magnetic stimulation or functional MRI can be used to delineate the course of the CST with fiber tracking. Nevertheless, the surgeon should have a basic concept of how to estimate the location of the CST in the corona radiata and the internal capsule. With a mass lesion, the anatomy is often distorted and one should keep in mind that a tumor can compress or shift brain tissue by several centimeters. Subcortical mapping remains the most reliable method for locating the CST and estimating its distance from the resection cavity.

Unlike for cortical landmarks, there are no direct signs for the location of the fiber tracts within the white matter. Their position therefore has to be determined by indirect signs and landmarks. ▶ Fig. 2.31, ▶ Fig. 2.32, and ▶ Fig. 2.33 illustrate signs used to localize the CST on sagittal and axial images. When applying the methods described below to localize the CST in the corona radiata and the internal capsule, two important limitations must be kept in mind.

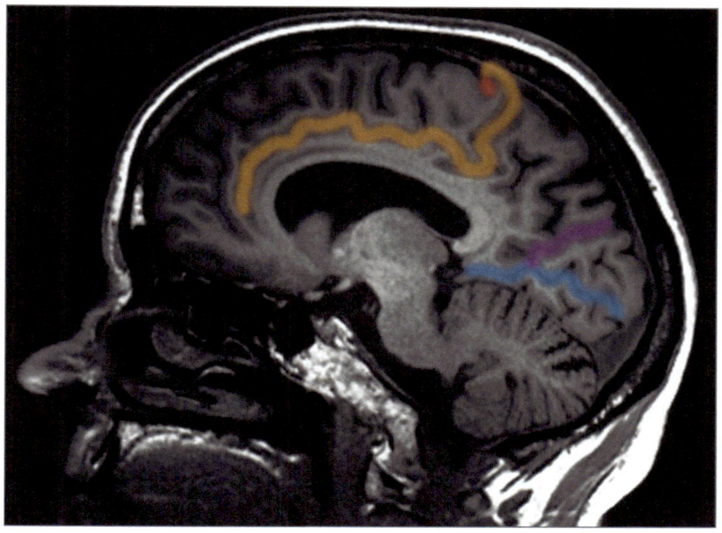

Fig. 2.30 Visual cortex on paramedian sagittal MRI sections. Cingulate gyrus with ascending marginal part (*orange*) indicating the bracket sign and the central sulcus immediately anterior to it (*red dot*), and the lazy-Y-sign, which is composed of the parieto-occipital sulcus (*purple*) and the calcarine sulcus (*blue*).

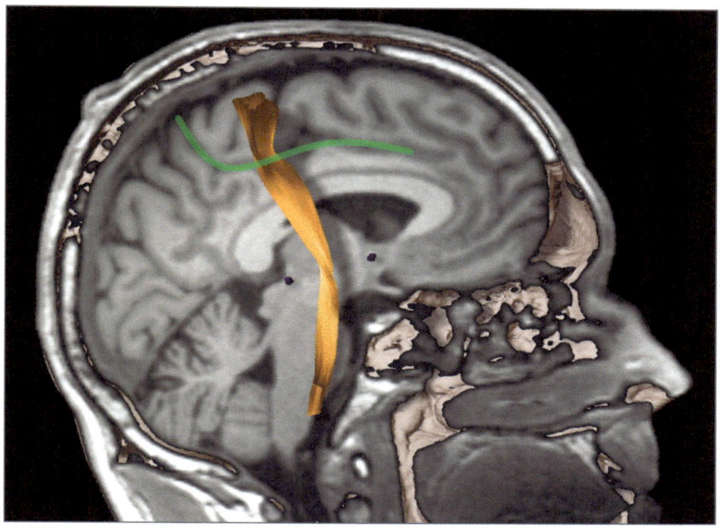

Fig. 2.31 On a sagittal image, the central sulcus is the first sulcus anterior to the marginal ramus of the cingulate sulcus (*green line*). From the precentral gyrus, the CST follows a line that can be drawn to a point midway between the anterior and posterior commissure (*violet dots*).[2]

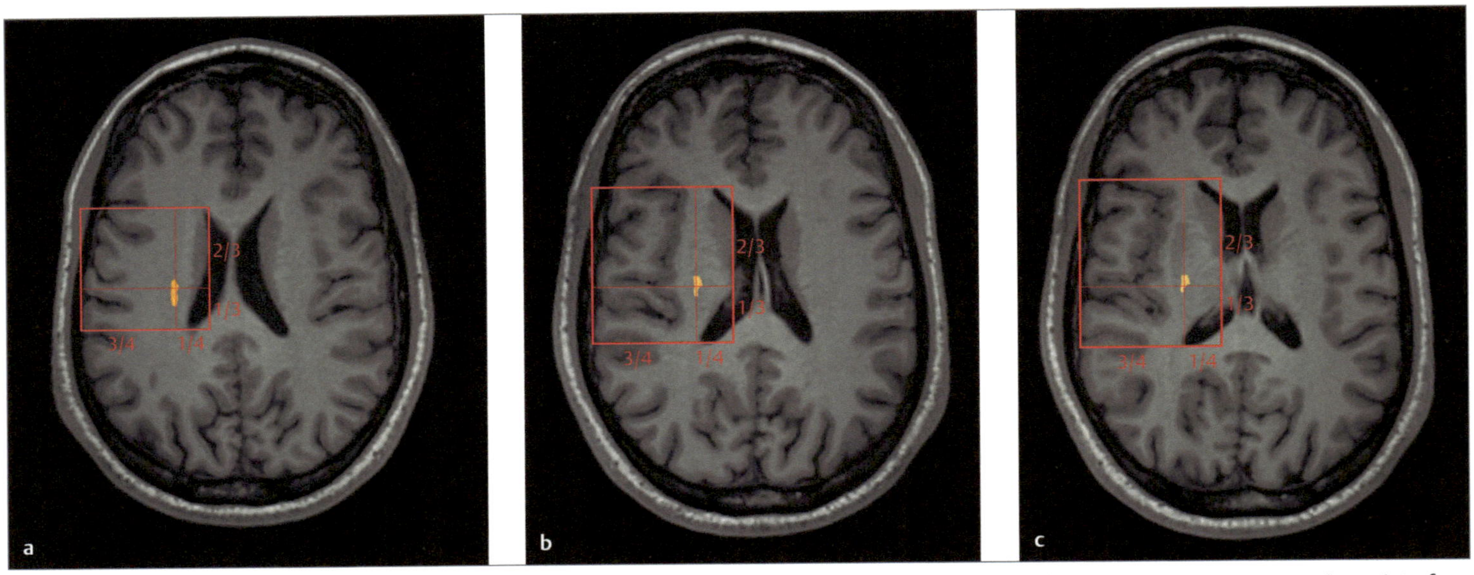

Fig. 2.32 (a–c) The CST in the white matter can be localized by drawing a rectangle along the most medial, most anterior, most posterior point of the lateral ventricle, and the most lateral point of the cerebral cortex. The CST (*yellow*) can be localized on different axial levels at the crossing point of a horizontal line drawn in the lower one-third and a vertical line drawn at the medial one-fourth of this rectangle.[3]

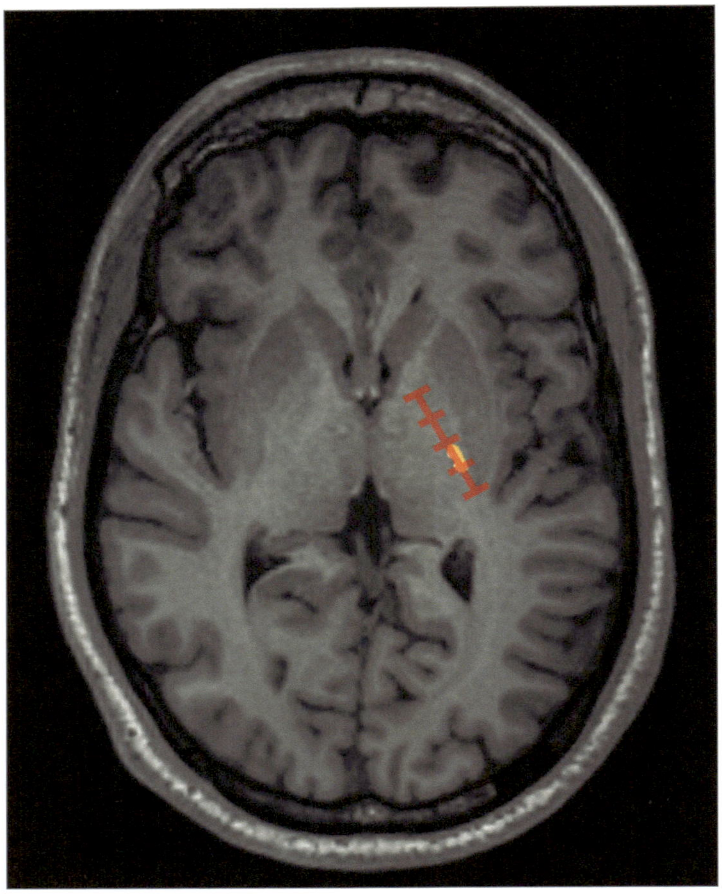

Fig. 2.33 Following its descent through the corona radiata, the fibers of the CST run through the posterior limb of the internal capsule toward the midbrain. The average location of the CST fibers in the posterior limb of the internal capsule is at one-half to three-fourths of the distance from the most medial point to the most posterior point of the lentiform nucleus.[4]

First, these landmarks indicate the location of fibers originating in the hand region of the primary motor cortex. The location of the fibers from the leg and face region diverges from that. In the corona radiata and the internal capsule, the CST shows a somatotopic organization, with the face fibers running more anteriorly and the leg fibers more posteriorly than the hand fibers. Since the precentral gyrus runs from medial to lateral in an anterior direction, with the face region being anterolateral to the hand and leg, the subcortical somatotopy can be easily remembered by the mnemonic "anterior stays anterior." Secondly, one should remember that even if most monosynaptically projecting corticomotoneurons can be found in the primary motor cortex, the corticospinal tract originates not only from the primary motor cortex, but also from a wide variety of precentral and parietal cortical areas. The above-mentioned methods are based on modern DTI studies using the primary motor cortex as sole origin and do not take this variety into account.

2.3.6 Determining the Position of Important Fiber Tracts on MRI—Arcuate Fascicle

See ▶ Fig. 2.34, ▶ Fig. 2.35, and ▶ Fig. 2.36.

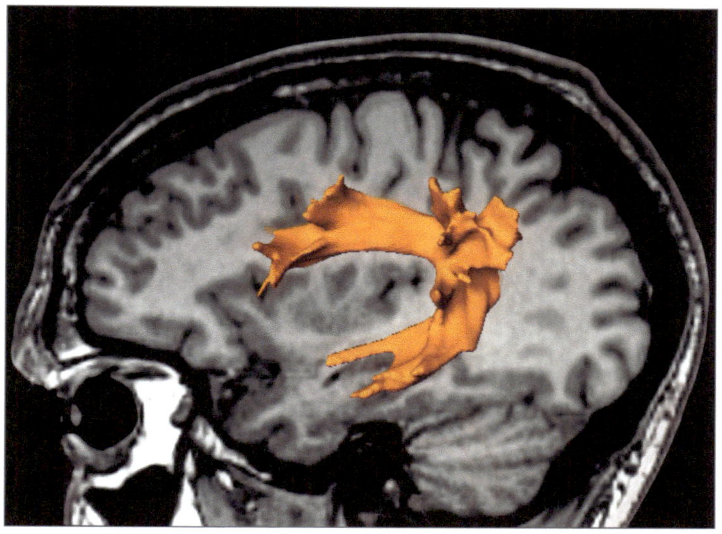

Fig. 2.34 Sagittal MRI showing the arcuate fascicle after DTI imaging and fiber tracking. It connects cortical language sites in the inferior frontal gyrus (F3) and posterior temporal lobe (T1) in the dominant hemisphere, which are commonly referred to as Broca's and Wernicke's area. The appearance is similar to an arch surrounding the insula and the circular sulci.

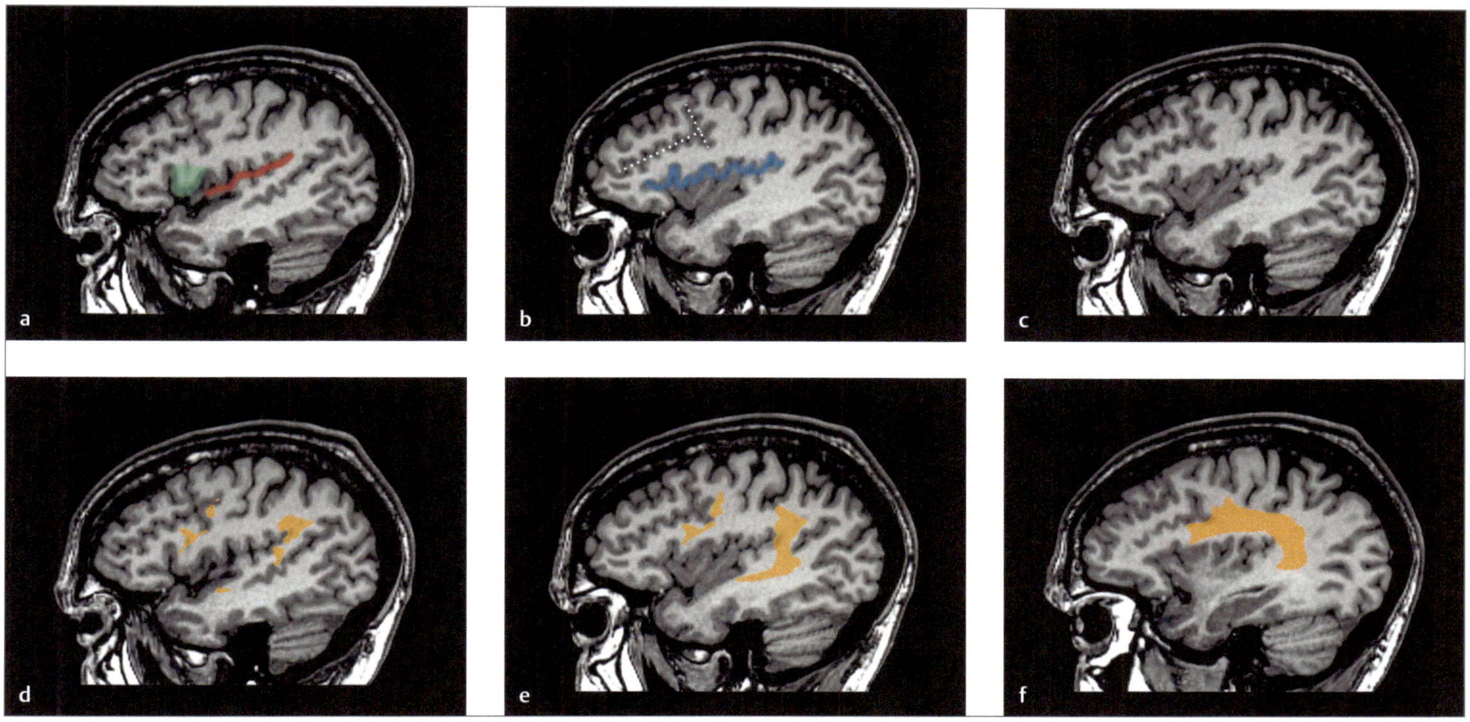

Fig. 2.35 Determining the location of the arcuate fascicle without DTI imaging and fiber tracking on sagittal MRIs. The indirect landmarks for the arcuate fascicle are: pars opercularis (*green*), the superior circular sulcus (*blue*), and the sylvian fissure (*red*). After marking the position of the pars opercularis and the sylvian fissure on cortical sagittal MRI sections **(a)**, the MR images are scrolled toward the subcortical white matter **(b, c)**. This reveals a white matter tract between the inferior frontal sulcus (*dotted line*: the T-sign) and the superior circular sulcus inferiorly (*blue*). It is this band of white matter that continues around the superior circular sulcus and around the sylvian fissure in the depth below the supramarginal sulcus. In this white matter band, the arcuate fascicle travels from frontally to temporally. **(d–f)** The result of the fiber tracking.

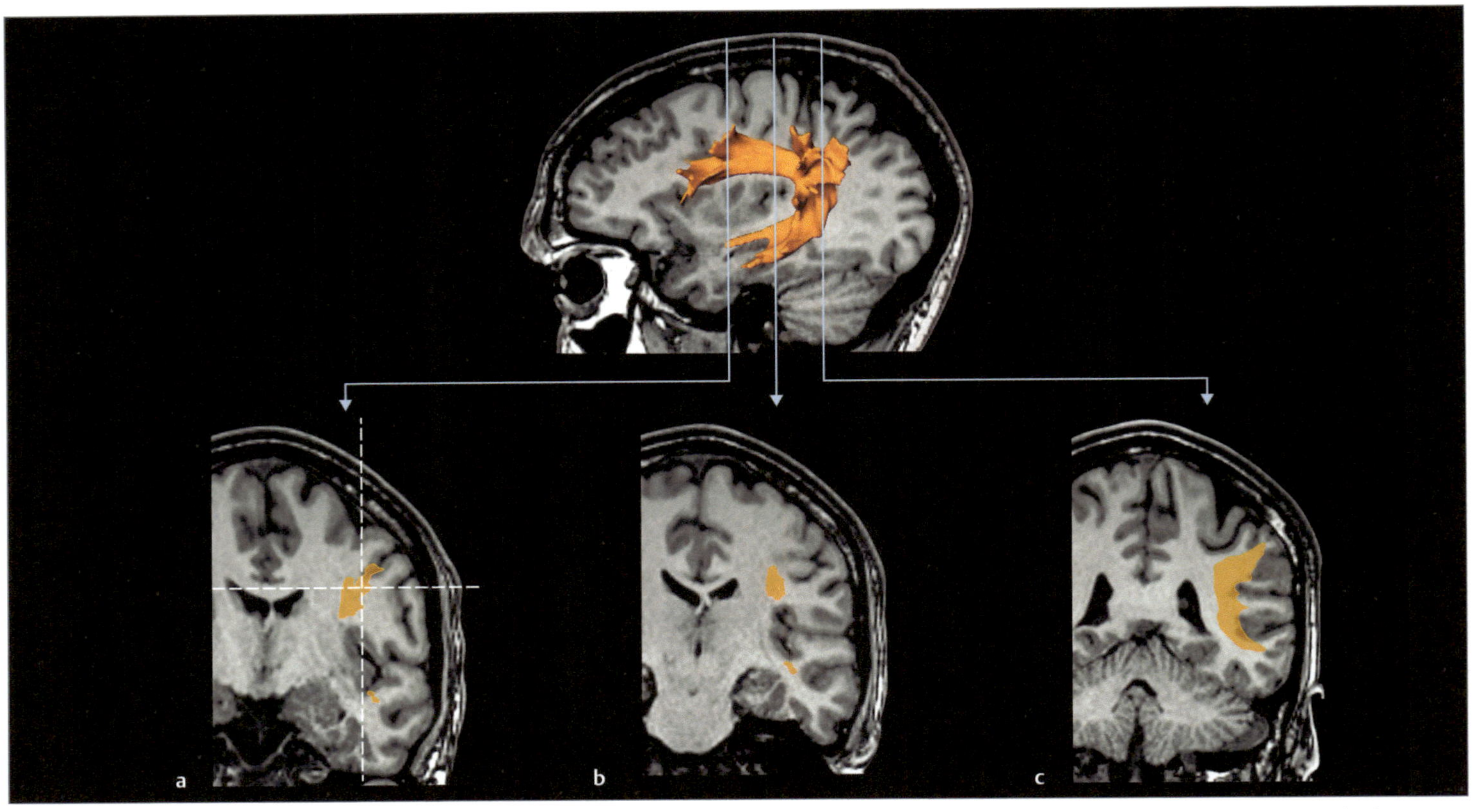

Fig. 2.36 **Determining the location of the arcuate fascicle without DTI imaging and fiber tracking on coronal MRIs.** On coronal MRIs, the location of the arcuate fascicle can be estimated by (1) the intersection of a horizontal line parallel to the lateral ventricles and a vertical line tangential to the insular cortex **(a)**. (2) Alternatively, the superior and inferior sulcus limitans of the insula can be used: the fascicle is situated just outside the superior and below the inferior circular sulcus **(b)**. In the posterior transition zone between the frontal and the temporal lobe (the posterior, more vertical part of the "b"), the arcuate fascicle can be identified lateral to the trigone of the lateral ventricle where the anterior horn continues into the temporal horn **(c)**.

2.3.7 Determining the Position of Important Fiber Tracts on MRI—Optical Tract

See ▶ Fig. 2.37, ▶ Fig. 2.38, and ▶ Fig. 2.39.

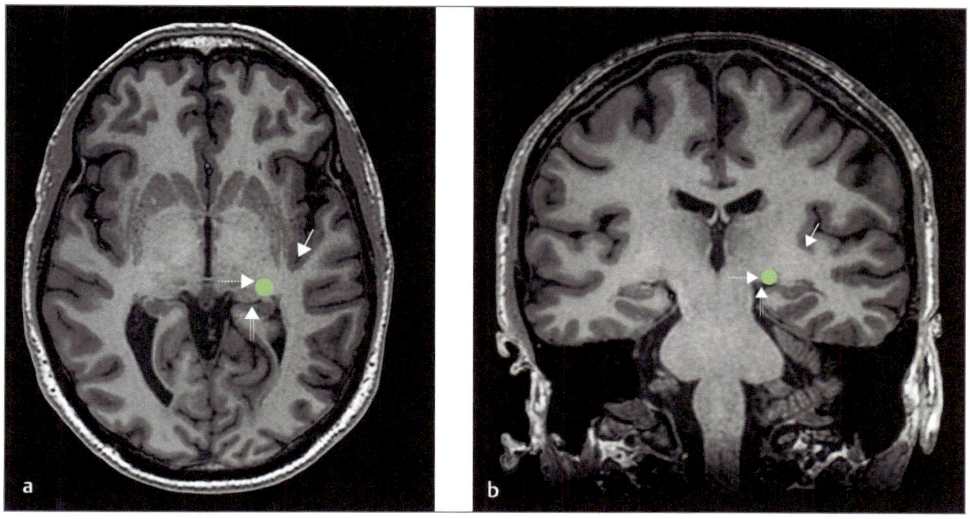

Fig. 2.37 Determining the position of the beginning of the optic tract. The origin of the optic tract at the lateral geniculate nucleus can be identified on axial MRI and coronal MRI sections. On axial MRI **(a)**, it is located roughly between the most posterior and inferior end of the circular sulcus of the insula (*white arrow*), the most inferior and lateral part of the thalamus (*dotted arrow*), and the most lateral superior extension of the ambient cistern (*white double arrow*). On coronal images **(b)**, it is located at the base of the white matter temporal stem (*dotted arrow*) between the most posterior and inferior end of the circular sulcus of the insula (*white arrow*) and the most lateral superior extension of the ambient cistern (*white double arrow*).

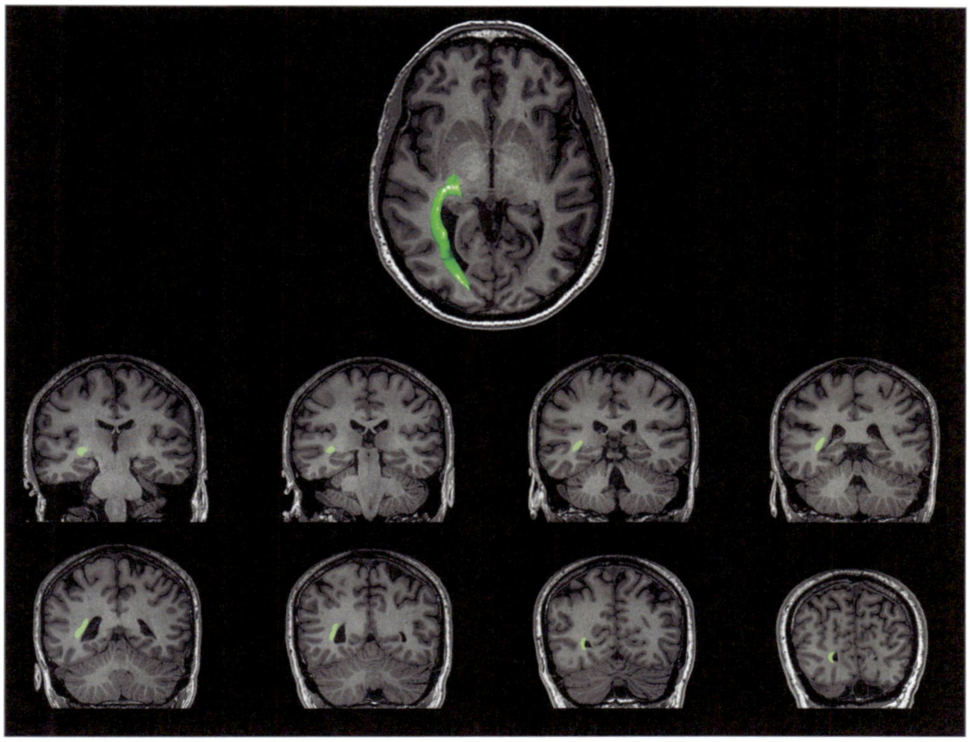

Fig. 2.38 Identifying the optic tract by its relation to the temporal horn, the atrium, and the occipital horn of the ventricle. Browsing MR images in either sagittal, coronal, or axial directions, the optic tract is identified by the position in relation to the wall of the lateral ventricle, i.e., the temporal horn, the atrium, and the occipital horn. From the lateral geniculate body, the optic tract courses 90° laterally to cross the roof of the temporal horn of the ventricle, except the fibers of the Meyer loop, which course anteriorly to cross beyond the tip of the temporal horn. The optic tract is situated above the entire temporal horn, beside the superior half of the lateral wall of the tip of the temporal horn, and the entire superior and lateral wall of the rest of the temporal horn. Posteriorly, the optic tract covers the lower two-thirds of the lateral wall of the trigone of the lateral ventricle, and the entire superior, lateral, and inferior wall of the occipital horn.

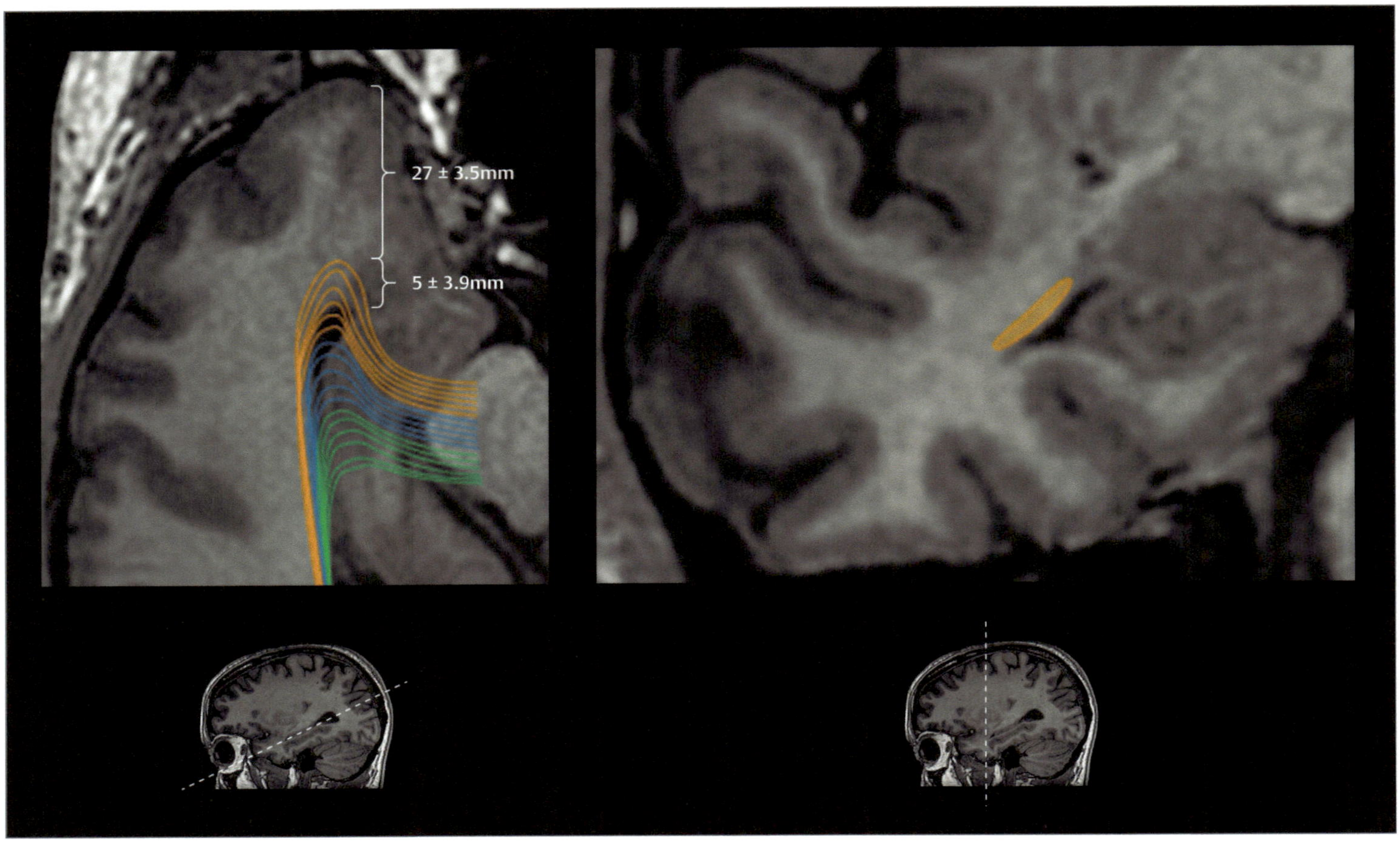

Fig. 2.39 Meyer loop. The optic radiation is composed of three main fiber bundles: the inferior bundle (*orange*), central bundle (*blue*), and upper bundle (*green*). The inferior bundle is also known as Meyer's loop and runs anteriorly and laterally from the lateral geniculate body fan-like above the tip of the temporal horn before turning sharply posteriorly to join the other fibers of the optic tract. This anatomical course relates to the growth of the temporal horn during embryogenesis. The fibers of the Meyer loop cover the roof of the tip of the temporal horn, the temporal horn, the upper half of the lateral wall of the tip of the temporal horn, and the entire lateral wall of the temporal horn posterior to the tip. The most anterior extension of the Meyer loop is situated on average 5 ± 3.9 mm anterior to the tip of the temporal horn or 27 ± 3.5 mm posterior to the tip of the temporal lobe. The fibers of the Meyer loop are difficult to identify with standard DTI imaging and fiber tracking.

References

[1] Naidich TP, Castillo M, Cha S, Smirniotopoulos JG. Imaging of the Brain: Expert Radiology. Elsevier Health Sciences; 2012

[2] Yamada K, Kizu O, Kubota T, et al. The pyramidal tract has a predictable course through the centrum semiovale: a diffusion-tensor based tractography study. J Magn Reson Imaging 2007;26(3):519–524

[3] Han BS, Hong JH, Hong C, et al. Location of the corticospinal tract at the corona radiata in human brain. Brain Res 2010;1326:75–80

[4] Kim Y-H, Kim D-S, Hong JH, et al. Corticospinal tract location in internal capsule of human brain: diffusion tensor tractography and functional MRI study. Neuroreport 2008;19(8):817–820

Further Readings

Catani M, de Schotten MT. Atlas of Human Brain Connections. Oxford University Press; 2012

Devlin JT, Poldrack RA. In praise of tedious anatomy. Neuroimage 2007;37(4):1033–1041, discussion 1050–1058

Ebeling U, Huber P, Reulen HJ. Localization of the precentral gyrus in the computed tomogram and its clinical application. J Neurol 1986;233(2):73–76

Ebeling U, Reulen H-J. Neurosurgical topography of the optic radiation in the temporal lobe. Acta Neurochir (Wien) 1988;92(1–4):29–36

Eberstaller O. Das Stirnhirn: ein Beitrag zur Anatomie der Oberfläche des Grosshirns. Urban & Schwarzenberg; 1890

Gonzalez LF, Smith K. Meyer's loop. BNI Q 2001;18:4–7

Kido DK, LeMay M, Levinson AW, Benson WE. Computed tomographic localization of the precentral gyrus. Radiology 1980;135(2):373–377

Meyer A. The connections of the occipital lobes and the present status of the cerebral visual affections. Trans Assoc Am Physicians 1907;22:7–16

Meyer JR, Roychowdhury S, Russell EJ, Callahan C, Gitelman D, Mesulam MM. Location of the central sulcus via cortical thickness of the precentral and postcentral gyri on MR. AJNR Am J Neuroradiol 1996;17(9):1699–1706

Mukamel R, Gelbard H, Arieli A, Hasson U, Fried I, Malach R. Coupling between neuronal firing, field potentials, and FMRI in human auditory cortex. Science 2005;309(5736):951–954

Naidich T, Brightbill T. Systems for localizing fronto-parietal gyri and sulci on axial CT and MRI. Int J Neuroradiol 1996;2(4):313–338

Naidich TP, Kang E, Fatterpekar GM, et al. The insula: anatomic study and MR imaging display at 1.5 T. AJNR Am J Neuroradiol 2004;25(2):222–232

Naidich TP, Valavanis AG, Kubik S. Anatomic relationships along the low-middle convexity: Part I--Normal specimens and magnetic resonance imaging. Neurosurgery 1995;36(3):517–532

Ono M, Kubik S, Abernathey C. Atlas of Cerebral Sulci. Georg Thieme Verlag; 1990

Shapleske J, Rossell SL, Woodruff PW, David AS. The planum temporale: a systematic, quantitative review of its structural, functional and clinical significance. Brain Res Brain Res Rev 1999;29(1):26–49

Ulmer S. Neuroanatomy and cortical landmarks. In: Ulmer S, Jansen O, eds. fMRI. Springer; 2010:5–13

Wagner M, Jurcoane A, Hattingen E. The U sign: tenth landmark to the central region on brain surface reformatted MR imaging. AJNR Am J Neuroradiol 2013;34(2):323–326

Welniarz Q, Dusart I, Roze E. The corticospinal tract: evolution, development, and human disorders. Dev Neurobiol 2017;77(7):810–829

Yousry TA, Schmid UD, Alkadhi H, et al. Localization of the motor hand area to a knob on the precentral gyrus. A new landmark. Brain 1997;120(Pt 1):141–157

Yousry TA, Schmid UD, Jassoy AG, et al. Topography of the cortical motor hand area: prospective study with functional MR imaging and direct motor mapping at surgery. Radiology 1995;195(1):23–29

3 Convexity Craniotomies

3.1 Convexity Craniotomy Planning

Andreas Raabe and Jens Fichtner

Inside-out Planning

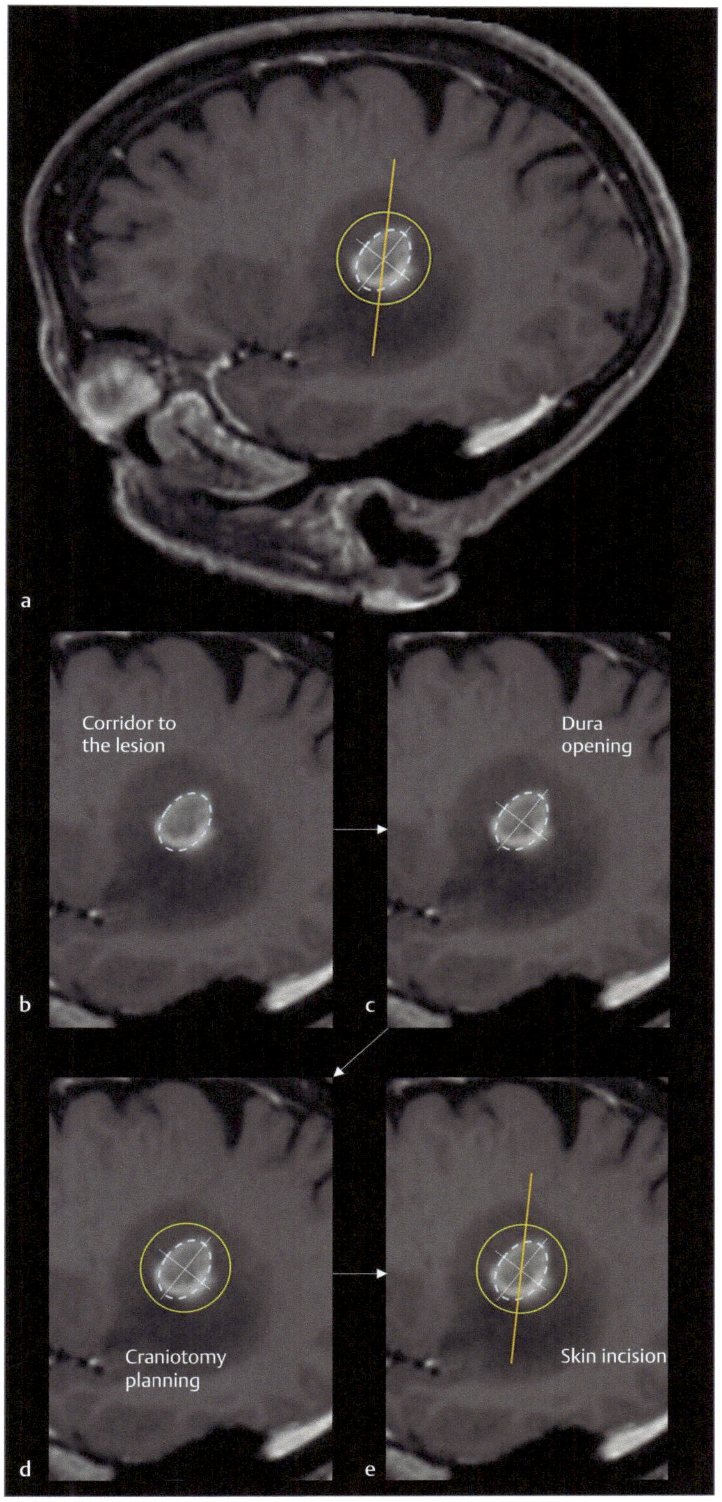

Fig. 3.1 Approach planning. Inside-out planning of craniotomy and skin incision in convexity craniotomies **(a)**. The location and size of the lesion determines the intraparenchymal or subdural corridor of the approach **(b)**. The corridor defines the size and shape of the dural opening **(c)**, which in turn determines the size and location of the craniotomy **(d)**. Finally, the skin incision is planned according to the location of the craniotomy **(e)**.

Planning of a convexity craniotomy is performed in the opposite direction to the surgery. Whereas the surgery starts with the skin incision, the craniotomy planning starts with the lesion (see ▶ Fig. 3.1 and ▶ Fig. 3.2).

1. First, the location of the lesion and the trajectory to the lesion has to be determined (which, of course, has already taken place in the mind of the surgeon during positioning of the patient).
2. There is a starting point for the trajectory, namely the subdural beginning of the corridor to the surgical target. This is the same whether a skull base approach or a transsulcal/transcortical approach is chosen.
3. The location of the corridor's beginning (not its end) determines where the dura has to be opened. This can be marked on the patient's skin.
4. When the site of the dura opening and the corridor have been determined, the craniotomy can be outlined. This applies not only to convexity craniotomies, but also to skull base craniotomies where the bony opening is determined by the location of other structures such as the transverse and sigmoid sinus (for retrosigmoid craniotomy) or the sagittal sinus (for midline craniotomies). These structures are drawn on the skin first, and then the craniotomy outline is drawn, taking the position of these structures into account.
5. When the contour of the craniotomy has been outlined on the patient's skin, the length and shape of the skin incision can be determined.

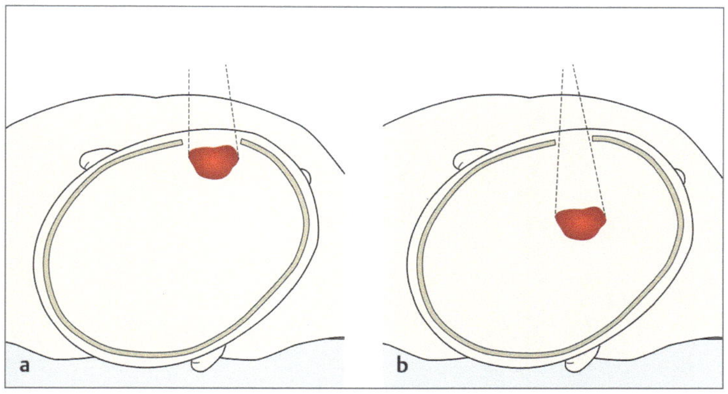

Fig. 3.2 The keyhole principle. The width of the surgical corridor depends on the depth and location of the lesion. In superficial tumors, the corridor, dural opening, and craniotomy are usually the same size or larger than the lesion **(a)**. For deeper lesions, the corridor, dural opening, and craniotomy can be much smaller because tilting of the microscope can reach the entire lesion, which is the principle of keyhole surgery **(b)**.

3.2 Planning of Craniotomies at the Skull Convexity without the Use of Navigation

Florian Ringel and Andreas Kramer

Introduction

Convexity lesions are poorly defined by landmarks. Craniotomies in these regions are usually performed with the help of a navigation system allowing the exact placement of the craniotomy above a given pathology. Certain circumstances, e.g., emergency treatment, unavailability of sufficient imaging data, or technical failures, among others, might hamper the use of navigation systems and require alternative strategies to place an ideal convexity craniotomy over a given pathology such as the left frontoparietal epidural hematoma shown in ▶Fig. 3.3. Exact localization and

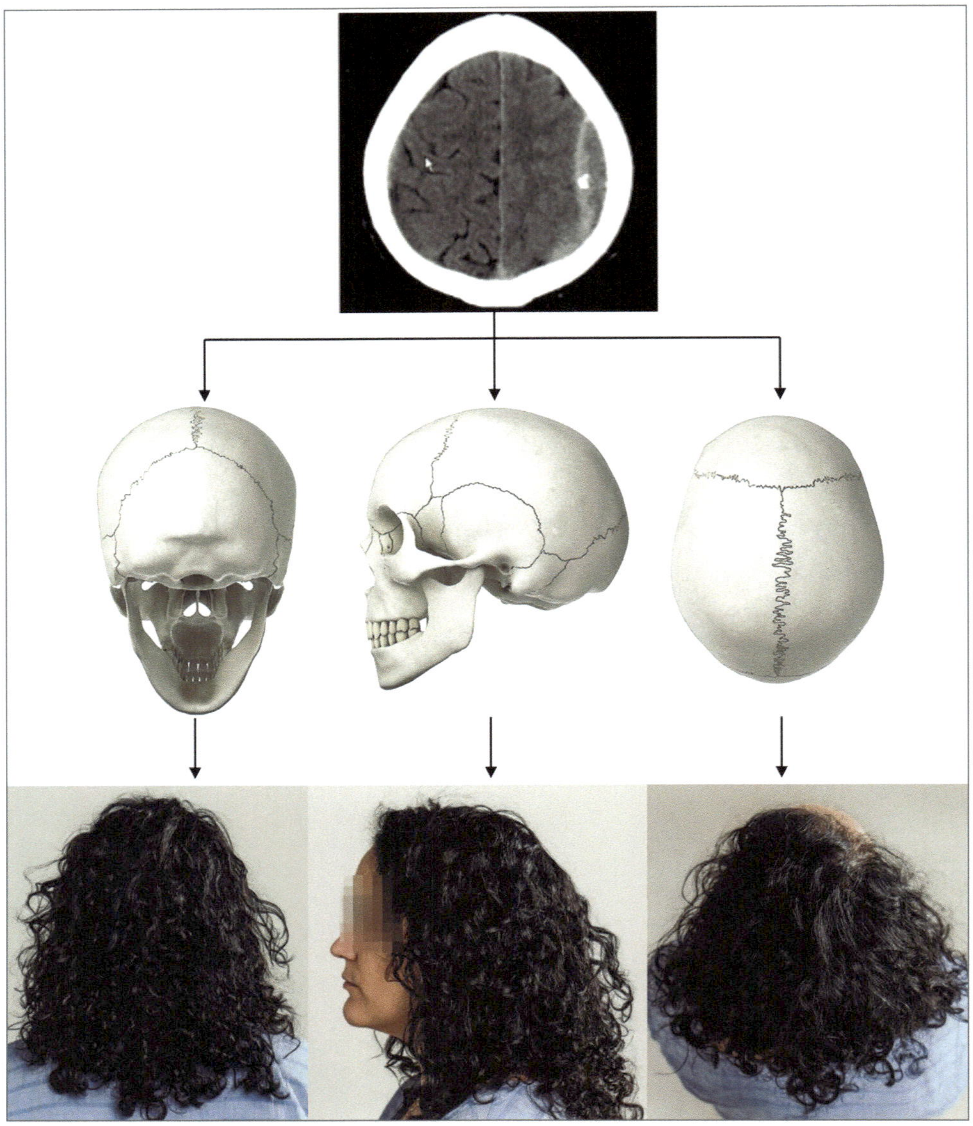

Fig. 3.3 From image to reality. Transferring a lesion visible on CT or MRI to the patient's anatomy can be challenging.

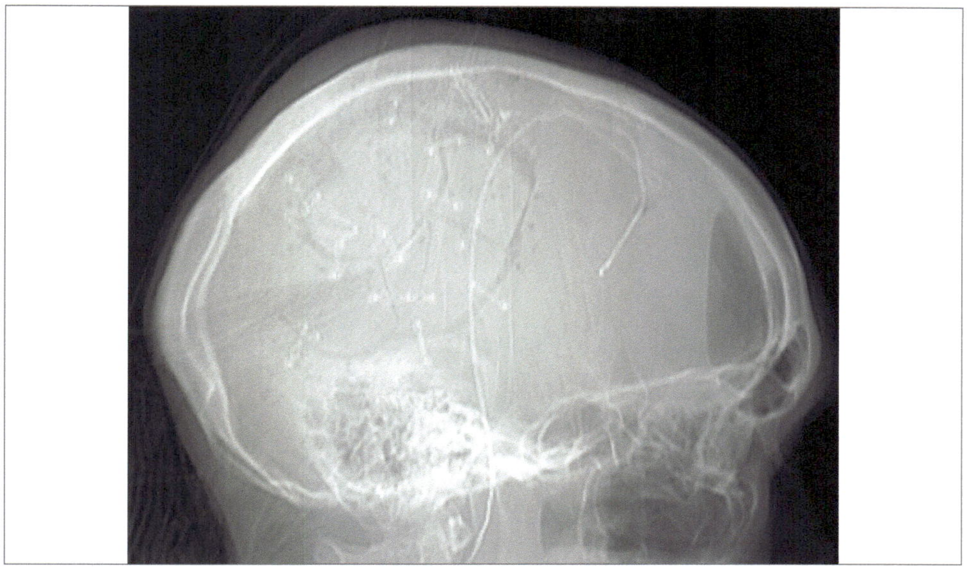

Fig. 3.4 Failure to localize a convexity lesion. Orientation and localizing of nonnavigated convexity craniotomy can lead to extension of the initial craniotomy. In this case, several bone flaps were required before the pathology was sufficiently exposed.

projection to the skull can be difficult without the use of a navigation system (▶ Fig. 3.4). When neuronavigation is not available, planning of convexity craniotomies in a standardized fashion is possible with the aid of a standard CT scan or MR images. The aim is to assess the relationship of the center and borders of a given pathology to recognizable anatomical landmarks such as the bregma or external auditory canal, among others. The examples below illustrate the necessary steps for a frontoparietal epidural hematoma using data from a CT scan for an emergency situation, and a frontoparietal meningioma using MR images for an elective case (▶ Fig. 3.5, ▶ Fig. 3.6, ▶ Fig. 3.7, ▶ Fig. 3.8, ▶ Fig. 3.9, ▶ Fig. 3.10, ▶ Fig. 3.11, ▶ Fig. 3.12, Fig. 3.13, and ▶ Fig. 3.14).)

Standardized Planning of a Craniotomy at the Convexity Using CT Images

The prerequisite for standardized planning of a convexity craniotomy using CT images is the knowledge of the CT slice thickness (which is usually given in the images), a DICOM viewer with the option to measure distances in the images, and the availability of a CT scout. ▶ Fig. 3.5, ▶ Fig. 3.6, ▶ Fig. 3.7, ▶ Fig. 3.8, and ▶ Fig. 3.9 outline the steps of planning.

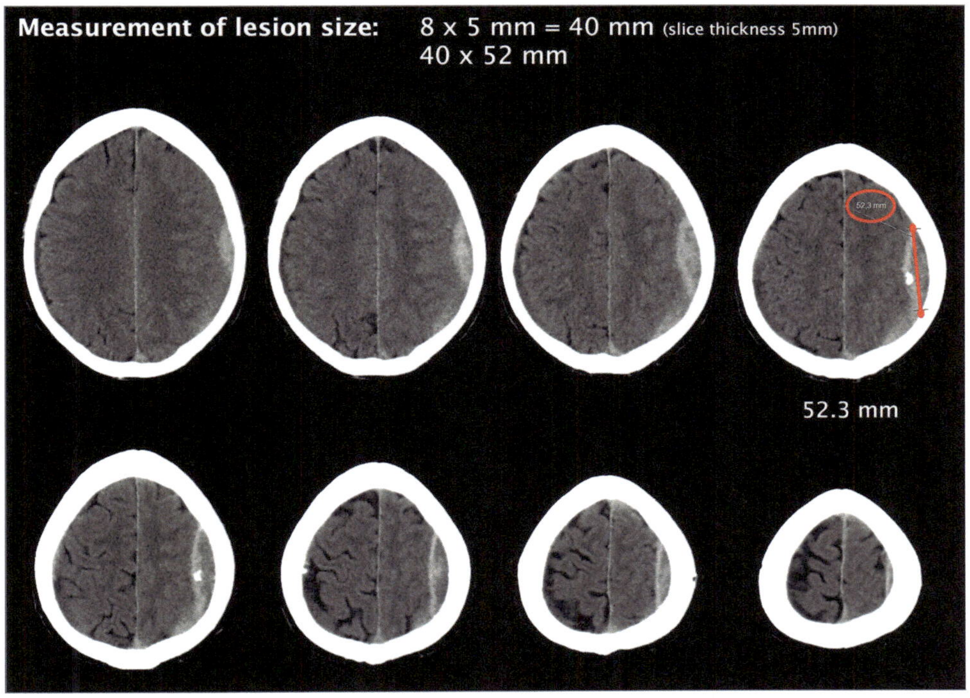

Fig. 3.5 CT image–based freehand planning: determining the size of the lesion. CT slice thickness in this case is 5 mm. The epidural hematoma is visible on eight slices, resulting in a calculated anteroposterior size of 8 × 5 mm = 40 mm. The superoinferior diameter measured on the slice with the largest diameter is 52 mm. Thus, the whole lesion has a size of 40 mm × 52 mm.

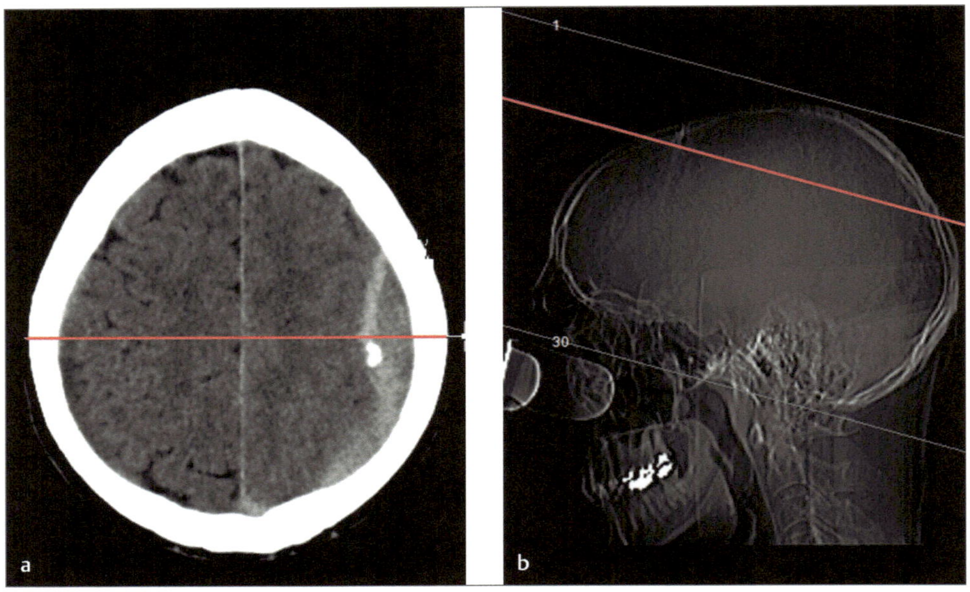

Fig. 3.6 Localizing the slice with the largest lesion diameter. The CT scout is used to mark the level of the slice with the maximal diameter of the lesion **(b)**. A line through the center of the lesion, perpendicular to the midline, is drawn **(a)**.

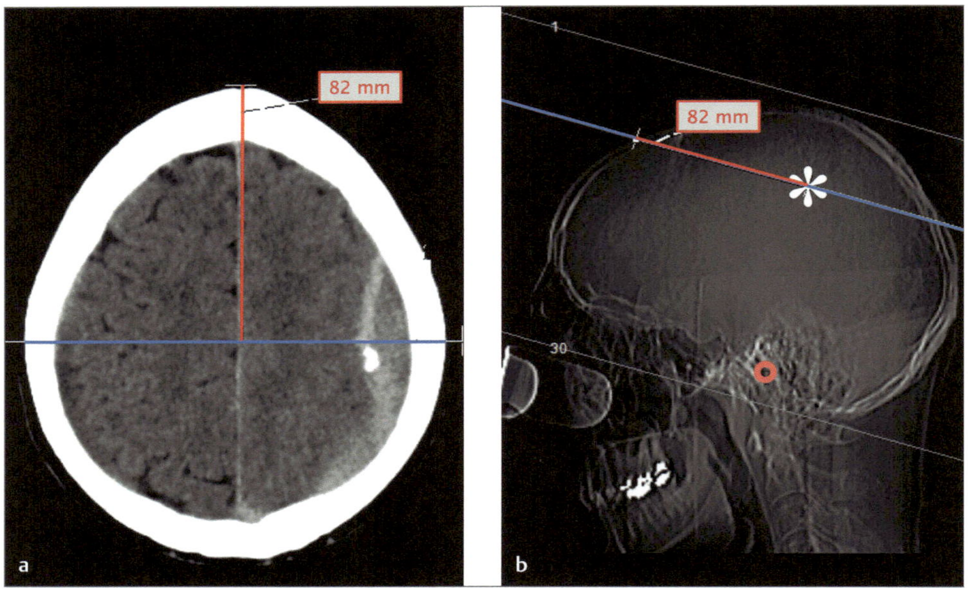

Fig. 3.7 Localizing the center of the lesion. The distance from the line through the center of the lesion to the rostral border of the skull in the axial slice is measured (**a**, *red line*) and this distance is translated to the CT scout (*right red line*) onto the level of the slice (**b**, *blue line*). The ∗ at the end of the line represents the position of the center of the lesion projected onto the skull. The external auditory canal is marked (**b**, *red circle*).

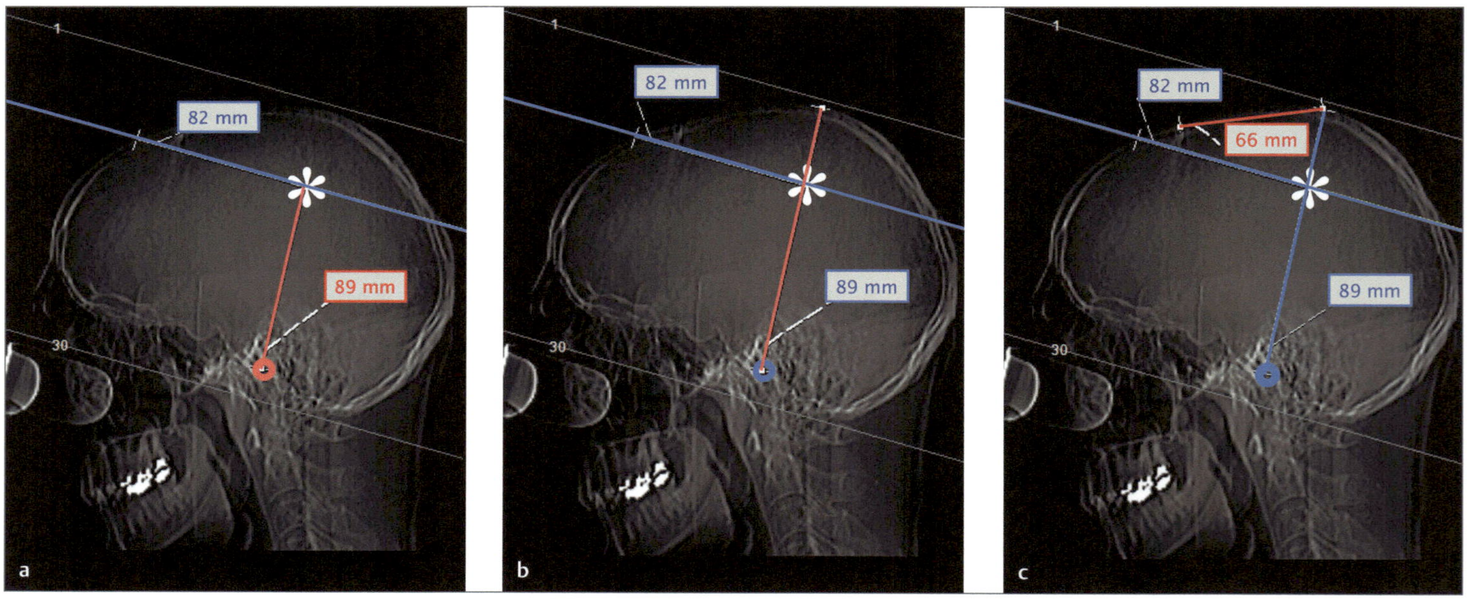

Fig. 3.8 Determining the external auditory canal reference line. The distance from the external auditory canal to the center of the lesion (∗) is measured (**a**, *red line*) and this line is extended to the limit of the bony skull (**b**, *red line*). From the crossing point of the line and the limit of the bony skull, the distance to the bregma rostrally is measured (**c**, *red line*).

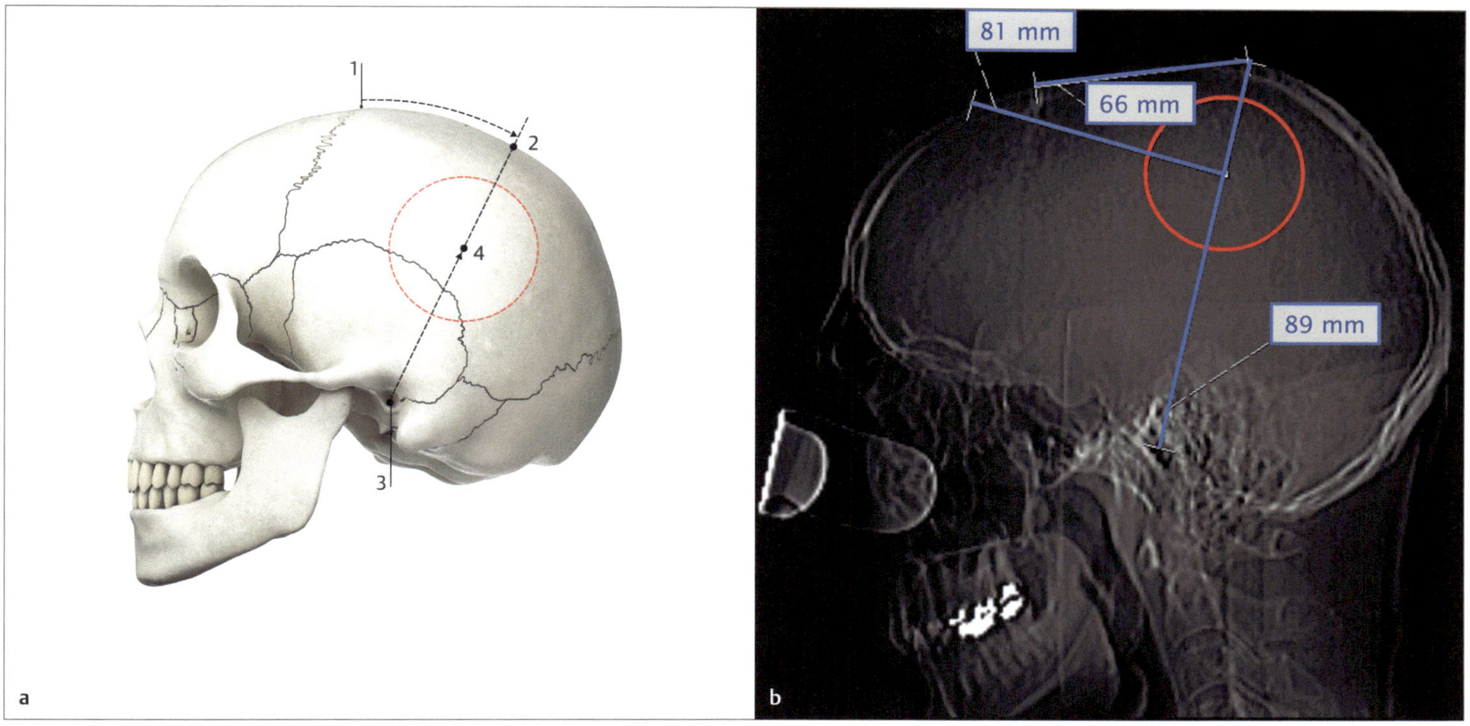

Fig. 3.9 Transferring the two measurements onto the patient's head. These measurements can be transferred to the head of the patient. The bregma (1) is palpated or measured 13 cm from the nasion. From the bregma, 66 mm is measured posteriorly and marked (2). From this point, a connecting line to the eternal auditory canal (3) is drawn. The center of the lesion (4) is on this line, 89 mm superior to the external auditory canal. Finally, a craniotomy according to the diameter of the lesion around the center and ideally with a linear skin incision at least twice the length of the diameter of the craniotomy is prepared. This method is not exactly accurate for high parietal lesions because it does not take the curve of the skull into account. For high parietal lesions, a second measurement from the midline to the midpoint of the lesion on axial slices can help to better localize the target.

Standardized Planning of a Craniotomy of the Convexity Using MR Images

The prerequisite for standardized planning of a convexity craniotomy using MR images is the knowledge of the MR slice thickness (which is usually given in the images), a DICOM viewer with the option to measure distances in the images, and images in at least two planes—in axial and coronal orientations.

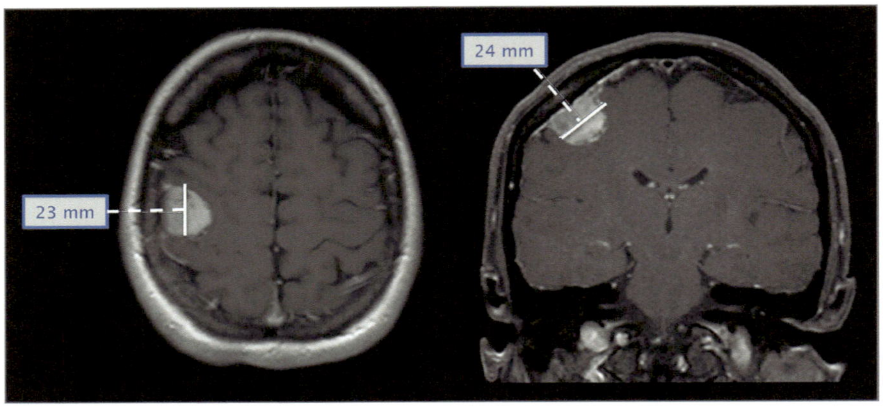

Fig. 3.10 MRI image–based freehand planning: determining the size of the lesion. The size of the lesion is determined. Measurements are performed in the axial and coronal plane.

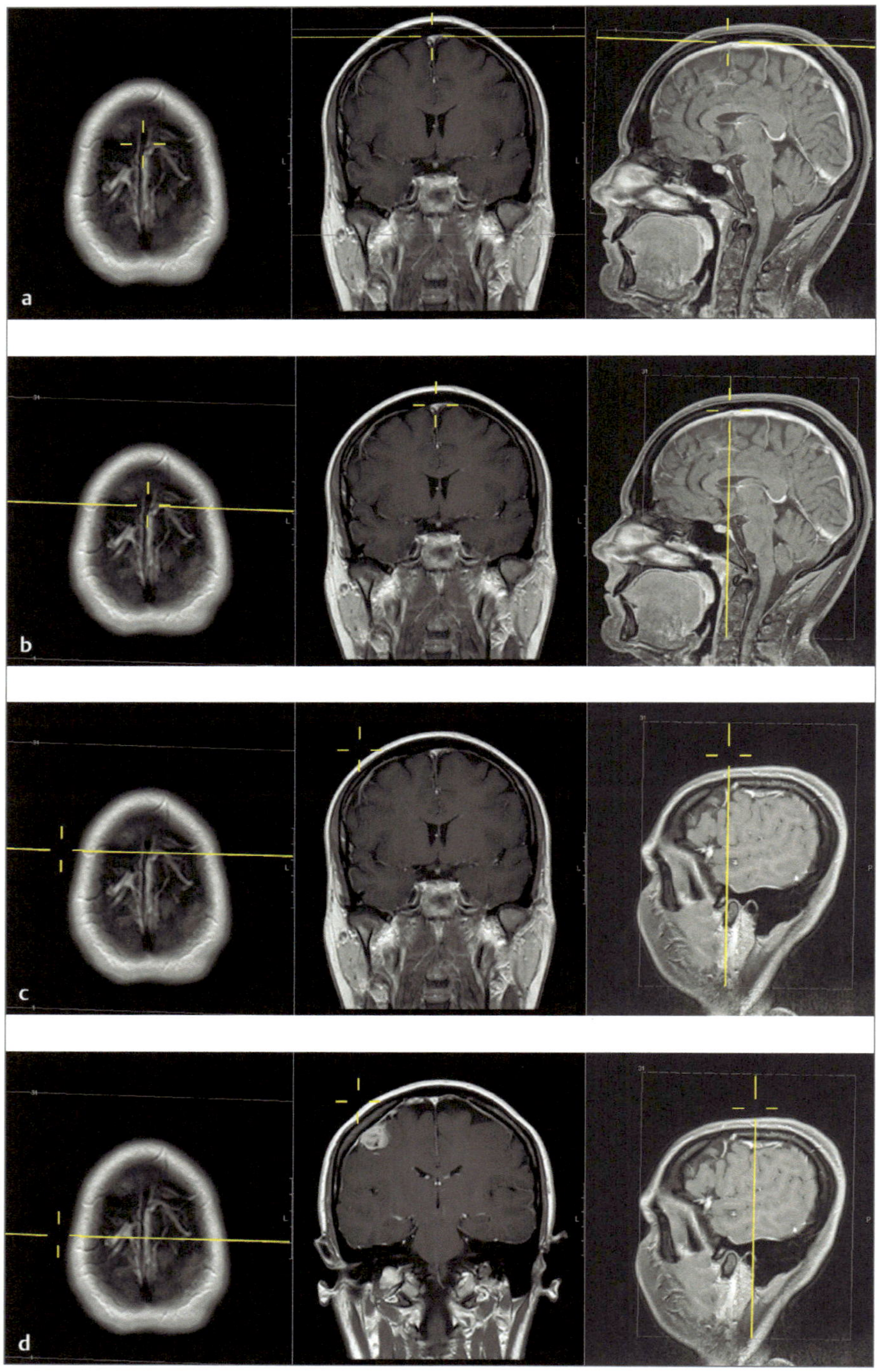

Fig. 3.11 Determination of the tilt of the coronal plane. The bregma is identified on axial, coronal, and sagittal images. Axial as well as coronal images are brought to the level of the bregma, and sagittal images are positioned to the midline. The angle of the coronal images can be estimated already **(a, b)**. The sagittal images are positioned to the external auditory meatus of the side of the lesion **(c)**. The coronal plane cutting the bregma is brought from the bregma to the posterior border of the external auditory canal and the necessary slices are counted (in this case four slices → 4 × 5 mm = 20 mm) **(d)**. Thereby, the coronal plane of the images is determined to cut the bregma and a point 20 mm anterior to the posterior rim of the external auditory canal perpendicular to the coronal plane.

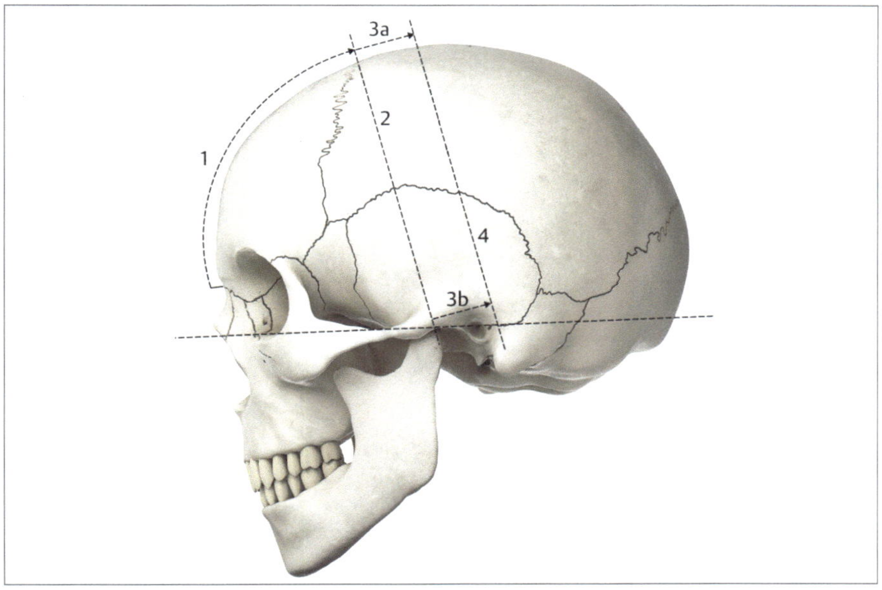

Fig. 3.12 Determination of the tilt of the coronal plane. The bregma is palpated or measured 13 cm from the nasion (1). The external auditory canal is identified. The coronal plane is identified from the bregma (see ▶ Fig. 3.13). In our example, the bregma corresponds to a point 2 cm anterior to the external auditory canal (2) in the sagittal view along the coronal tilt. The tumor is on a line parallel to this "coronal tilt" plane 25 mm posteriorly to the bregma line (▶ Fig. 3.11). The tumor borders are located on this line 52 mm lateroinferiorly from the midline (3.14) and 86 mm above the Frankfort horizontal plane (3.14). Finally, a craniotomy according to the diameter of the lesion around the center using an ideally linear skin incision at least twice the length of the diameter of the craniotomy is prepared.

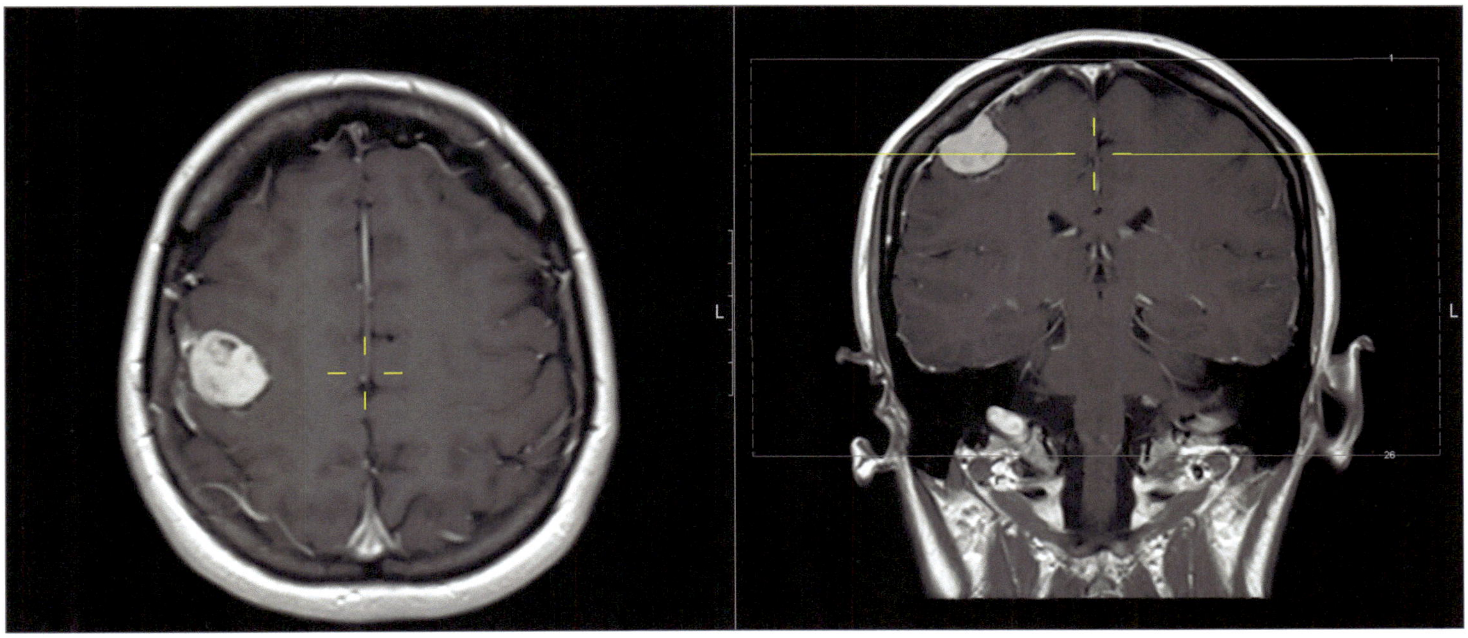

Fig. 3.13 Position of the center of the tumor in the coronal plane. The coronal plane is moved from the plane cutting the bregma backward to the center of the tumor and the number of slices necessary to reach the center of the tumor are counted, in this case five slices → 5 × 5 mm = 25 mm. Therefore, the tumor is on a line 25 mm behind and parallel to the line from the bregma to a point 20 mm anterior to the posterior rim of the external auditory canal.

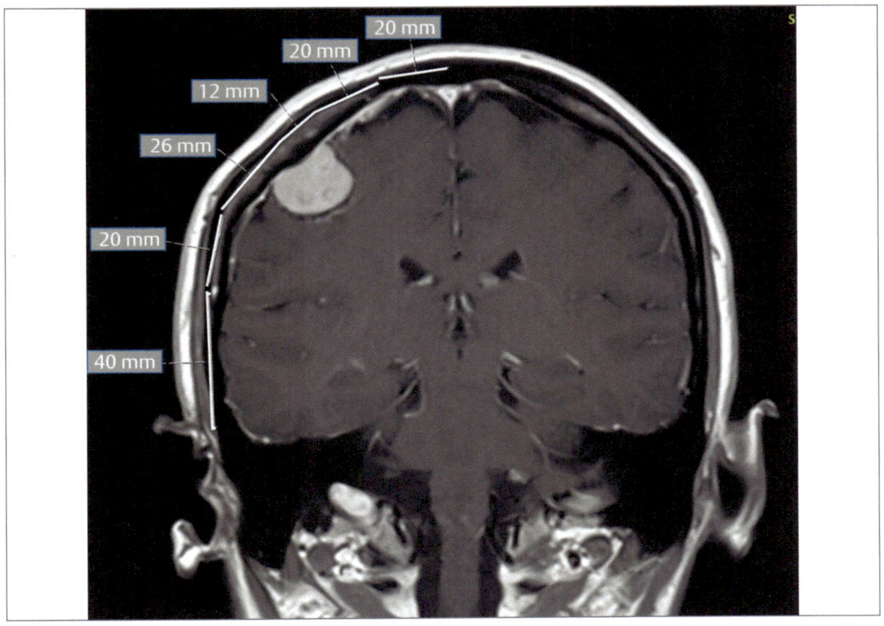

Fig. 3.14 Distance of the tumor center from the midline and the skull base on the curved skull surface. The distance of the center of the tumor from the sagittal midline and the base is measured in the coronal plane through the maximum diameter of the tumor. As most DICOM viewers do not allow measuring curved lines, several straight lines covering the convexity of the head need to be added. The borders of the tumor of this case are 86 mm above the base and 52 mm from the midline. Finally these measurements are transferred to the patient's head.

3.3 Supratentorial Convexity Craniotomy

Philippe Schucht

Generally speaking, craniotomies should be made as small as you are comfortable with. A smaller craniotomy may reduce soft tissue damage and postoperative pain, and improves healing. It also reduces the amount of brain exposed to dehydration, heat from the microscope's light source, and incidental injury during surgery.

One of the main sources of trouble in minimally invasive surgery is misplacement of the craniotomy. Because the convexity itself has no reliable landmarks, neuronavigation should be used for correct placement of the craniotomy. In the case of technical failure, the images of the patient can be used to determine the site of the craniotomy (see Chapter 3.2, Planning of Craniotomies at the Skull Convexity without the Use of Navigation, by Ringel and Kramer).

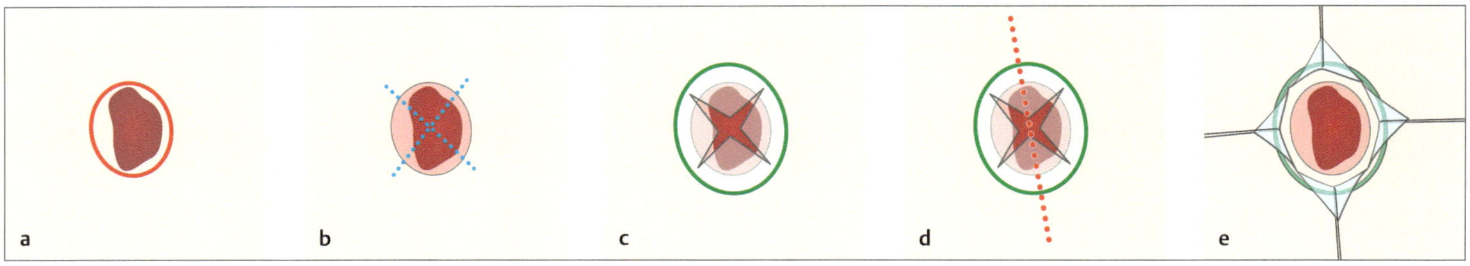

Fig. 3.15 Planning from inside-out. The approach planning is inside-out. First, the tumor and the area of cortical exposure are sketched on the skin, based on landmarks and confirmed by neuronavigation **(a)**. Using these marks, the required dural opening **(b)** and craniotomy **(c)** is sketched, and the drawing of the craniotomy is then used to draw the required skin incision **(d)** and the access to the lesion is performed **(e)**.

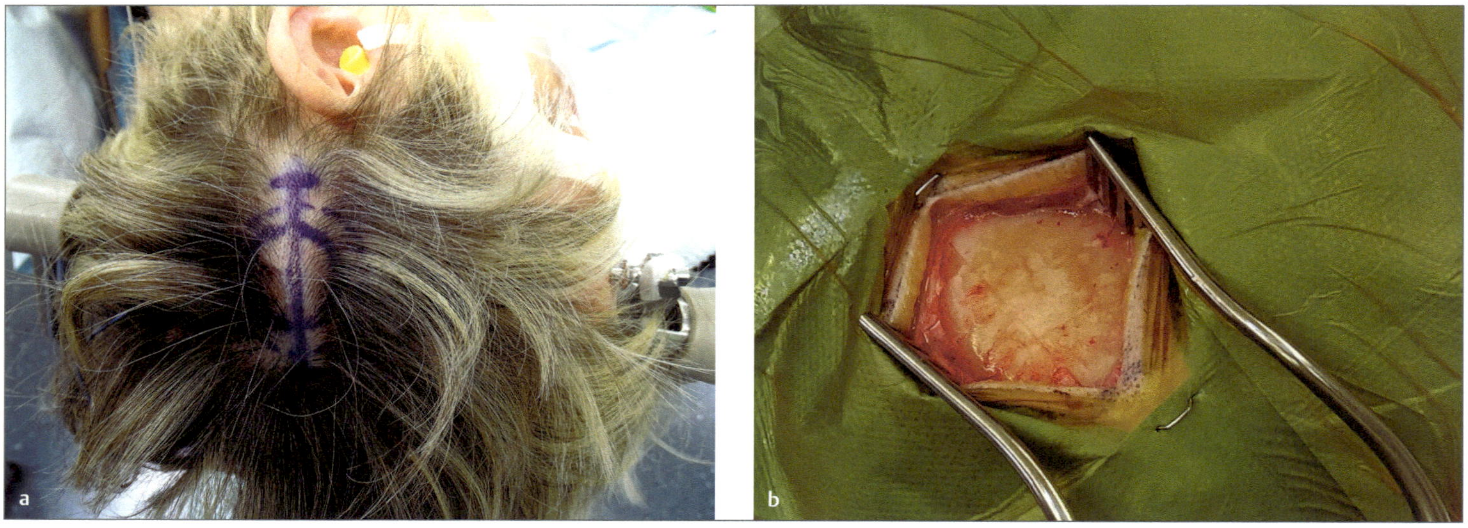

Fig. 3.16 (a, b) Skin incision. Straight skin incisions are preferred for small- and medium-sized craniotomies over the convexity. Straight incisions have the advantage of reduced oozing from the subcutaneous tissue once the skin retractors are applied. In addition, closure time is generally shorter because straight incisions require fewer stitches than curved incisions and thus avoid the risk of hypoperfused skin areas, which are inherent to curved incisions. The skin incision is drawn perpendicular to the sagittal sinus near the vertex, and perpendicular to the cranial base in most cases. The area of the skin incision is infiltrated with local anesthetic mixed with epinephrine (1:100,000 = 1 mL of epinephrine 1:1,000 diluted with 100 mL of saline or anesthetic) in order to reduce the need for coagulation and to reduce pain reaction with the associated increase in systolic blood pressure following skin incision. Choosing a long-lasting local anesthetic has the additional benefit of early postoperative pain reduction.

After planning from inside to outside, the skin is incised with a scalpel down to the bone and, together with the underlying periosteum, is pushed sideways with the help of a rasp (▶Fig. 3.15 and ▶Fig. 3.16). A retractor is used to keep the skin edges apart. Any bleeding from the larger vessels running below the subcutis should be coagulated. Bleeding from the smaller vessels within the cutis stops once self-retractors are applied: the tension created by self-retractors is preferred to the use of coagulation or Raney clips. Coagulation within the subcutis needs to be avoided because it irrevocably destroys hair follicles and increases the size of the scar.

Larger craniotomies or those on visible skin anterior to the hairline require a curved or a question-mark-shaped skin flap. To avoid injury to the facial nerve, the skin incision should not go lower than the zygoma.

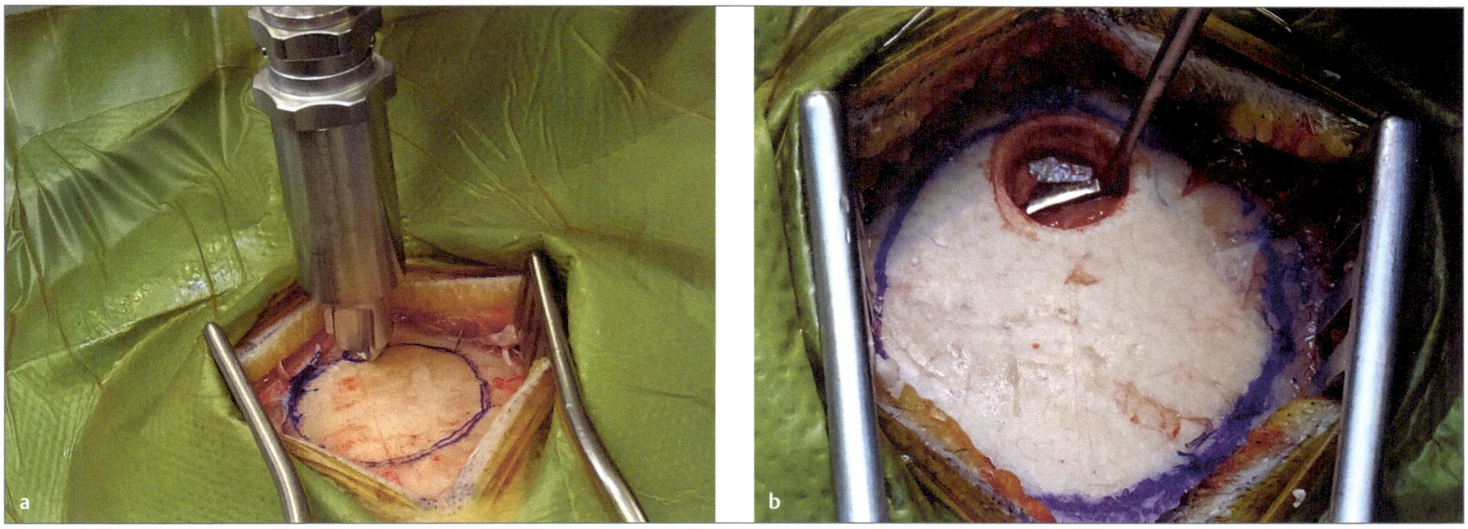

Fig. 3.17 (a, b) Burr hole and detachment of dura. One of the major risks of craniotomy is injury to a neighboring sinus. Because injury to a sinus is less likely with a trephine than a craniotome, the burr hole(s) should be made at the planned craniotomy site(s) closest to the sinus. Usually, one burr hole is sufficient.

The dura is detached from the skull at the burr holes, preferably with a 90° angled dissector (▶Fig. 3.17). The head may move slightly during trepanation and craniotomy and the accuracy of neuronavigation may decrease. Small marks drilled in the periphery before making the burr hole and performing the craniotomy may be used as rescue reference points for neuronavigation. They need to be outside the planned craniotomy. They are usually registered clockwise as landmarks for the navigation system and may be used as rescue points to restore the accuracy of the image guidance. This procedure takes less than 60 seconds and may save the entire operation (▶Fig. 3.18).

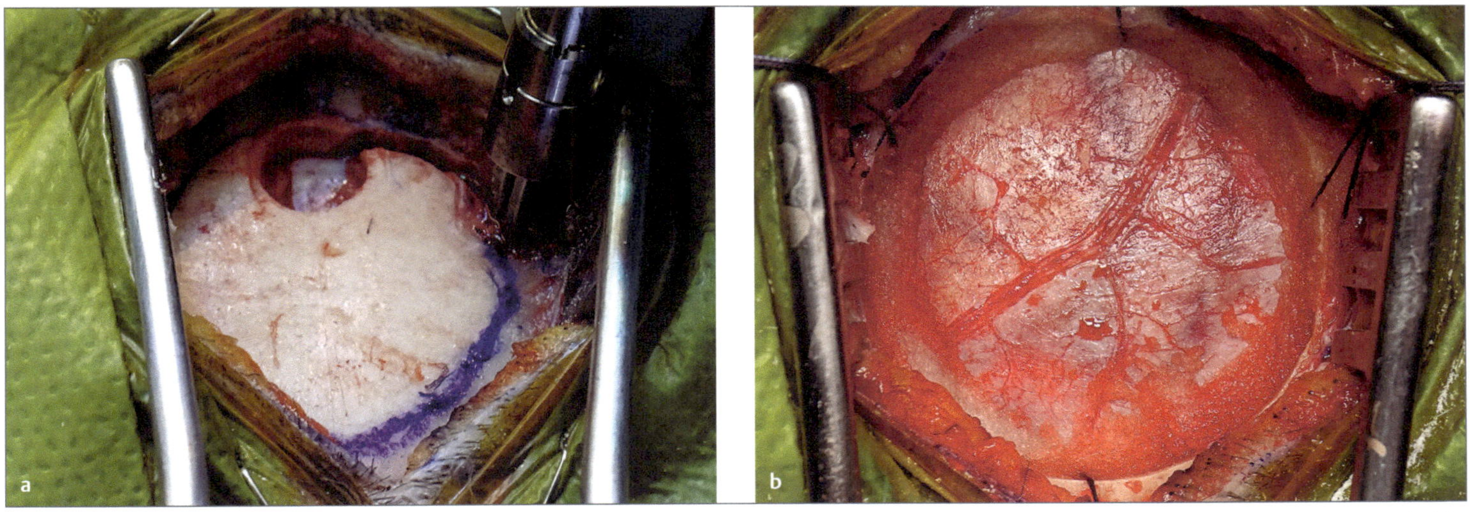

Fig. 3.18 (a, b) Craniotomy. Craniotomy is always performed away from the sinus (the burr holes being closest to the sinus). The craniotome is held like a pencil with one hand and gently pushed forward with the other applying little force. Every few centimeters the craniotomy should be stopped, the craniotome is drawn back, and advanced again to avoid dural laceration. After completion of the craniotomy, the bone flap is elevated with the help of dissectors. The underlying dura is carefully detached from the bone. Especially in older patients the dura may be tenaciously adherent to the bone and may easily be lacerated if not handled carefully.

Bleeding after craniotomy should be treated according to the type of bleeding: bleeding from the skull's spongiosa is stopped with bone wax, from dural vessels with bipolar coagulation (use low power and avoid dural shrinkage through overuse), and from venous sinuses with fibrin glue and Gelfoam. For diffuse bleeding from under the dural edge, Gelfoam powder may be applied and compressed. Superfluous powder is rinsed away (▶Fig. 3.19).

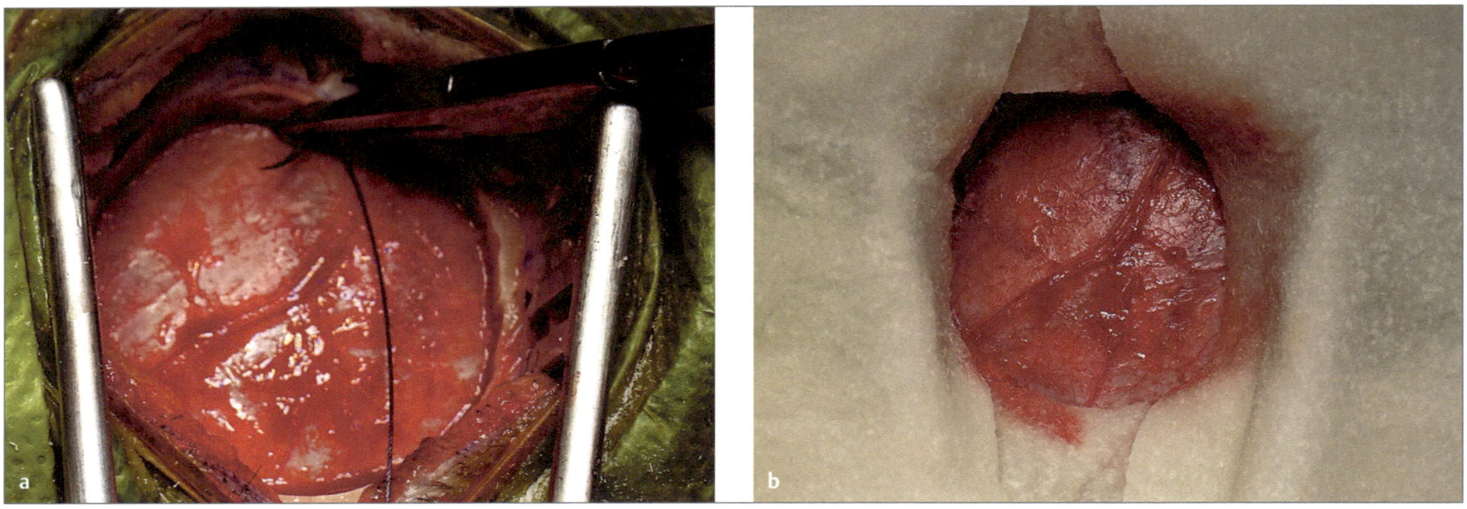

Fig. 3.19 (a, b) Dural tenting sutures and preparation for dural opening. We use dural tenting sutures inserted before dural opening (1) to decrease the risk of intraoperative epidural bleeding or oozing and (2) to prevent postoperative epidural hematoma. The dural suture is inserted before opening because any cortical bleeding caused by an epidural stich will become visible after dural opening. These sutures attach the dura to the skull at 1–5 cm intervals along the edge of the craniotomy: the sutures should not be tied as this leads to tightening of the dura and may result in difficulties in suturing the dura at the end of surgery. Rather, the sutures should then be clamped to the draping, and sutured after dura closure.

The edges of the craniotomy are covered with sterile pads soaked in an antibiotic solution. Covering with cottonoids should not obstruct the field. They should be squeezed to the craniotomy edge or, in small craniotomies, should only cover the bone (▶ Fig. 3.20, ▶ Fig. 3.21, ▶ Fig. 3.22, and Fig. 3.23).

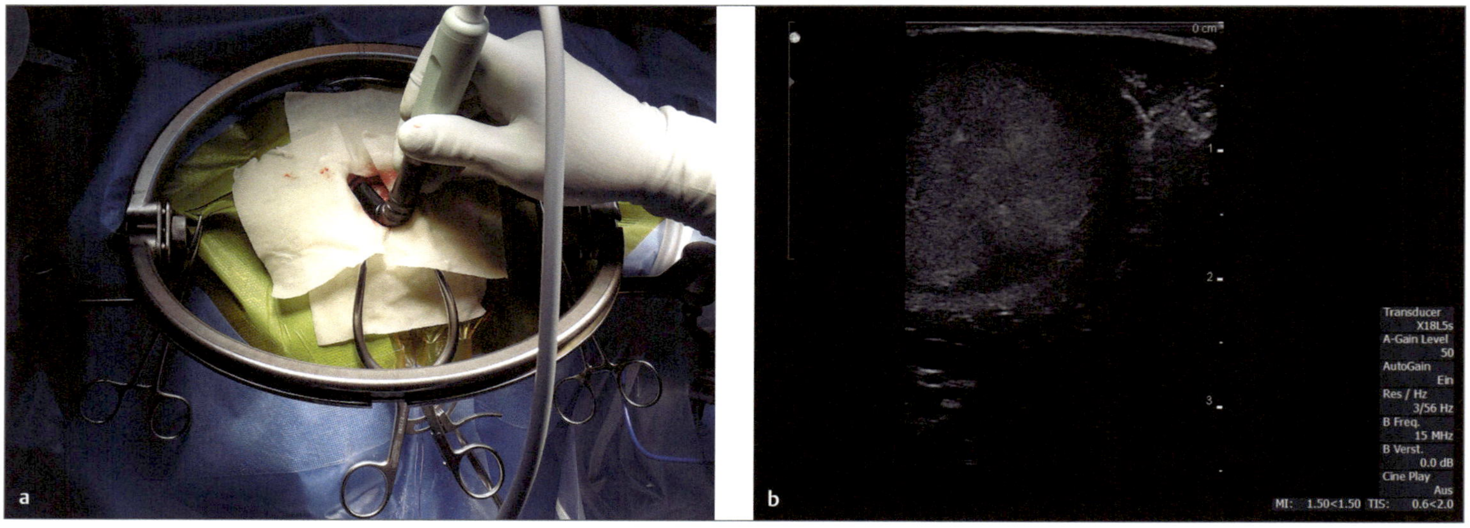

Fig. 3.20 (a, b) Localizing the lesion with navigation and ultrasound. At this stage, the location of the lesion can be verified. Navigation is a valuable tool for spatial orientation, especially at the beginning of surgery, provided that the accuracy of registration is high and is not altered during the procedure. Ultrasound gives additional real-time information on the spatial relationship between the opening, the lesion (left-hand side of the figure), and sulci and vessels (right-hand side of the figure).

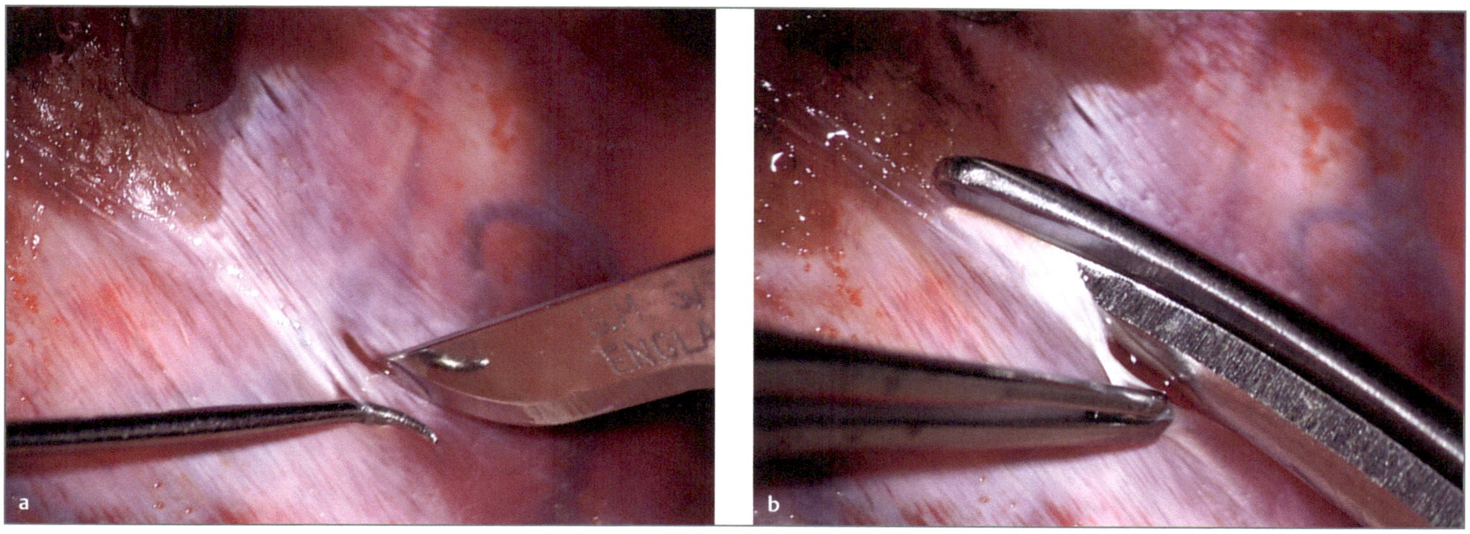

Fig. 3.21 (a, b) Dura opening. The dura is first lifted with a hook and cut open with a small scalpel. One edge of the dura is then lifted with forceps and the dural opening is enlarged with small scissors or a knife.

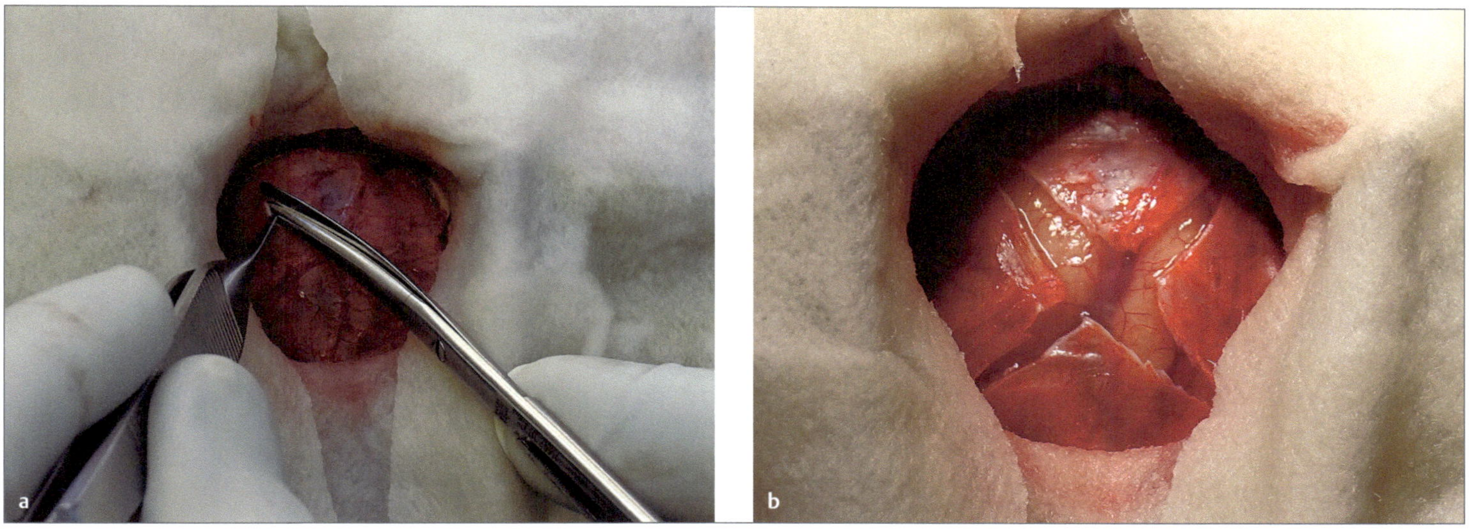

Fig. 3.22 (a, b) Dura opening. The dura may be opened either as a flap or cross-wise, and the dura leaflets are lifted and fixed with additional sutures. Dural vessels are located between the two dural sheets. When coagulating bleeding from dural vessels, the inner dural sheet should be spared to prevent shrinkage of the dura (and therefore to prevent difficulties in closure of the dura).

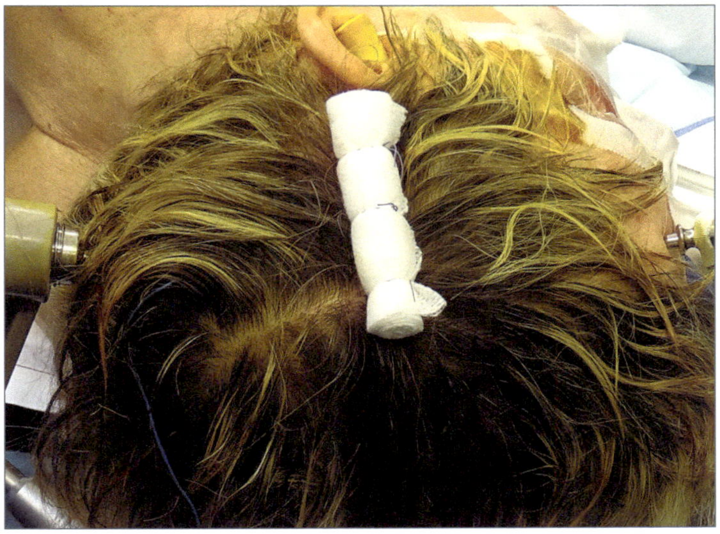

Fig. 3.23 Closure. The dressing is attached by means of sutures to avoid displacement.

Checklist

- Center the planned craniotomy on the tumor based on external landmarks or neuronavigation.
- Use an inside-out approach to plan corticotomy, durotomy, craniotomy, and skin incision.
- Use local anesthetics with epinephrine, and self-retractors on a straight skin incision to avoid bipolar coagulation; coagulate only larger vessels below the subcutis.
- Mobilize the skin and the periosteum with a rasp; use retractors to spread the skin.
- Make the burr holes at the site closest to the venous sinus.
- Always direct the craniotome away from the sinus, never toward it.
- Check correct positioning of the craniotomy prior to dura opening; preferably with an ultrasound probe.

4 Midline Craniotomies

Ulrich Sure and Philipp Dammann

See ▸ Fig. 4.1.

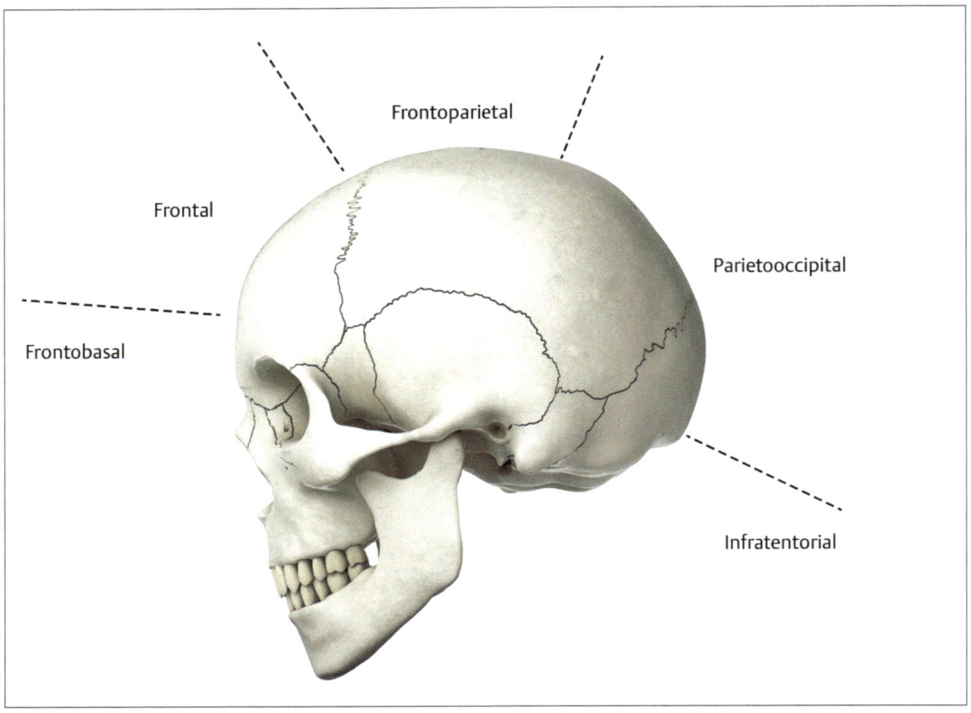

Fig. 4.1 Overview. Depending on the brain regions the surgeon wishes to access via a midline approach, the positioning of the patient and craniotomy technique have to be adapted accordingly. This diagram gives an overview of the standard approaches commonly used in neurosurgery.

4.1 Sinus-Crossing Craniotomies—Basic Principles

Ulrich Sure and Philipp Dammann

See ▶ Fig. 4.2, ▶ Fig. 4.3, and ▶ Fig. 4.4.

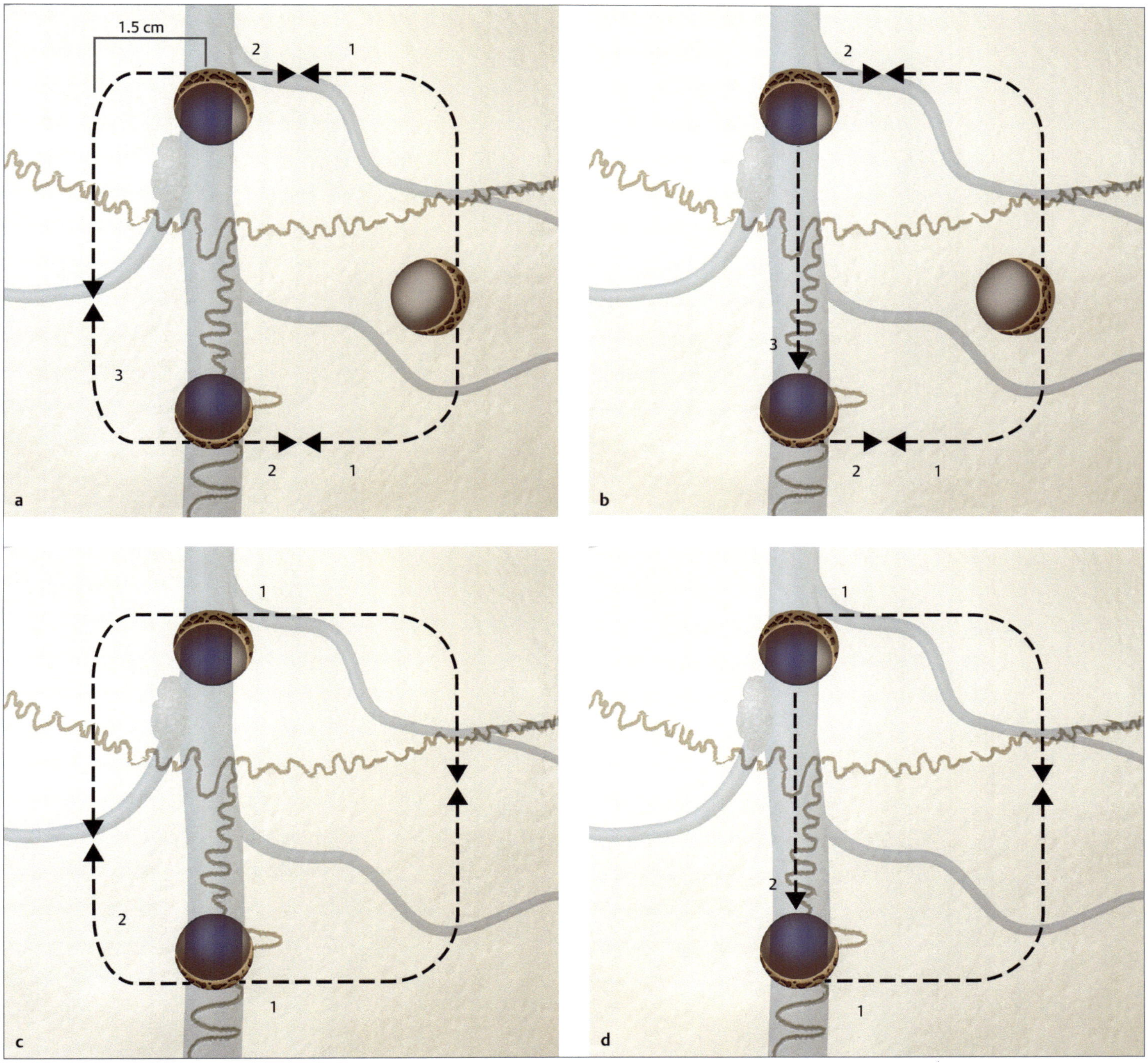

Fig. 4.2 Small bone flaps. Sinus-crossing craniotomies can be performed in various ways. We adhere to the following principles to assure sufficient exposure and avoid sinus injury. In small (<5 cm sagittal dimension) craniotomies, we make two burr holes on the sinus and one burr hole laterally (**a** or **b**). The craniotomy starts at the lateral burr hole reaching medially and stopping approximately 1.5 cm lateral to the sinus. From the medial burr holes, the craniotomy is then interconnected from medial to lateral. Depending on the amount of retraction of midline structures to the contralateral side that is necessary (e.g., in superficial tumors), the sinus is crossed 1.5 cm contralaterally **(a)** or the craniotomy is performed on the sinus in the most contralateral aspect of the burr hole **(b)**. The same procedure may also be performed without a lateral burr hole (**c**, **d**, young patients, better cosmesis).

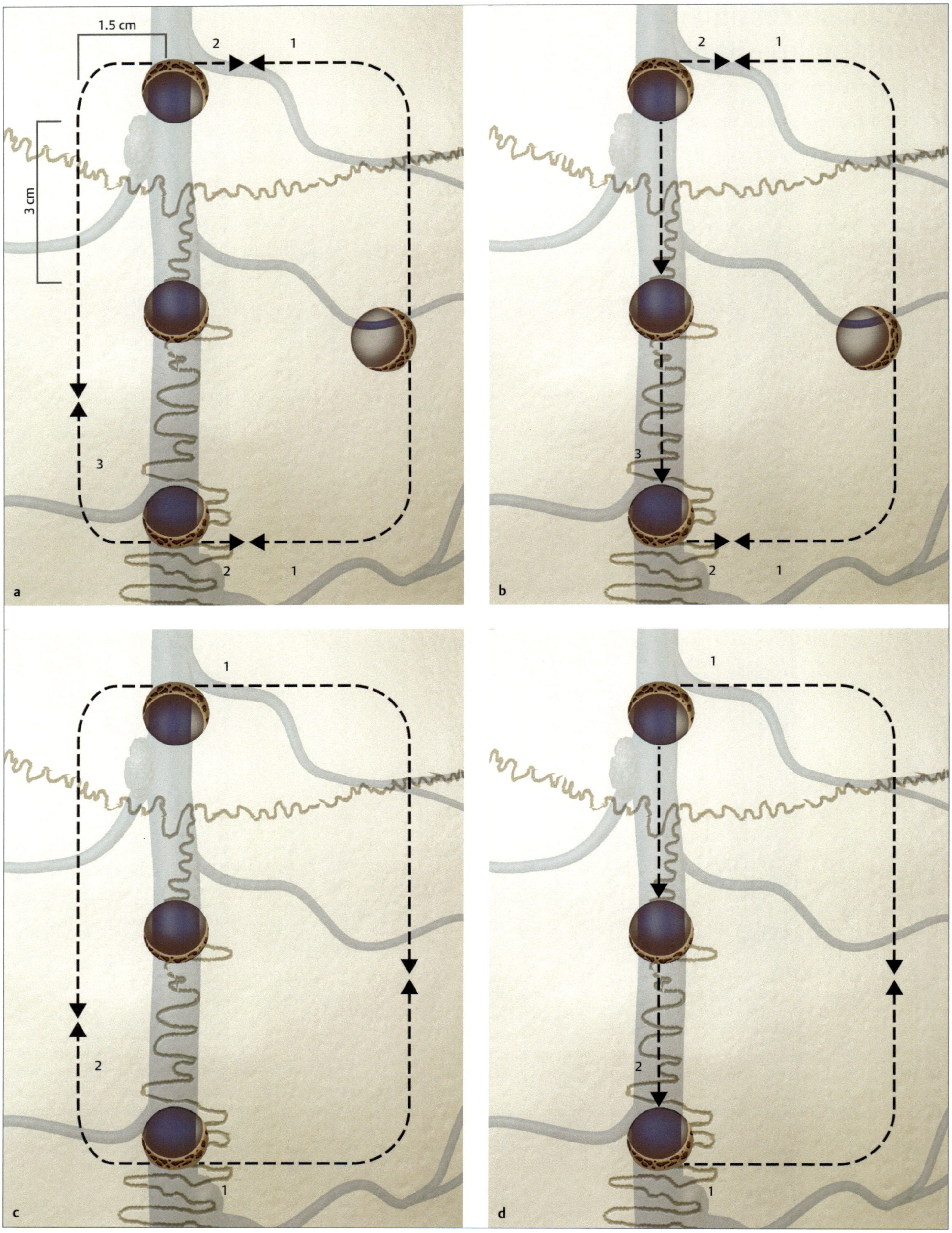

Fig. 4.3 Medium **and large bone flaps.** For larger bone flaps, we make burr holes every 3–4 cm along the sinus **(a–d)**. Again, a lateral burr hole is optional **(a, b)**. In large bone flaps (>9 cm sagittal dimension), we always cross the sinus and cut contralateral to the sinus **(a, c)**. Despite crossing to the contralateral side and not interconnecting all burr holes, the number of burr holes on the sinus may remain the same. They are used to detach the dura mater from the bone flap above the sinus to prevent sinus injury during removal of the bone flap.

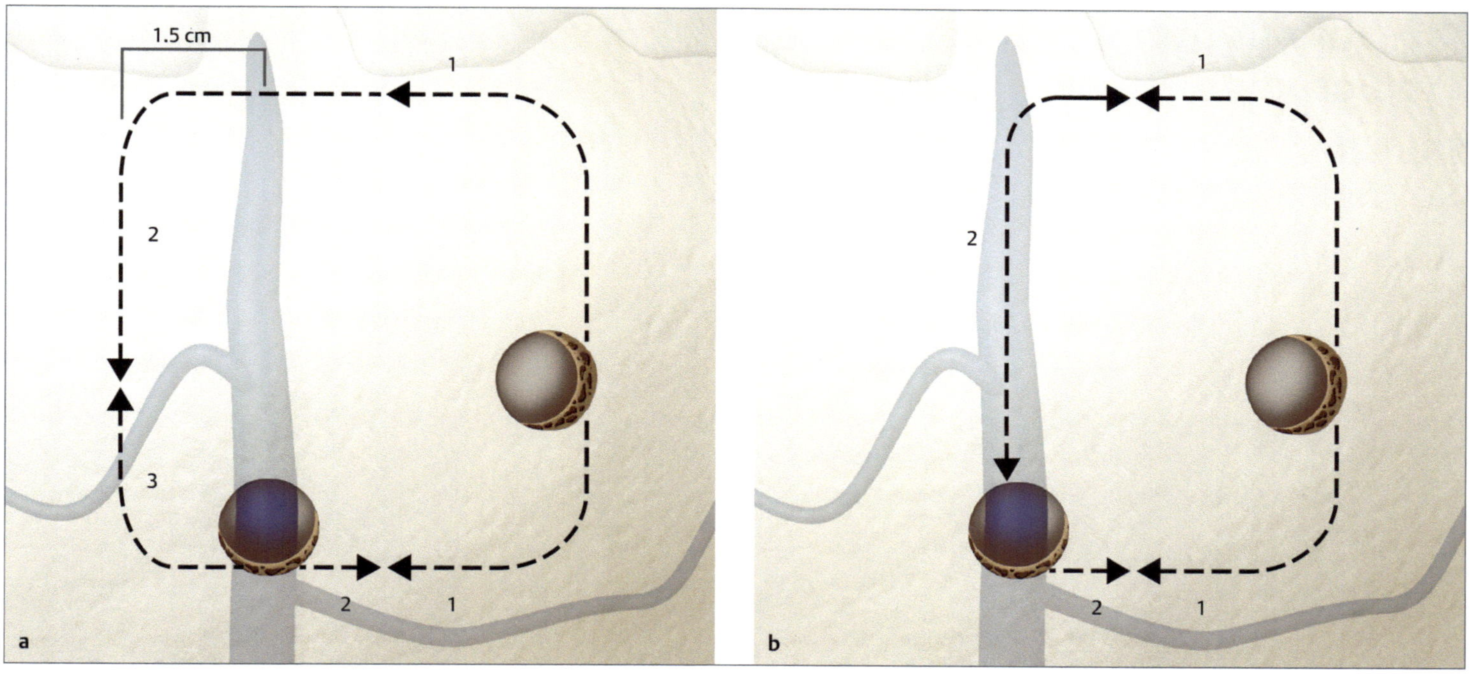

Fig. 4.4 Frontal or subfrontal approaches. For frontal approaches above the frontal skull base, we do not make an anterior burr hole (cosmesis, lower risk of sinus injury). Whether the sinus is crossed **(a)** or not **(b)** depends on the surgical target. Remnant bony structures (frontal sinus) may be resected using a drill. Opening of the frontal sinus should be avoided unless indicated (e.g., frontal skull base fracture).

4.2 Supratentorial Midline Craniotomy

Frontal

Ulrich Sure and Philipp Dammann

See ▶ Fig. 4.5, ▶ Fig. 4.6, ▶ Fig. 4.7, ▶ Fig. 4.8, ▶ Fig. 4.9, ▶ Fig. 4.10, ▶ Fig. 4.11, ▶ Fig. 4.12, ▶ Fig. 4.13, ▶ Fig. 4.14, ▶ Fig. 4.15, ▶ Fig. 4.16, ▶ Fig. 4.17, ▶ Fig. 4.18, ▶ Fig. 4.19, ▶ Fig. 4.20, and ▶ Fig. 4.21.

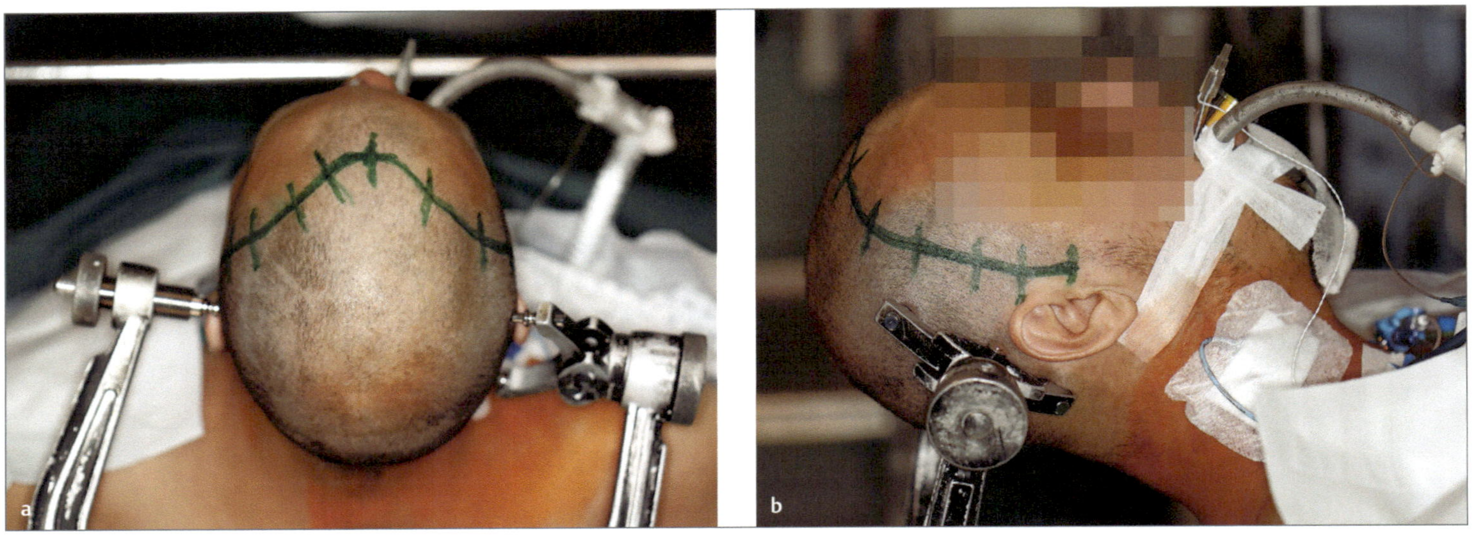

Fig. 4.5 (a, b) Positioning. The (anterior) frontal midline approach is used to access structures near, in, or via the frontal part of the interhemispheric fissure, frontal skull base, or orbital roof. It can be performed either unilaterally or bilaterally. Normally, the head is positioned straight without any rotation and is slightly elevated. In unilateral approaches, the head may be slightly tilted to the contralateral side to facilitate access to the interhemispheric fissure. The degree of head flexion required depends on the planned surgical trajectory.

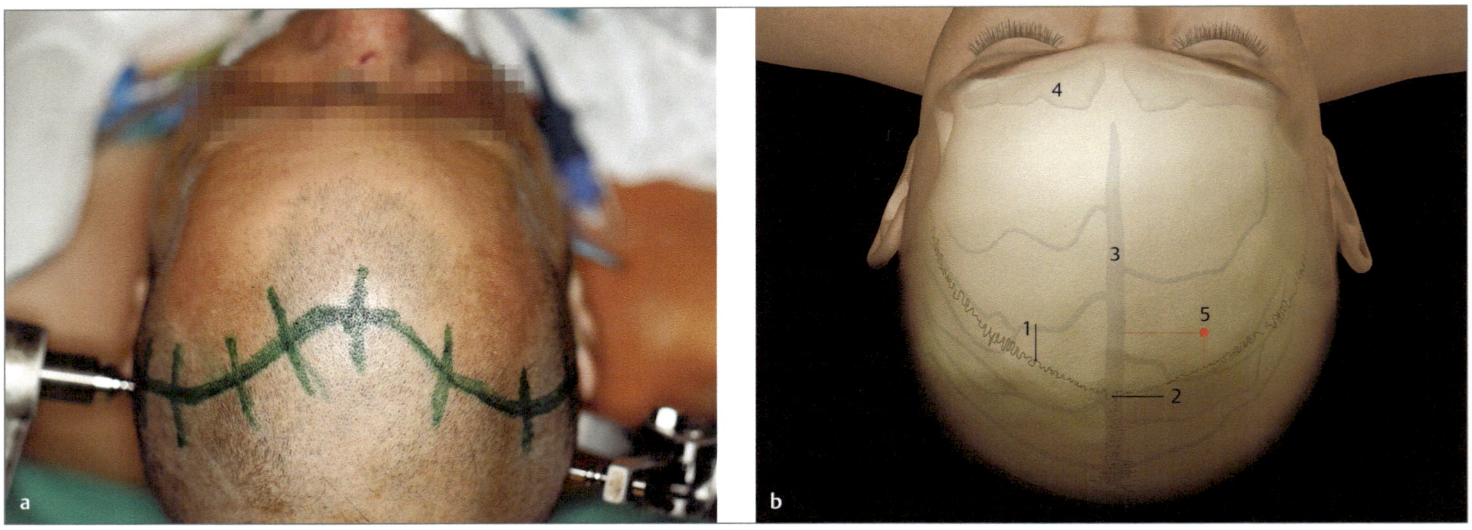

Fig. 4.6 (a, b) Anatomy overview. Important landmarks are (1) coronal suture, (2) sagittal suture and bregma, (3) superior sagittal sinus, and (4) frontal sinus. Another helpful orientation marker (placement of ventricular catheter) is (5) Kocher's point (1 cm anterior to the coronal suture, 2.5 cm lateral to the midline).

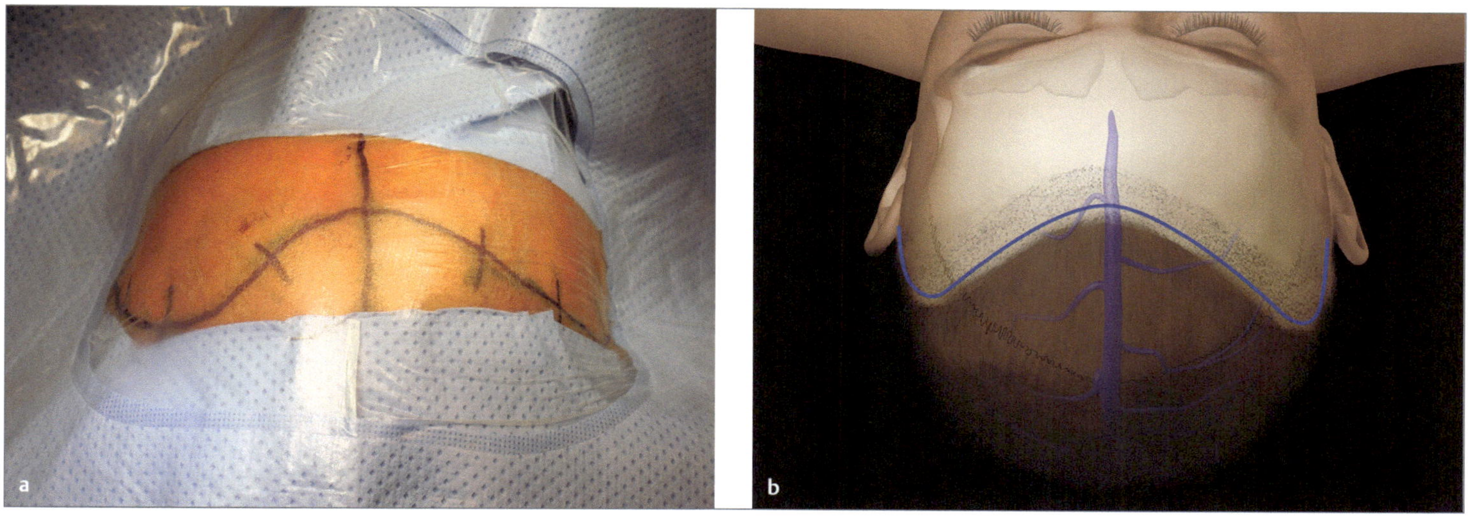

Fig. 4.7 (a, b) Draped position before skin incision. The skin incision for a large bilateral craniotomy runs from tragus to tragus, starting roughly 1 cm anteriorly after locating the main branch of the superficial temporal artery by palpation to avoid injury. The incision should usually cross the midline approximately 1 cm anterior to the bregma. However, the size of the skin flap can be adapted according to the size of the craniotomy. In unilateral craniotomies, the incision may end on the contralateral side 2–3 cm above the tragus. The more anterior the planned access, the larger the incision. It should allow the frontal skin flap to be completely folded over without putting it under too much tension (skin color!). The incision line is made behind the hairline for cosmesis. Usually, we shave the hair at a minimum 1 cm anterior and posteriorly to the incision. We prefer a slightly curved incision in the midline. This avoids asymmetry of the forehead skin after wound healing.

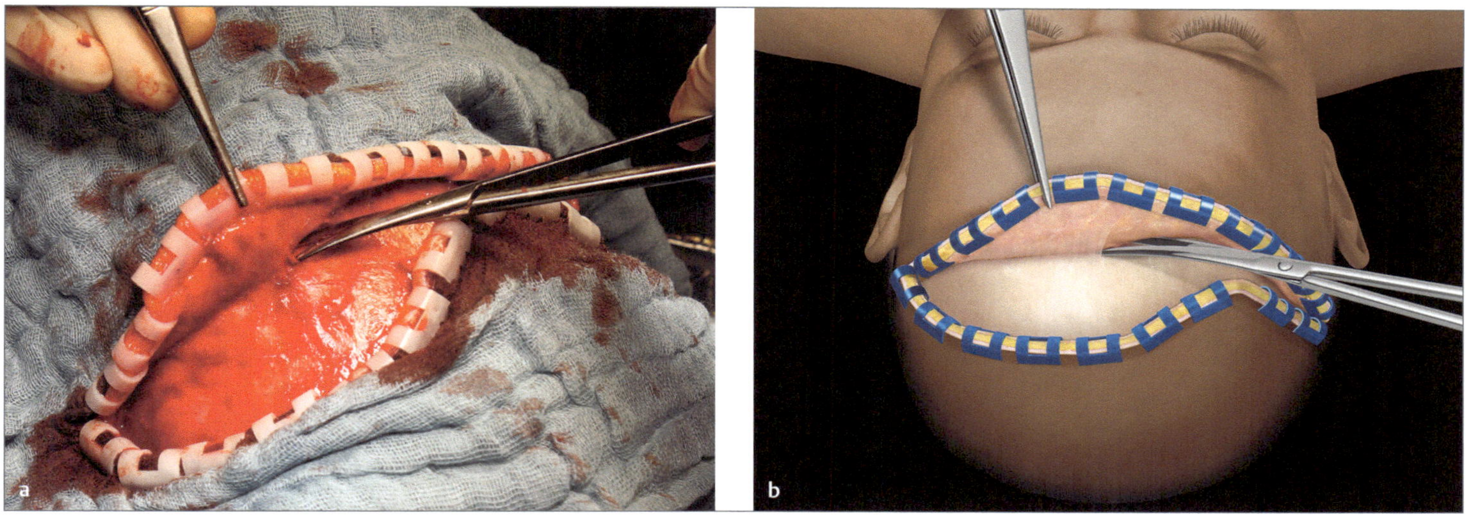

Fig. 4.8 (a, b) Skin incision. The skin incision spares the periosteum because in most scenarios using such an approach requires a galeal flap. A long incision should be started on one side first. Especially above the tragus, it is sometimes not possible to preserve small branches of the superficial temporal artery. After careful (sparing the superficial layers of the scalp) coagulation of arterial oozing, bleeding from the scalp is controlled with scalp clips covering the entire length of the incision. To place the scalp clips correctly, the subcutaneous scalp layer should be sharply dissected from the periosteum anterior and posteriorly. Fine white tissue adhesions indicate the correct layer.

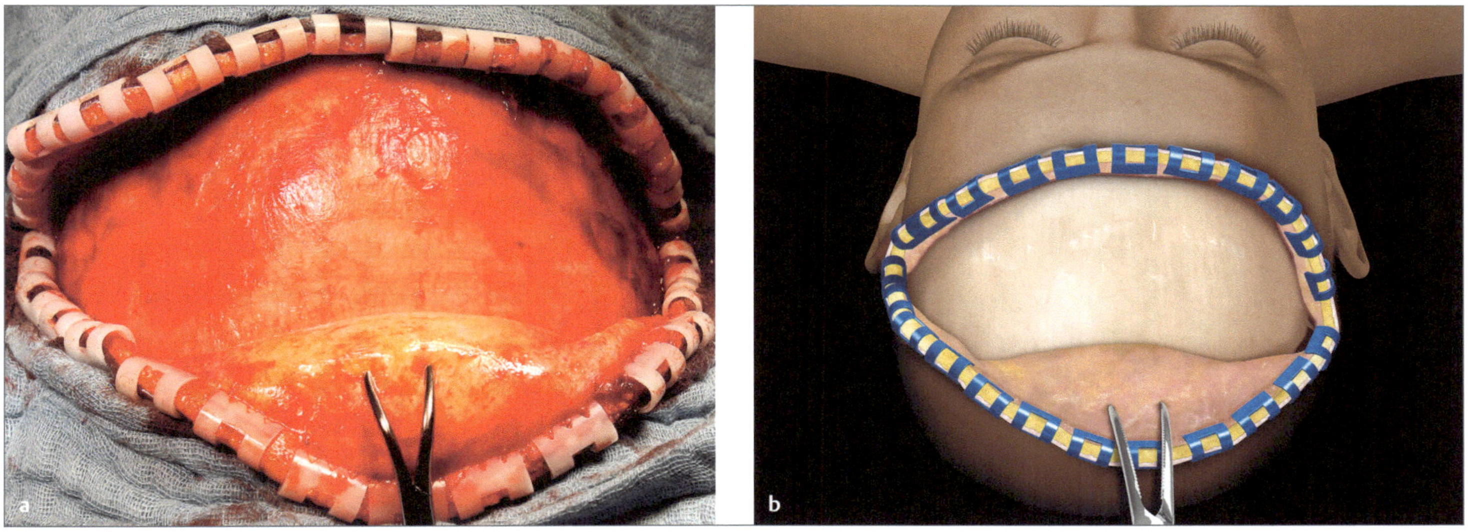

Fig. 4.9 (a, b) Subgaleal flap preparation. The posterior skin flap is pulled back (e.g., using a clamp). Depending on the planned surgery, the anterior skin flap is then dissected to the desired extent using sharp, and careful blunt, dissection.

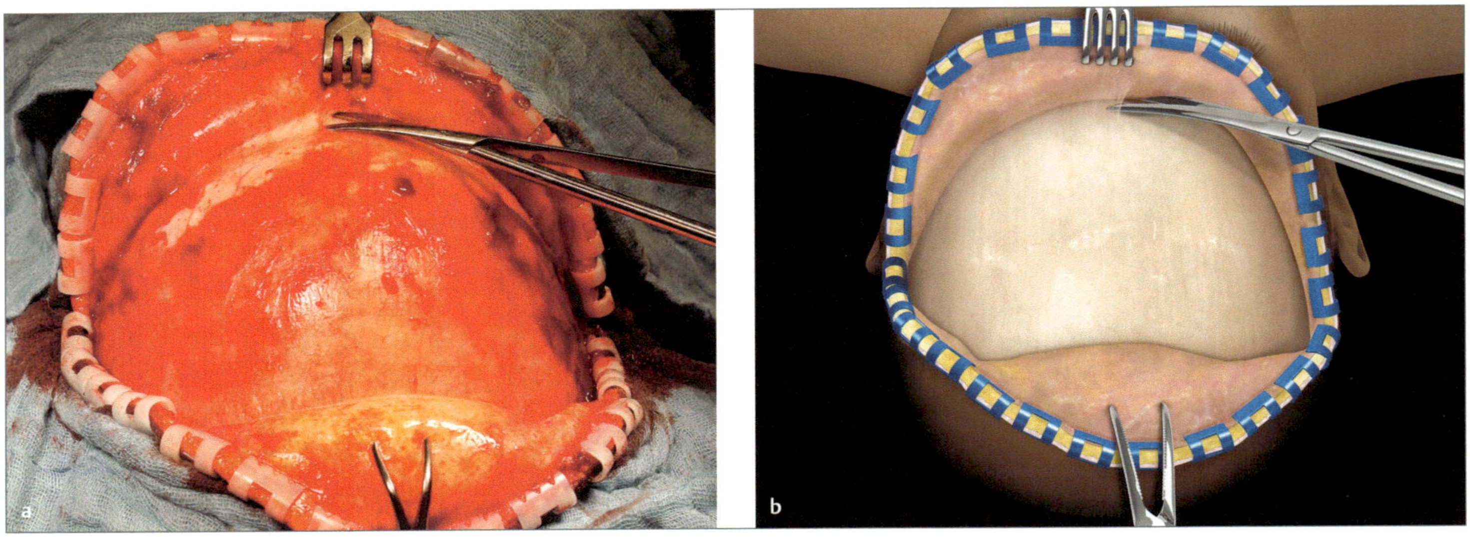

Fig. 4.10 (a, b) Subgaleal flap preparation. While further dissecting the scalp from the periosteum, the assistant pulls back the skin flap with a retractor and completely folds over the flap in a stepwise manner. Particularly above the temporal muscle fascia, adhesion to the scalp might be very tight.

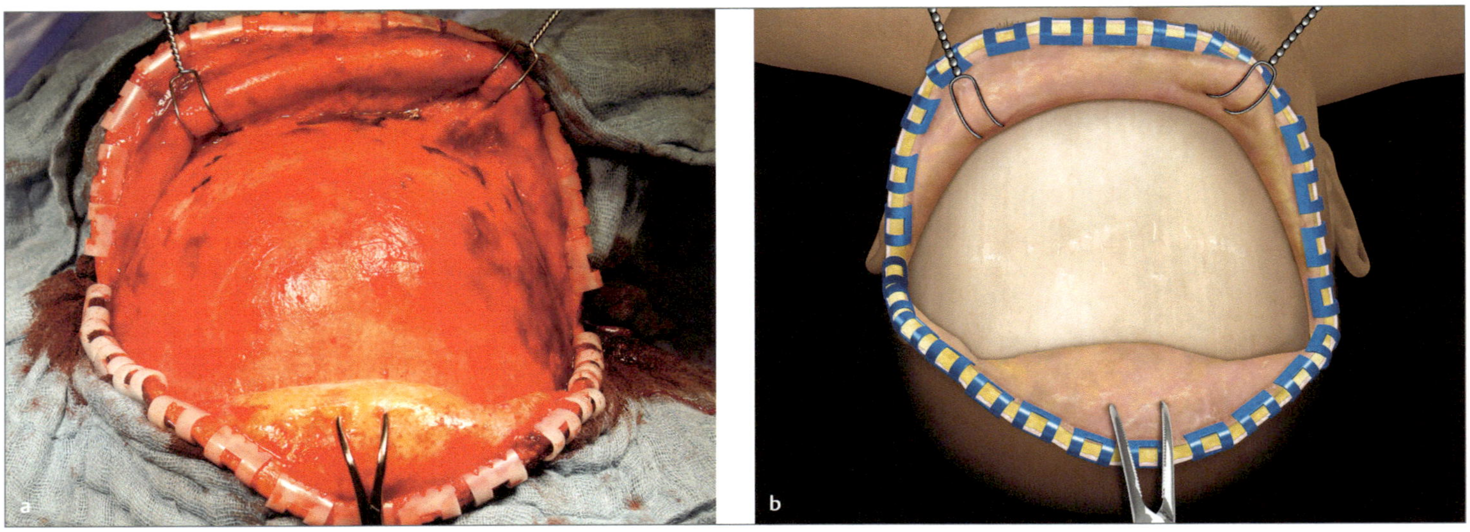

Fig. 4.11 (a, b) Subgaleal flap preparation. The skin flap is then held in position with retractors (e.g., Yasargil spring hooks). Bleeding from the skin flap or periosteum is localized and coagulated. Depending on the extent of dissection toward the frontal base, the supraorbital nerve with its accompanying artery and vein passing the supraorbital foramen should be located and spared.

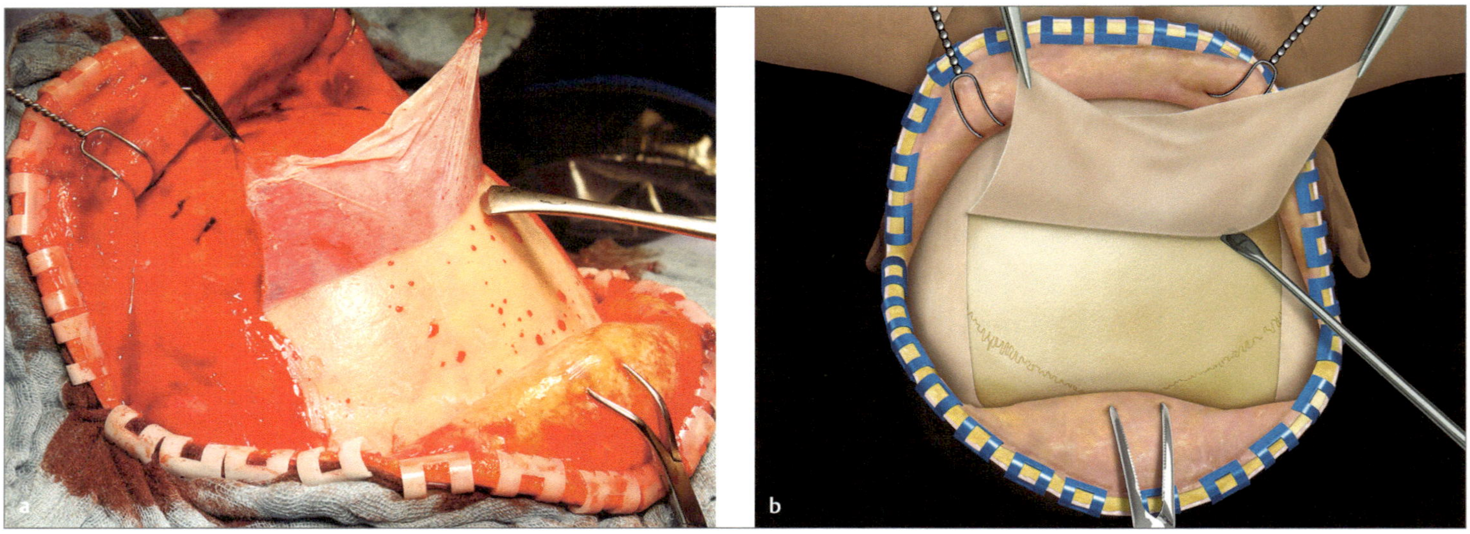

Fig. 4.12 (a, b) Subgaleal flap preparation. Finally, the periosteum is individually incised, staying above the temporal line bilaterally and preserving the frontal stalk of the flap. The flap is then dissected stepwise from the bone using a rasp (supraorbital nerve!).

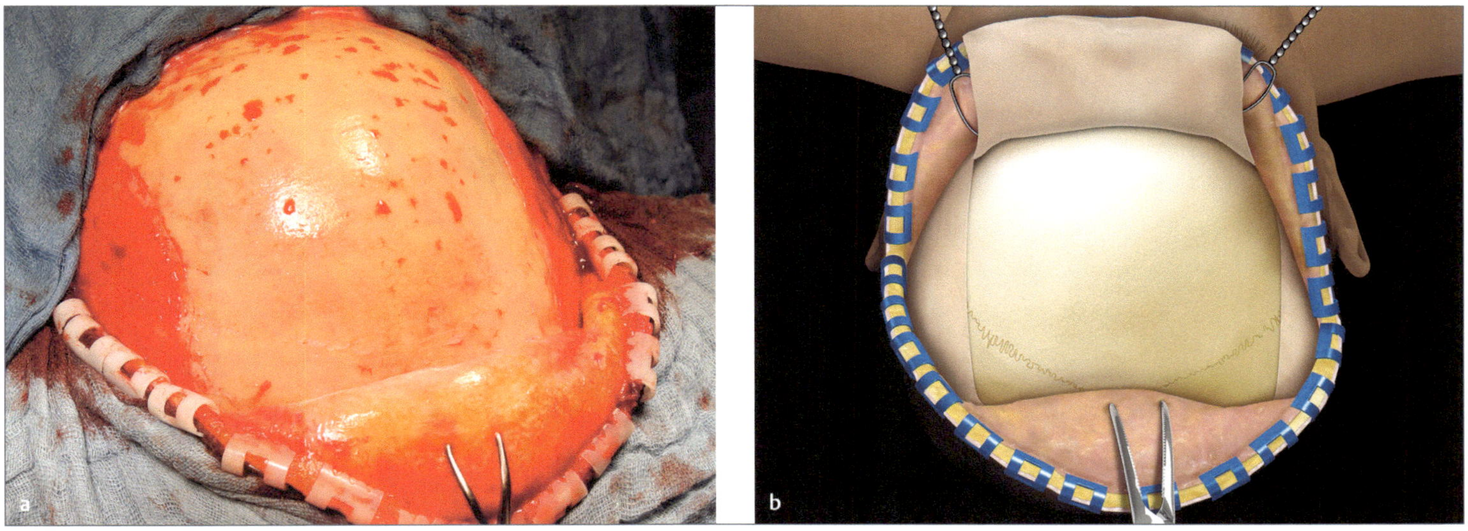

Fig. 4.13 (a, b) Subgaleal flap preparation. After dissection, the periosteum is positioned and kept rostrally. For better conservation, it is covered with wet surgical cottonoids or towels.

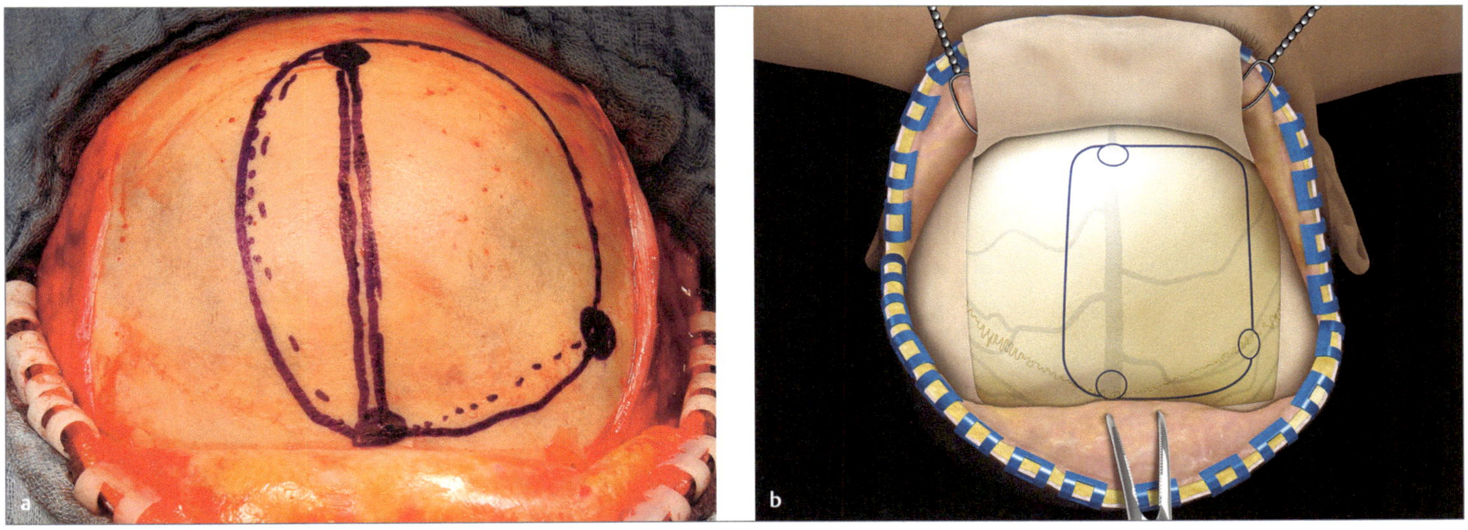

Fig. 4.14 (a, b) Craniotomy planning. The cranial sutures indicate midline structures and intracranial localization of a target lesion. The planning of burr hole placement and craniotomy depends on various parameters such as the target lesion, age of the patient, previous surgery, etc. In this illustration, a large unilateral craniotomy to the midline was necessary. To allow gentle retraction of the midline structure to the contralateral side, the sinus was crossed and exposed 1.5 cm contralaterally. To prevent wound healing problems, the burr holes should not be directly underneath the skin incision. For beginners, it may be helpful to draw the planned craniotomy on the skull with a surgical pen. If performing an extended frontal craniotomy, the borders of the frontal sinus should be respected (see measurements from CT or using navigation to localize the borders) unless opening of the sinus is desired (e.g., for fractures of the frontal skull base). In these cases, an anterior burr hole on the midline can also be avoided for better cosmesis. The risks of injuring the sagittal sinus are very low in this region.

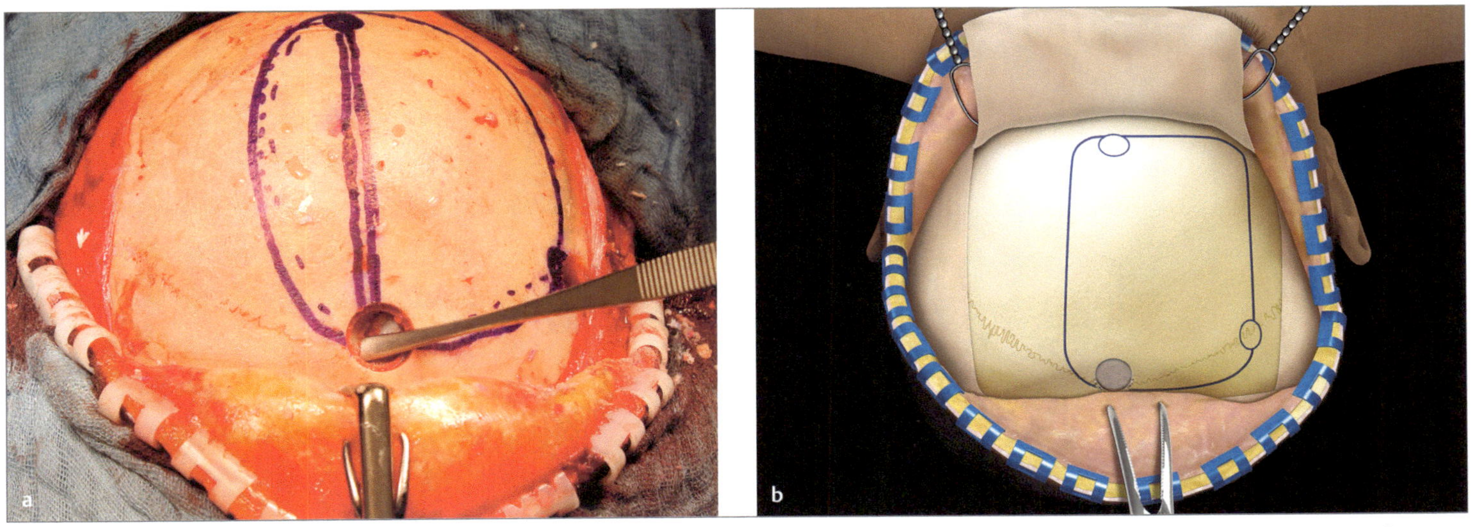

Fig. 4.15 (a, b) Burr holes. The burr hole(s) on the sinus should be drilled with a large trephine (18 mm) which may offer a better protection for injury of the sinus. The direction is strictly perpendicular to the skull. Residual bone chips should then be removed using a blunt dissector. If the dura adheres to the bone, a small punch sometimes helps to detach the structures and provide an entry for the craniotome. The lateral burr holes can be drilled with a smaller trephine.

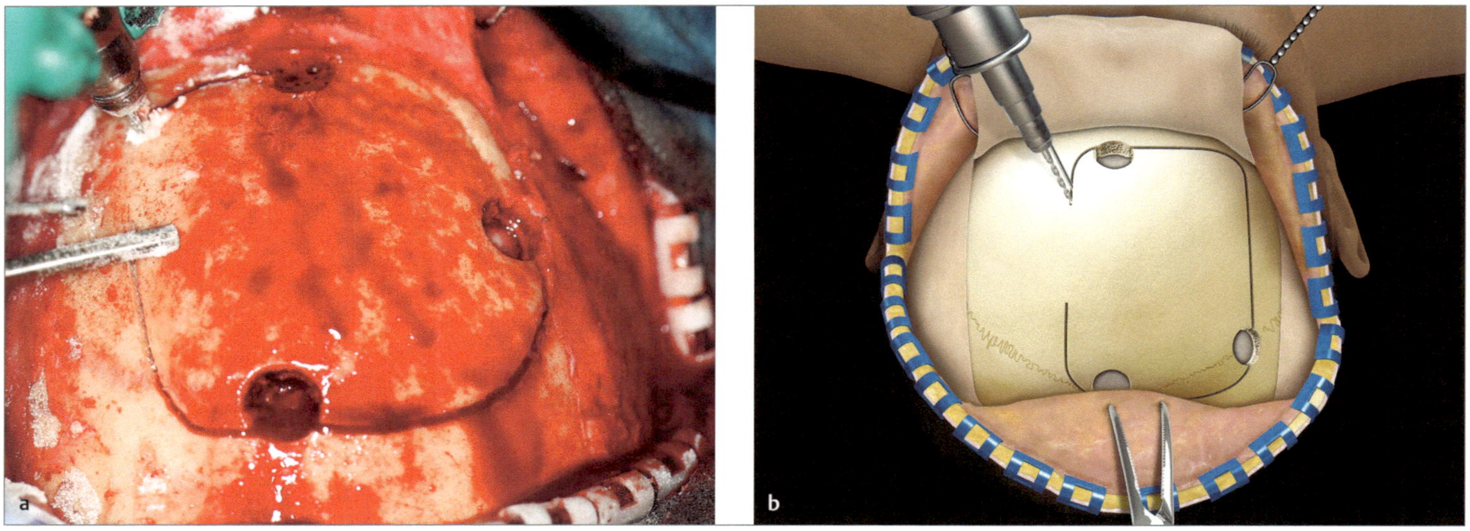

Fig. 4.16 (a, b) Craniotomy. The craniotomy is usually performed starting from a lateral burr hole and stopping 2 cm lateral to the midline. From the burr hole on top of the sinus, we then cut from medially to laterally interconnecting the craniotomy. When no lateral burr hole is present, the craniotomy starts in the midline, cutting away from it and interconnecting the craniotomy laterally. The assistant uses the flush to cool the craniotome and tissue structures and the sucker to provide optimal visibility for the surgeon.

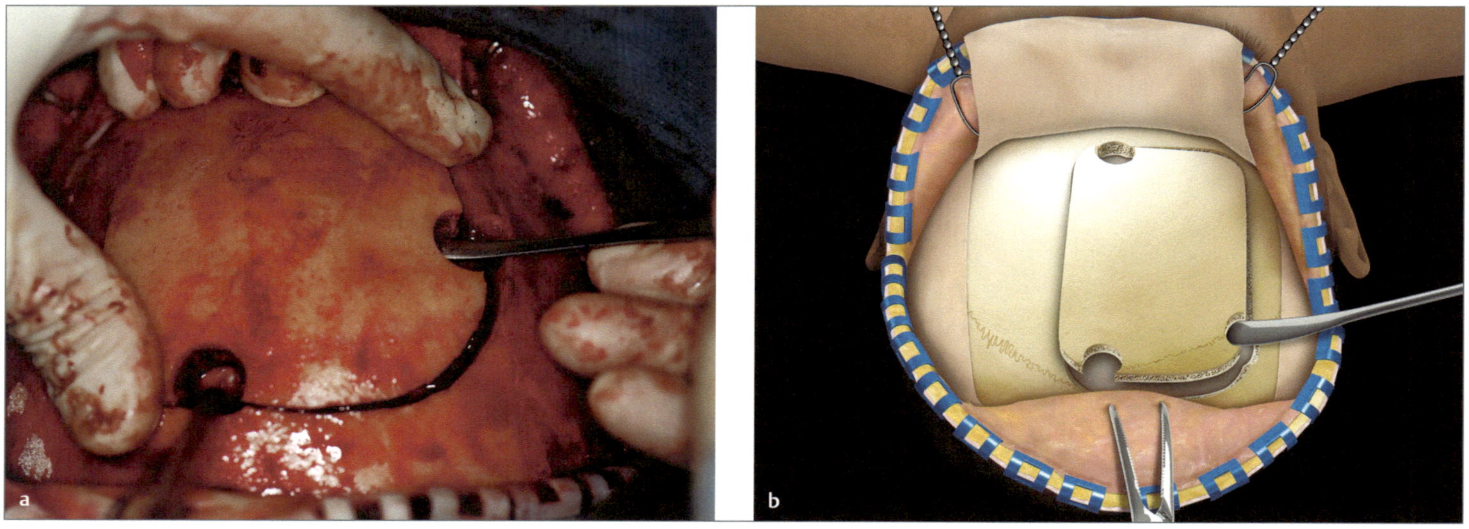

Fig. 4.17 (a, b) Craniotomy. After complete circumferential craniotomy, the bone flap is gently elevated with an elevator and the dural layer dissected stepwise from the bone. This is performed with special care in the midline to prevent injury of the sinus. The bone flap should always (!) be secured manually by the assistant or surgeon. During this step, the team should be prepared for a potential sinus laceration. In the case of an injury, the sinus is covered with prepared cottonoids before the injury is sutured or sealed with fibrin glue or a hemostasis patch.

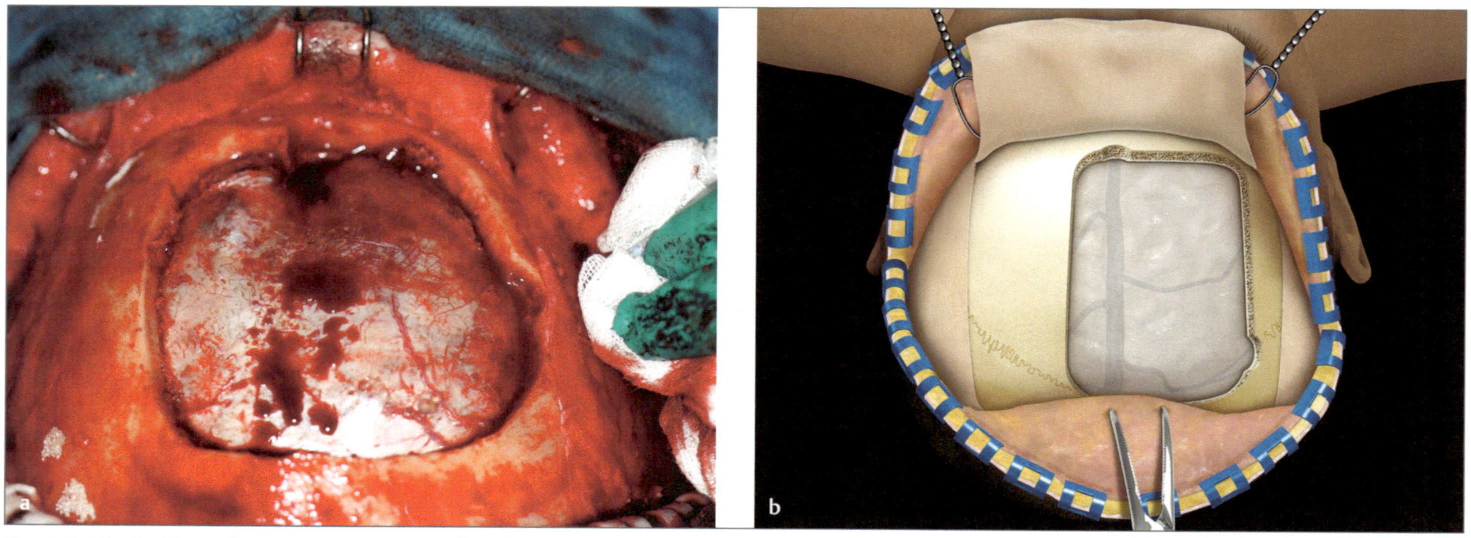

Fig. 4.18 (a, b) Situs after craniotomy. Typically, after elevation of the bone flap, some minor venous bleeding occurs in the area of the sagittal sinus from pacchionian granulations. This can normally be controlled by coagulation and compression with cottonoids. Further bleeding from dural vessels more laterally should also be coagulated. The whole site then has to be meticulously cleared of bone dust using irrigation.

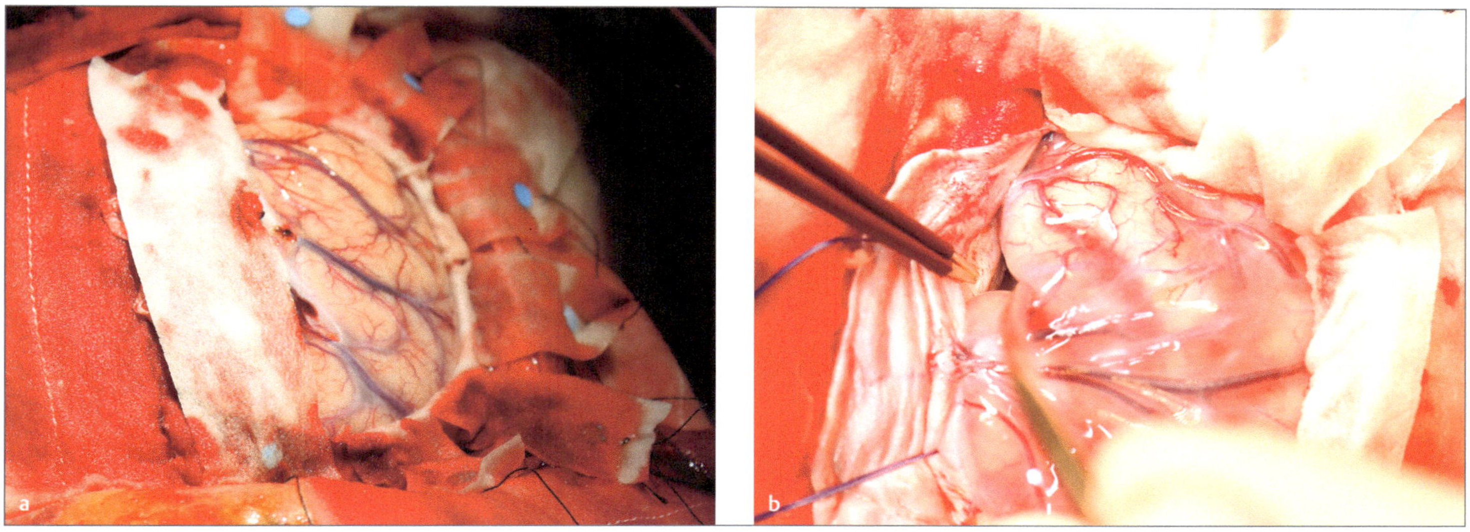

Fig. 4.19 (a, b) **Dura opening.** After placing surgical cotton around the circumference to protect the brain tissue, the dura is opened from laterally to medially with the base at the sagittal sinus. It is essential to avoid injury of bridging veins whose position should be known from preoperative imaging. Sometimes, small lacunae of the sinus extend laterally. If injured, these can be easily closed using small clips or sutures. Stitches in the dura lateral to the sinus or in the falx inferior of the sinus can be used to gently retract the falx and sinus contralaterally to allow better access to the interhemispheric fissure.

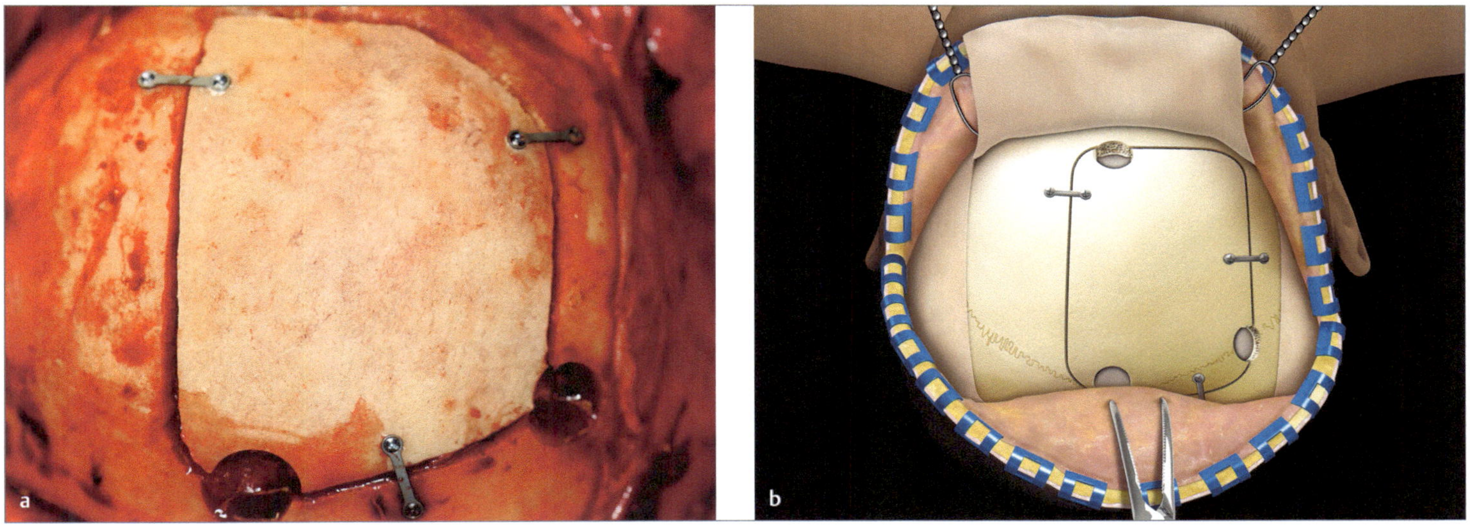

Fig. 4.20 (a, b) **Closure: bone flap refixation.** The bone flap is fixed to the skull using titanium mini-plates with a distance of roughly 120° between the plates. The bone flap is positioned so that the anterior part adjoins the frontal skull without any gap. If a rostral burr hole is placed within the cosmetically sensitive area of the forehead, it should be covered with a burr hole mini-plate or filled with bone cement.

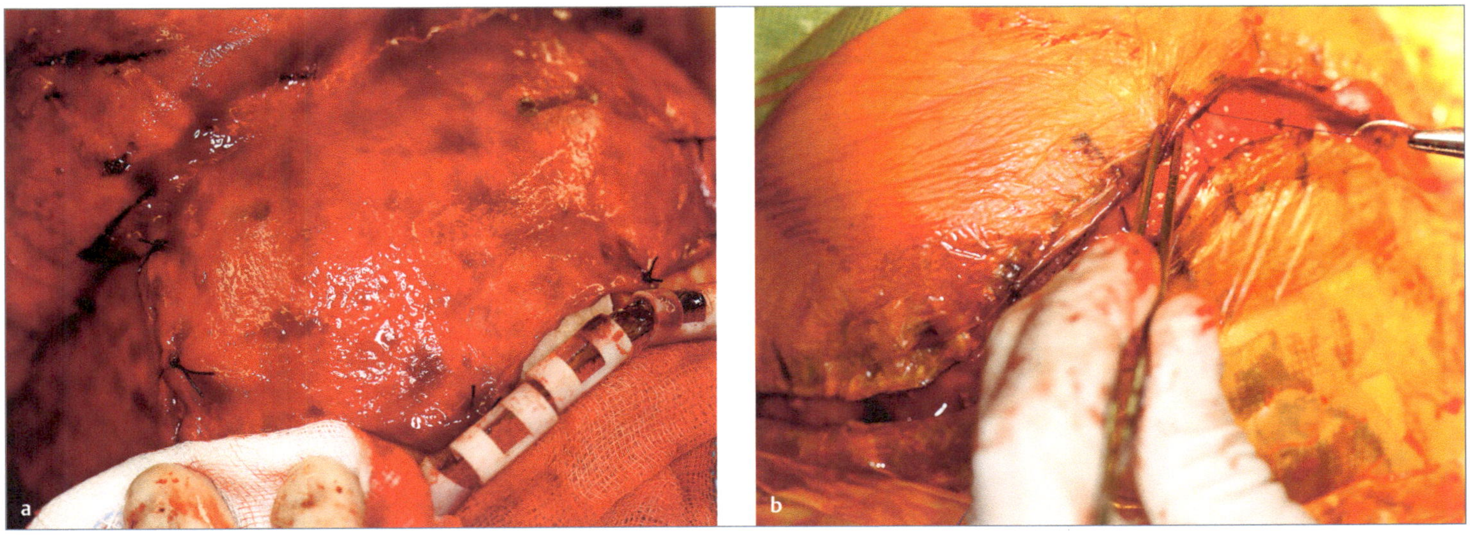

Fig. 4.21 (a, b) **Closure: subgaleal flap handling and skin closure.** If not used as a patch, the subgaleal flap can be reattached to the periosteum. The skin is closed in typical manner using subcutaneous sutures (each 1 cm distance apart) and running or single skin suture. Usually, a subcutaneous drain is inserted.

Checklist

- Position the Mayfield clamp in such a way that it does not obstruct you during opening and closure of the skin.
- Try to preserve the whole galeal flap (if needed, also preserve its base).
- Make sure (in frontal skull base approaches) to preserve supraorbital nerves.
- Make sure not to open the frontal sinus unless it is necessary (neuronavigation may be helpful in difficult cases).
- Ligation of the first third of the sagittal superior sinus is normally possible in the case of an injury that cannot otherwise be remedied.
- Cosmesis in this area of the skull is very important! Respect the hairline, make a curved incision, avoid (if possible) and cover burr holes, replace the bone flap achieving a minimum gap at the anterior and medial borders, and close the wound very carefully.

Frontoparietal

Ulrich Sure and Philipp Dammann

See ▸Fig. 4.22, ▸Fig. 4.23, ▸Fig. 4.24, ▸Fig. 4.25, ▸Fig. 4.26, ▸Fig. 4.27, ▸Fig. 4.28, ▸Fig. 4.29,▸Fig. 4.30, ▸Fig. 4.31,▸Fig. 4.32, ▸Fig. 4.33, and ▸Fig. 4.34.

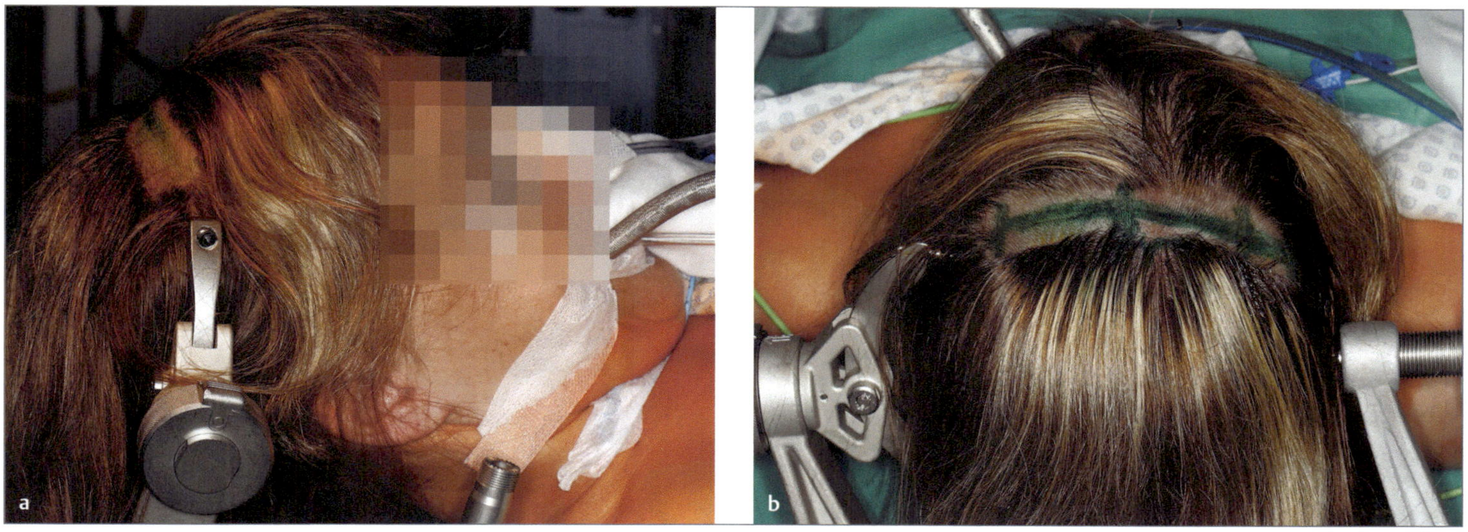

Fig. 4.22 (a, b) Positioning. The frontal midline approach is used to access structures near, via, or in the interhemispheric fissure located from 5 cm anterior to the bregma up to the superior parietal lobule. It can be performed in a unilateral or a bilateral way. The patient is in the supine position. Normally, the head is straight, but sometimes (in unilateral approaches) it is slightly tilted to the contralateral side to facilitate access to the midline. The head is elevated and flexed, with the bregma being the highest point. At least a finger's width space should be left between the chin and jugulum.

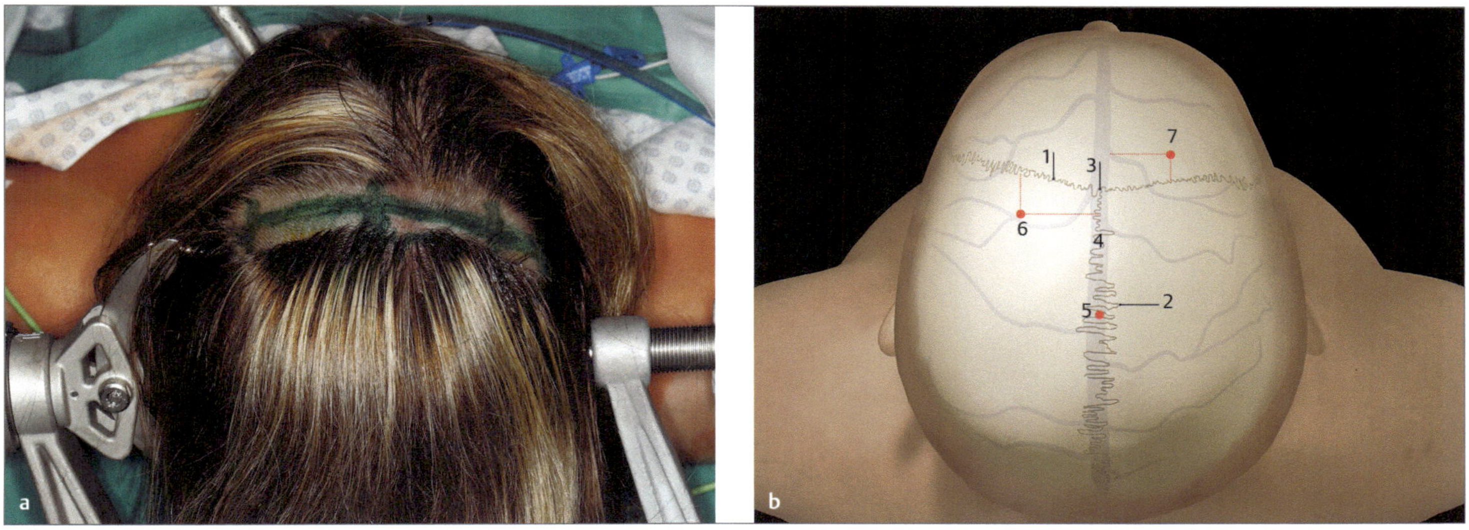

Fig. 4.23 (a, b) Anatomy overview. Important landmarks are (1) coronal suture, (2) sagittal suture and (3) bregma, the (4) superior sagittal sinus, (5) the superior rolandic point (5 cm posterior to the bregma, indicating the central sulcus), and (6) the posterior coronal point (3 cm lateral to the sagittal suture, 1 cm posterior to the coronal suture, indicating the anterior border of the hand motor cortex). Another helpful orientation aid (for placement of a ventricular catheter) is (7) Kocher's point (10 mm anterior to the coronal suture, 25 mm lateral to the midline).

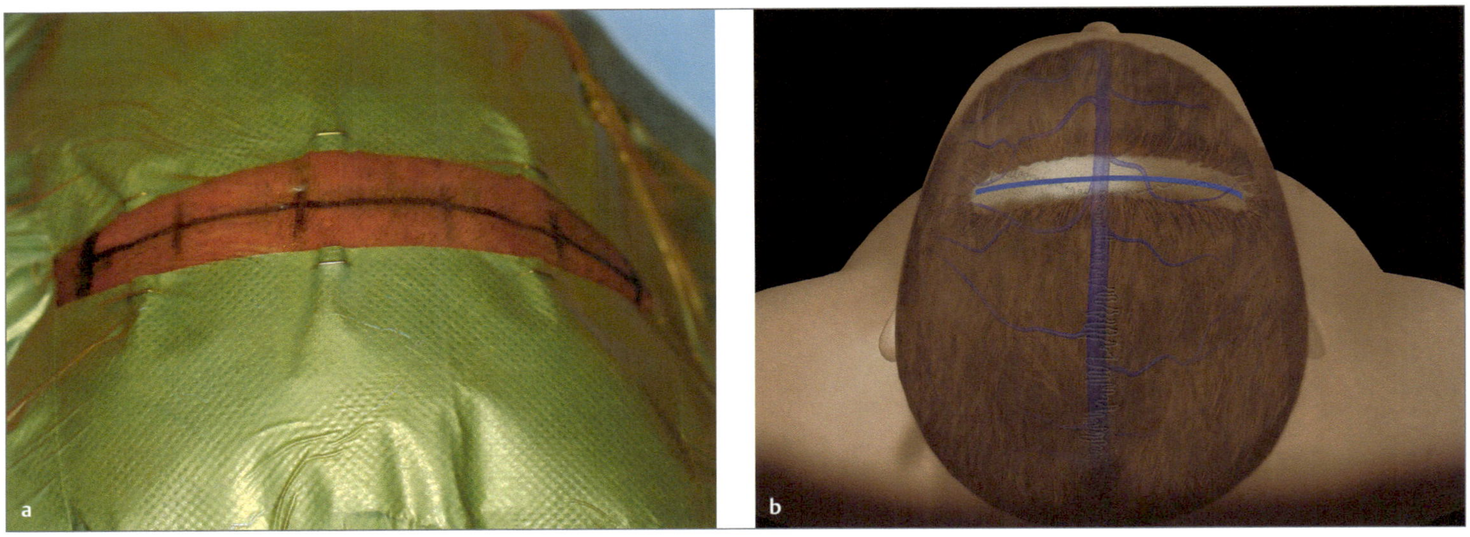

Fig. 4.24 (a, b) **Draped position before skin incision.** The skin incision (straight, coronal for a bilateral approach) extends approximately 5 cm bilaterally to the midline, depending on the desired size of the craniotomy. Even in large bone flaps, it should normally not cross the superior temporal line. For unilateral approaches, the incision extends the midline approximately 3 cm on the contralateral side and 5 cm on the ipsilateral side, again depending on the planned size of the craniotomy. An incision that is too small limits the exposure of the midline in the sagittal plane. In very anterior approaches, the incision line may be modified (curved) to respect the hairline for better cosmesis. Usually, we shave the hair 1 cm anterior and posterior to the incision.

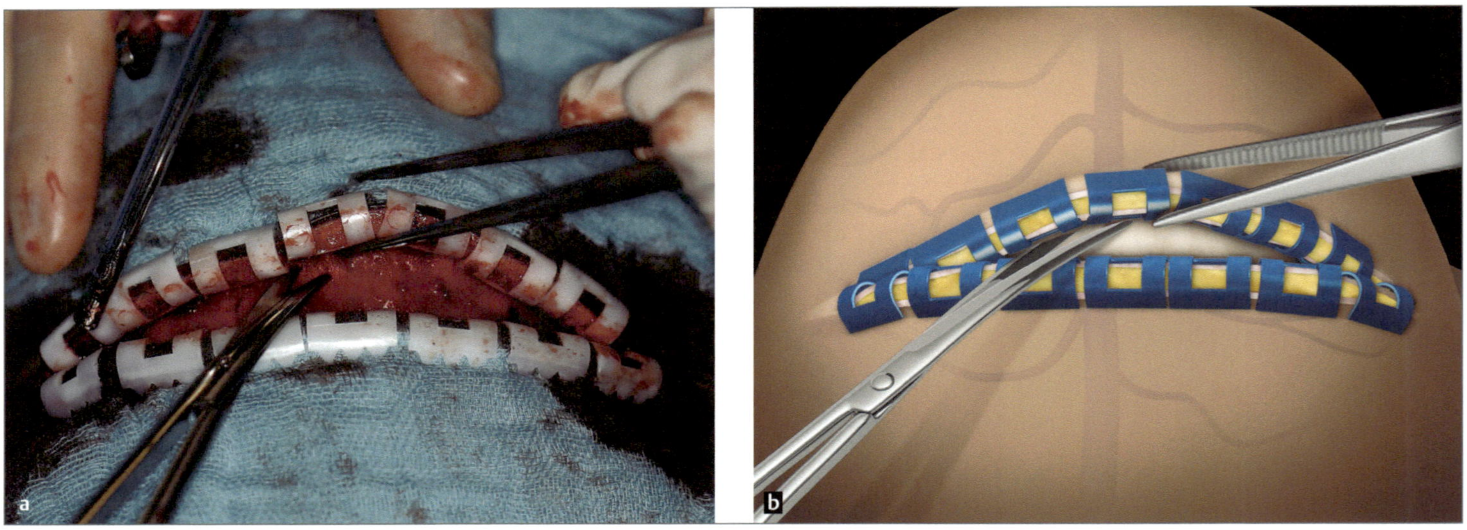

Fig. 4.25 (a, b) **Skin incision.** The skin incision spares the periosteum if a galea flap is desired. After careful coagulation of arterial oozing (sparing the superficial layers of the scalp), bleeding from the scalp is controlled with scalp clips covering the entire length of the incision. To place the scalp clips properly, the subcutaneous scalp layer has to be sharply dissected from the periosteum, i.e., the incision needs to extend to the periosteum and the skin–galea flap needs to be mobilized a few millimeters.

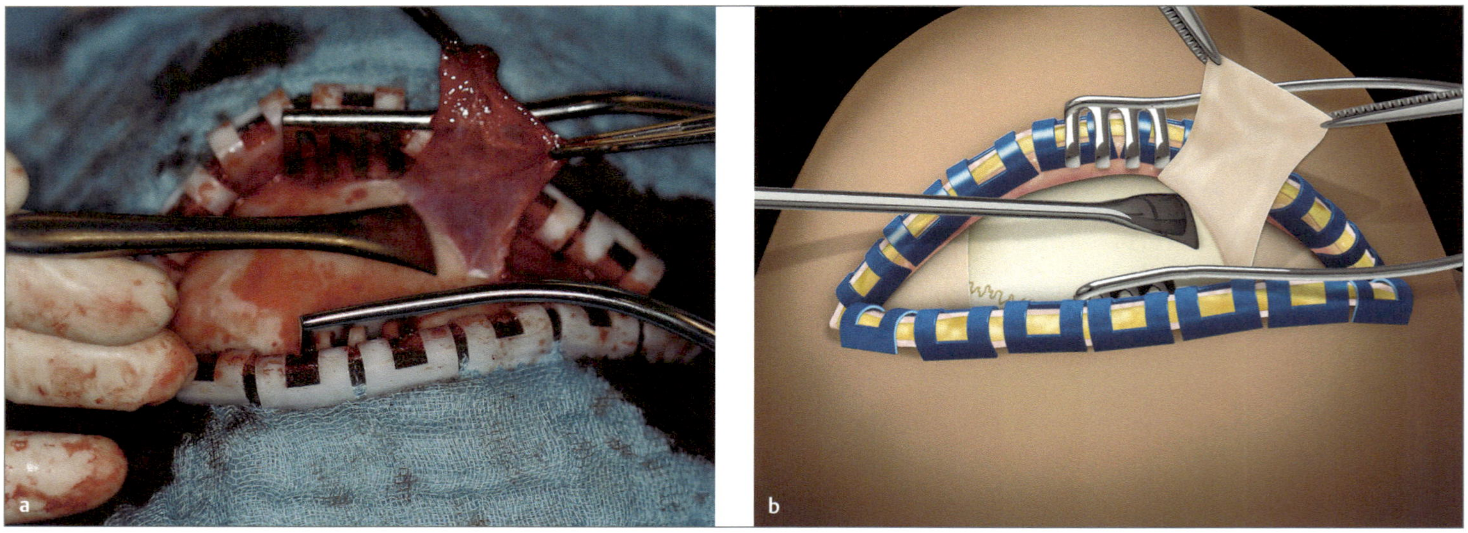

Fig. 4.26 (a, b) **Subgaleal flap preparation.** If a subgaleal flap is desired, the periosteum is incised circumferentially after placement of a skin retractor. The flap is carefully dissected from the bone using a raspatorium. The assistant retracts the flap using anatomical forceps. The flap should be preserved in wet cottonoids.

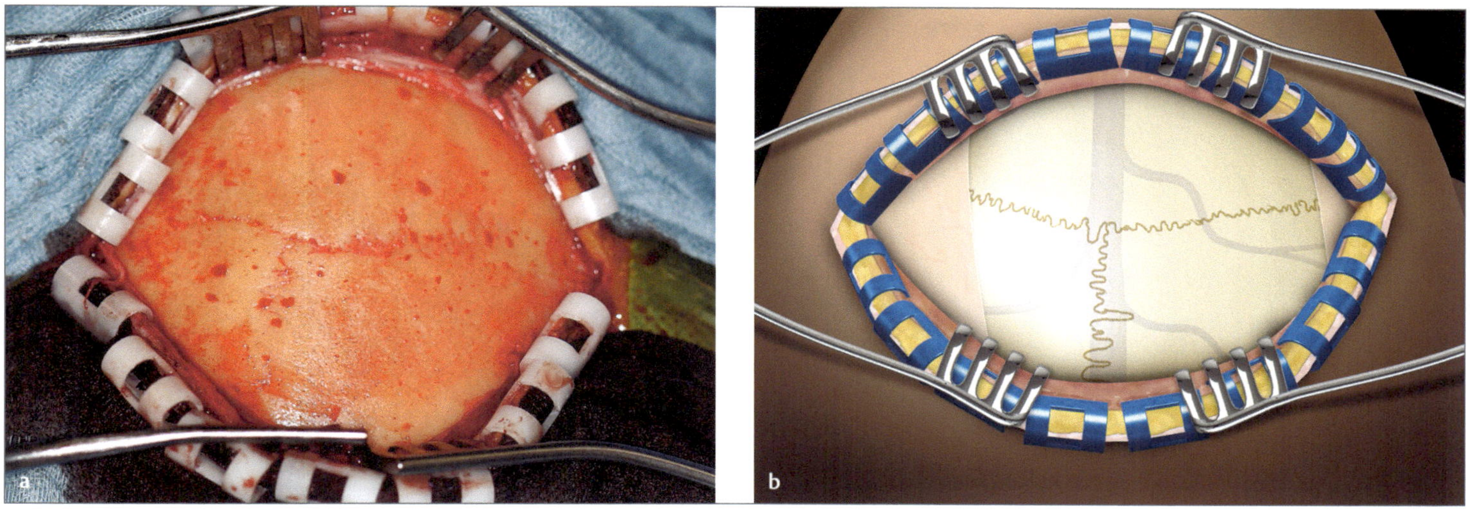

Fig. 4.27 (a, b) **Craniotomy planning.** The cranial sutures indicate midline structures and intracranial localization of a target lesion (x cm anterior/posterior to the coronal suture). The planning of burr hole placement and craniotomy depends on various parameters such as the target lesion, age of the patient, and previous surgery. For the basic principles of the craniotomy, see Chapter 4.1, Sinus-Crossing Craniotomies. In the scenario illustrated here, we made three burr holes on the midline to control the superior sagittal sinus, and one lateral burr hole.

Several craniometric points are helpful for orientation. Besides the bregma, the superior rolandic point and posterior coronal point are helpful as indicators of the projection of the motor cortex. When an interhemispheric approach is desired, it is helpful to know that fewer bridging veins are encountered in the zone 5 cm anterior to the bregma. Before making the burr holes, the anterior course of the midline (not indicated by the sagittal suture) has to be traced.

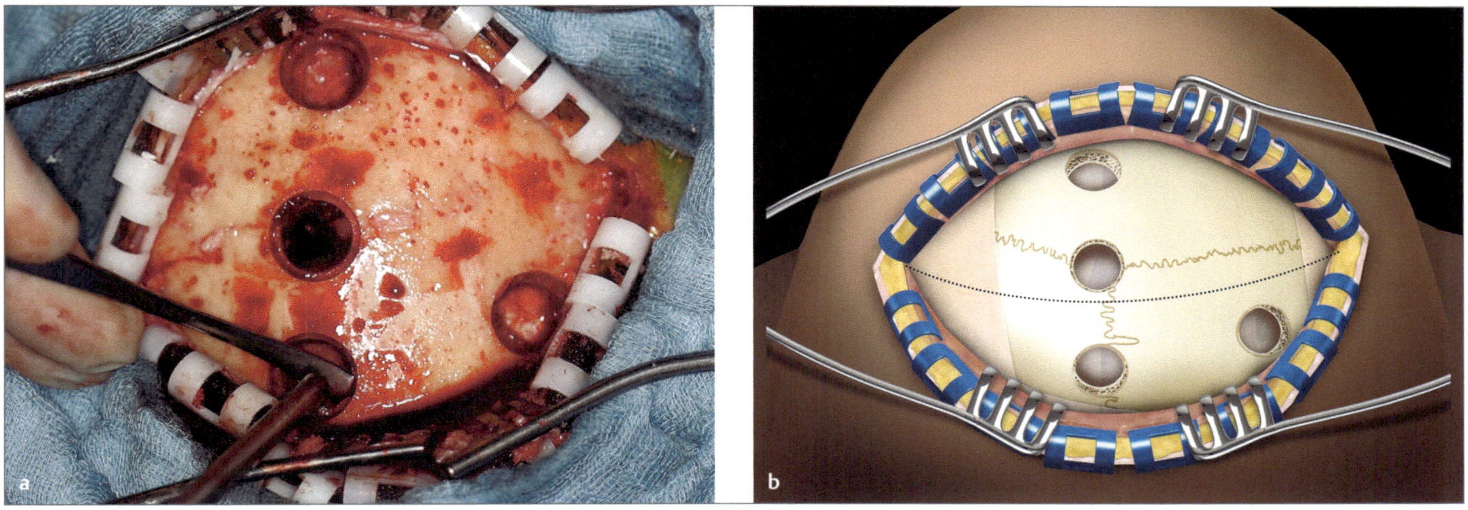

Fig. 4.28 (a, b) **Burr holes.** The burr holes on the sinus should be drilled with a large trephine (18 mm) to ensure sufficient control. The direction is strictly perpendicular to the skull. Residual bone chips should be removed using a blunt dissector. In the case of dural adhesion to the bone, a small punch can sometimes help to detach the structures and provide an entry for the craniotome. The epidural space is then carefully dissected from the sinus surface using a dissector. If the burr holes are located close enough together, the sinus surface can be detached from the bone along the entire border of the craniotomy. Cave: particularly in patients with very thin skin or wound-healing problems, the burr holes should not be made directly beneath the skin incision (*dotted line*).

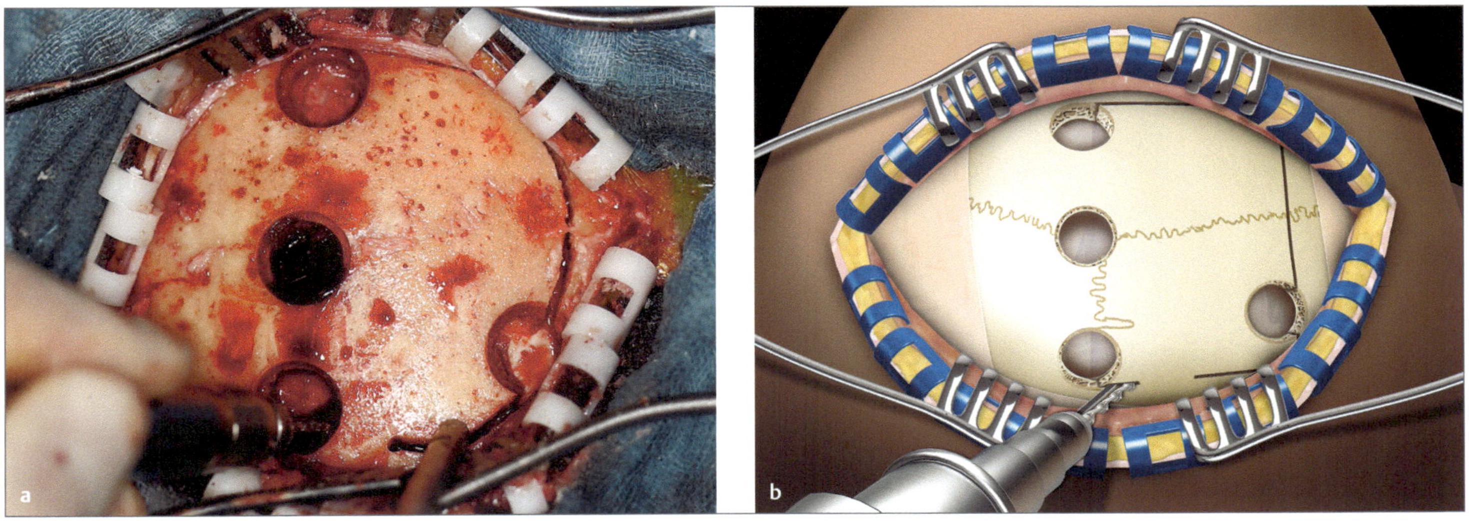

Fig. 4.29 (a, b) **Craniotomy: beginning.** The craniotomy starts at the lateral burr hole extending medially and ends approximately 2 cm lateral to the sinus. The craniotomy is then continued from the sinus burr hole in a medial-to-lateral direction. Caution: never cut from a lateral directing toward the sinus and on to the sinus, because this creates a much higher risk of injuring the sinus by slippage into a lateral lacuna. Particularly for beginners, it may be helpful to outline the planned craniotomy on the bone with a surgical pen.

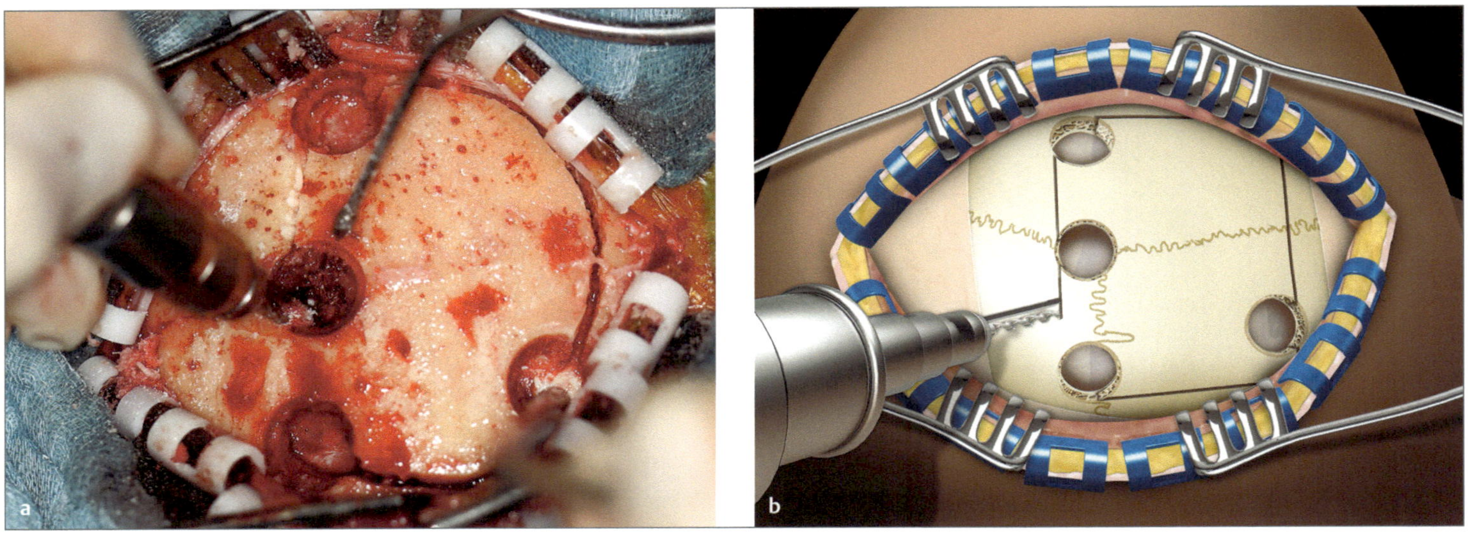

Fig. 4.30 (a, b) Craniotomy: completion. The craniotomy is then completed by interconnecting the burr holes on the sinus at its most contralateral aspect, starting at the most anterior burr hole before going dorsally.

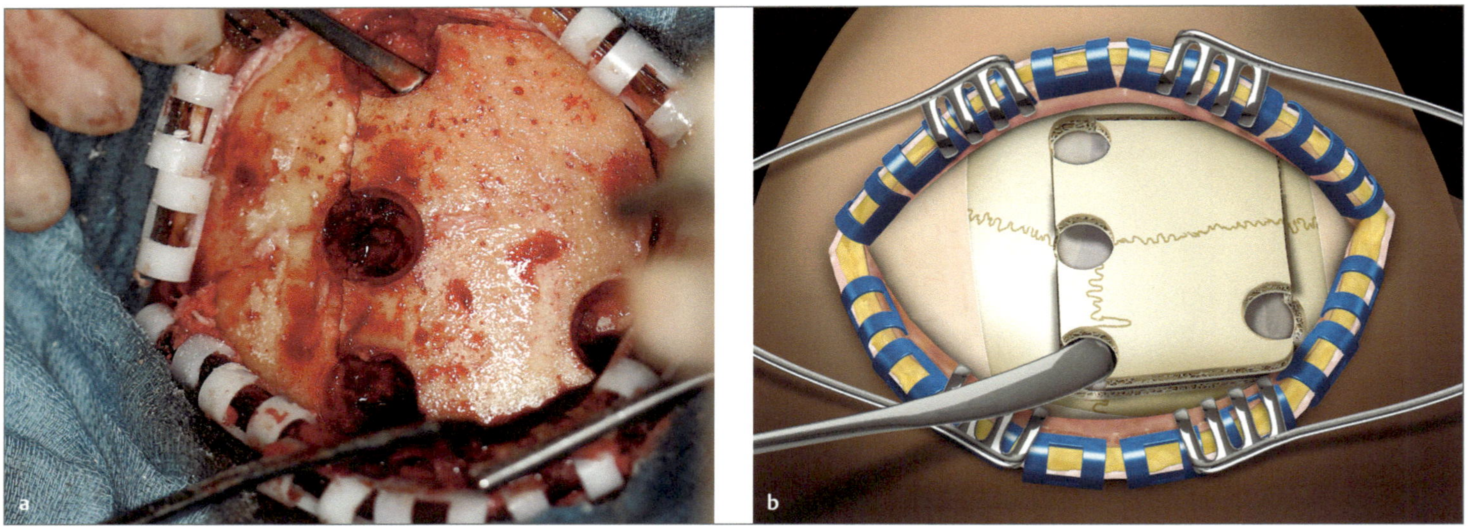

Fig. 4.31 (a, b) Craniotomy: completion. After complete circumferential craniotomy, the bone flap is gently removed with an elevator and the dural layer is dissected stepwise from the bone. This is performed with special care in the midline to prevent injury of the sinus. The bone flap should always be secured manually by the assistant or surgeon. During this step, the team should be prepared for sinus laceration. If such an injury does occur, the sinus is covered with prepared cottonoids before being sutured or sealed with fibrin glue or a hemostasis patch.

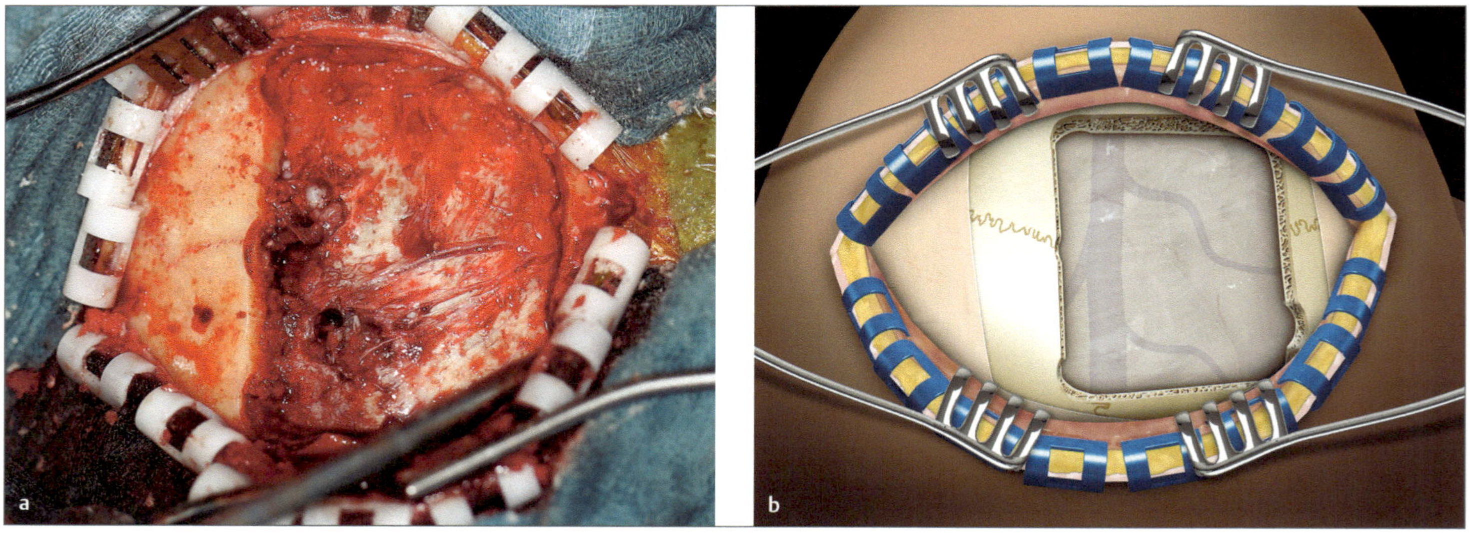

Fig. 4.32 (a, b) Situs after craniotomy. Typically after elevation of the bone flap, some minor venous bleeding occurs in the area of the sagittal sinus from pacchionian granulations (very large in this case). Bleeding can normally be controlled by coagulation and compression with cottonoids. Further bleeding from dural vessels situated more laterally should also be coagulated. The whole situs then has to be meticulously cleared of bone dust using irrigation. Particularly in deep-seated lesions or if there is complex bridging vein anatomy, additional verification of the planned trajectory and interhemispheric approach is helpful at this stage of surgery (with neuronavigation or ultrasound).

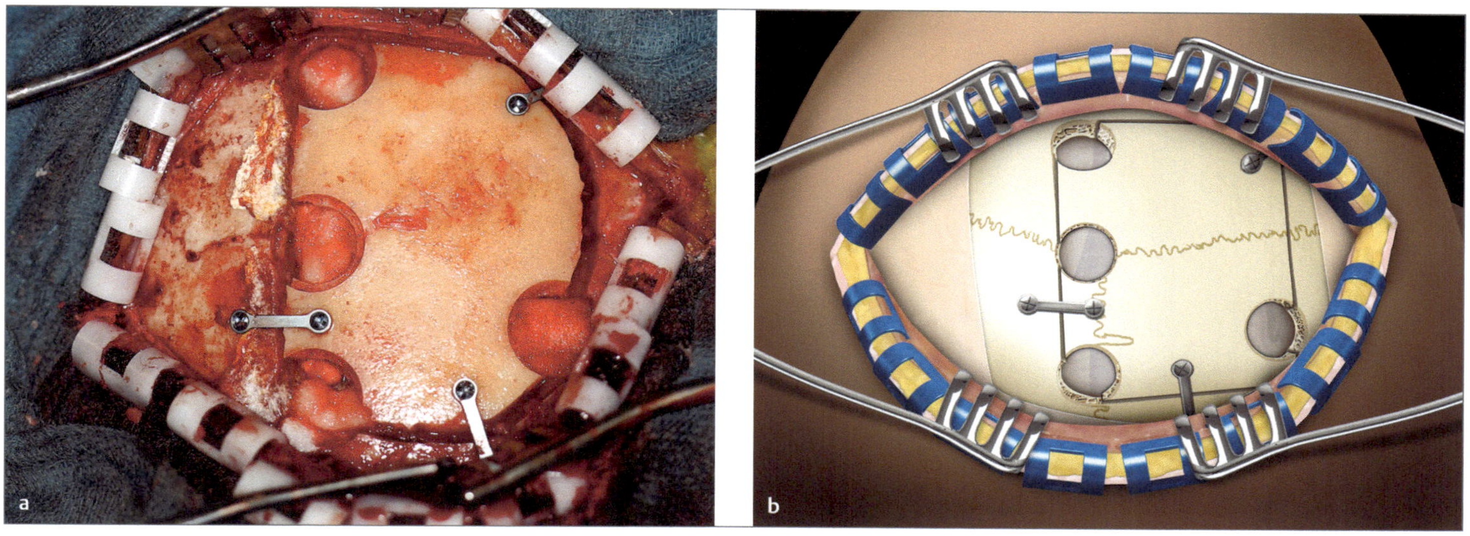

Fig. 4.33 (a, b) Closure: bone flap refixation. The bone flap is positioned so that the anterior part adjoins the frontal skull without any gap. If a rostral burr hole is located within the cosmetically relevant area of the forehead, it should be covered with a burr hole mini-plate device or filled with bone cement.

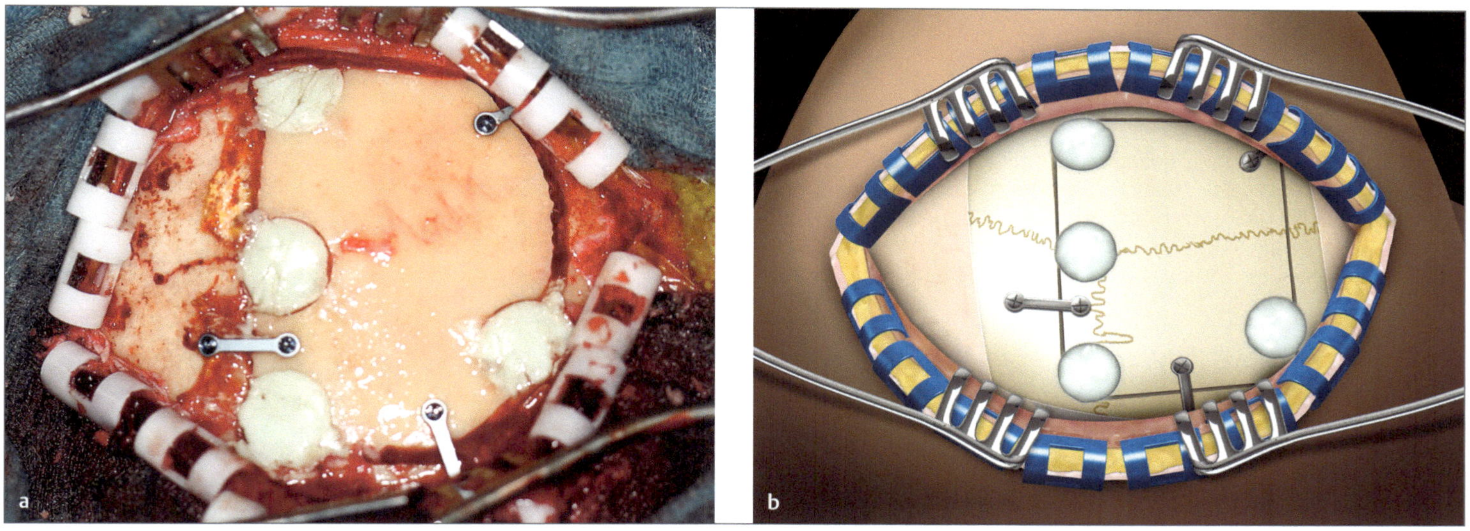

Fig. 4.34 (a, b) Closure: bone flap refixation. Covering the burr holes with, e.g., bone cement or titanium plates for cosmesis is optional. The skin is then closed in a typical two-layer manner. Usually, a subcutaneous drain is inserted.

Checklist

- Pinpoint the midline prior to positioning of the patient.
- Preserve the galea for a potential flap.
- Identify craniometric points for better orientation.
- Use a large craniotome to make burr holes on the sinus.
- Make sure to detach dural adhesions at the rims of the burr hole before performing the craniotomy.
- Never cut toward the sinus.
- Be prepared for potential sinus injury before elevating the bone flap.
- When closing, take care to avoid bony defects. Cover the burr holes in the forehead area for better cosmesis.

Parieto-occipital

Ulrich Sure and Philipp Dammann

See ▶ Fig. 4.35, ▶ Fig. 4.36, ▶ Fig. 4.37, ▶ Fig. 4.38, ▶ Fig. 4.39, ▶ Fig. 4.40, ▶ Fig. 4.41, ▶ Fig. 4.42, ▶ Fig. 4.43, ▶ Fig. 4.44, ▶ Fig. 4.45, ▶ Fig. 4.46, ▶ Fig. 4.47, ▶ Fig. 4.48, and ▶ Fig. 4.49.

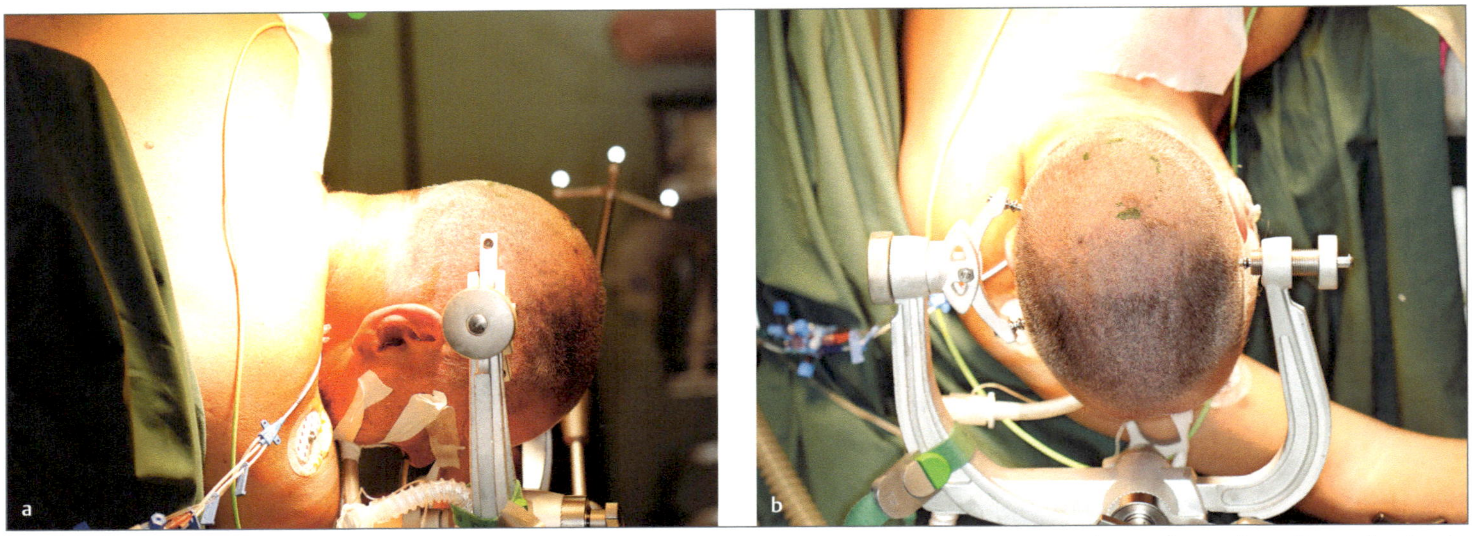

Fig. 4.35 (a, b) Positioning. The parieto-occipital midline approach is used to access structures near, via, or in the interhemispheric fissure, localized in the area of or posterior to the superior parietal lobule. It can be performed in a unilateral or bilateral way. The patient is placed in the lateral or prone position. Normally, the head is rotated to face perpendicularly downward with a slight degree of flexion, depending on the target lesion. Extensive rotation should be avoided to ensure sufficient venous flow and so as not to compromise the jugular veins. At least a finger-sized space should be left between the chin and scapula. Exact localization of the midline prior to draping is crucial.

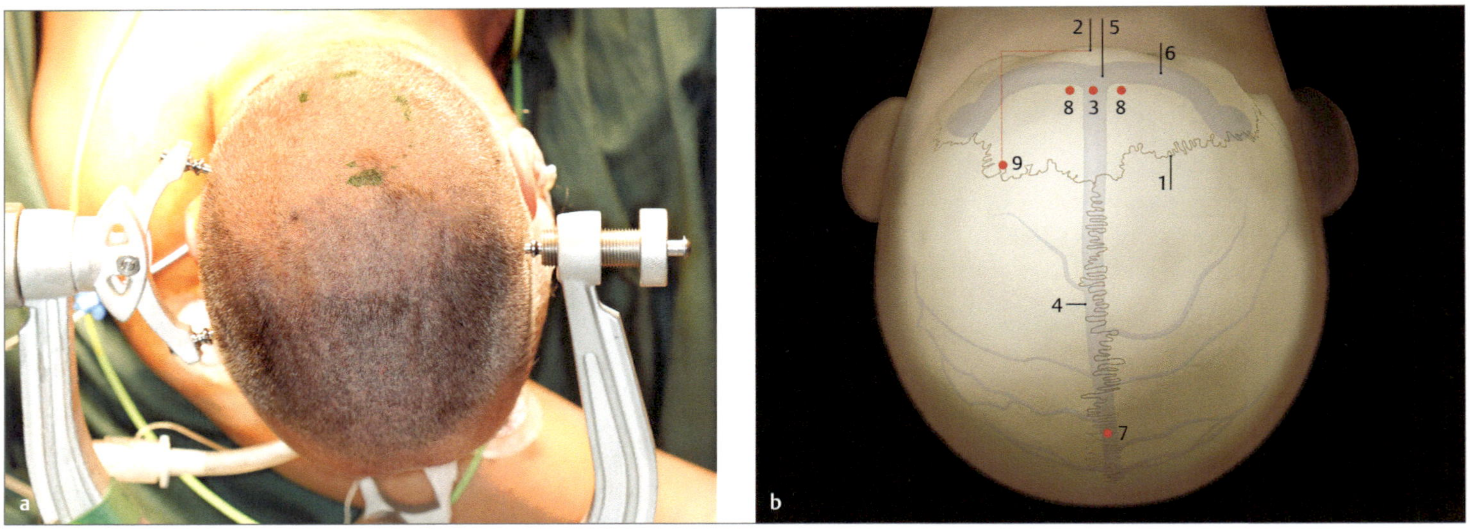

Fig. 4.36 (a, b) Anatomy overview. Important landmarks are (1) lambdoid suture (13 cm posterior to the bregma—usually corresponds with the parieto-occipital sulcus), (2) the inion, (3) the opisthocranion, (4) the superior sagittal sinus, (5) confluence of sinuses (torcular herophili), and (6) the transverse sinus. The surgeon should also be aware of (7) the projection of the central sulcus on the parietal bone (superior margin, superior to the rolandic point, approximately 5 cm posterior to the bregma) and (8) the primary visual cortex on the occipital bone. Another helpful orientation (placement of ventricular catheter) is (9) Frazier's point (6 cm superior to the inion, 3–4 cm lateral to the midline).

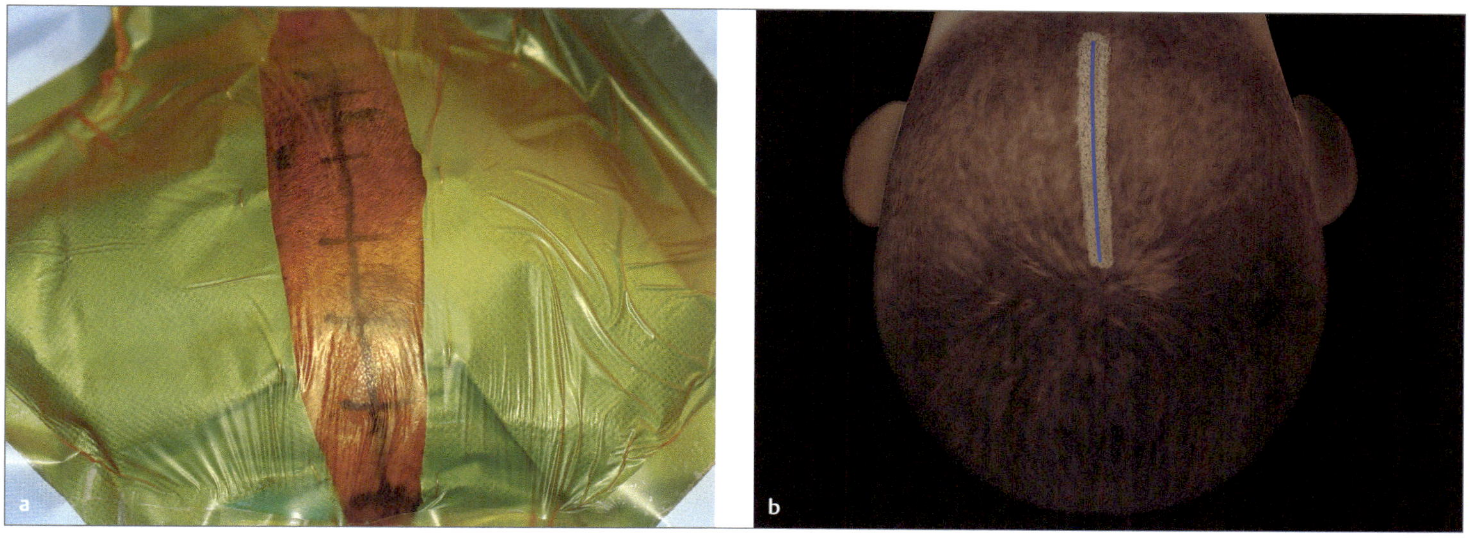

Fig. 4.37 **(a, b) Draped position before skin incision.** The skin incision is made slightly (bilateral or very small craniotomies) or approximately 2 cm parallel (unilateral craniotomies) to the midline. We usually try not to make incisions directly on the midline to avoid placement of all burr holes underneath the skin incision. We nearly always use straight incisions. However, in very large craniotomies, a curved incision with its base directed to the transverse sinus may be suitable. The length and exact position of the incision depends on the planned craniotomy. Usually, we shave the hair 1 cm laterally to the incision in each direction.

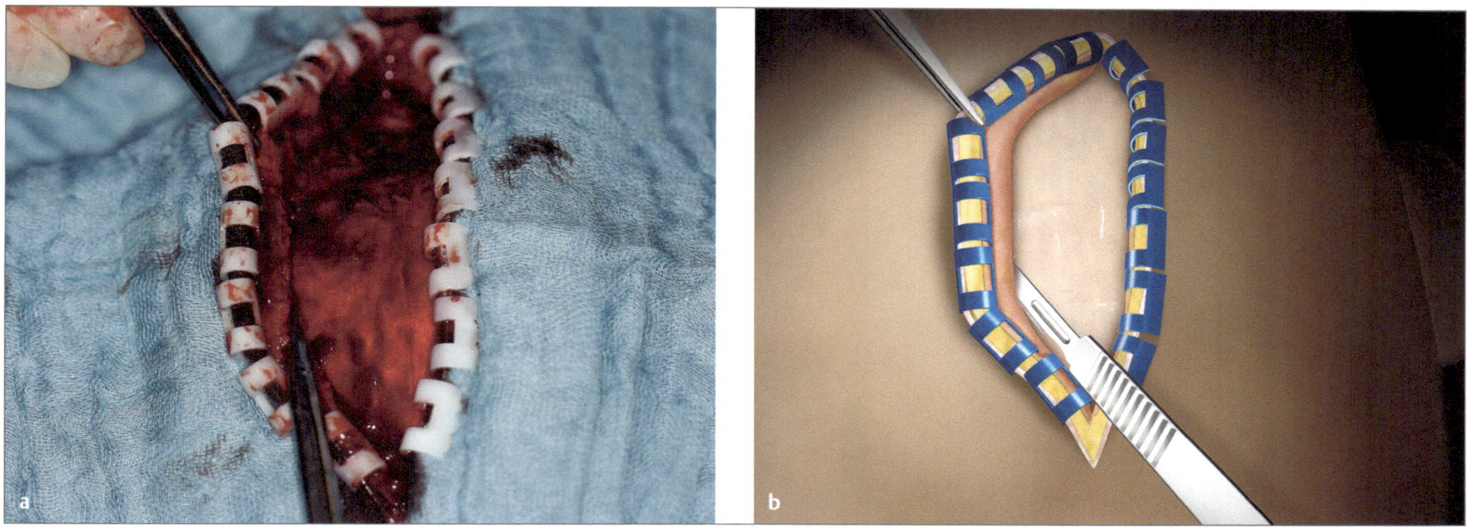

Fig. 4.38 **(a, b) Skin incision.** The skin incision spares the periosteum if a galea flap is desired. In very lateral incisions, larger peripheral branches of the occipital artery (crossing the lambdoid suture 2–4 cm lateral to the midline) may be encountered. After careful (sparing superficial layers of the scalp) coagulation of arterial oozing, bleeding from the scalp is controlled with scalp clips covering the entire length of the incision. To place the scalp clips correctly, the subcutaneous scalp layer has to be sharply dissected from the periosteum bilaterally.

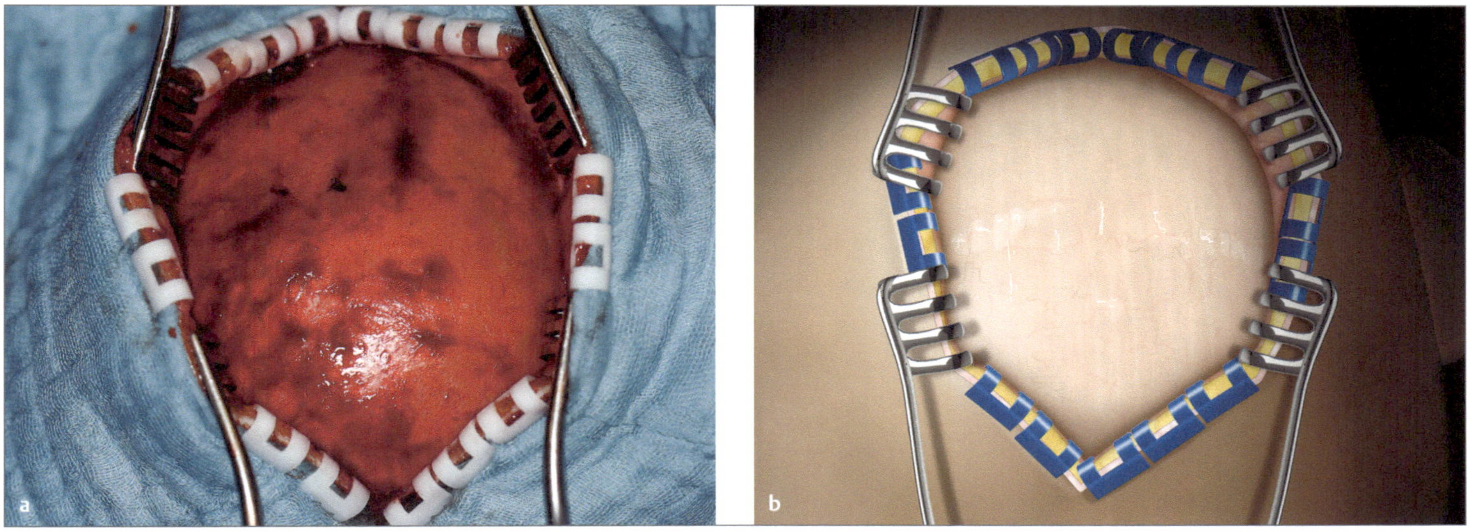

Fig. 4.39 **(a, b) Subgaleal flap preparation.** If a subgaleal flap is desired, the periosteum is incised in a circumferential way after placement of a skin retractor.

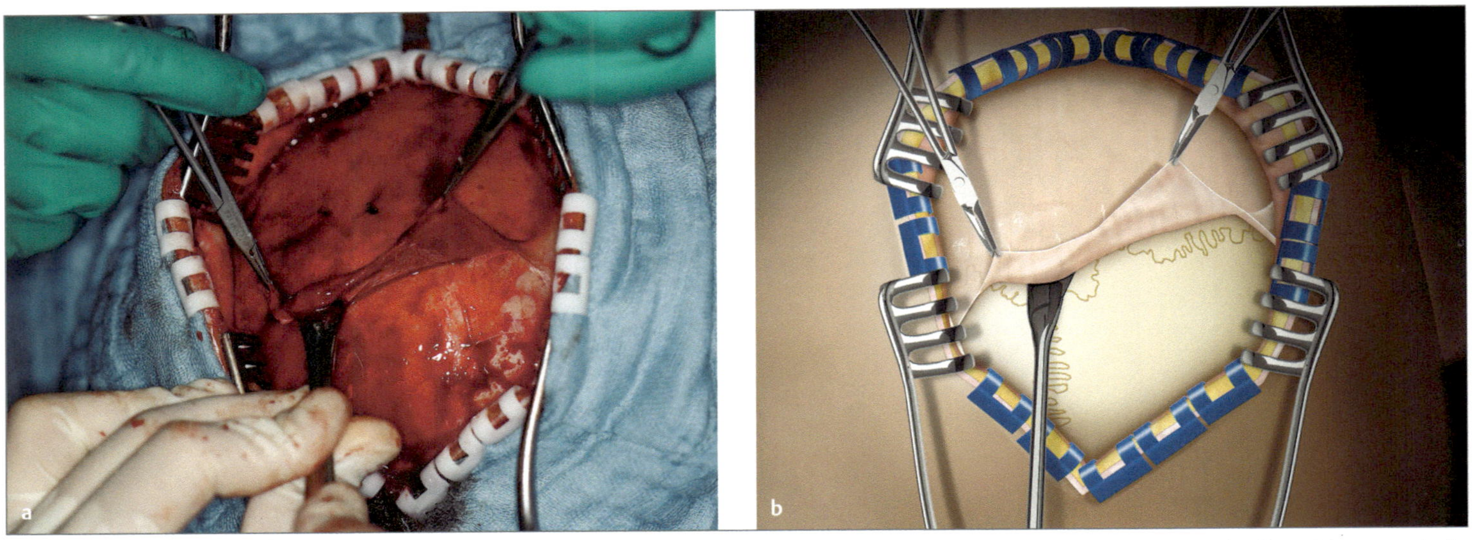

Fig. 4.40 (a, b) Subgaleal flap preparation. The flap is carefully dissected from the bone using a rasp. The assistant retracts the flap with anatomical forceps. The flap has to be preserved in wet surgical cottonoids. During this stage of surgery, the identification of the sutures help to orientate.

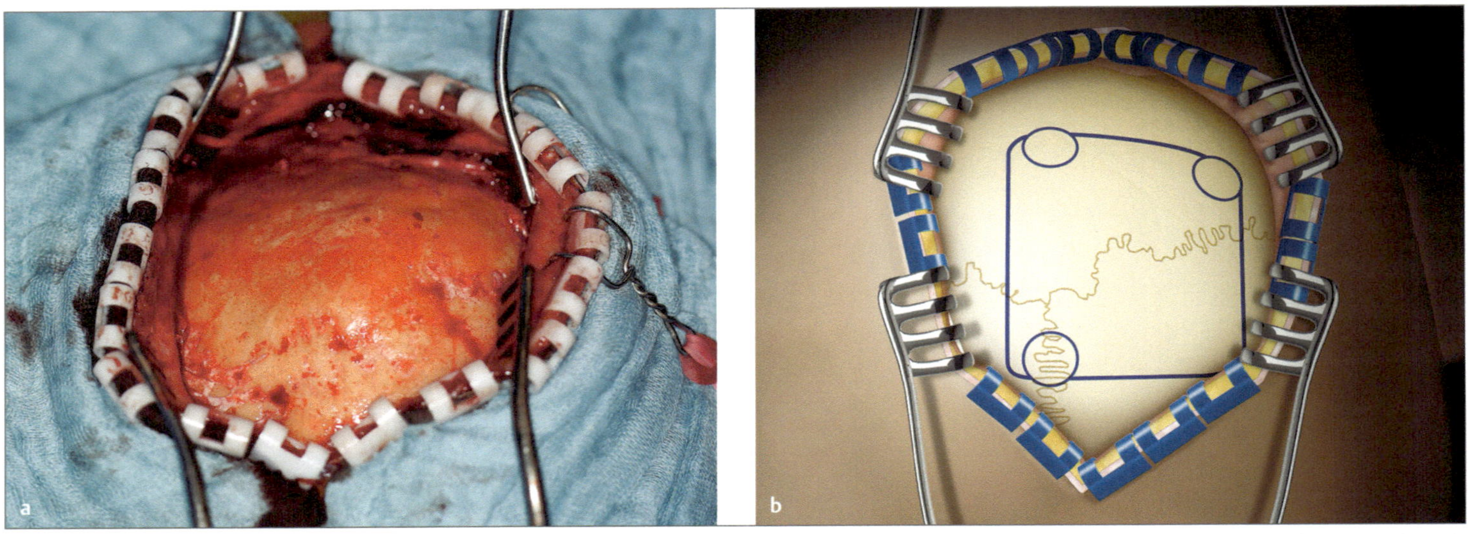

Fig. 4.41 (a, b) Craniotomy planning. The cranial sutures indicate midline structures and intracranial localization of a target lesion (distance inferior/superior to the lambda). The planning of burr hole placement and craniotomy depends on various considerations including target lesion, age of the patient, and previous surgery, among others. For basic principles of the craniotomy, see Chapter 4.1, Sinus-Crossing Craniotomies. In this scenario, two burr holes were made on the sinus. Another may be placed laterally. If the craniotomy extends to the transverse sinus, an additional burr hole should be made on the sinus (inferolateral corner of craniotomy).

Several craniometric points are helpful for orientation. The lambda usually corresponds to the meeting point of the external occipital fissure/parieto-occipital sulcus, indicating the borders of precuneus (parietal) and cuneus (occipital) in the midline. The opisthocranion (approximately 2 cm superior to the inion, 2–4 cm inferior to the lambda) is related to the superior aspect of the calcarine fissure. It divides the occipital cuneus and the occipital lingual gyrus. When interhemispheric approaches are desirable, it is helpful to be aware that fewer bridging veins are encountered inferior to the lambda.

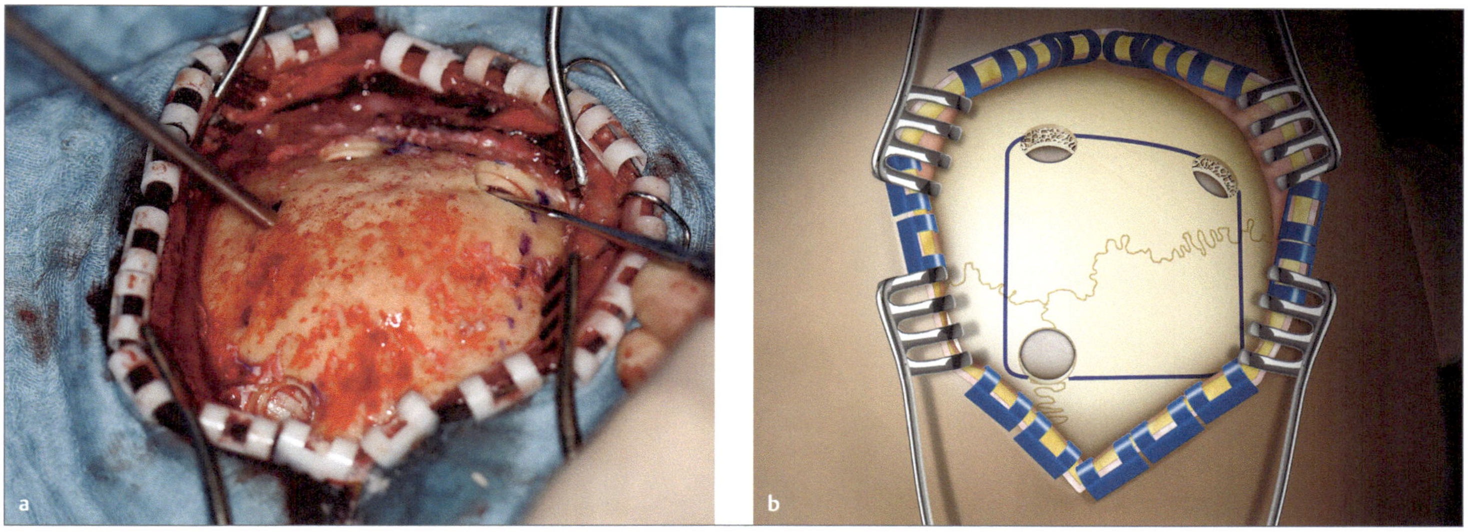

Fig. 4.42 (a, b) Burr holes. The burr holes on the sinus should be drilled with a large trephine (18 mm) to maintain sufficient control. The direction is strictly perpendicular to the skull. Residual bone chips are then removed using a blunt dissector. In cases of dural adhesion to the bone, a small punch sometimes helps to detach the structures and provide an entry for the craniotome. The epidural space is then carefully dissected from the sinus surface using a dissector. If the burr holes are located close enough together, the sinus surface can be detached from the bone along the entire border of the craniotomy.

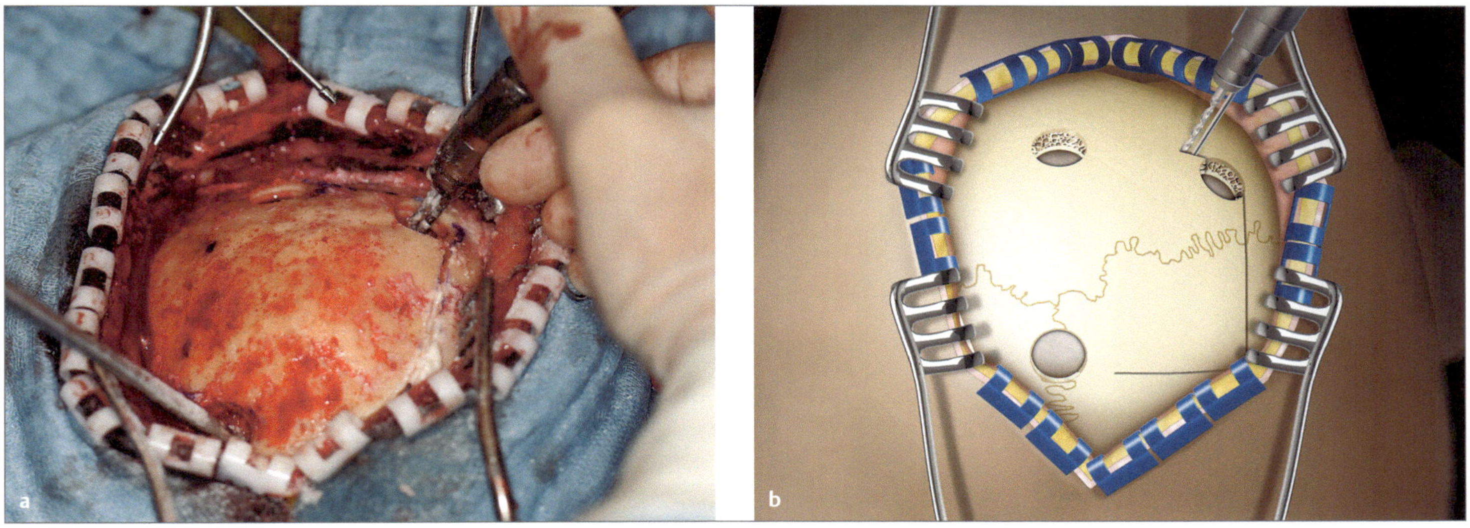

Fig. 4.43 (a, b) Craniotomy. The craniotomy starts at the lateral burr hole reaching medially and stopping approximately 2 cm lateral the sinus. **Caution:** never cut from the lateral direction toward the sinus, because this leads to a much higher risk of injuring the sinus. From the medial burr holes, the craniotomy is then interconnected from medial to lateral. Again, especially for beginners, it may be helpful to outline the planned craniotomy on the bone with a surgical pen.

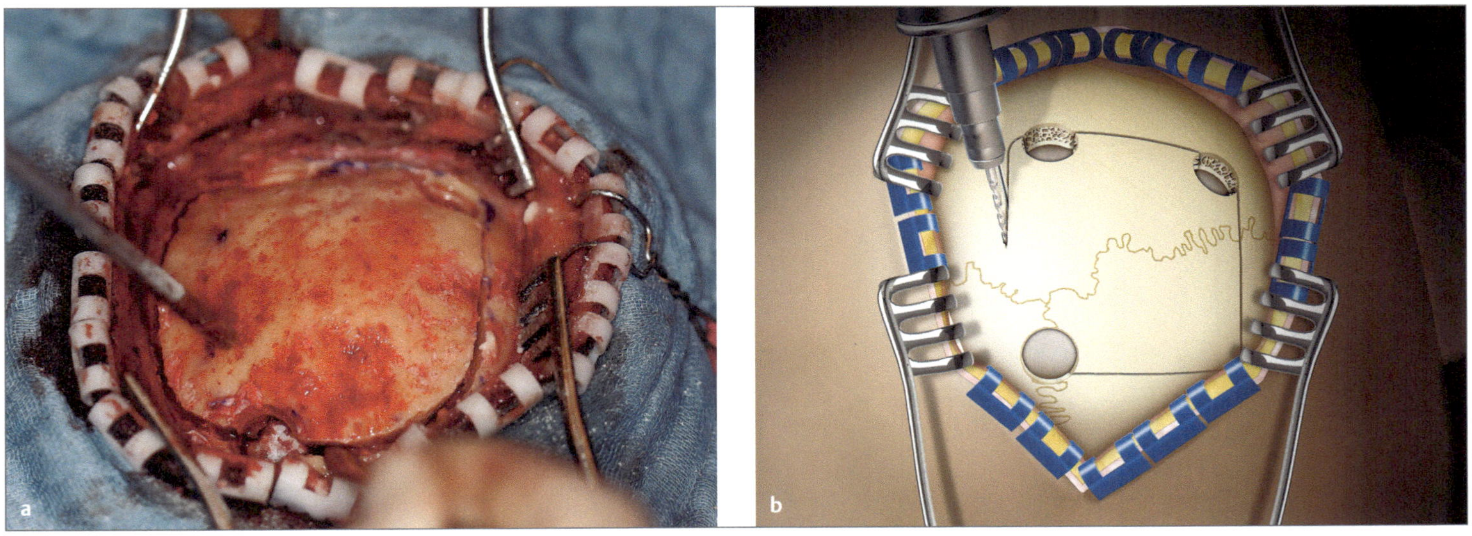

Fig. 4.44 (a, b) Craniotomy. Finally, the craniotomy is extended to the contralateral side, crossing the sinus. The surgeon cuts away from the midline burr hole, at a distance of approximately 1.5 cm parallel to the midline. This is performed from the inferior and superior burr hole with the cuts meeting halfway.

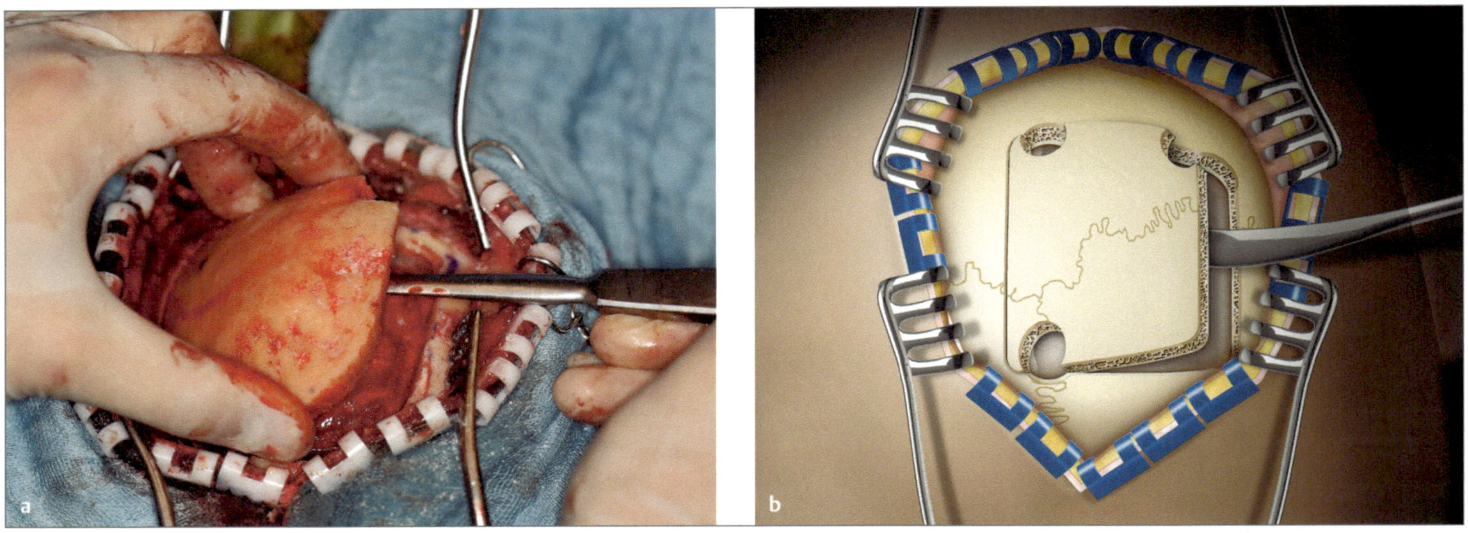

Fig. 4.45 (a, b) **Craniotomy.** After complete circumferential craniotomy, the bone flap is gently removed with an elevator and the dural layer dissected stepwise from the bone. This is performed with particular care in the midline to prevent injury of the sinus. The bone flap should always (!) be secured manually by the assistant or surgeon. During this step the team should be prepared for a possible sinus laceration. If an injury occurs, the sinus is covered with prepared cottonoids before being sutured or sealed with fibrin glue or a hemostasis patch.

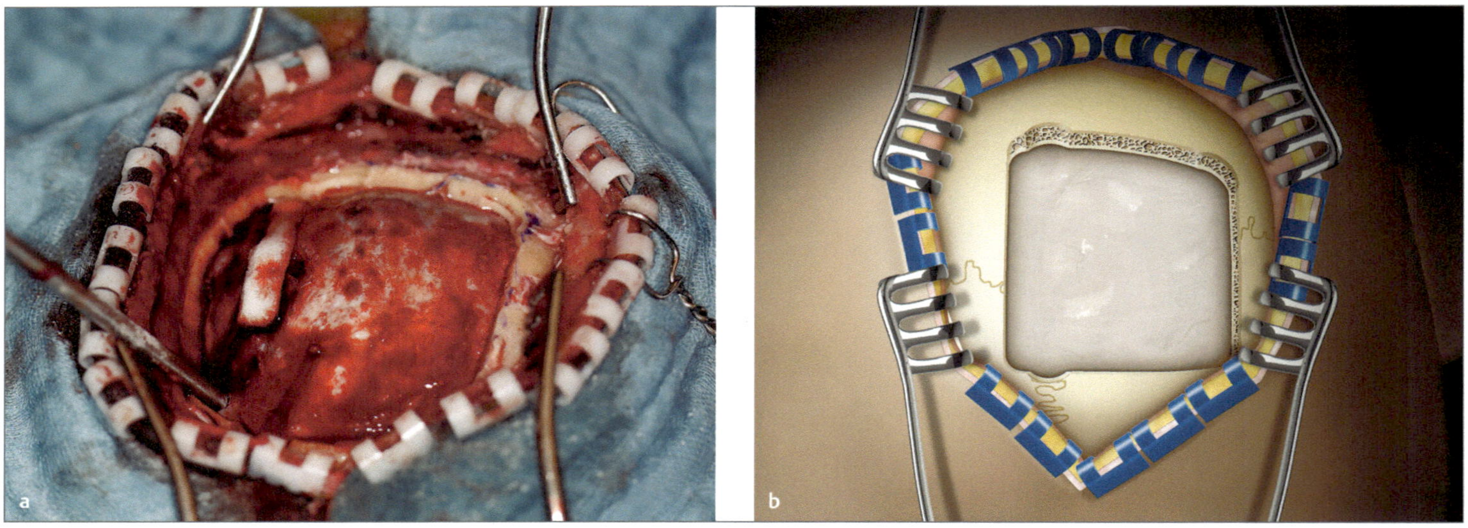

Fig. 4.46 (a, b) **Situs after craniotomy.** Typically, after elevation of the bone flap, some minor venous bleeding occurs in the area of the sagittal sinus from pacchionian granulations. Bleeding can normally be controlled by coagulation and compression with cottonoids. Further bleeding from dural vessels more laterally should also be coagulated. The whole situs then has to be meticulously cleared of bone dust using irrigation.

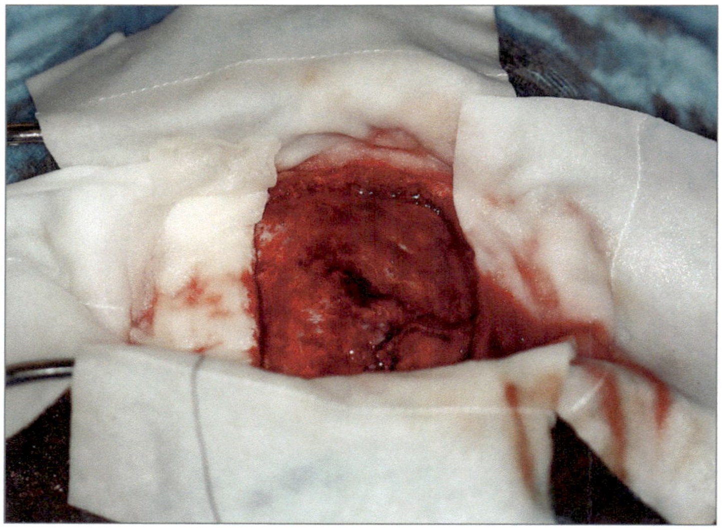

Fig. 4.47 **Situs after craniotomy.** Particularly in deep-seated lesions or complex bridging vein anatomy, additional verification of the planned trajectory and interhemispheric approach is helpful at this stage of surgery (using neuronavigation or ultrasound).

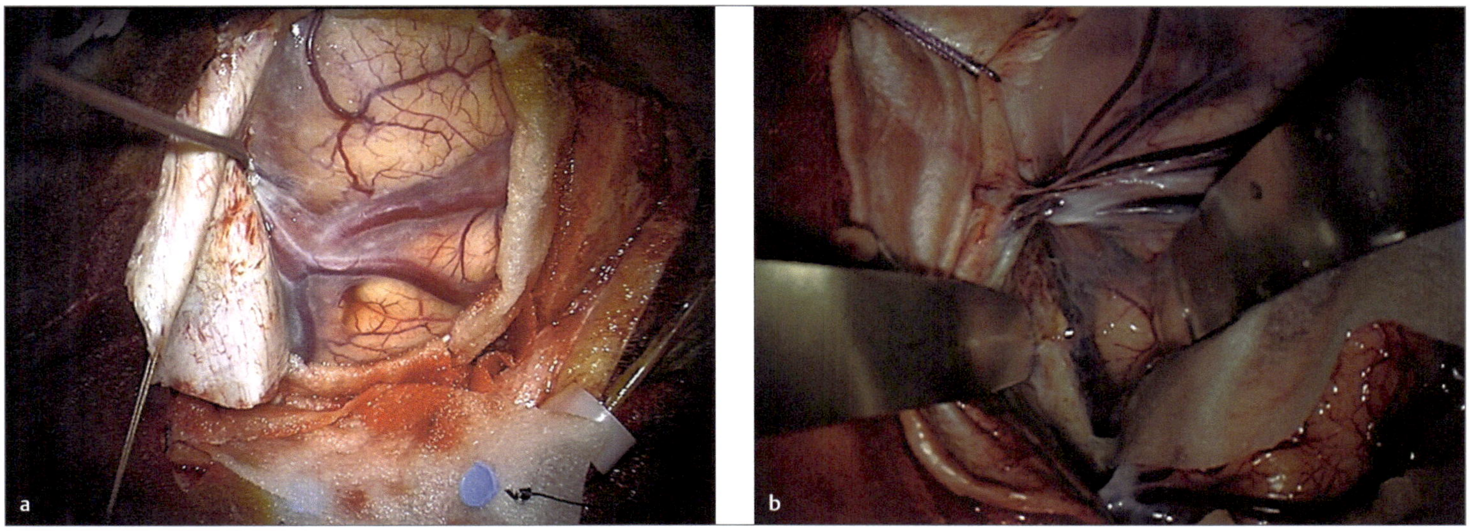

Fig. 4.48 (a, b) Dura opening. After placing surgical cotton around the circumference to protect the brain tissue, the dura is opened with the base at the sagittal sinus. Injury of bridging veins, whose position should already be known from preoperative imaging, must be avoided at all costs. Sometimes, small lacunae of the sinus extend laterally. If injured, these can be easily closed using small clips or sutures. Stitches to the dura lateral to the sinus or in the falx inferior of the sinus can be used to gently retract the falx and sinus contralaterally to enable better access to the interhemispheric fissure.

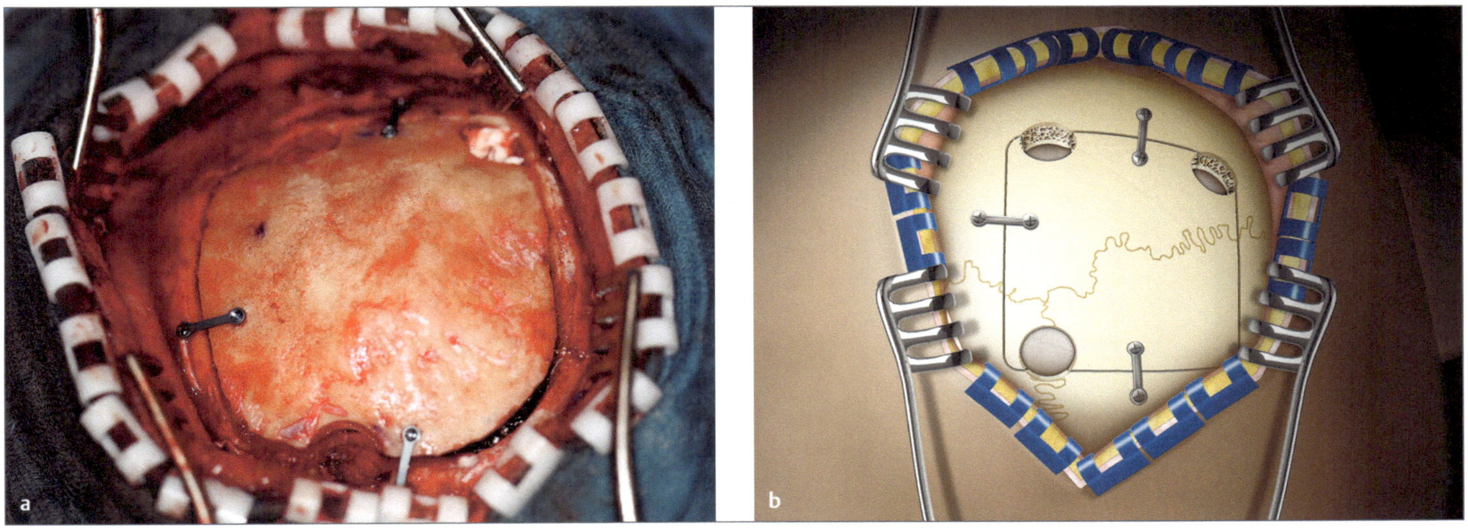

Fig. 4.49 (a, b) Closure: bone flap refixation and skin closure. The bone flap is fixed to the skull using titanium mini-plates with roughly 120° distance between them. The burr holes are covered with a burr hole mini-plate or filled with bone cement. The skin is then closed in a typical two-layer manner. Usually, a subcutaneous drain is inserted.

Checklist

- Avoid incision directly on the midline.
- Anticipate localization of visual cortex.
- Remember that there are fewer bridging veins inferior to the lambda.
- Always be prepared for potential sinus laceration.

4.3 Infratentorial Midline Craniotomy

Infratentorial Supracerebellar

Ulrich Sure and Philipp Dammann

See ► Fig. 4.50, ► Fig. 4.51, ► Fig. 4.52, ► Fig. 4.53, ► Fig. 4.54, ► Fig. 4.55, ► Fig. 4.56, ► Fig. 4.57, ► Fig. 4.58, ► Fig. 4.59, ► Fig. 4.60, and ► Fig. 4.61.

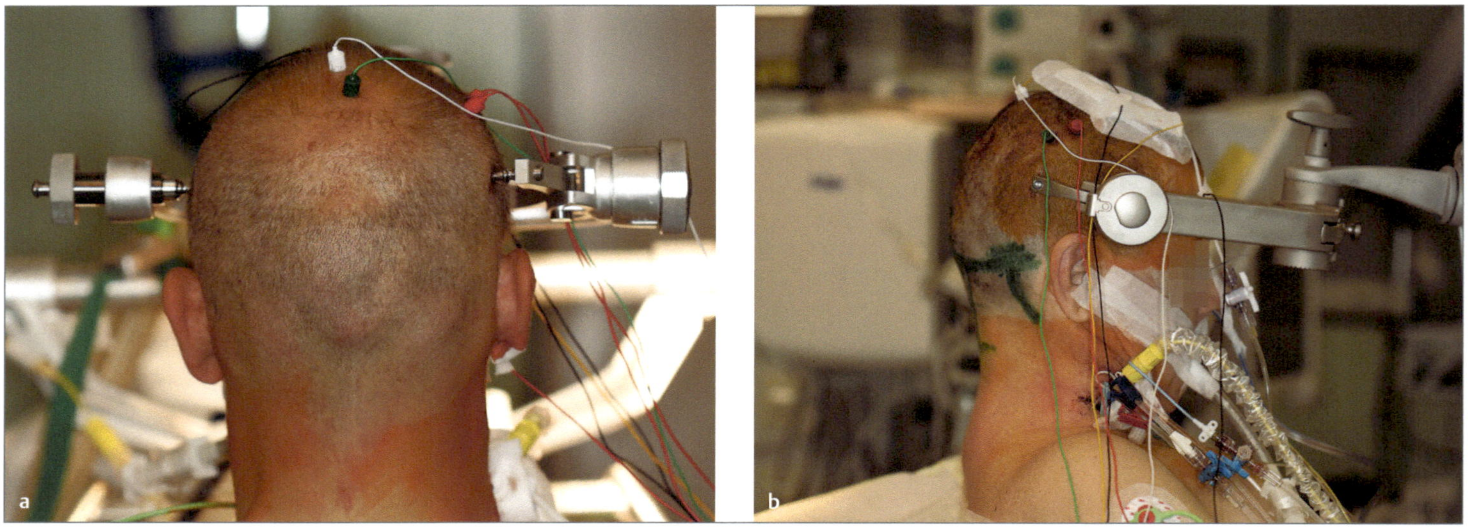

Fig. 4.50 (a, b) Positioning. The infratentorial supracerebellar approach is used for lesions of the pineal region, cerebellum, or tentorium. We always perform this operation with the patient in a semisitting position. Prone or lateral positioning is an alternative. The head is straight—no rotation, no tilting, but significant flexion. Flexion should be carried out with extra care in patients with degenerative disease of the cervical spine. Between the chin and jugulum, a space of at least a finger's width should be left (to avoid bruising of the skin and impairment of venous drainage).

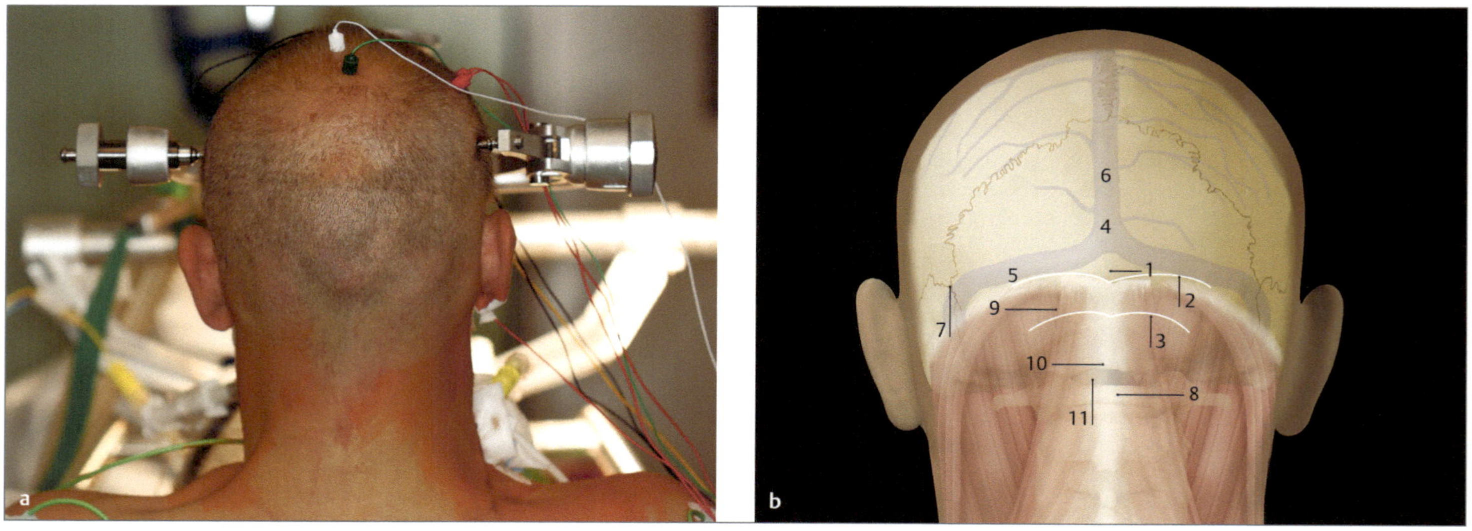

Fig. 4.51 (a, b) Anatomy overview. Important landmarks are (1) inion, (2) superior nuchal line (normally palpable), (3) inferior nuchal line, (4) confluence of sinuses, (5) transverse sinus, (6) sagittal sinus, (7) asterion, (8) C1, (9) nuchal musculature, (10) nuchal ligament (inion to C7), and (11) foramen magnum. It is important to correctly identify the midline for skin incision. Slight tilting or rotation of the head can significantly displace the nuchal ligament.

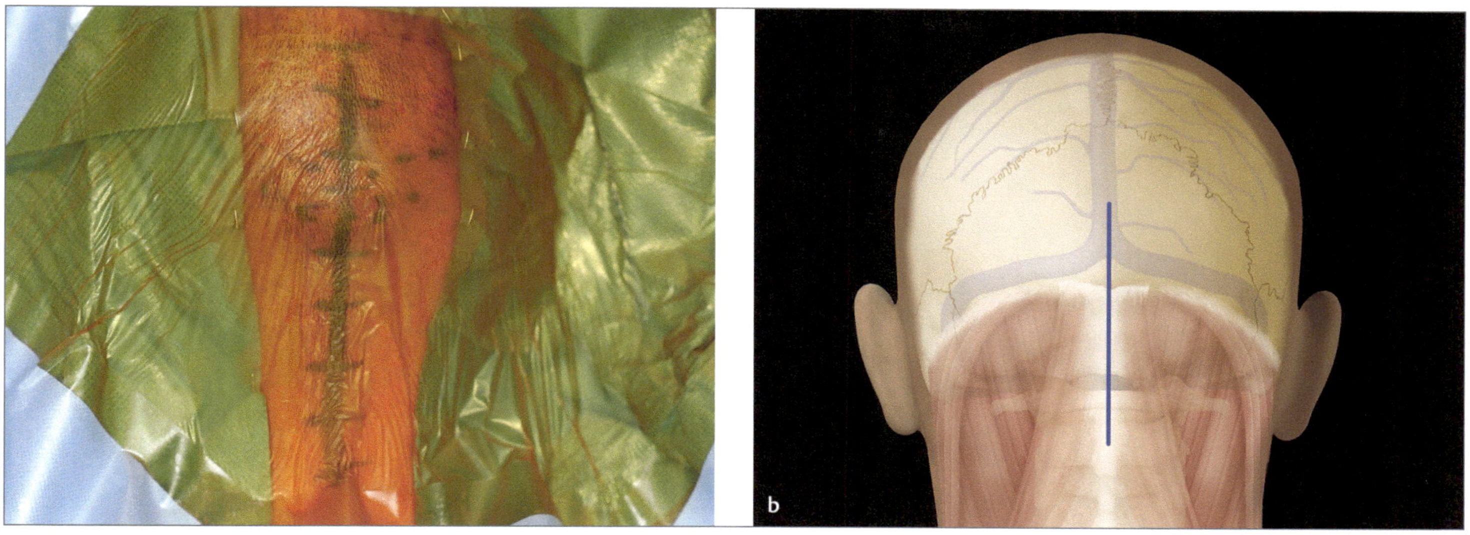

Fig. 4.52 (a, b) Draped position before skin incision. The skin incision ranges from 2–3 cm superior to the inion to the level of C2. In patients with very strong nuchal musculature, the incision may be extended inferiorly (retraction).

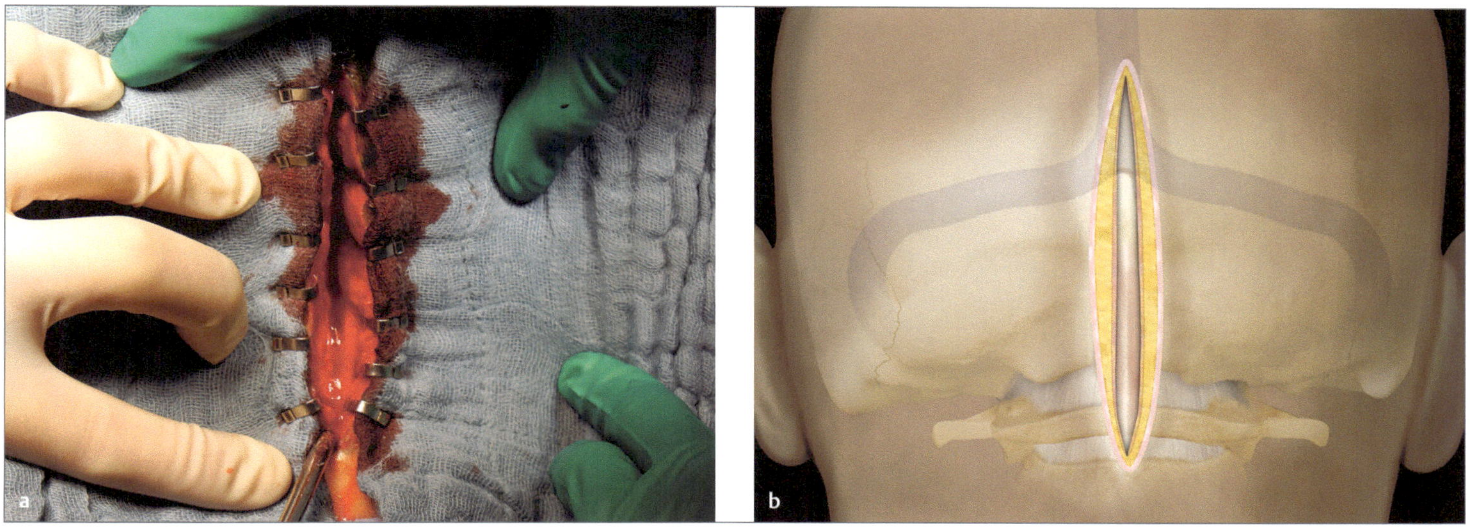

Fig. 4.53 (a, b) Skin incision. The skin incision spares the nuchal ligament. After coagulation of arterial oozing, any further bleeding from the scalp is controlled with scalp clips covering the entire length of the incision. To place the scalp clips correctly, the subcutaneous scalp layer has to be sharply dissected from the nuchal ligament and fascia of the trapezius muscle.

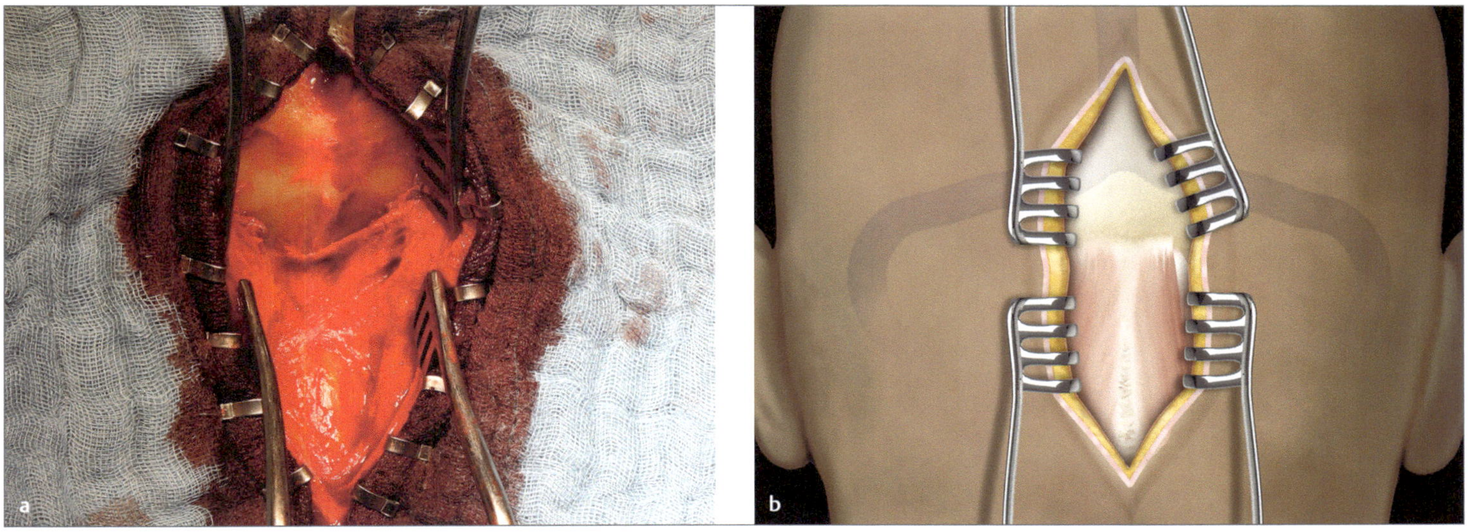

Fig. 4.54 (a, b) Nuchal ligament incision. The nuchal ligament is followed through the muscle layers taking care to stay in the midline until the suboccipital surface is reached. In this zone, bleeding is minimal and muscle integrity is preserved. The retractor is repositioned stepwise until all muscle layers are lateralized. Muscle attachments to the inion are sharply dissected (a small stub may be left for later reattachment if desired). Muscle attachments to the occiput are dissected using a raspatorium monopolar knife. Exposure of the subocciput depends on the desired size of the craniotomy. For a standard infratentorial suboccipital approach, the craniotomy extends 1 cm superior to the inion and does not go beyond the inferior nuchal line. Normally, the widest lateral exposure is needed at the level of the transverse sinus.

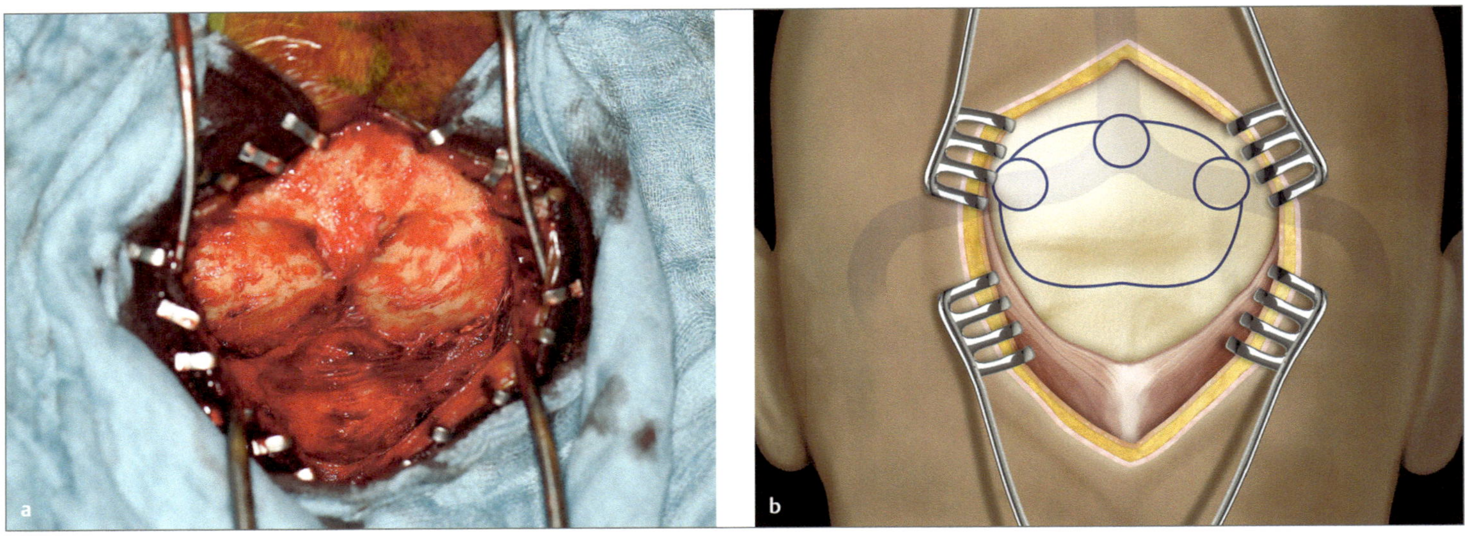

Fig. 4.55 (a, b) Craniotomy planning. We prefer to make two burr holes laterally on the predicted position of the transverse sinus and—especially in older patients with adherent dura mater—one burr hole on the superior sagittal sinus just above the inion. A fourth burr hole central on the inferior nuchal line is optional. At least on one side, the craniotomy is extended as far laterally as possible. This is to provide paramedian access above the cerebellum, as the trajectory to the pineal region is steepest in the midline.

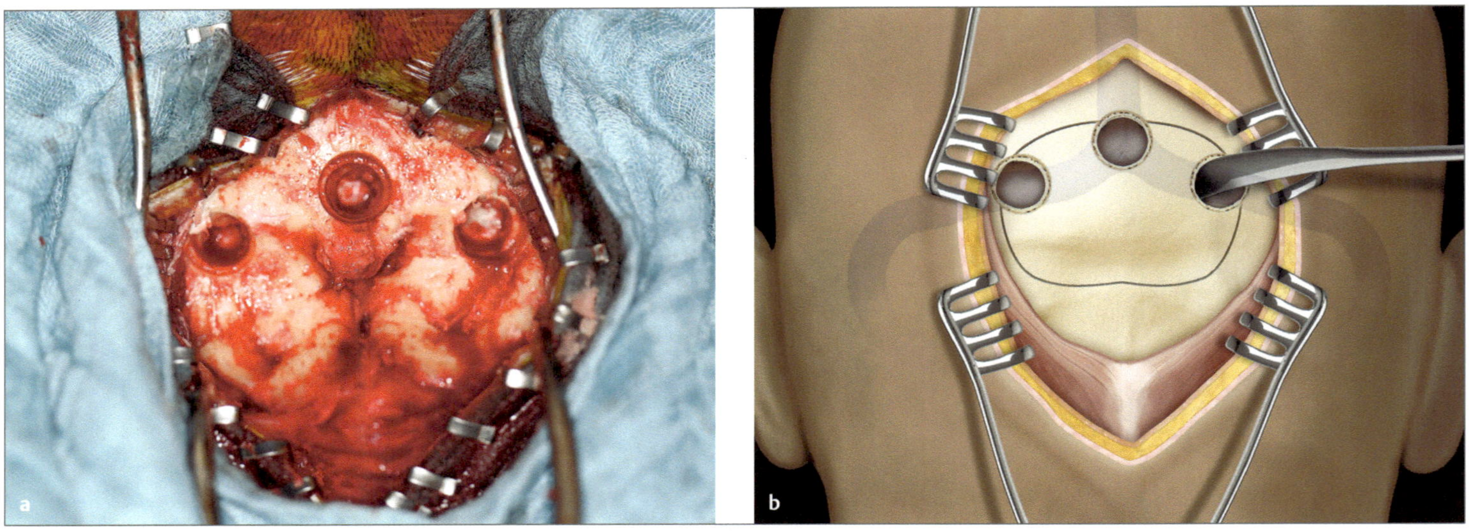

Fig. 4.56 (a, b) Burr holes. The burr holes on the sinuses should be drilled with large trephine (18 mm). The direction is strictly perpendicular to the skull. Residual bone chips should then be removed using a blunt dissector or nerve hook. If the dura adheres to the bone, a small punch sometimes helps to detach the structures and provide an entry point for the craniotome.

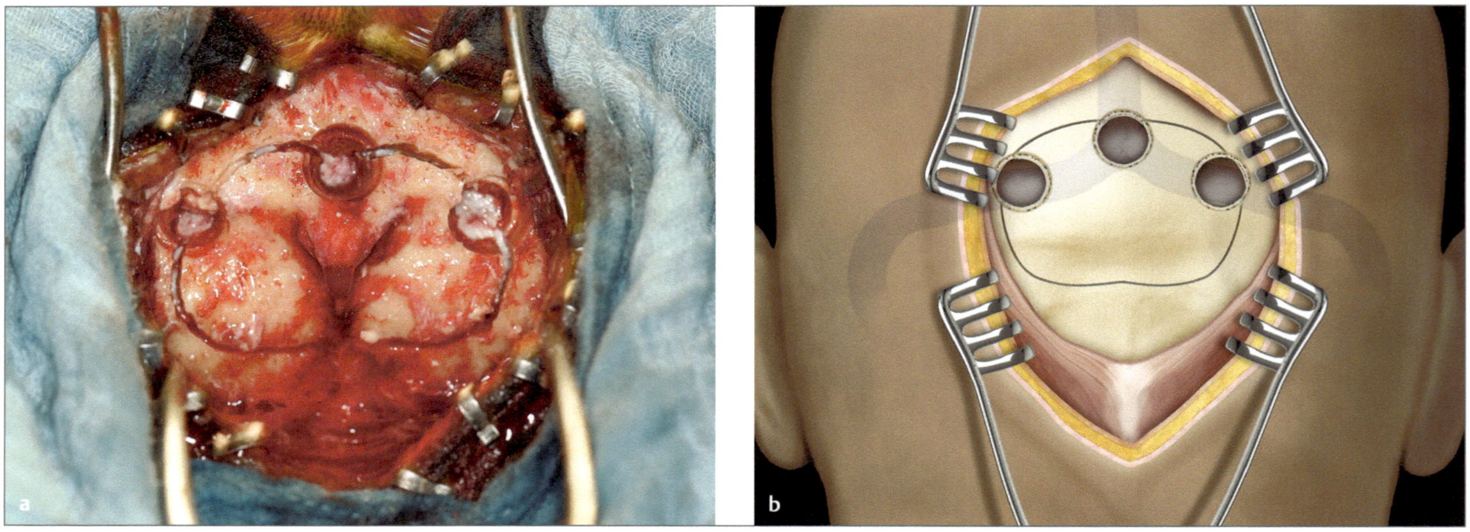

Fig. 4.57 (a, b) Craniotomy. The craniotomy is performed by connecting all the burr holes and creating an ellipsoid bone flap. First, the inferior borders of the craniotomy are cut, directing away from the sinus. Secondly, the superior borders are cut, interconnecting the three burr holes, again moving away from the sinuses. The assistant uses the flush to cool the craniotome and tissue structures and the sucker to provide optimal visibility for the surgeon.

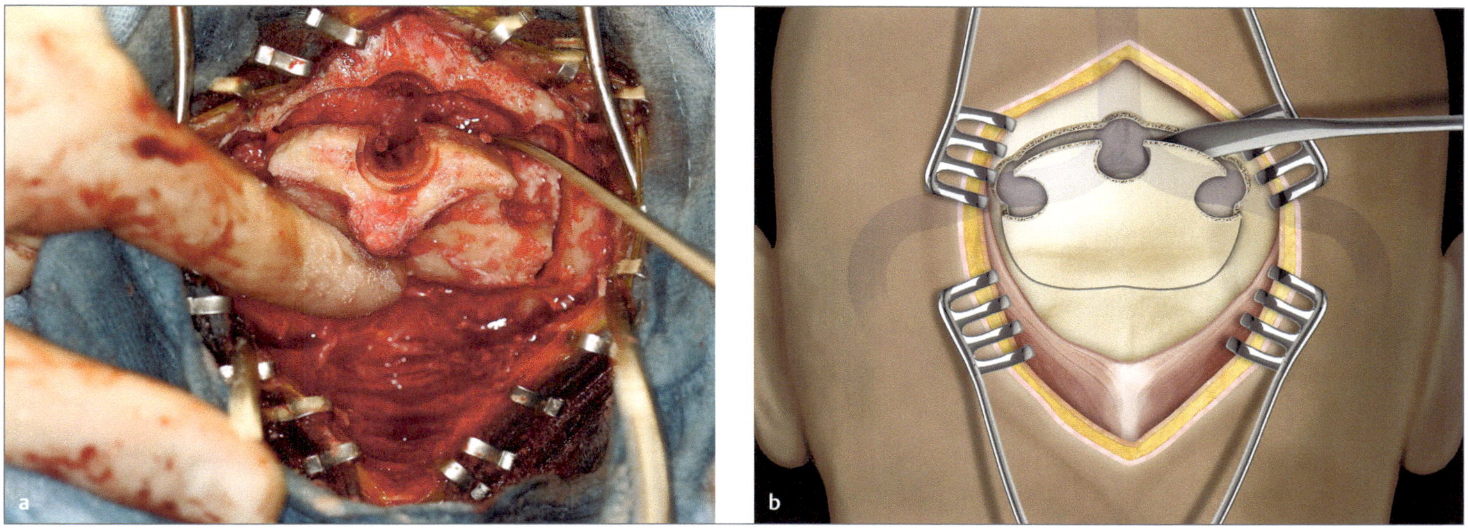

Fig. 4.58 (a, b) **Craniotomy.** After complete circumferential craniotomy, the bone flap is gently elevated with an elevator and the dural layer dissected from the bone in a stepwise manner. This requires special attention in the area of the transverse and sagittal sinus to prevent injury of the sinus. The bone flap should always be secured manually by the assistant or surgeon. While performing this step, the team should be prepared for a potential sinus laceration. If an injury does occur, the sinus is covered with prepared cottonoids before the injury is sealed with fibrin glue, a hemostasis patch, or sutured.

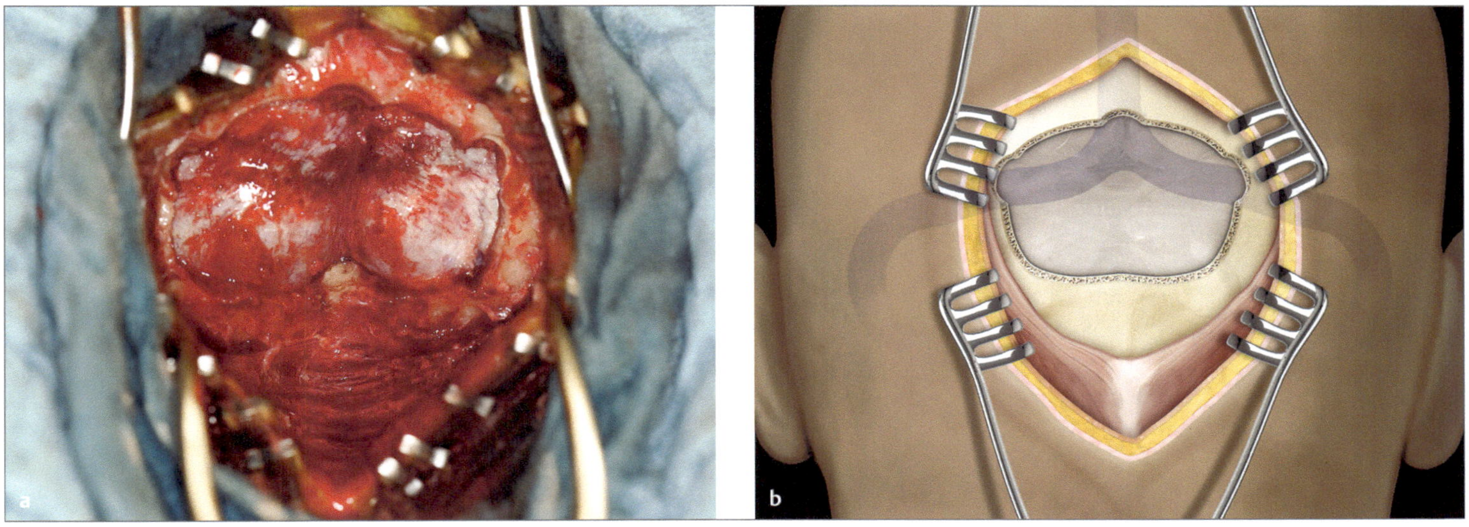

Fig. 4.59 (a, b) **Situs after craniotomy.** Typically, some dural bleeding will occur after elevation of the bone flap. This can be controlled by coagulation. The whole site then has to be meticulously cleared of bone dust using irrigation. The sinus surface is covered with a hemostasis patch and surgical cottonoids.

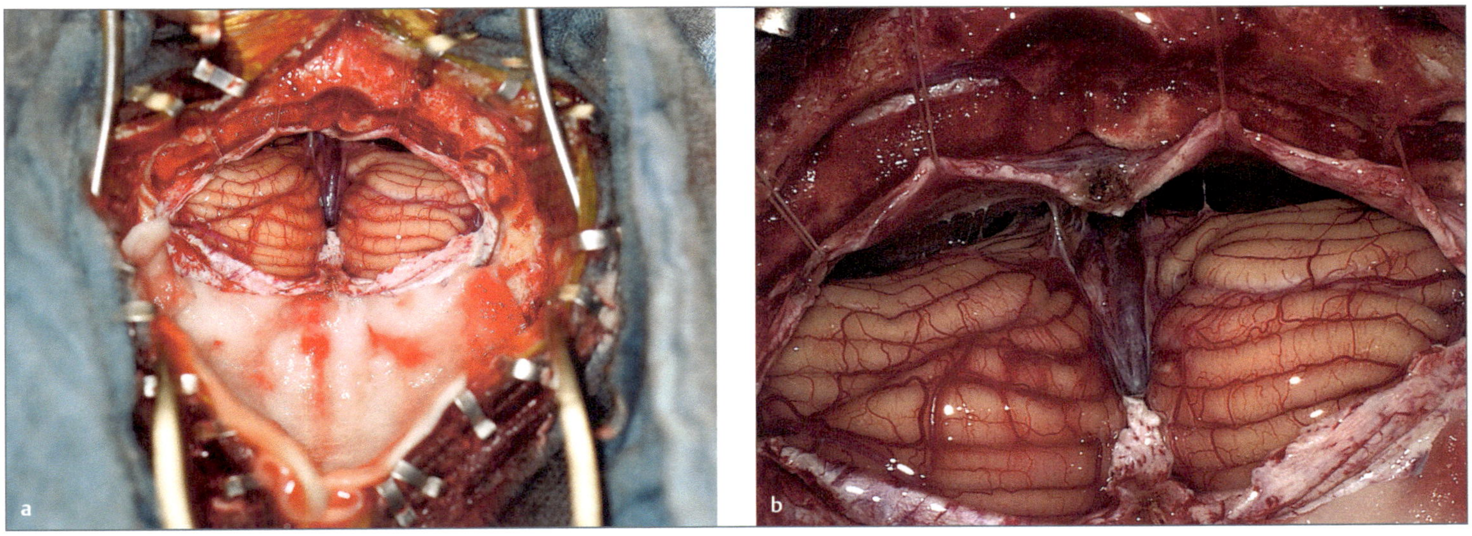

Fig. 4.60 (a, b) **Dura opening.** A large bilateral incision of the dura is shown here. The dura is opened parallel to the transverse sinus in a slightly curved fashion. The (sometimes present) suboccipital sinus is ligated proximally and distally where the incision crosses the midline. Stitches to the dura at the inferior borders are attached to skin or previously drilled holes in the occiput to gently retract the dura and transverse sinus and expose the supracerebellar trajectory.

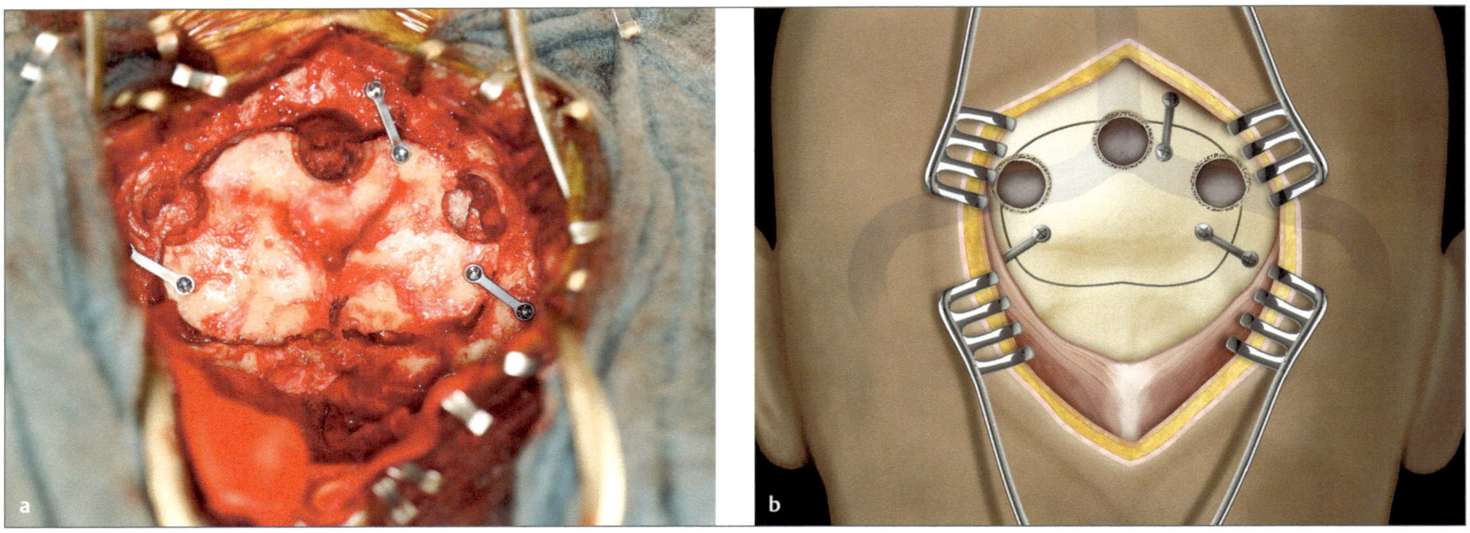

Fig. 4.61 (a, b) Closure: bone flap refixation. The bone flap is fixed to the skull using titanium mini-plates with a distance of roughly 120° between the plates. Try to avoid placing material directly underneath the skin incision. The muscles are closed in two layers in typical manner using single sutures (spaced about 1 cm apart). The skin is also closed in a typical manner using subcutaneous sutures (spaced about 1 cm apart) and a running or single skin suture.

Checklist

- Avoid tilting and rotating of the head so as not to displace the nuchal ligament.
- Use a large craniotome to make burr holes on the sinus.
- Be prepared for potential sinus injury prior to elevation of the bone flap.
- Make sure to extend the craniotomy far enough laterally if the tentorium is very steep (to access pineal region).

Median Suboccipital (Involving Foramen Magnum)

Ulrich Sure and Philipp Dammann

See ▶ Fig. 4.62, ▶ Fig. 4.63, ▶ Fig. 4.64, ▶ Fig. 4.65, ▶ Fig. 4.66, ▶ Fig. 4.67, ▶ Fig. 4.68, ▶ Fig. 4.69, ▶ Fig. 4.70, ▶ Fig. 4.71, ▶ Fig. 4.72, and ▶ Fig. 4.73.

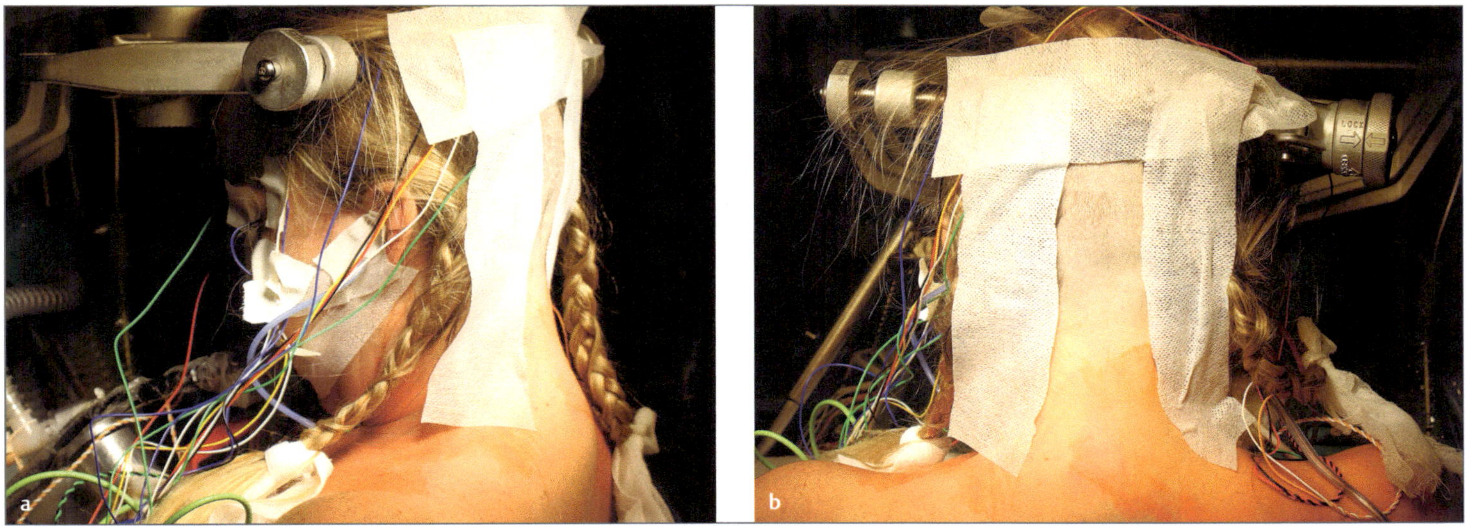

Fig. 4.62 (a, b) Positioning. The suboccipital bihemispheric midline approach (including or excluding foramen magnum access) is used to approach midline lesions of the cerebellum or lesions of the fourth ventricle or medulla oblongata. It can be performed with the patient in the prone or semisitting position. Both positions have specific pros and cons. We prefer the semisitting position. The head is straight, with no rotation and no tilting, but significant flexion. Careful flexion is necessary in patients with degenerative disease of the cervical spine. At least a finger-sized space should be left between the chin and jugulum (to avoid skin bruising and compromised venous drainage).

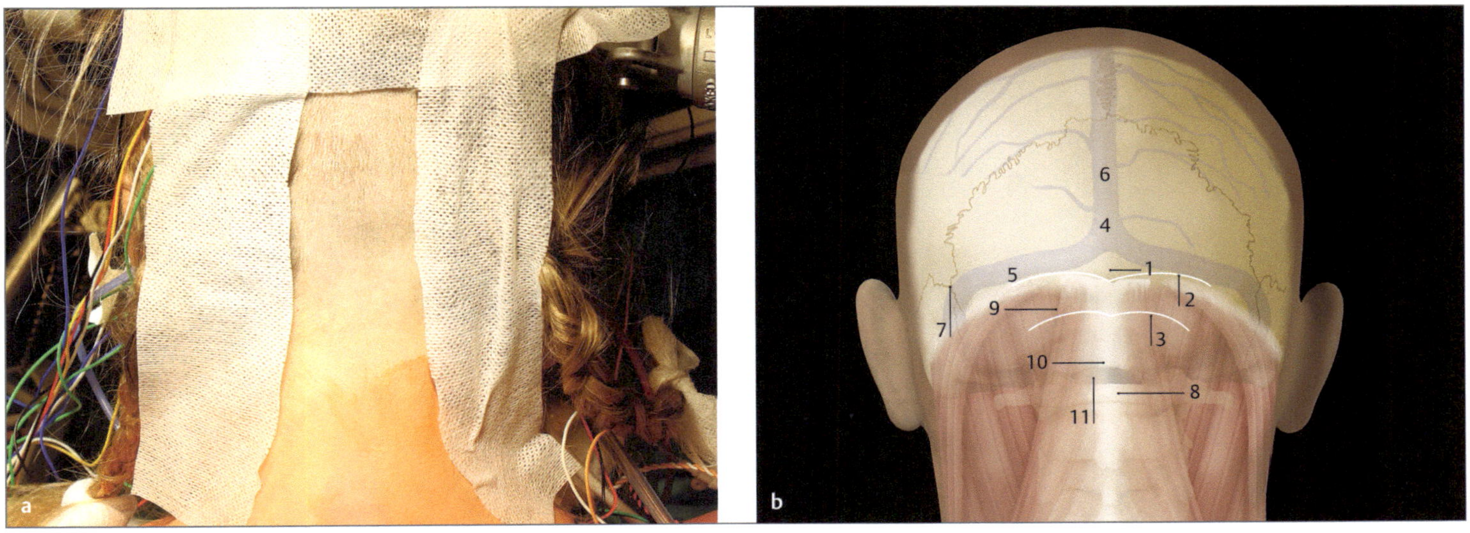

Fig. 4.63 (a, b) Anatomy overview. Important landmarks are (1) inion, (2) superior nuchal line (normally palpable), (3) inferior nuchal line, (4) confluence of sinuses, (5) transverse sinus, (6) sagittal sinus, (7) asterion, (8) posterior arch of C1, (9) nuchal musculature, (10) nuchal ligament (inion to C7), and (11) foramen magnum. It is crucial to correctly identify the midline for skin incision. Note that slight tilting or rotation of the head can significantly displace the nuchal ligament.

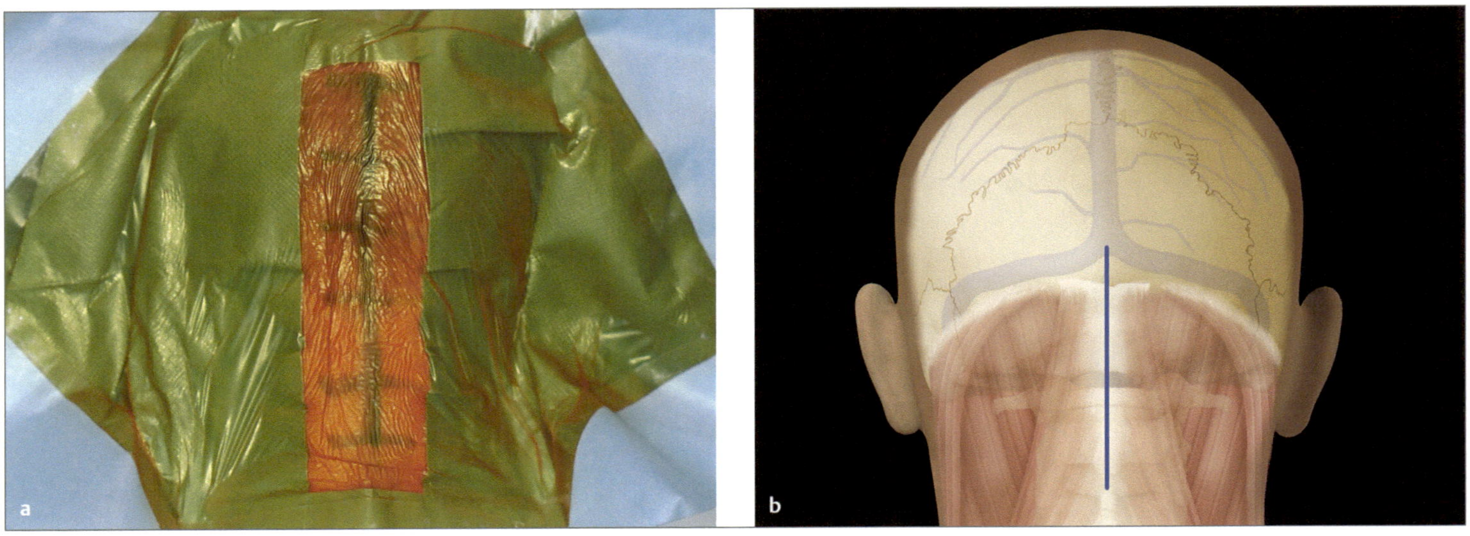

Fig. 4.64 (a, b) Draped position before skin incision. The skin incision extends from 1 cm superior to the inion to the level of C3 (C5 if the foramen magnum is approached). If the nuchal musculature is very strong, the incision may be extended inferiorly (retraction). In **b**, the head is flexed as described in ▶ Fig. 4.62.

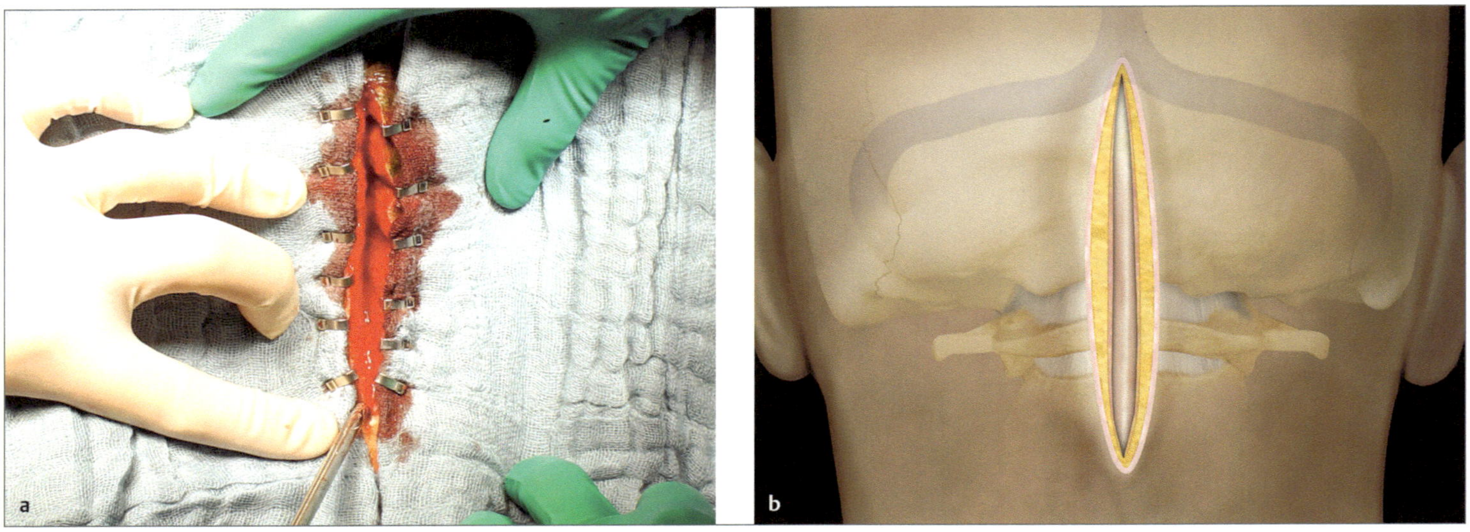

Fig. 4.65 (a, b) Skin incision. The skin incision spares the nuchal ligament. After careful coagulation of arterial oozing, bleeding from the scalp is controlled with scalp clips covering the entire length of the incision. To place the scalp clips properly, the subcutaneous scalp layer has to be sharply dissected from the nuchal ligament and fascia of the trapezius muscle.

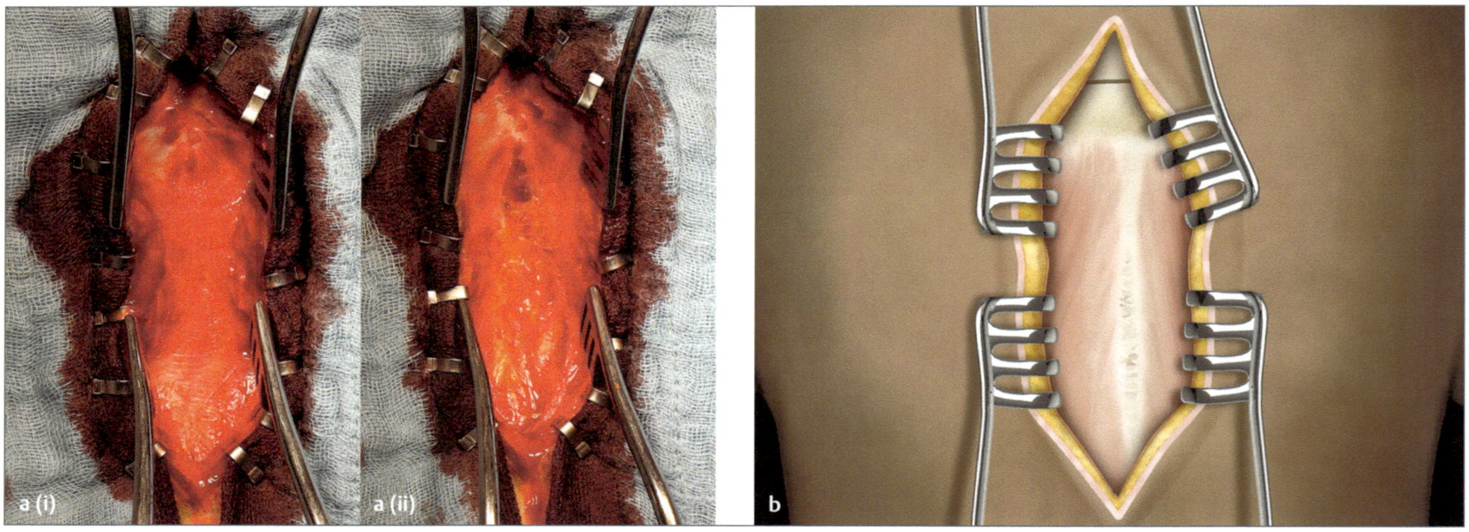

Fig. 4.66 (a, b) Nuchal ligament incision. The nuchal ligament is followed through the muscle layers taking care to stay in the midline until you reach the suboccipital surface and arch of C1 (the spinous process of C2 is palpable early during dissection and serves as a landmark for C1). In this zone, bleeding is minimal and muscle integrity is preserved. The retractor is repositioned stepwise until all muscle layers are lateralized. Muscle attachments to the inion are sharply dissected (a small stub for later reattachment can be left if desired). Muscle attachments to the subocciput are dissected using a rasp. Exposure of the suboccipital bone depends on the desired size of the craniotomy. Normally, the widest exposure is needed between the superior and inferior nuchal line.

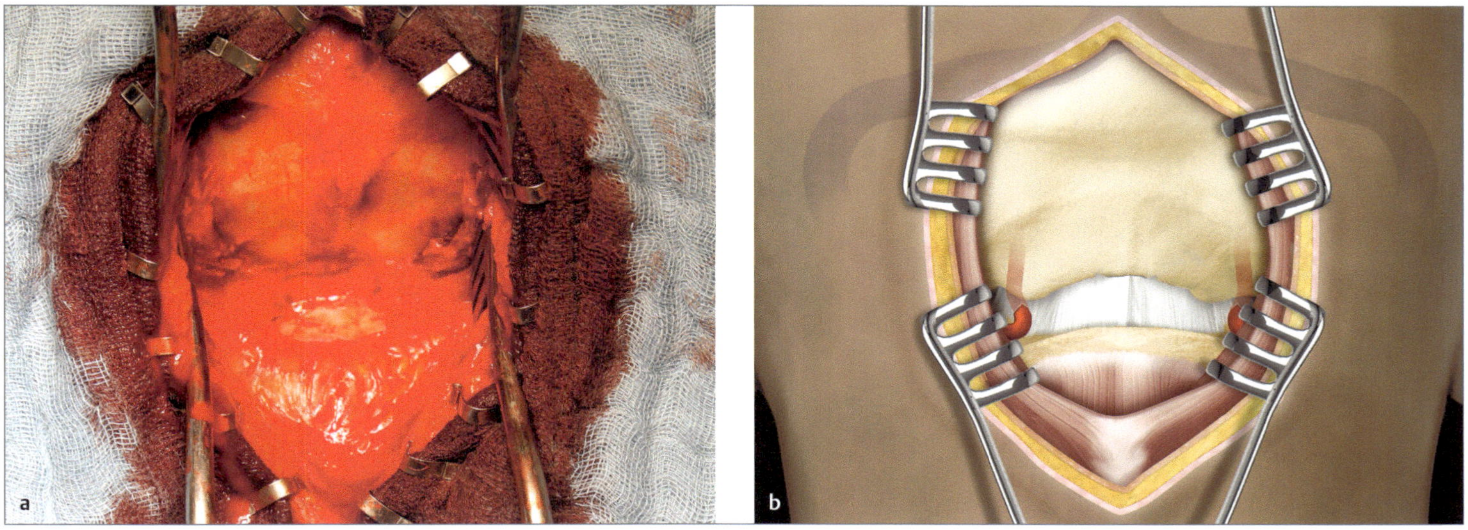

Fig. 4.67 **(a, b) Exposure of C1 arch.** Upon reaching the C1 arch in the midline, a finger rasp is used to detach the rectus capitis posterior minor muscle and parts of the posterior atlanto-occipital membrane: 15 mm lateral exposure is normally safe (the course of the vertebral artery must be checked preoperatively). For craniotomies not involving the foramen magnum, the exposure of C1 is not necessary.

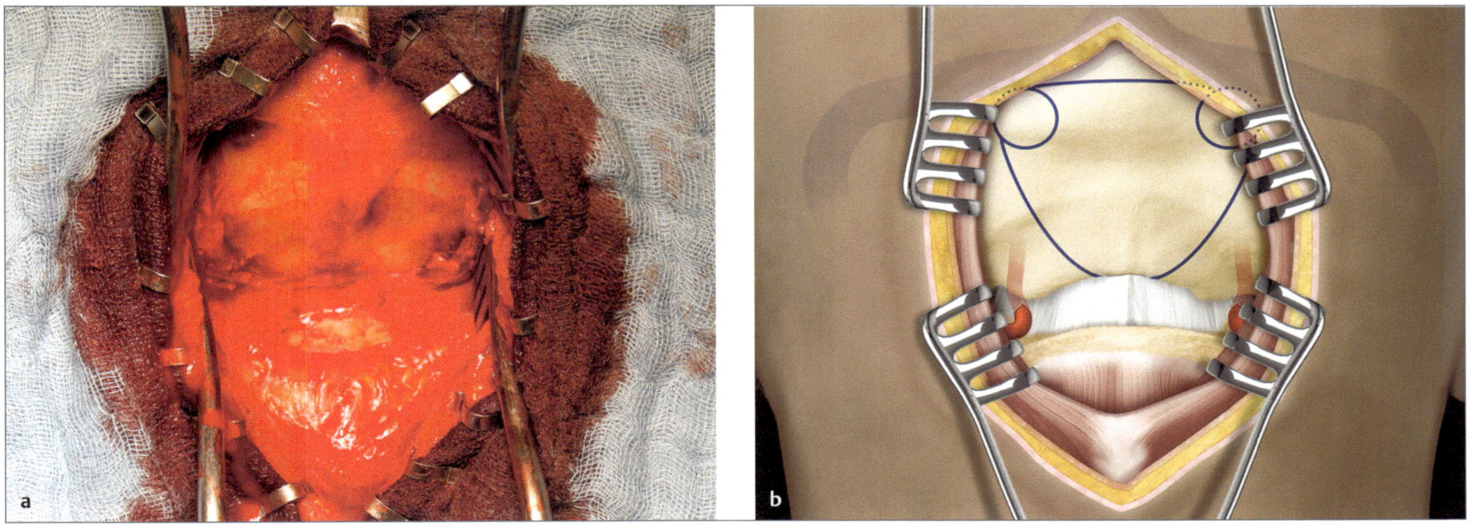

Fig. 4.68 **(a, b) Craniotomy planning.** To approach the hemispheres of the cerebellum in the midline, it is not necessary to expose the transverse sinus. We prefer to make two burr holes laterally, just below the anticipated transverse sinus, with the superior margin of the burr holes interconnecting just below the inion. If no approach to the foramen magnum is planned, a third burr hole in the midline, 1 cm superior to the foramen, may be made. In some cases, a larger craniotomy involving the transverse sinus may be necessary.

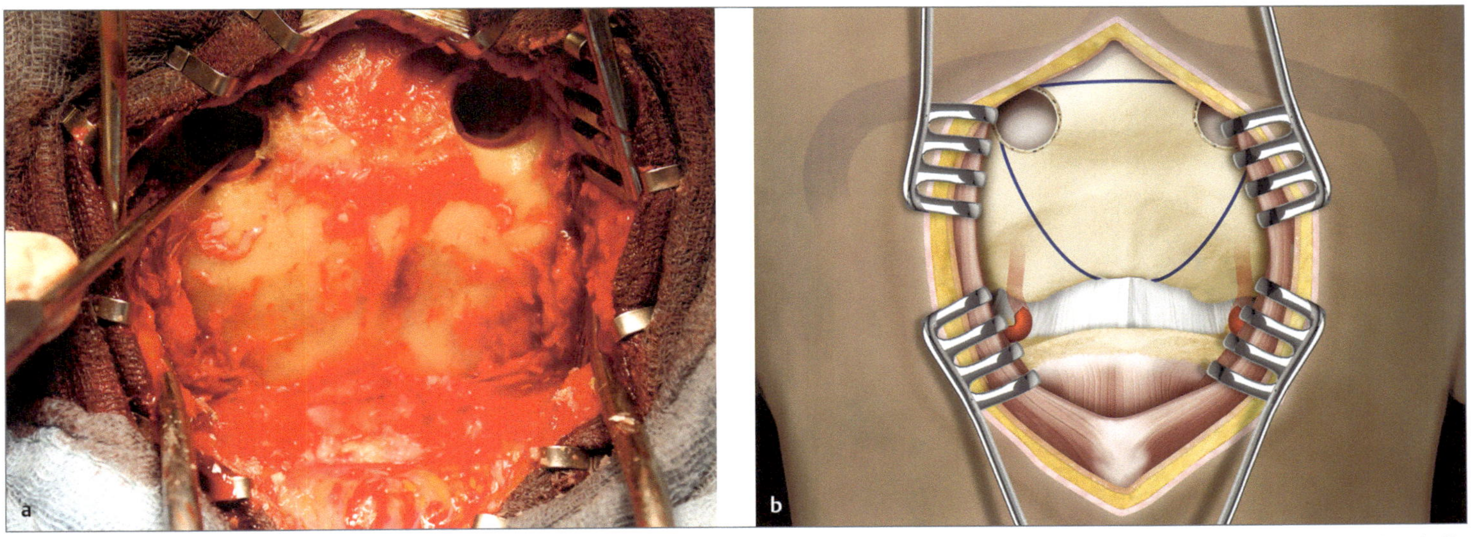

Fig. 4.69 **(a, b) Burr holes.** The burr holes can be drilled with a medium or large trephine (18 mm). The direction is strictly perpendicular to the skull. Residual bone chips are then removed using a blunt dissector or nerve hook. In the case of dural adhesion to the bone, a small punch sometimes helps to detach the structures and provide an entry for the craniotome. At the level of the foramen magnum, the bone is carefully detached from the posterior atlanto-occipital membrane to enable access for the craniotome.

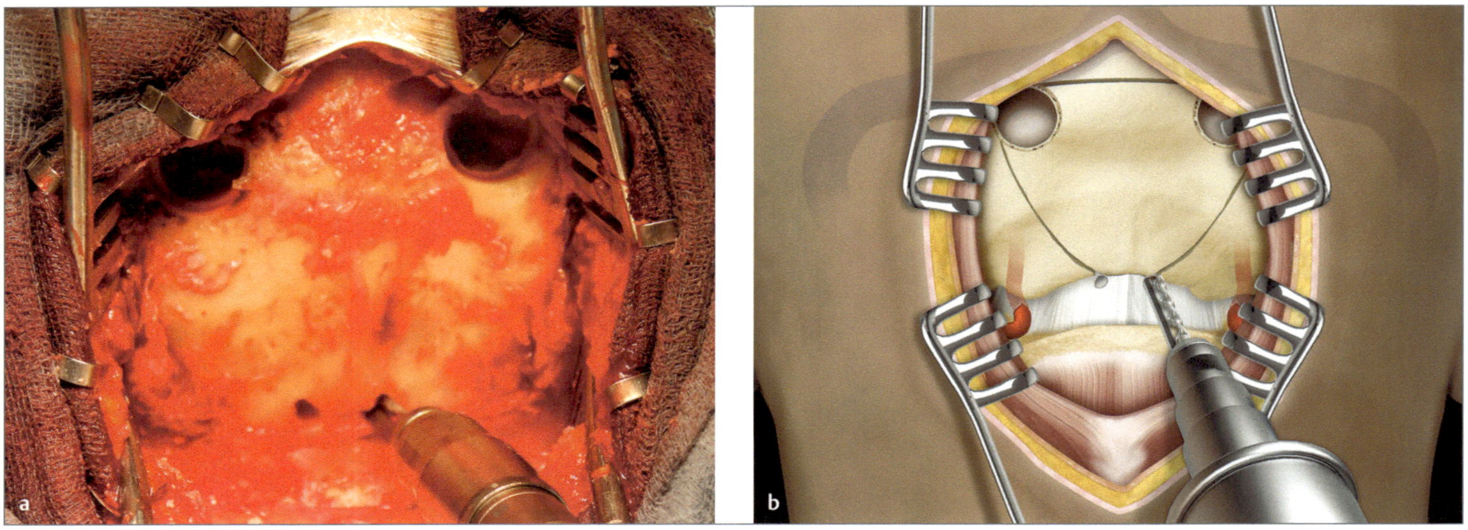

Fig. 4.70 (a, b) Craniotomy. The craniotomy is performed by interconnecting all burr holes and creating a slightly heart-shaped bone flap. While connecting the two superior burr holes, very thick bone can sometimes be present in the midline (inion). A long craniotome should be used. Sometimes residual bone here has to be removed with a diamond drill. Caution is needed because some individuals might have a preserved occipital sinus that should not be compromised by the craniotomy. The assistant uses the flush to cool the craniotome and tissue structures, and the sucker to provide optimal visibility for the surgeon.

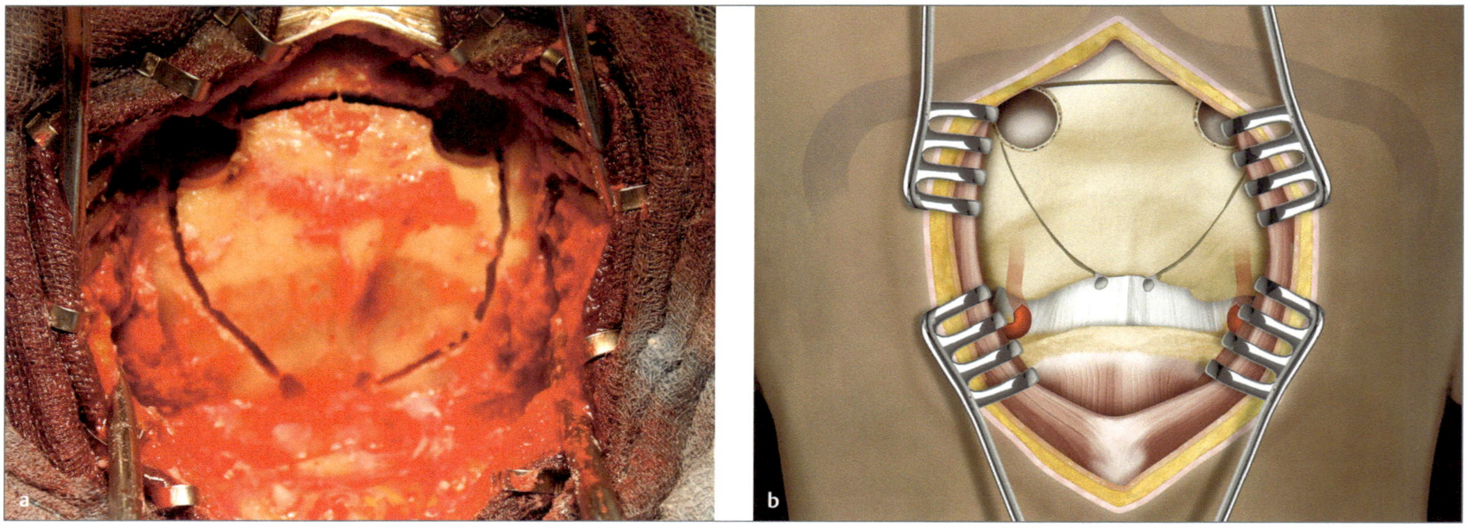

Fig. 4.71 (a, b) Craniotomy. After complete circumferential craniotomy, the bone flap is gently elevated and the dural layer is dissected from the bone in a stepwise manner. At the inferior border, attachments of the posterior atlanto-occipital membrane often have to be dissected using surgical scissors.

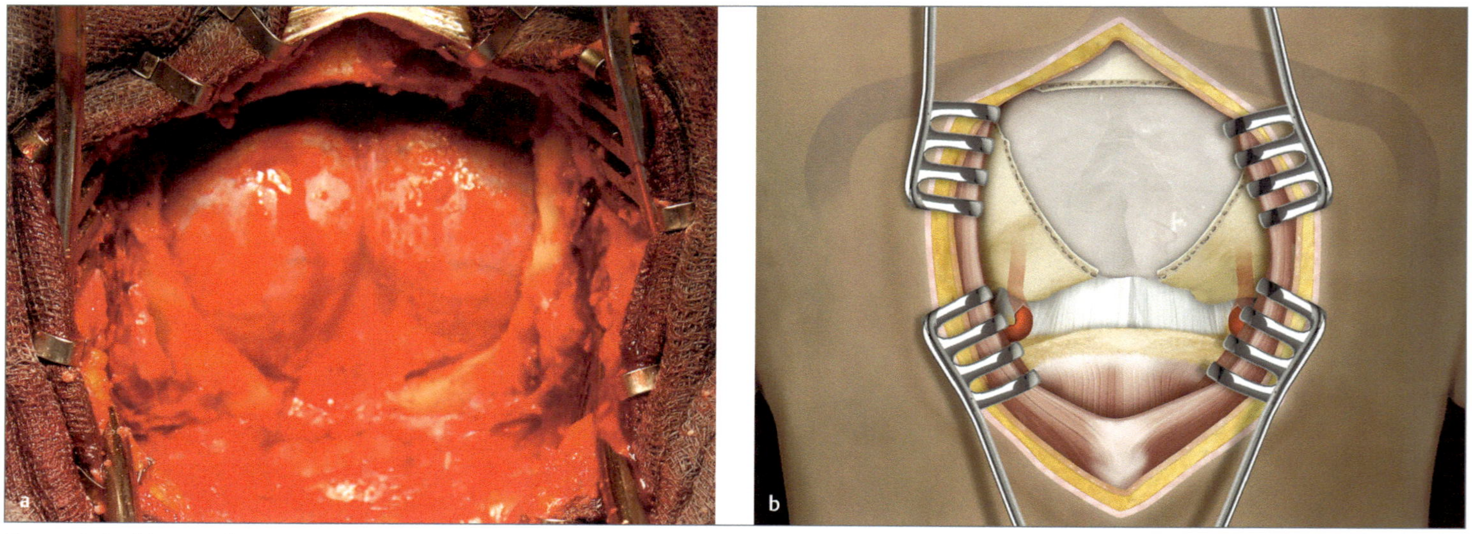

Fig. 4.72 (a, b) Situs after craniotomy and dura opening. After elevation of the bone flap, there is typically some dural bleeding. This can be controlled by coagulation. Depending on the planned surgery, further bony decompression in the area of the foramen magnum may be necessary. The whole situs then has to be meticulously cleared of bone dust using irrigation.

After circumferential placement of surgical cotton to protect the brain tissue, the dura is opened in a Y-shape. The (sometimes present) suboccipital sinus is ligated proximally and distally where the incision crosses the midline. Inferiorly, the incision is then performed slightly off but parallel to the midline on one side. Stitches in the dura at the outer borders of the dural flap help to gently retract the dura and expose the cerebellar surface.

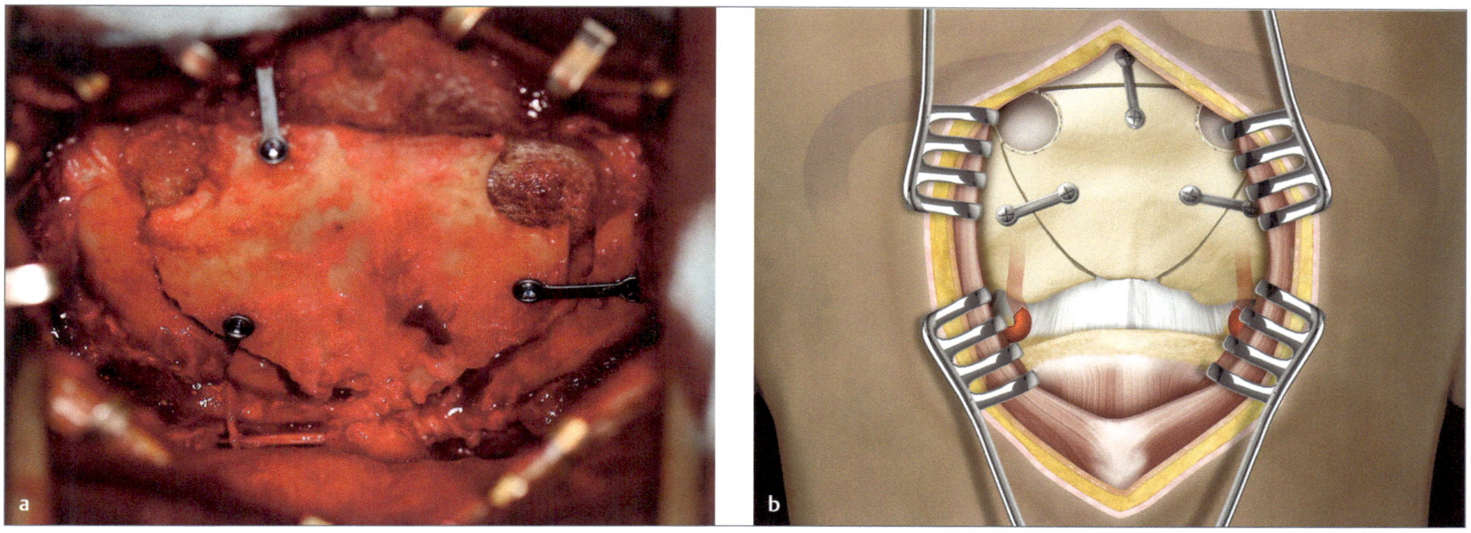

Fig. 4.73 (a, b) Closure: bone flap refixation and wound closure. The bone flap is fixed to the skull using titanium mini-plates with a distance of roughly 120° between the plates. The muscles are closed in two layers in typical manner using single sutures (1 cm distance between the stiches).

Checklist

- Avoid tilting and rotating of the head and thus displacing the nuchal ligament from the midline.
- Stay in the midline during soft tissue dissection.
- Anticipate the course of the vertebral artery when exposing the arch of C1.

5 Skull Base Craniotomies

5.1 Frontal Craniotomies

5.1.1 Bifrontal

Torstein R. Meling and Marton König

The bifrontal approach was first described by Horsley and Cushing. A bifrontal craniotomy can be used for pathologies in the anterior skull base, those that extend into the nasal cavity, and those that extend back to the suprasellar region. This craniotomy allows a low approach to one or both frontal fossae. It is considered a traditional skull base approach used to target difficult tumors toward the front of the brain, based on the concept that it is safer to remove extra bone than to unnecessarily manipulate the brain. This approach is typically used for tumors that are not suitable for removal by minimally invasive approaches because of their anatomy, their possible pathology, or the goals of surgery (see ▶ Fig. 5.1, ▶ Fig. 5.2, ▶ Fig. 5.3, ▶ Fig. 5.4, ▶ Fig. 5.5 ▶ Fig. 5.6, ▶ Fig. 5.7, ▶ Fig. 5.8, ▶ Fig. 5.9, ▶ Fig. 5.10, ▶ Fig. 5.11, ▶ Fig. 5.12, ▶ Fig. 5.13, and ▶ Fig. 5.14).

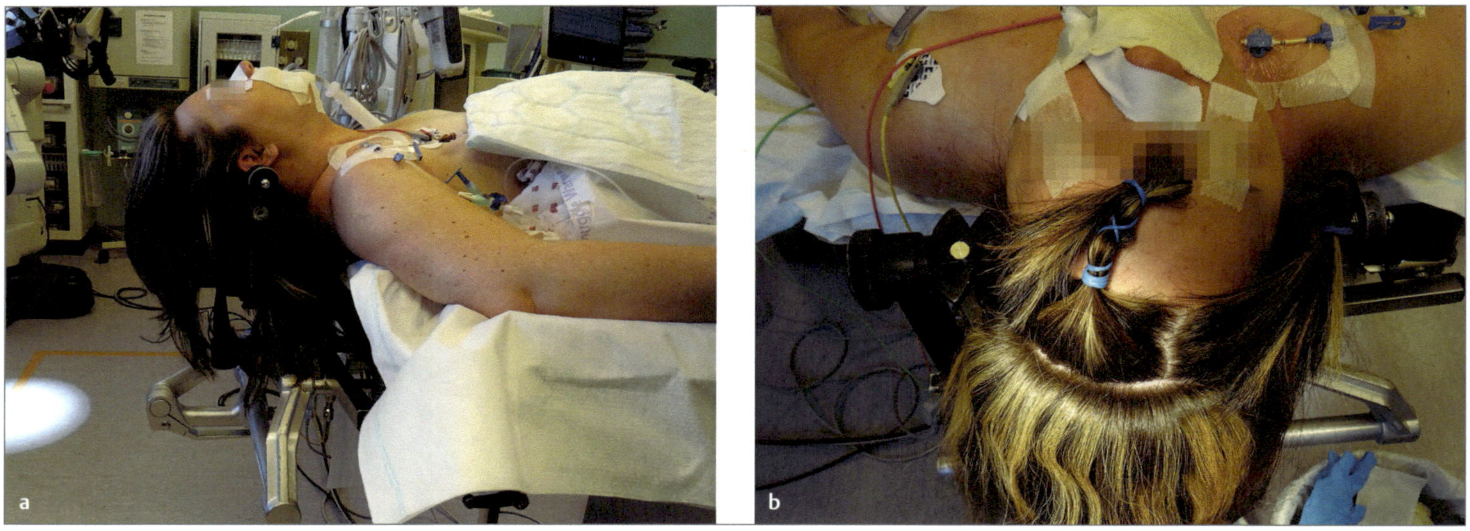

Fig. 5.1 (a, b) Positioning. The patient is in a supine position with the body slightly elevated. The head is fixed in a three-pin headrest and elevated above the level of the heart. The head is extended 15° with no sideways rotation or flexion, so that gravity causes the frontal lobe to fall away from the anterior cranial fossa, allowing retractor-free intracranial dissection.

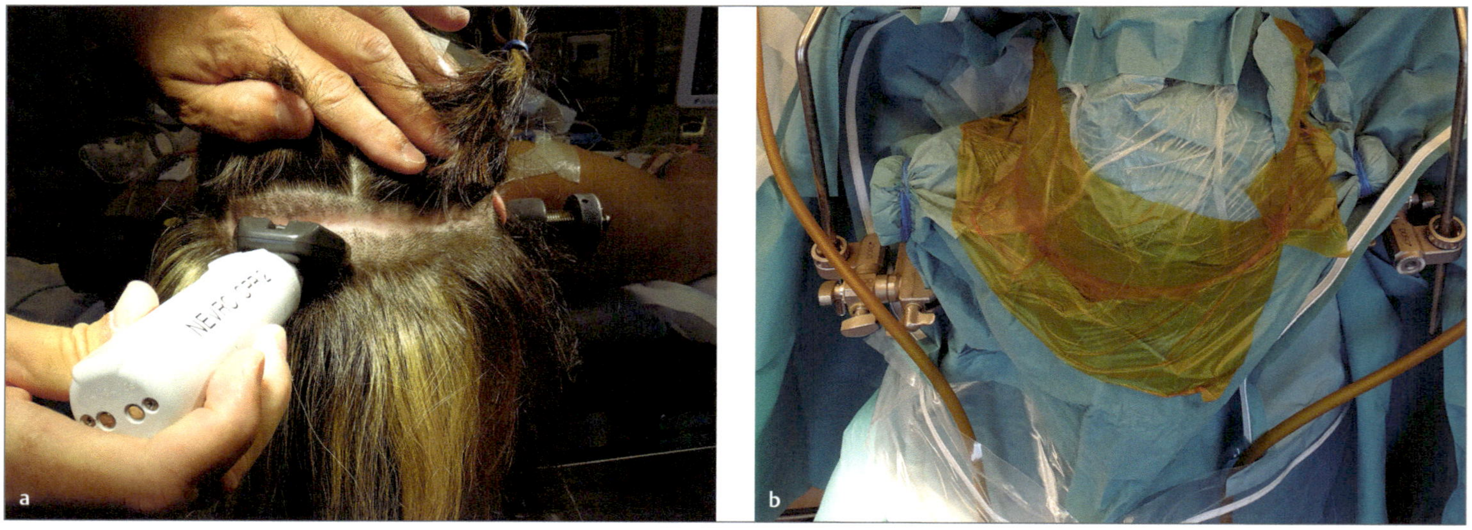

Fig. 5.2 (a, b) Shaving and draping. Once the patient has been correctly positioned, the hair is washed meticulously to reduce the risk of infection. The skin is minimally shaved, just behind the hairline. The skin incision line is infiltrated using 1% Xylocaine with 1:200,000 epinephrine. The hair is kept out of the surgical field—when necessary using hair ties and tape with underlying dressing (to avoid pulling of the patient's hair during removal).

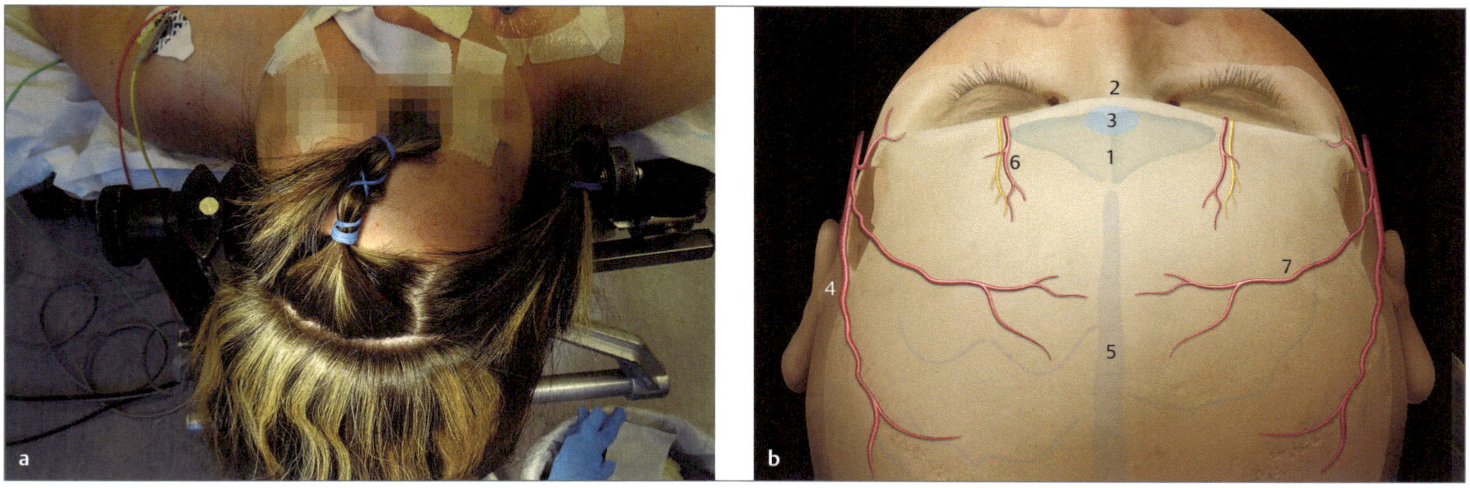

Fig. 5.3 (a,b) Anatomy overview. Important anatomical landmarks are: (1) the frontal sinus, (2) nasion, (3) glabella, (4) tragus, (5) superior sagittal sinus (SSS), (6) supraorbital artery, vein, and nerve, and (7) the superficial temporal artery (frontal and parietal branches).

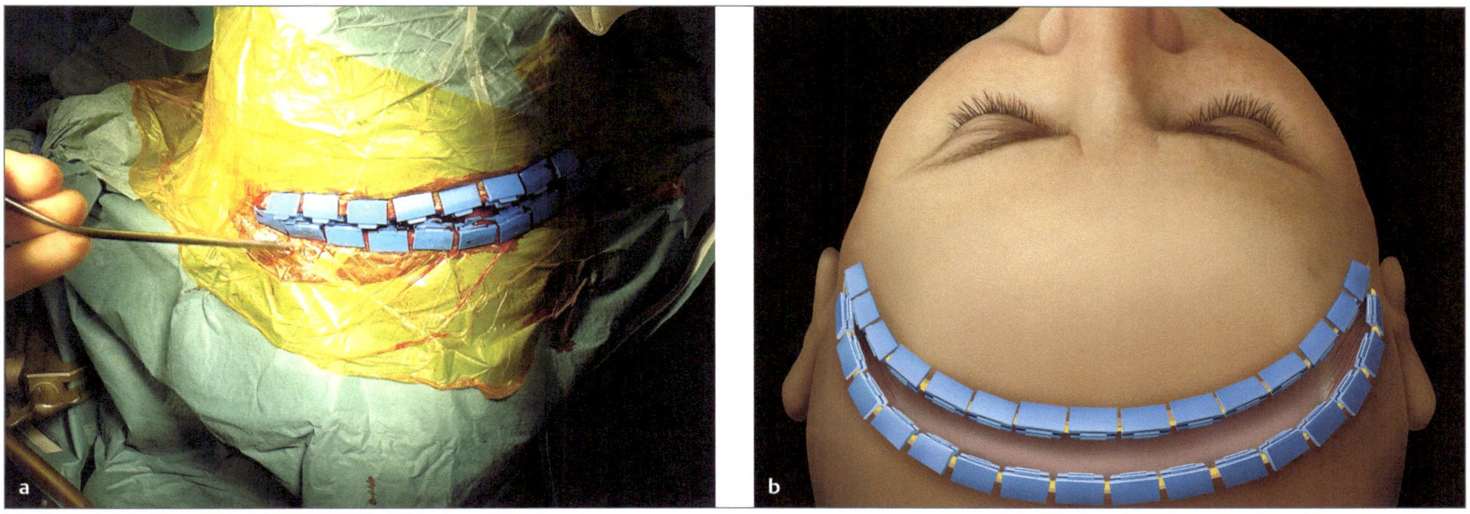

Fig. 5.4 (a, b) Skin incision. Typically, a bicoronal skin incision running from ear to ear (also known as a Souttar incision) is made just behind the hairline using a No. 20 knife blade. Note that only the epidermis and dermis are incised, leaving the galea aponeurotica over the bone and the temporal muscles intact. The skin incision starts 1 cm in front of the tragus, slightly above the level of the zygomatic arch (at the approximate level of the orbital roof), and is continued behind the hairline to the contralateral side. This incision spares the branches of the facial nerve and the parietal branch of the superficial temporal artery. After meticulous hemostasis, Raney hemostatic clips are placed along the margins of the skin incision in order to secure the draping and obtain hemostasis.

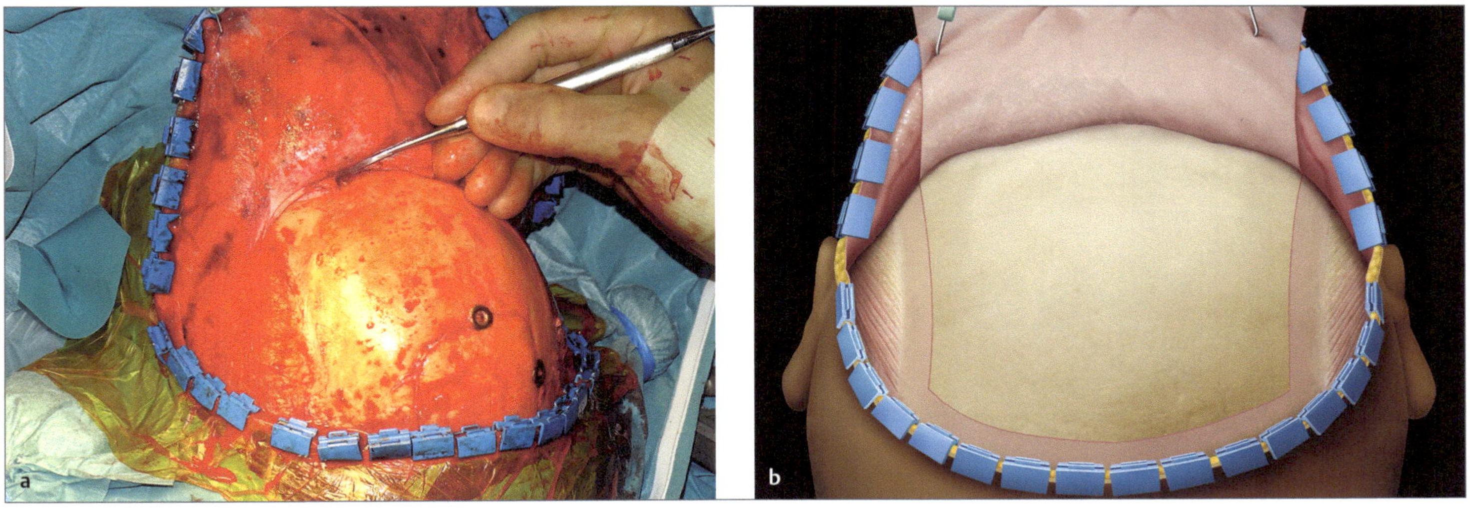

Fig. 5.5 (a, b) Flap preparation. The skin flap is retracted anteriorly using four small fishhooks with elastic bands. Particular attention is paid to the dissection of the superficial and deep fascia of the temporalis muscle to prevent injury to the facial nerve and maintain the arterial vascularization of the temporal muscle. Incision of the temporalis muscle and fascia is not necessary, as a standard interfascial dissection over the temporal muscle is adequate for exposure.

The galea and pericranium can now be harvested as a pedicled flap vascularized by the supratrochlear, supraorbital, and zygomaticotemporal arteries anteriorly. The posterior limit of the graft can be either at the level of the skin incision if a small graft is needed or all the way posteriorly to the superior nuchal line/lambda if a large pericranial flap is needed for reconstruction of large dural defects and/or defects in the anterior cranial fossa. In both cases, the lateral limit is along the superior temporal line. Great care should be taken to dissect the scalp in the subgaleal plane to avoid any defects in the flap as well as to avoid damaging the arterial blood supply to the pericranial flap. Sharp dissection is performed toward the superior orbital margins on both sides, paying particular attention to the supraorbital nerves. The nerve is dissected away, or freed, from its foramen.

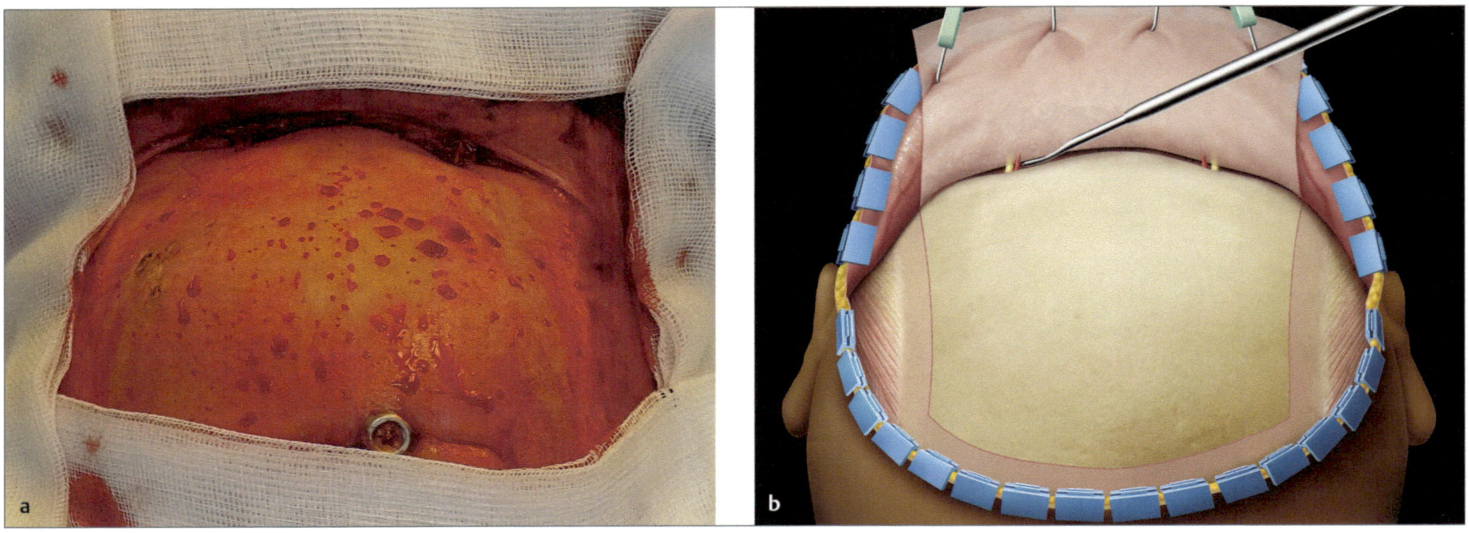

Fig. 5.6 (a, b) Preparing the surgical field. The flap is covered with wet dressings to prevent tissue damage due to desiccation and thermal injury from the xenon microscope lamp.

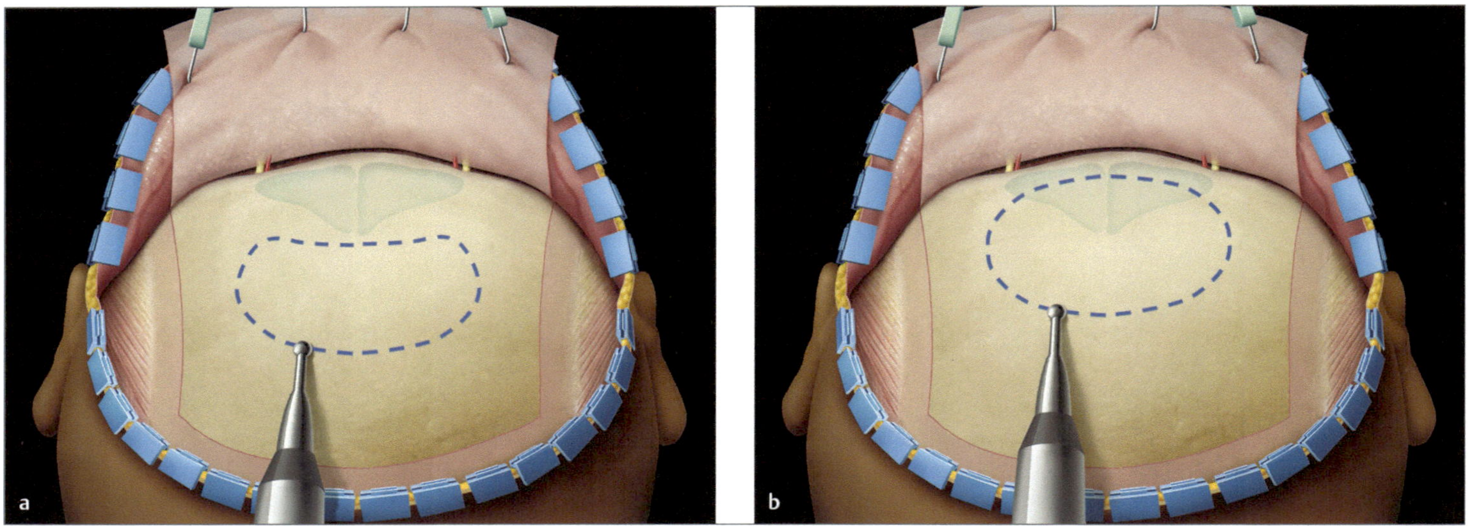

Fig. 5.7 (a, b) Craniotomy configuration and landmarks. Important anatomical bony landmarks such as the nasion, glabella, supraorbital fissure, frontotemporal suture, stephanion, and bregma must be exposed, and serve as major orientation points. In addition to such landmarks, neuronavigation assists in exact placement of the craniotomy. If the approach is above the frontal sinus, the craniotomy is more kidney-shaped; if the craniotomy needs to be low and to cross the sinus, it is more superelliptic.

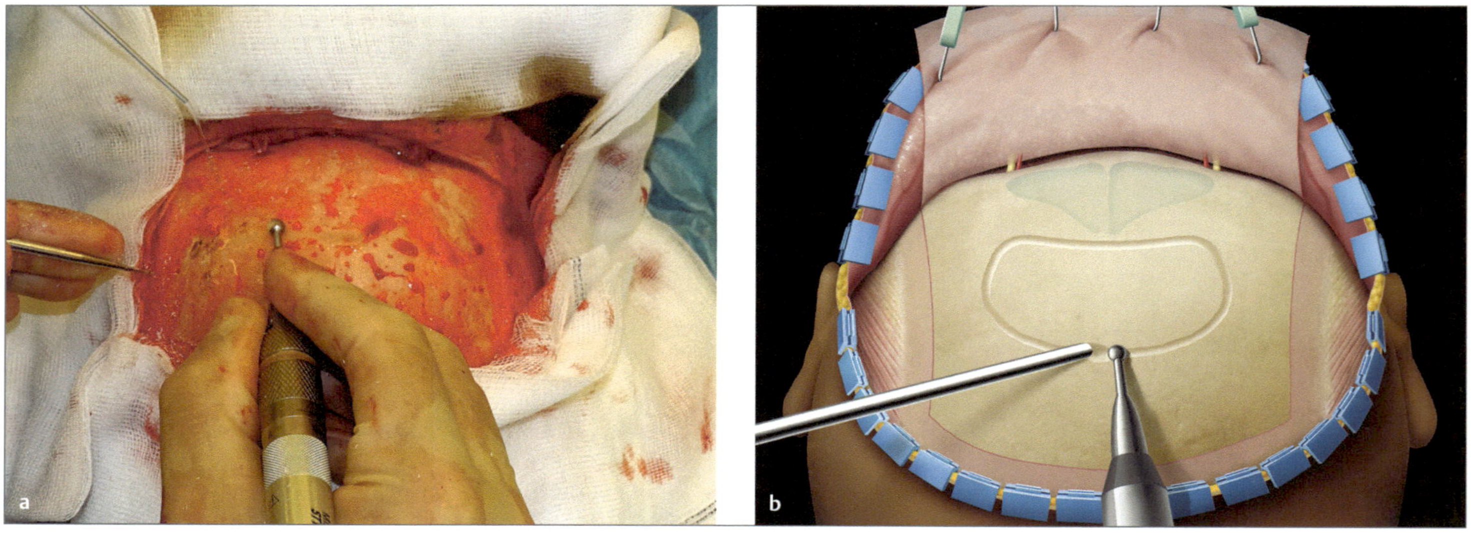

Fig. 5.8 (a, b) Craniotomy outline. A bifrontal craniotomy is made using a high-speed electric craniotome. The bone flap is usually 8–10 cm wide (coronal plane) and 3 cm deep (sagittal plane). The superior margin of the craniotomy is marked by the posterior burr hole placed over the SSS. The lateral borders of the craniotomy are approximately at the midpupillary line. The inferior margin of the craniotomy is planned according to the intracranial target. Using the drill and the navigation pointer, the craniotomy outline is engraved into the bone.

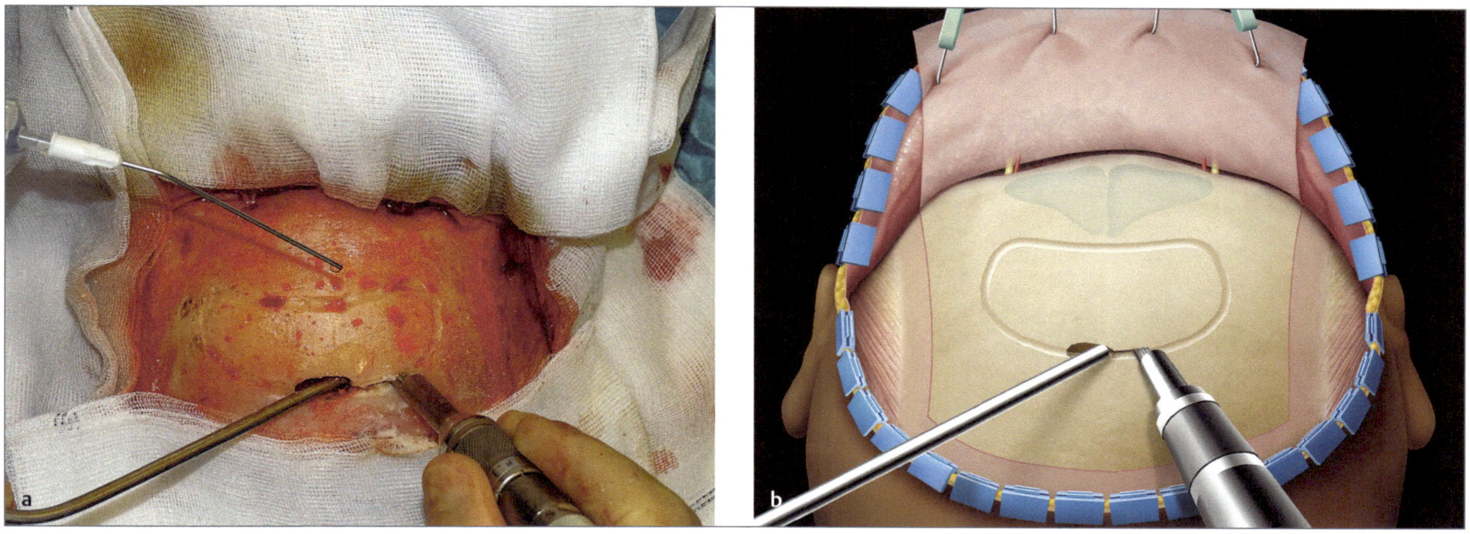

Fig. 5.9 (a, b) Craniotomy. A single 5 × 10 mm oval burr hole is made 6 cm behind the glabella using a high-speed drill with a sharp 4-mm drill bit. It is situated directly over the SSS and oriented transversely to avoid burr hole defects in the forehead. The craniotomy is performed away from the SSS. If the frontal sinus can be avoided, care should be taken to prevent inadvertently entering it, by using a neuronavigation system or taking into account the position of the lateral border of the frontal sinus as measured on preoperative imaging (CT scan and/or MRI).

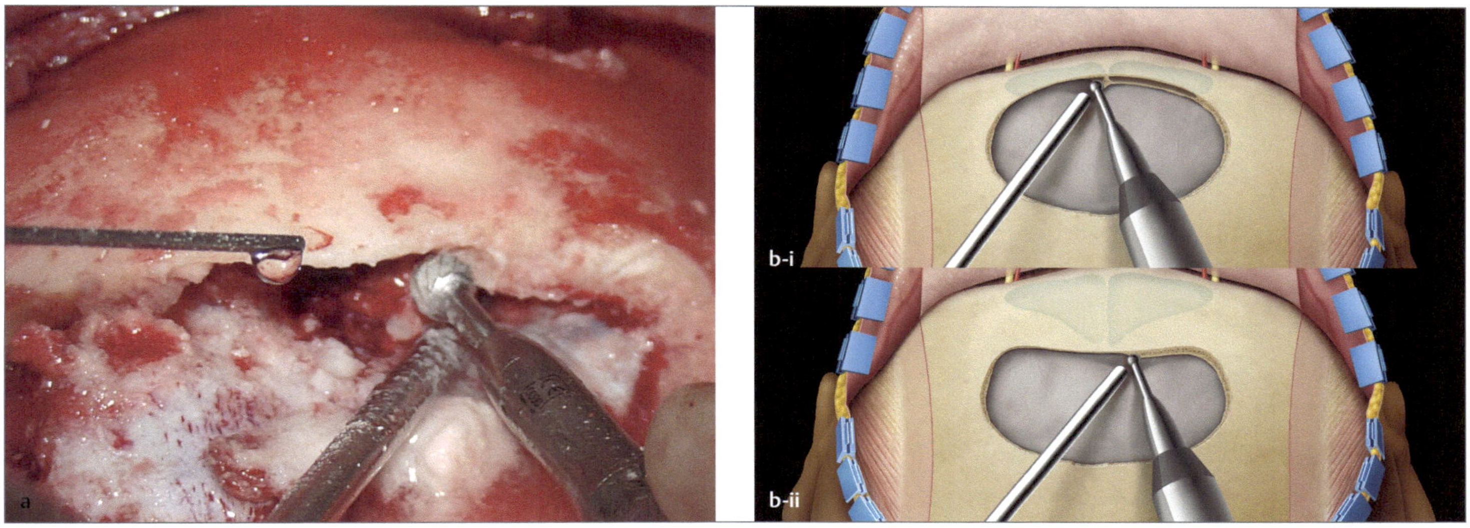

Fig. 5.10 (a, b) Bone drilling. If the frontal sinus can be spared, the tabula interna and frontal bone crest are removed using a high-speed drill with a sharp 4-mm drill bit. If the approach needs to traverse the frontal sinuses (e.g., for a transbasal approach, for a low angle of attack, or in patients with large frontal sinuses), the frontal sinuses may be cranialized by complete removal of the posterior wall of the frontal sinus and eversion of the mucosa down to the frontonasal duct. Opening of the frontal sinuses, either inadvertently or deliberately, may increase the risk of postoperative meningitis.

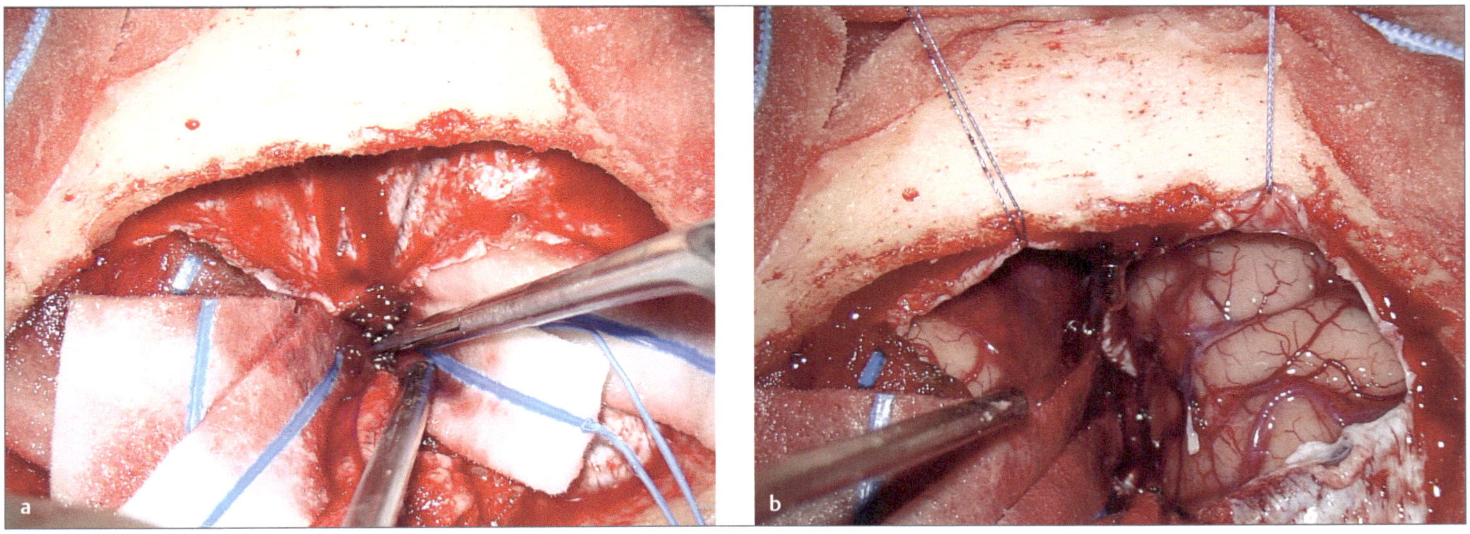

Fig. 5.11 (a, b) Dura opening. The dura is opened in a slightly curved form transversely in the midline. Surgicel is placed extradurally to support hemostasis. Tacking sutures in the dura are attached to skin or previously drilled holes in the frontal bone to gently retract the dura and expose the frontal brain surface. The SSS may be divided basally, by electrocoagulation, next to the crista galli, near the orbital roof, with little risk. The falx is cut until its deep edge.

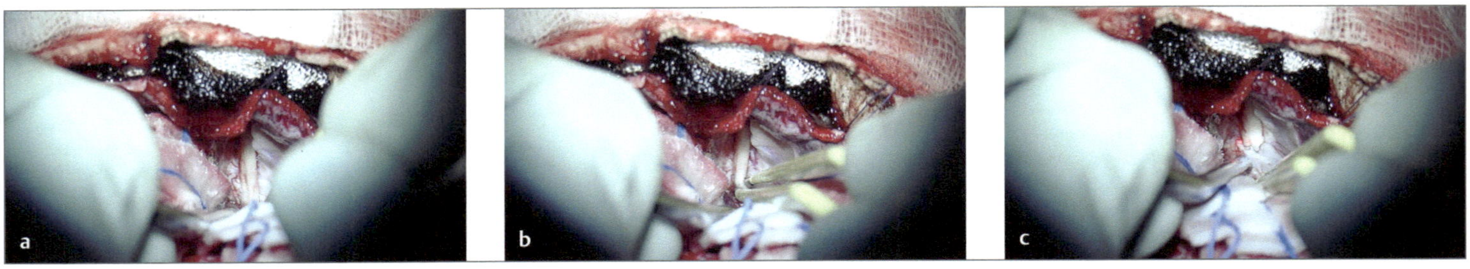

Fig. 5.12 (a–c) Intracranial dissection and targets. Further dissection beginning with the olfactory tracts is performed under the microscope. We try to preserve the olfactory tracts by careful, sharp dissection and by covering them with fibrin sealant. The tracts might be sacrificed if necessary, either unilaterally or bilaterally, allowing separation of the dura from the cribriform plate and the crista galli.

Frontal craniotomies provide surgical access to the frontal lobe(s) of the brain (e.g., for intrinsic brain tumors), to the third ventricle via lamina terminalis (e.g., craniopharyngiomas or brainstem cavernomas), to the parasellar region (e.g., tuberculum sella or planum sphenoidale meningiomas), to the anterior skull base (e.g., olfactory groove meningiomas), to the ethmoid region (e.g., transbasal resection of ethmoidal tumors), and for repair of ethmoidal cerebrospinal fluid (CSF) fistulas.

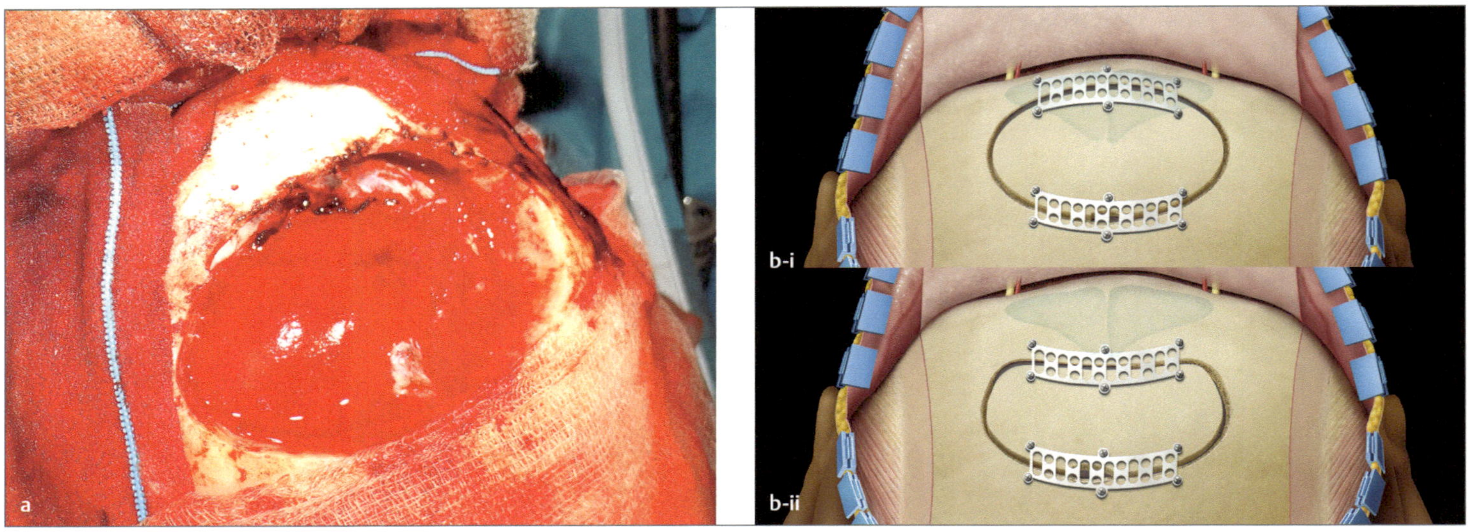

Fig. 5.13 (a, b) Closure. Meticulous hemostasis is performed both intra- and extradurally. The dura is closed using a PDS 5–0 running suture. A sheath of TachoSil is placed over the dura mater to reduce the risk of CSF leaks, if deemed necessary. The bone flap is refixed and plates are used to cover large and cosmetically relevant bone gaps.

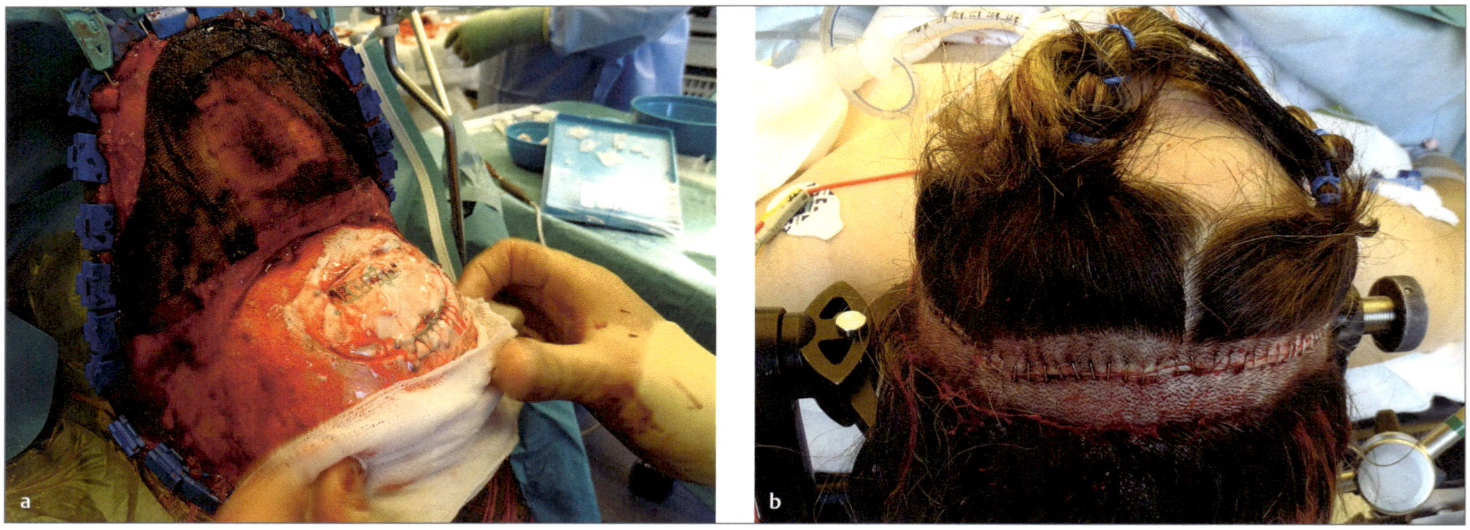

Fig. 5.14 (a, b) Galea and skin closure. Care should be taken to level bony structures so that they are flush with the surrounding cranium during the replacement of the bone flap. Any remaining irregularities and larger gaps are filled using hydroxyapatite cement. The galea is closed with a running Monocryl 3–0 suture. The skin is closed using skin staples. The wound is dressed using Steri-Strips.

Checklist

- Use neuronavigation planning to familiarize yourself with your trajectory relative to the frontal sinus anatomy. Cave: very lateral extensions.
- Before skin incision, make sure the head is retroflexed enough to enable the frontal lobe to fall away from the anterior cranial fossa and allow for retractor-free intracranial dissection.
- Make the bicoronal skin incision > 1 cm behind the hairline, starting just anterior to the tragus. Note that only the epidermis and dermis are incised, leaving the pericranium over the bone and the temporal muscles intact.
- Continue to dissect the skin flap in the loose areolar skin layer in a posterior-to-anterior fashion all the way to the superior orbital rim area, preserving the pericranium on the bone and preserving the supraorbital arteries anteriorly.
- When performing the interfascial dissection laterally, stay directly on the superficial layer of the deep temporal fascia *at all times* to avoid injury to the temporal branch of the facial nerve.
- Harvest the pericranial flap from the bone by making a horizontal cut posteriorly, at the lambda if a large flap is needed or at the bregma if a smaller flap is sufficient, and along the linea temporalis superior laterally.
- Stay subperiosteally at all times and harvest the flap in a posterior-to-anterior fashion all the way to the superior orbital rim. Cover the pericranial flap in wet gauze. Cave: subperiosteal dissection of margo orbitalis superior can injure the supraorbital nerve if not properly detached from its canal/groove.
- Use neuronavigation to identify the borders of the frontal sinus.
- When a low trajectory is needed and the frontal sinuses are being cranialized, make a small, oval burr hole directly on the superior sagittal sinus, 5 cm posterior to the glabella.
- Make the first cut C-shaped, starting from the burr hole and running to the apex of the margo orbitalis superior, which defines the lateral extension.
- Make the last cut straight and run it as close to the superior orbital rim as possible in a lateral-to-medial direction.
- Repeat the same two steps on the contralateral side.
- Cranialize the frontal sinuses by removing the mucosa and posterior wall completely and drilling down all trabeculae, while leaving the tabula externa intact for cosmesis.
- Toward the frontonasal ducts, the residual mucosa is gently scraped off the tabula interna in a superior-to-inferior direction to preserve its blood supply, and is used to plug the duct.
- When a higher trajectory is needed and the frontal sinuses can be preserved, perform the craniotomy 3 cm further posteriorly and make the straight, basal cuts superior to the frontal sinus.
- Open the dura with a straight, horizontal incision on either side of the superior sagittal sinus 1 cm above the horizontal bone cuts, and retract the dura anteriorly. Use bipolar electrocoagulation or hemo-clips to ligate the superior sagittal sinus and make additional cuts to connect the two durotomies.
- Continue to open the falx cerebri toward the anterior cranial base and use bipolar electrocoagulation to ligate the inferior sagittal sinus. Cave: do not drift off too far posteriorly.
- Close the dura with a running monofilament 6–0 suture. Make sure that it is watertight, as any CSF leak here might cause rhinorrhea and/or infections. "Stress-test" your closure by injecting water subdurally via a venous catheter and close the puncture site.
- Fix the bone flap with 1-mm titanium mini-plates. Take care to level the bone flap flush with the surrounding cranium so as to avoid any irregularities, and use hydroxyapatite cement to fill any larger gaps.

5.2 Frontotemporal Craniotomies

5.2.1 Facial Nerve Anatomy and Protection

Andreas Raabe and Peter A. Winkler

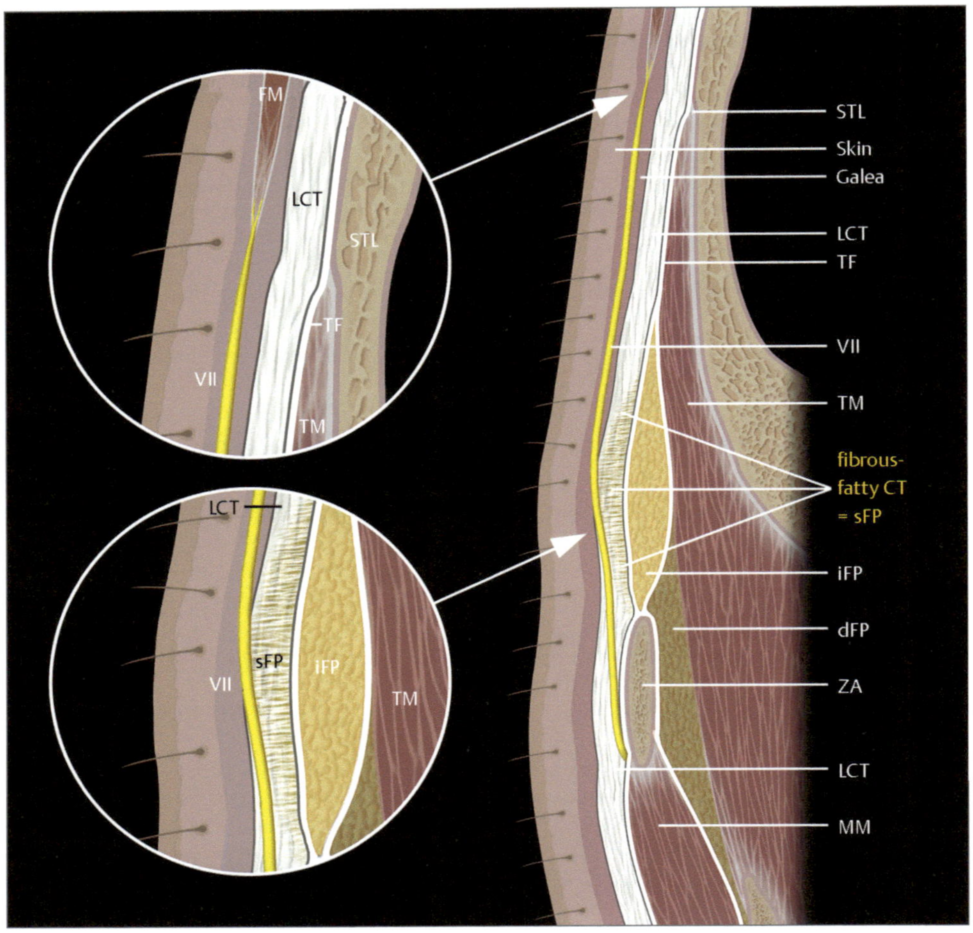

Fig. 5.15 Frontotemporal tissue layers.

dFP: deep fat pad;
FM: frontalis muscle;
iFP: interfascial fat pad;
LCT: loose connective tissue;
MM: masseter muscle;
sFP: suprafascial fat pad;
STL: superior temporal line;
TF: temporalis fascia;
VII: facial nerve;
ZA: zygomatic arch.

The branches of the facial nerve are at risk of mechanical or thermal injury when the skin–galea flap is separated from the temporalis muscle inferior to the superior temporal line (STL). In the lower half of the temporal region, between the STL and the zygomatic arch, the easy plane of dissection during elevation of the scalp (loose connective tissue = LCT) merges into the fibrous fatty connective tissue and becomes difficult to separate because fibrous adhesions bind the scalp to the superficial layer of the temporalis fascia. When dissection and elevation of the scalp flap is continued in this area, the facial nerve may be injured. Due to the presence of fatty tissue, this part of the LCT is also called the suprafascial fat pad (sFP). The size of the fat deposit in this subgaleal–suprafascial plane varies between individuals (▶ Fig. 5.15).

It is in this layer, between the STL and the zygoma, that the facial nerve is at highest risk of injury. Therefore, the galea should not be separated from the layers below in the lower half between the STL and the zygomatic arch (see ▶ Fig. 5.16, ▶ Fig. 5.17, ▶ Fig. 5.18, and ▶ Fig. 5.19).

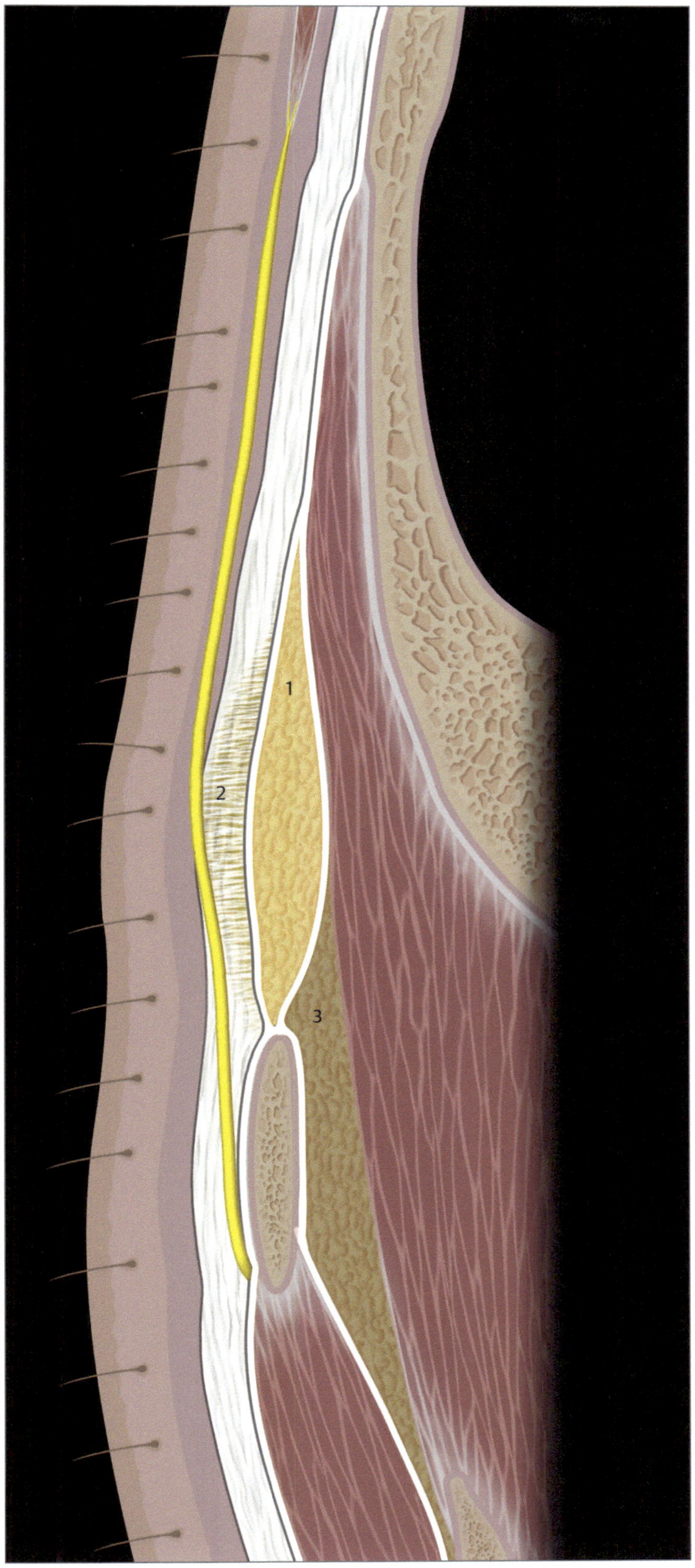

Fig. 5.16 The three temporal fat pads and their significance. There are three fat pads in relation to the layers of the temporalis fascia:

1. Interfascial (iFP): between the superior and the deep layers of the temporal fat pad lies the interfascial fat pad. There is no facial nerve running in this layer. This is the first fat pad that becomes visible through the superficial temporalis fascia when the scalp flap is turned anteriorly and separated from the temporalis muscle.
2. Suprafascial (sFP): this is the middle part of the LCT plane but it is composed of fatty and fibrous tissue, as described above. It covers the lower half of the distance between the STL and the zygomatic arch, but varies in size and extension. It is through this layer that the facial nerve passes.
3. Deep fat pad (dFP): this is located below the deep layer of the temporalis fascia.

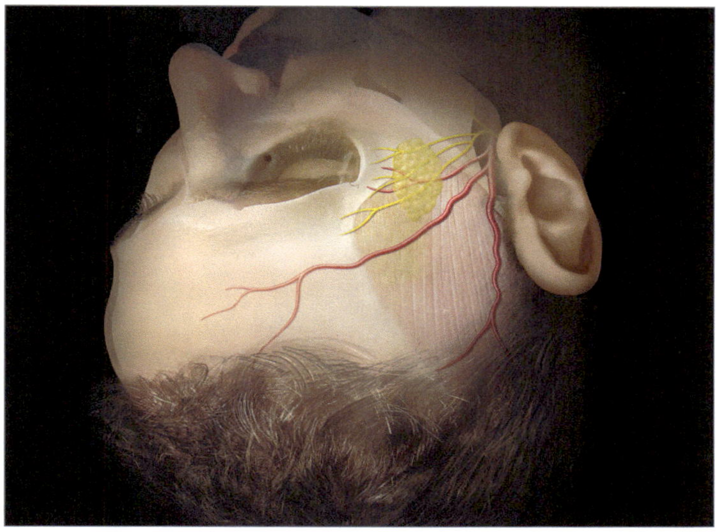

Fig. 5.17 Anatomical course of the temporal branches of the facial nerve and landmarks. There are typically two to four branches of the facial nerve crossing the zygomatic arch with a course that runs anteriorly and superiorly to innervate the orbicularis oculi, frontalis, and corrugator muscles. Below the level of the zygoma, these branches are located in the LCT layer. After crossing the zygomatic arch superficially, they enter the fibrous and fatty sFP. At the sFP, they enter the galeal or fascial layer of the skin and travel to their muscles.
The following landmarks help to avoid injury of the facial nerve:
1. The appearance of the yellowish interfascial fat pad (iFP) during lifting of the scalp flap indicates that the critical suprafascial fat pad (sFP) is close.
2. Subgaleal adhesions: the easy subgaleal plane ends when adhesions connect the galea to the superficial temporal fascia, indicating the sFP.
3. STA: the appearance of the frontal branch of the STA within the galea when elevating the flap.

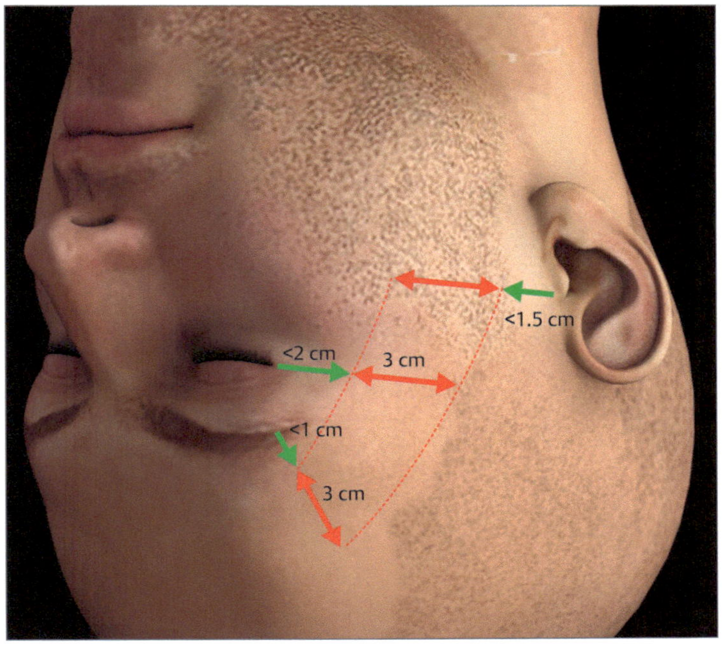

Fig. 5.18 Metric measurements for safe zones. Metric measurements for safe distances may also help to avoid the facial nerve.
Safe zones are:
1. At the level of the zygomatic arch: up to 1.5 cm anteriorly to the tragus.
2. At the level of the orbit: from the lateral cantus 2 cm laterally, parallel to the lid line.
3. At the level of the STL: from the middle of the eyebrow less than 1 cm above the eyebrow.
4. Posterior or superior to the danger zone corridor (see below).

Danger zones are:
1. At the level of the zygomatic arch: anteriorly to the safe 1.5 cm zone.
2. At the level of the orbit: a corridor of 3 cm posterior to the safe zone.
3. At the level of the STL: a corridor of 3 cm posterosuperior to the safe zone.

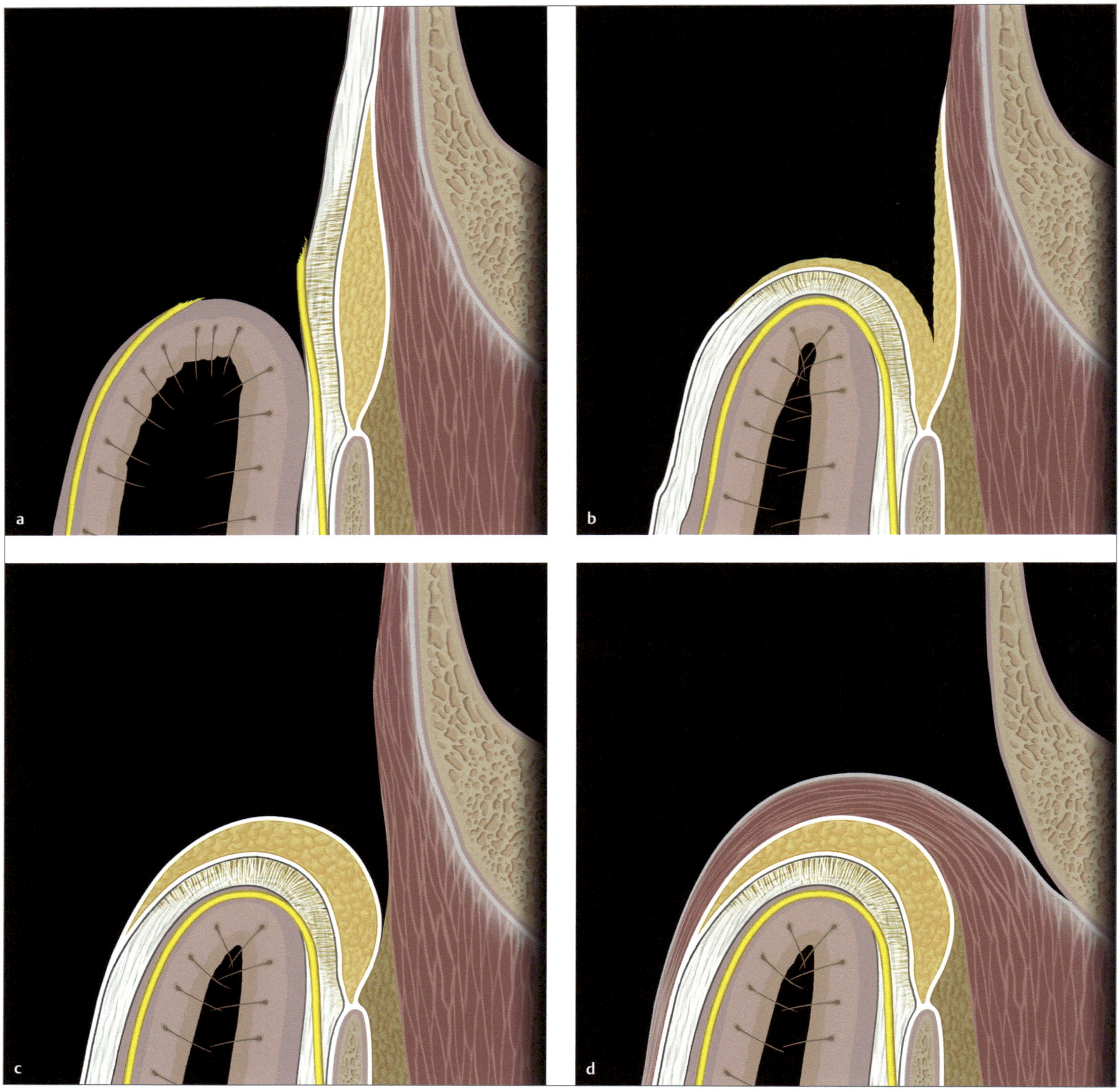

Fig. 5.19 (a–d) **Techniques for facial nerve preservation.** If the galea is separated from the temporalis muscle down to the zygoma without using a facial nerve preservation technique, the nerve is injured (a top left). There are three surgical techniques for facial nerve preservation: (**b**, top right) interfascial flap (for orbitocranial or orbitozygomatic approaches) and (**c**, bottom left) subfascial flap (for orbitocranial or orbitozygomatic approaches), and (**d**, bottom right) combined myocutaneous flap (for pterional craniotomy).

Combined Musculocutaneous Flap

In the combined musculocutaneous flap, the temporalis muscle is not separated from the galea. They are lifted together as a single flap (▶ Fig. 5.20 and ▶ Fig. 5.21).

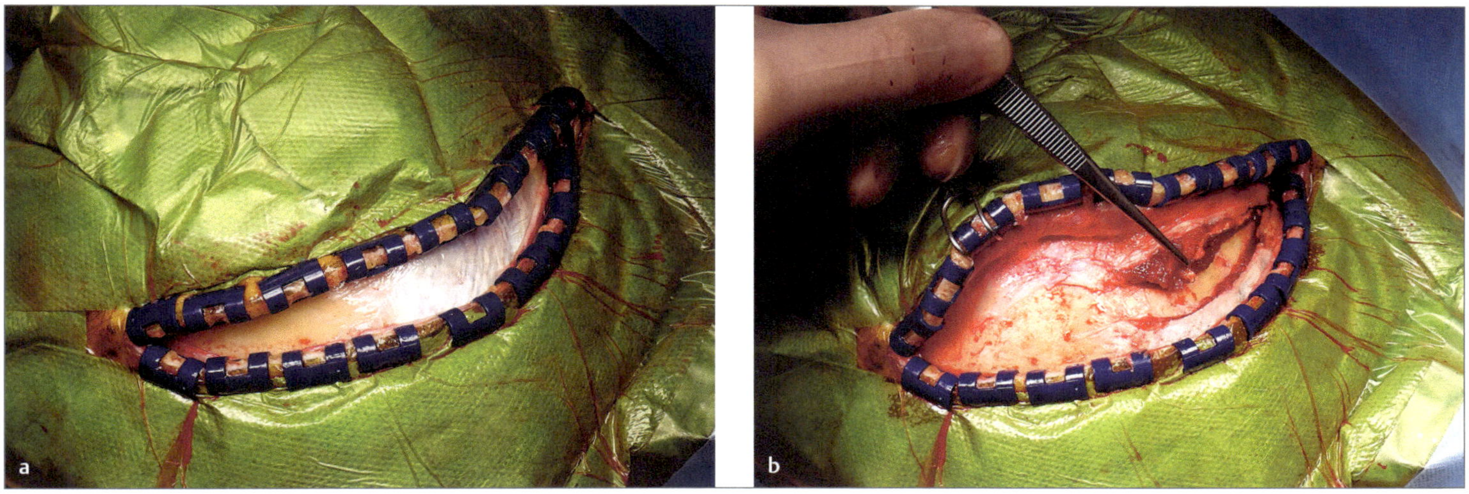

Fig. 5.20 (a, b) Combined musculocutaneous flap. After incision, the skin–galea flap is slightly elevated and the scalp clips are placed for hemostasis **(a)**. The temporalis fascia and muscle are cut down to the bone slightly anterior to the skin incision to facilitate suturing of the temporalis fascia when closing the layers **(b)**.

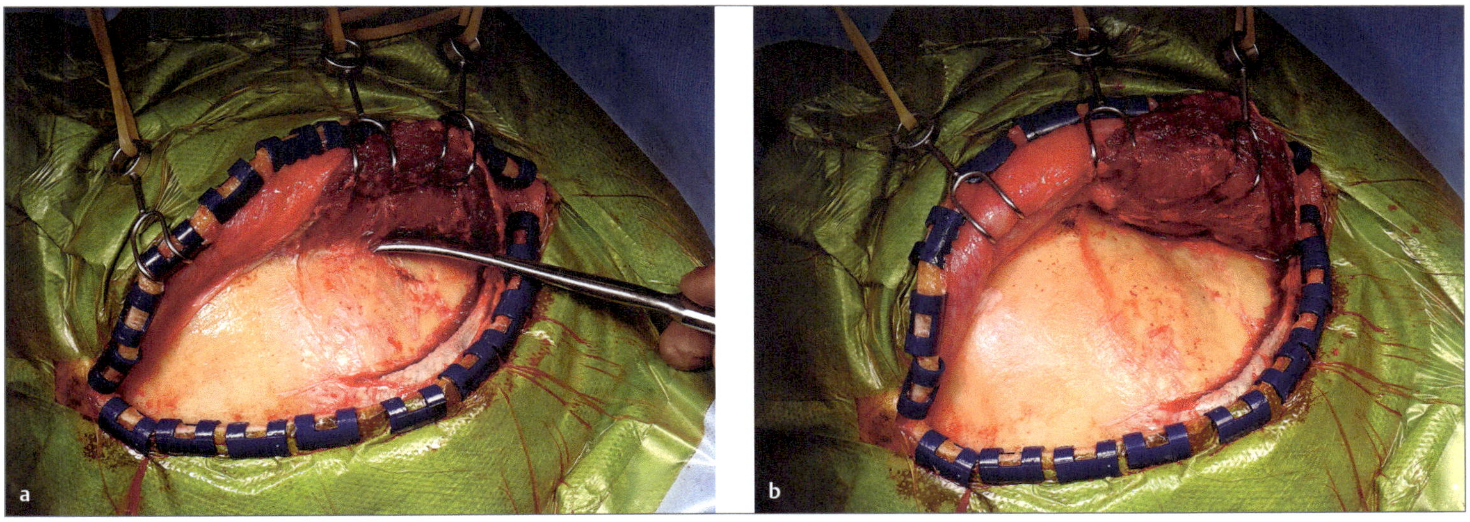

Fig. 5.21 (a, b) Combined musculocutaneous flap. The muscle is then sharply detached subperiostally from the bone in an inferior-to-superior direction that preserves the muscle fibers and vascularization **(a)**. All layers are also subperiostally detached from the STL and frontally until the frontotemporale (see Chapter 2, Landmarks) and the zygomatic process can be palpated with the finger. After elevating the myocutaneous flap, the entire flap is turned anteriorly to expose the frontal and temporal bone at the site of the craniotomy **(b)**. The advantage of the myocutaneous flap is its ease of use and excellent protection of the facial nerve. It is the standard technique for the pterional approach. The disadvantages are (1) the bulk of muscle that may narrow the working space and restrict the view along the sphenoid ridge and the lower margin of exposure for some approaches (i.e., for large anterior communicating [Acom] artery aneurysms) and (2) the fixation of the muscle at the zygoma. Thus, it is not suitable for an orbitozygomatic approach and provides only limited exposure of the lateral orbital rim during orbitocraniotomy or orbital extensions of other craniotomies.

Subfascial Dissection

In the subfascial dissection, the tissue is cut down including the deep layer of the temporalis fascia, but not the temporalis muscle. All layers above the muscle fibers are elevated with the flap (▶ Fig. 5.22 and ▶ Fig. 5.23).

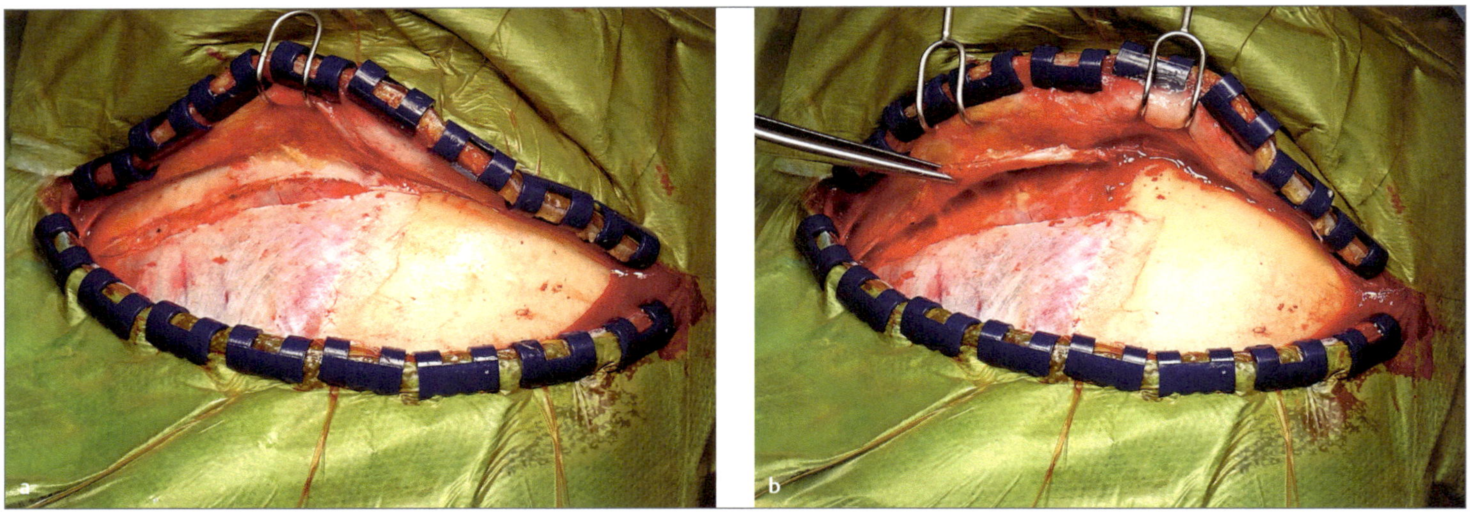

Fig. 5.22 (a, b) Subfascial dissection. The scalp (skin–galea) is cut. Scalp clips are placed. The superficial fascia of the temporalis muscle is exposed. The scalp flap is elevated until the interfascial yellow fat pad and/or the frontal branch of the STA are visible. The superficial layer of the temporalis muscle, the interfascial fat, and the deep layer of the temporalis muscle are cut **(a)**. Care has to be taken not to damage the surface of the temporalis muscle. The deep temporalis fascia is dissected from the temporalis muscle. All layers above the muscle fibers are elevated **(b)**.

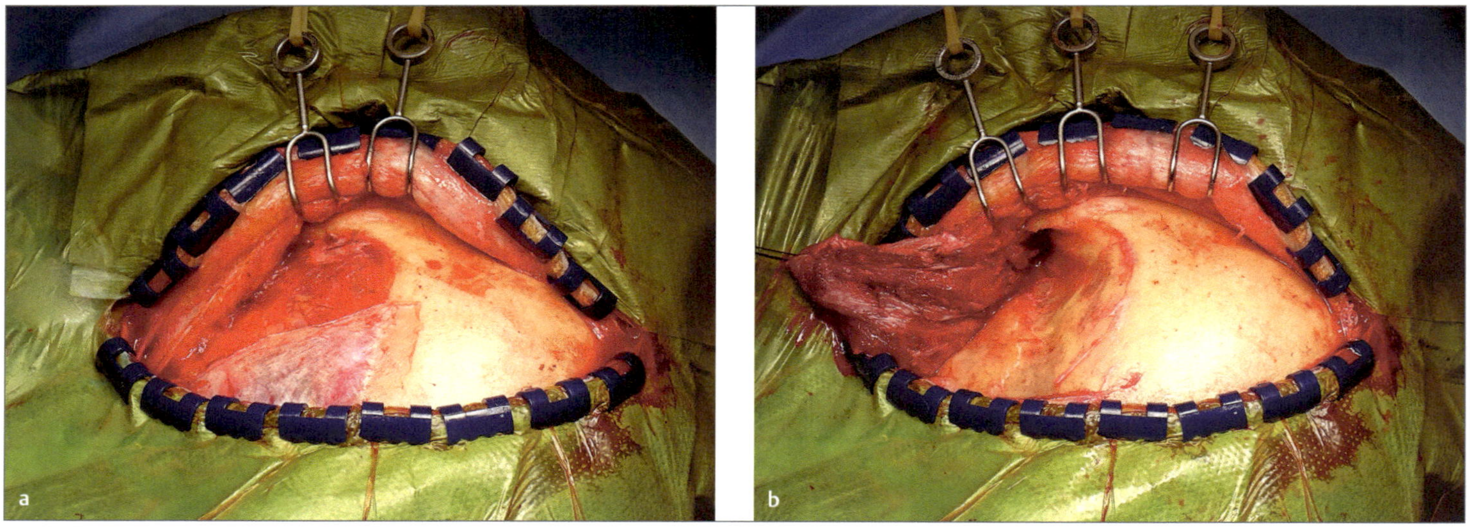

Fig. 5.23 (a, b) Subfascial dissection. The temporalis muscle and the orbital rim are exposed **(a)**. Fish hooks are used to retract the other layers of the flap. Care should be taken to apply only enough tension to hold the flap in place, because excessive traction may also injure the branches of the facial nerve. Now the temporalis muscle is cut at the posterior border parallel to the posterior skin incision line and detached from the bone in an inferior-to-superior direction **(b)**. It is also detached from the STL and the orbital rim and reflected inferiorly. A suture with loose tension holds the muscle in place. This maneuver moves the temporalis muscle away from the anterior cranial base as is required for orbital rim or orbitozygomatic approaches.

Interfascial Dissection

In 1984, Gazi Yaşargil described the interfascial dissection technique and how its use for pterional craniotomy allowed sufficient basal exposure and retraction of the temporalis muscle when needed. Use of the interfascial dissection technique has markedly reduced, but not eliminated, the incidence of frontal muscle palsy. This is because surgeons sometimes mixed up the fat pads or did not correctly follow the concept and description. Interfascial dissection is similar to subfascial dissection, but the deep layer of the temporalis fascia covering the temporalis muscle is left intact (▶ Fig. 5.24 and ▶ Fig. 5.25).

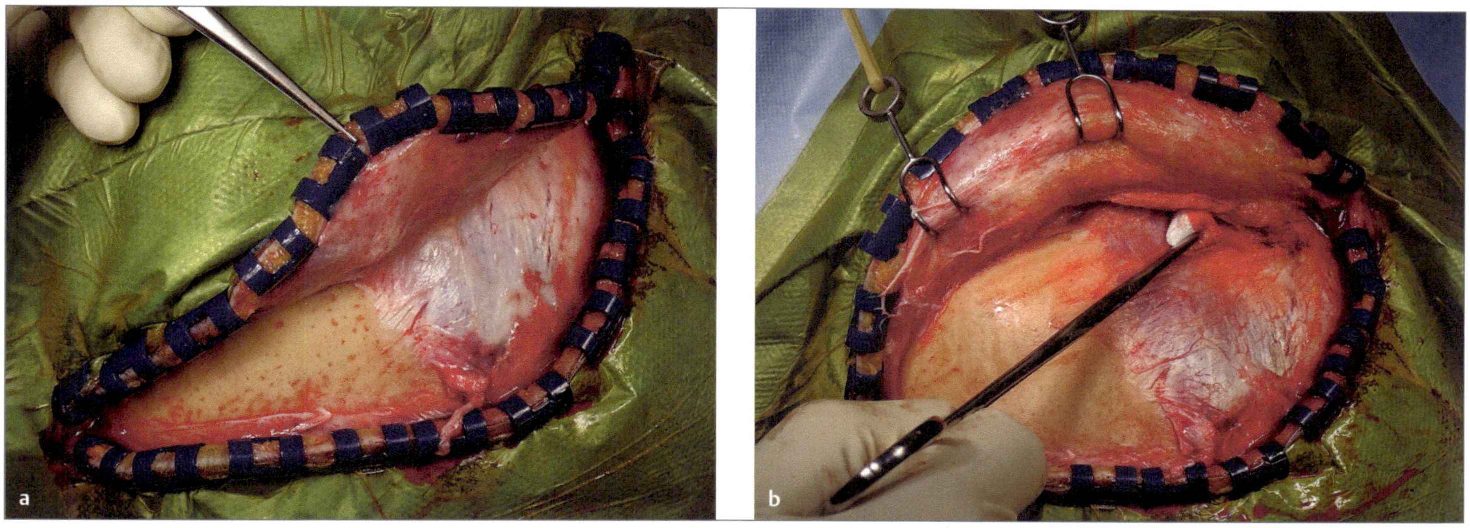

Fig. 5.24 (a, b) Interfascial dissection. After incision, the skin–galea flap is elevated until the yellowish fat pad appears **(a)**. The superficial layer of the temporalis fascia and the interfascial fat pad is incised. The deep temporalis fascia covering the muscle becomes visible. Now, the fat and the layers above are mobilized anteriorly using a swab. A typical error is to dissect too superficially within the suprafascial fat pad where the facial nerve runs. Therefore, the subfascial technique is preferred because dissection may be easier as there is a clear border between the deep layer of the temporalis fascia and the temporalis muscle. Interfascial or subfascial dissection is only required when the lateral orbit or the zygoma has to be exposed, or where the temporalis muscle is likely to obstruct the surgical field.

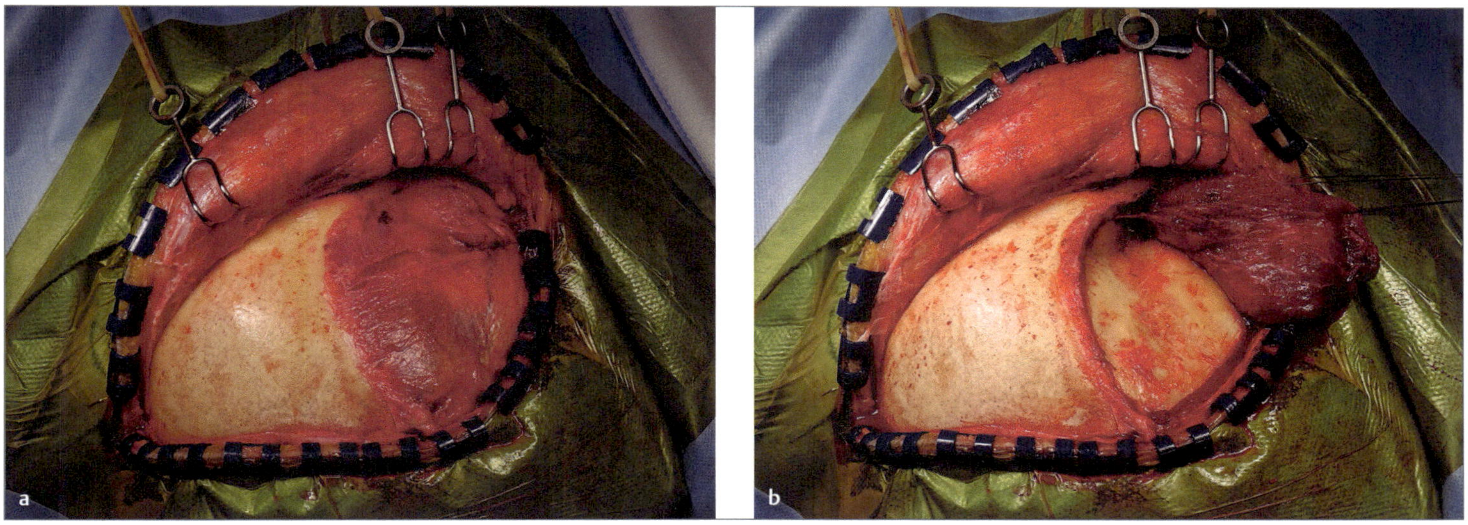

Fig. 5.25 (a, b) Interfascial dissection. The temporalis muscle and the orbital rim are exposed. Fish hooks are used to retract the combined flap. Care should be taken to apply only as much tension as is required to hold the flap in place, because excessive traction may also injure the branches of the facial nerve **(a)**. Now the temporalis muscle is cut at the posterior border parallel to the posterior skin incision line and detached from the bone in an inferior-to-superior direction **(b)**. It is then also detached behind the orbital rim and reflected inferiorly. A suture with loose tension holds the muscle in place. In this example, a muscle cuff is left at the STL to enable better refixation by suturing the muscle to this cuff during closure.

5.2.2 Superficial Temporal Artery Preservation during Frontolateral Approaches

Andreas Raabe and Peter Vajkoczy

See ▶Fig. 5.26, ▶Fig. 5.27, ▶Fig. 5.28, ▶Fig. 5.29, ▶Fig. 5.30, ▶Fig. 5.31, ▶Fig. 5.32, ▶Fig. 5.33, ▶Fig. 5.34, and ▶Fig. 5.35.

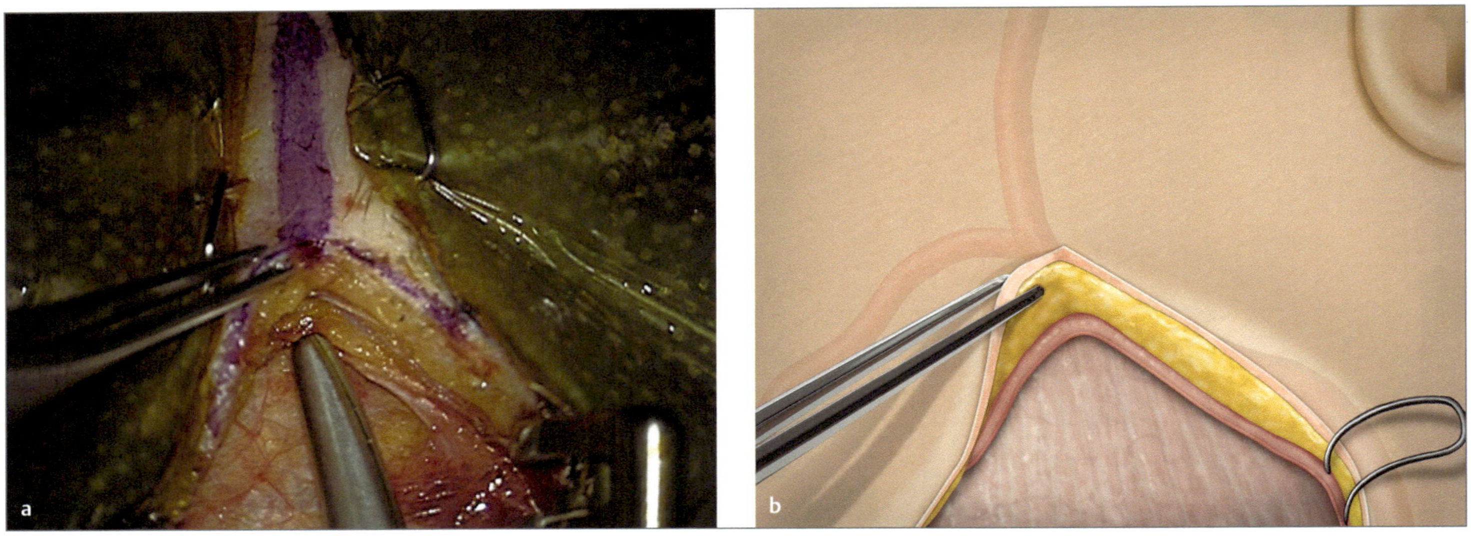

Fig. 5.26 (a,b) Preserving the superficial temporal artery: anatomy of the skin flap. When the lower (temporal preauricular) part of the frontotemporal skin incision is reached (e.g., pterional, frontolateral, or anterior temporal approaches), the surgical technique should be adapted to preserve the superficial temporal artery (STA). The skin flap above the fascia of the temporal muscle consists of two basic layers: the skin with the subcutaneous tissue (superficial layer) and the galea layer containing connective tissue where the STA is embedded above the galeal aponeurotic fascia.

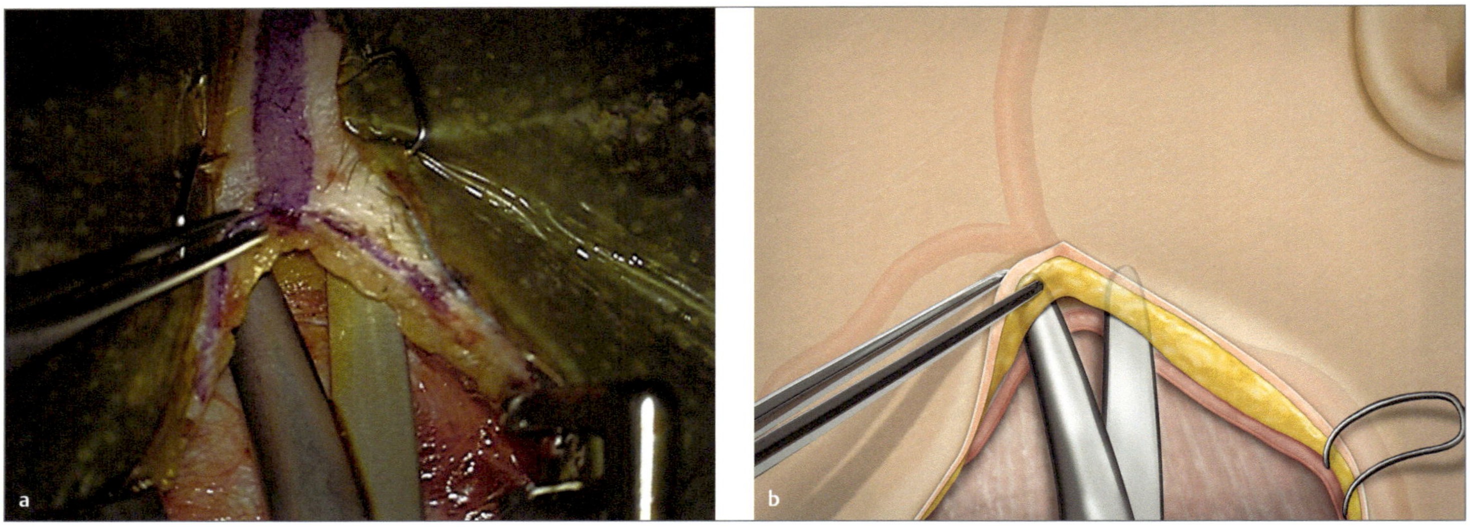

Fig. 5.27 (a, b) Subcutaneous dissection of the two skin flap layers. Using fine scissors, a horizontal dissection is done between the two layers. This creates a space allowing for separate incision of the superficial skin layer leaving the galeal layer with the STA intact.

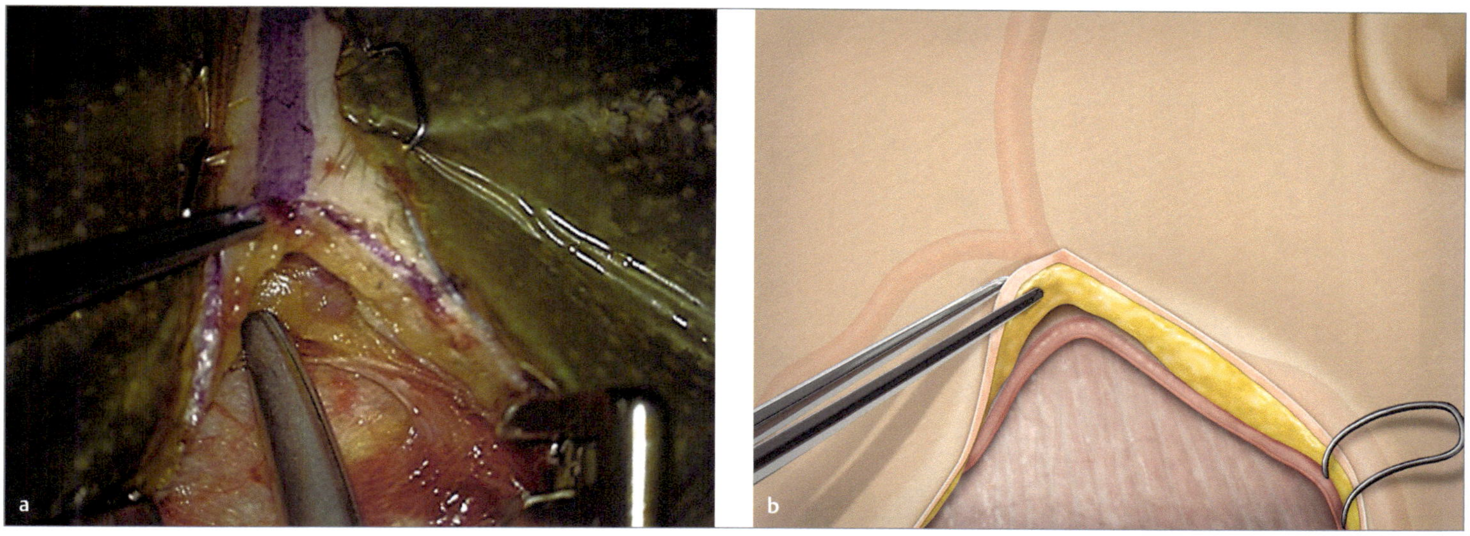

Fig. 5.28 (a, b) Exposing the deep galeal tissue layer. The deep layer is visualized. The connective tissue containing the STA and the galeal aponeurotic fascia is visible.

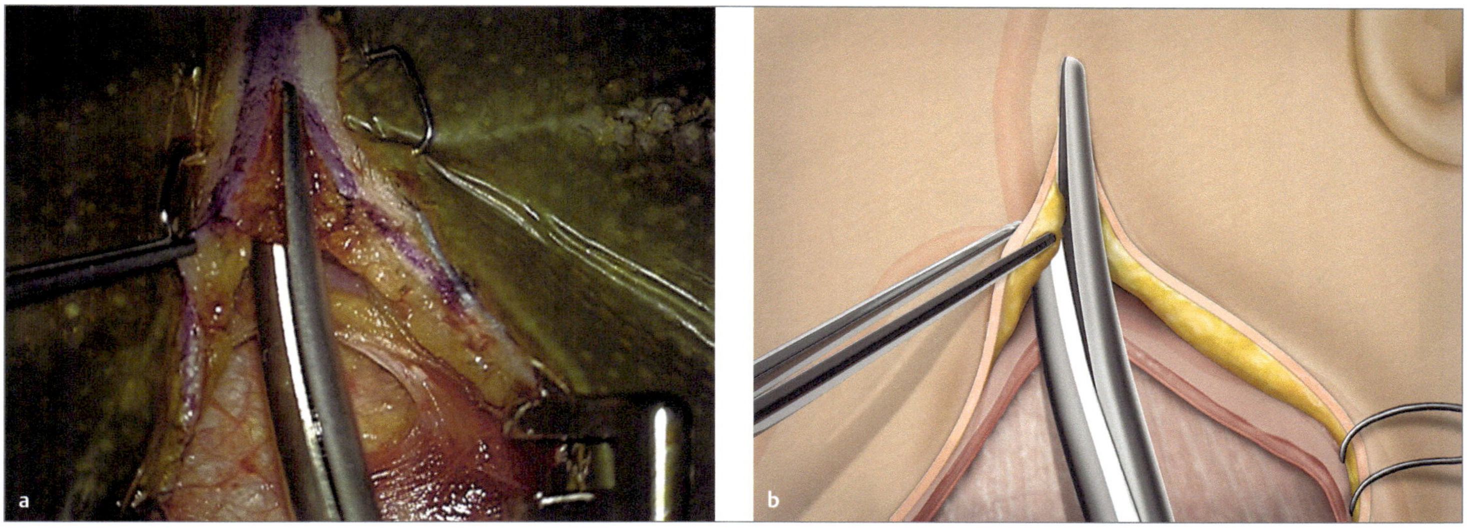

Fig. 5.29 (a, b) Selective supragaleal skin incision for preserving the superficial temporary artery. Now that the two layers are separated, the superficial subcutaneous tissue layer is cut. The STA is embedded in the deep layer.

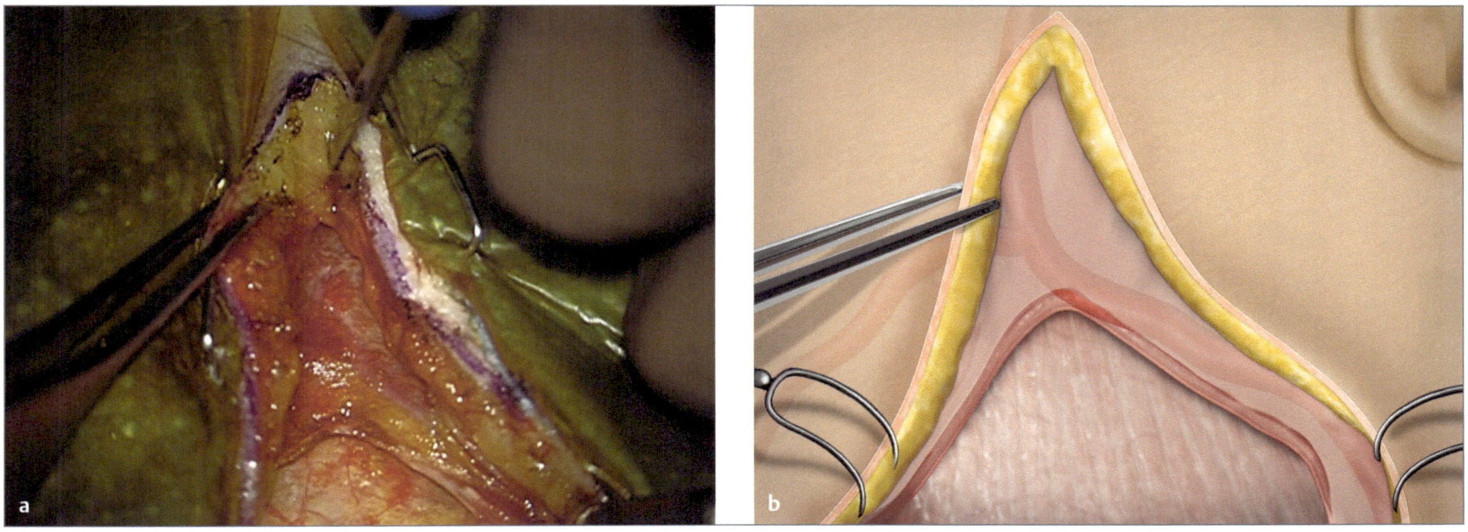

Fig. 5.30 (a, b) Exposing the deep galeal tissue layer with the STA. The deep layer containing connective tissue and the STA is visible.

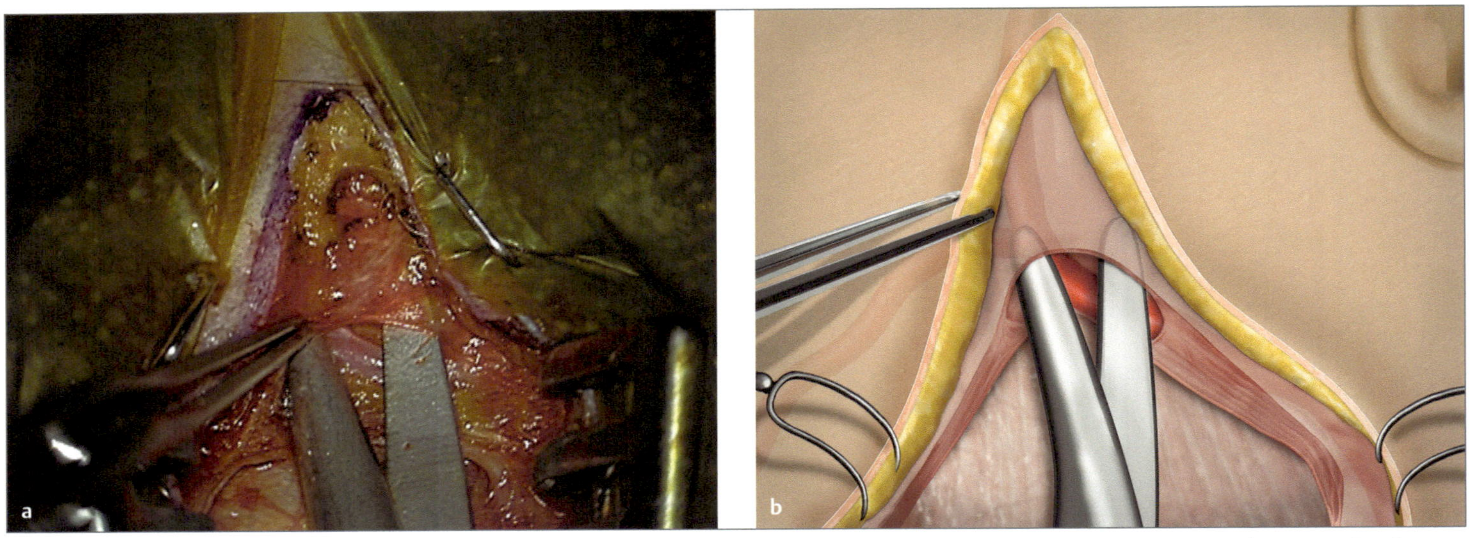

Fig. 5.31 (a, b) Freeing the superficial temporal artery. The scissors are used to dissect horizontally as described in ▶ Fig. 5.27 but immediately below the remaining connective tissue plane and above the STA. The artery is separated from the surrounding connective tissue.

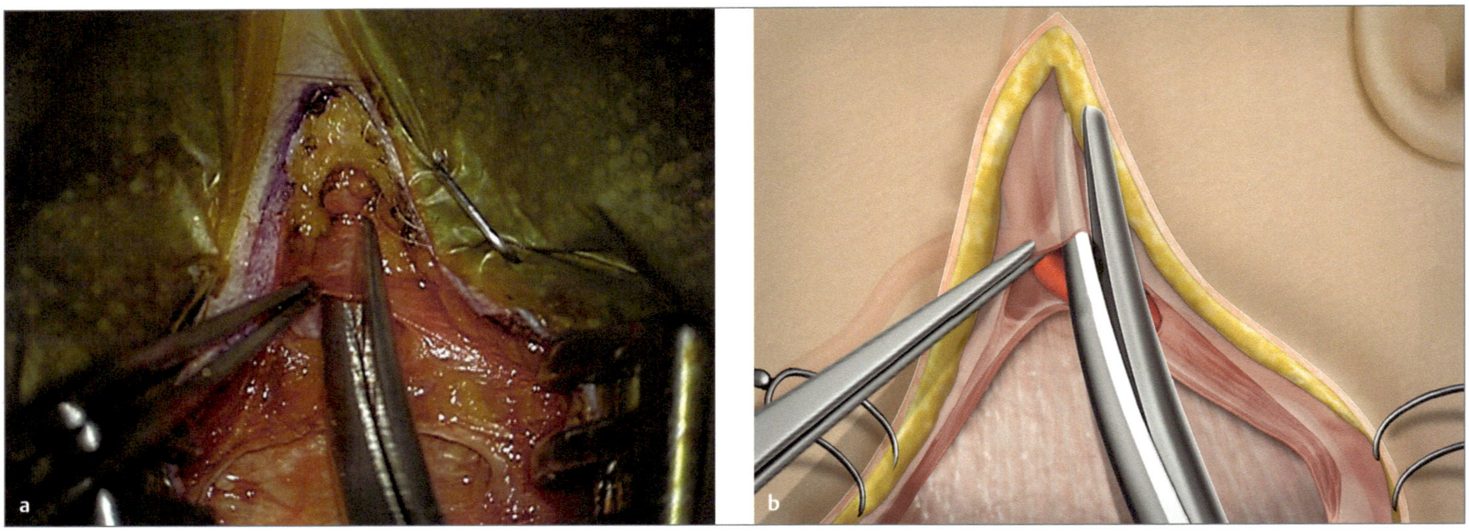

Fig. 5.32 (a, b) Exposure of the superficial temporal artery. The remaining connective tissue plane is cut above the STA.

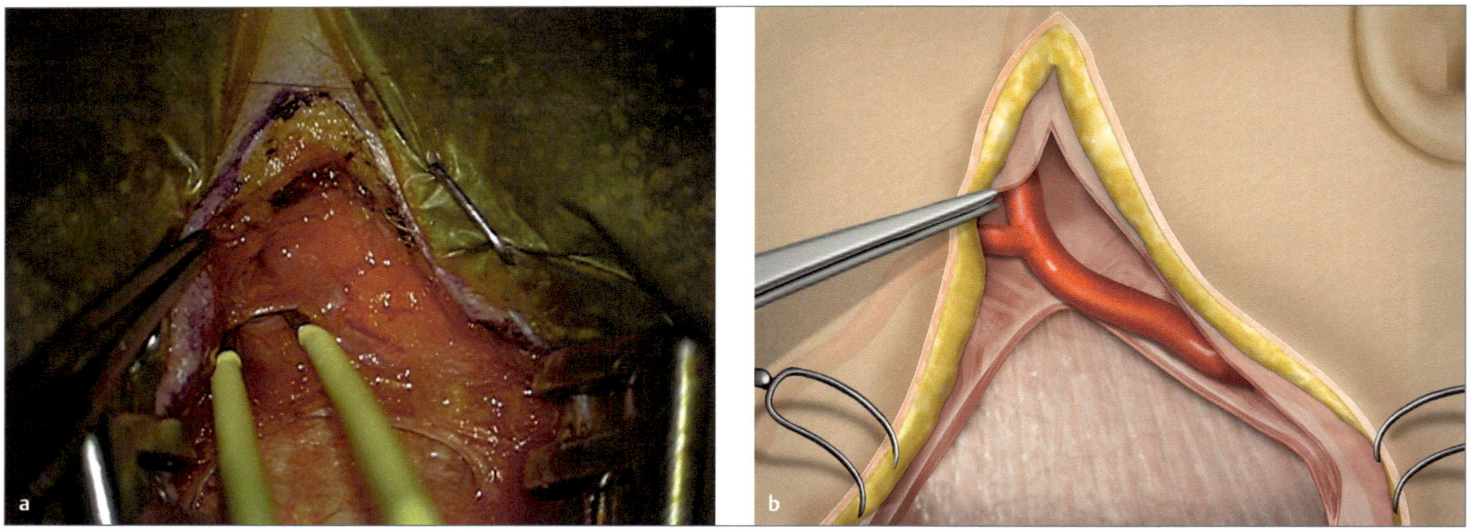

Fig. 5.33 (a ,b) Exposure of the superficial temporal artery bifurcation and the smaller branch. The STA bifurcation can sometimes be found at the level of the incision. To finish the incision, one branch has to be coagulated and divided. Usually the smaller branch or, if the branches have the same diameter, the shorter branch is sacrificed. In this illustration, the frontal branch is smaller.

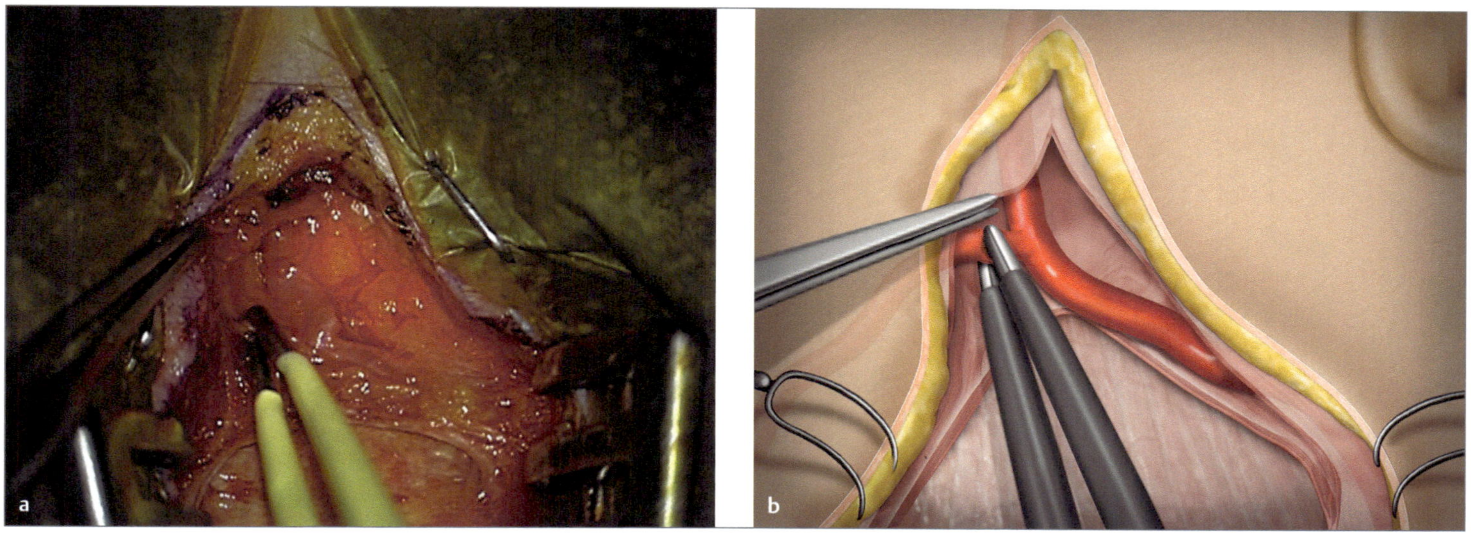

Fig. 5.34 (a, b) Exposure and coagulation of the smaller branch. The smaller branch—in this case, the frontal branch—is coagulated and cut a few millimeters away from the STA. Staying away with the bipolar coagulation from the bifurcation prevents it from shrinking during coagulation and allows for safe recoagulation of the stump of the frontal branch if bleeding occurs after cutting it.

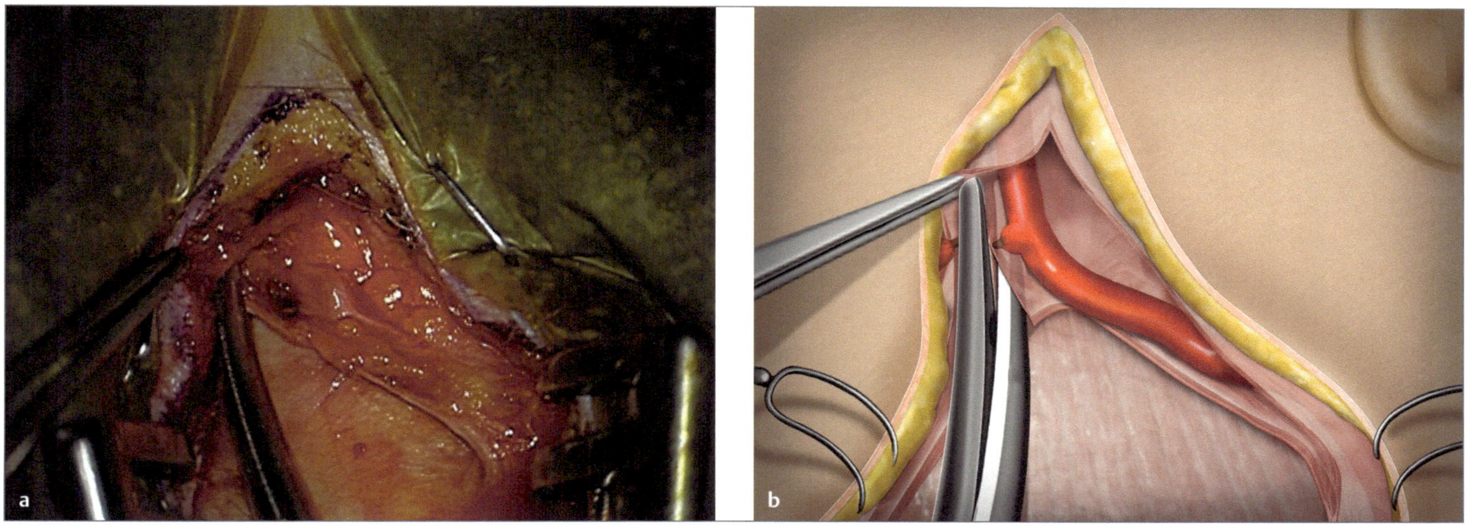

Fig. 5.35 (a, b) Finishing galea incision. The galea can now be cut to finish the incision. Although the situations requiring an emergency bypass is exceptionally rare, preserving the STA is required for maintaining optimal skin blood flow, a neat and gentle surgical approach, and a true microsurgical mindset.

Checklist

- Identify the deep galea layer of the skin flap.
- Dissect the space above the galea layer.
- Cut the superficial layer.
- Use the same technique to free the STA from connective tissue in the deep layer.
- Identify the smaller branch when one branch has to be sacrificed to continue skin incision.
- Keep 3 to 5 mm away from the main STA trunk when coagulating the smaller branch.

5.2.3 Supraorbital

Nikolai Hopf and Robert Reisch

See ▸Fig. 5.36, ▸Fig. 5.37, ▸Fig. 5.38, ▸Fig. 5.39, ▸Fig. 5.40, ▸Fig. 5.41, ▸Fig. 5.42, ▸Fig. 5.43, ▸Fig. 5.44, ▸Fig. 5.45, ▸Fig. 5.46, ▸Fig. 5.47, ▸Fig. 5.48, ▸Fig. 5.49, and ▸Fig. 5.50.

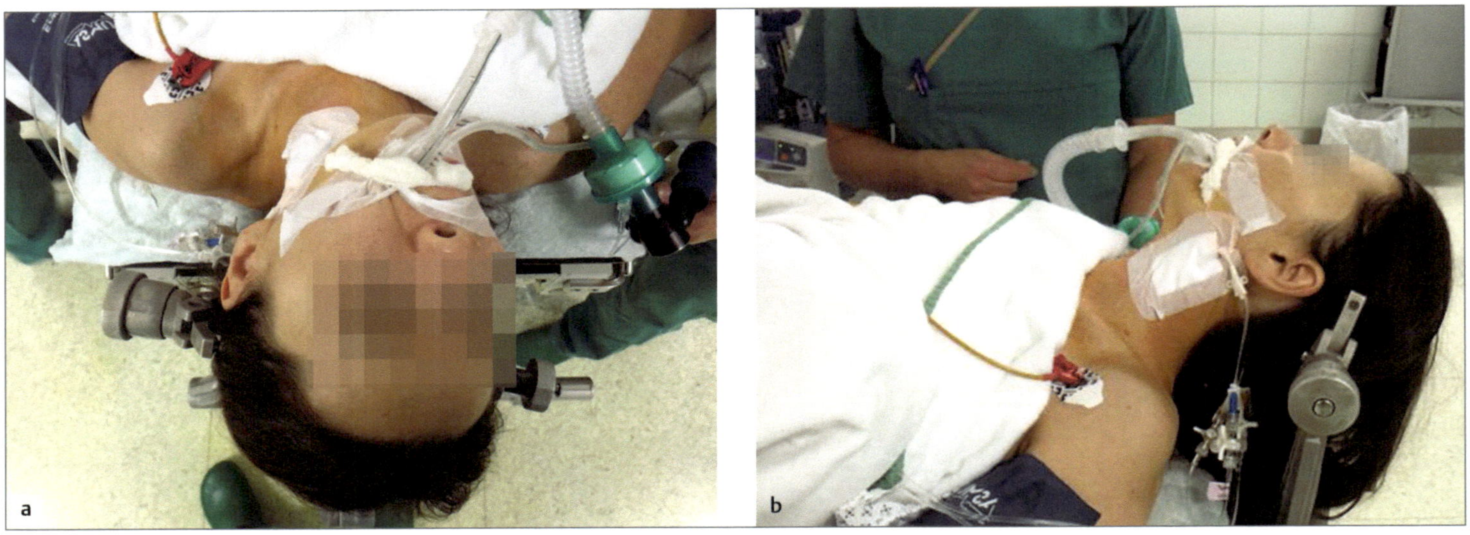

Fig. 5.36 (a, b) Positioning. The supraorbital approach is used for frontobasal, subfrontal, parasellar, temporomesial, and midline lesions including the contralateral side and intrasylvian pathologies. The head is in a slightly reclined position with the eyebrow being the highest point, and the head is rotated to the contralateral side to achieve a perpendicular view toward the target. The angle of head rotation varies accordingly between 15° and 45° (30° for most cases).

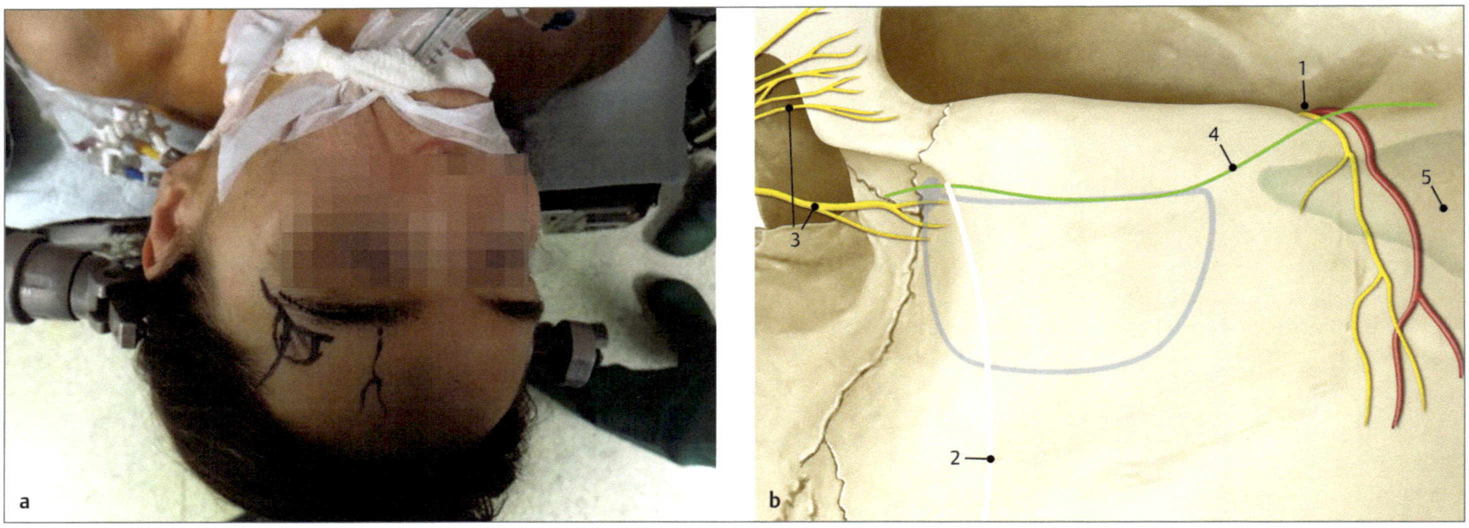

Fig. 5.37 (a, b) Anatomy overview. Important landmarks are (1) the supraorbital foramen with the supraorbital nerve and artery, (2) the temporal line, (3) the frontal branch of the facial nerve, (4) the level of the frontolateral skull base, and (5) the frontal sinus.

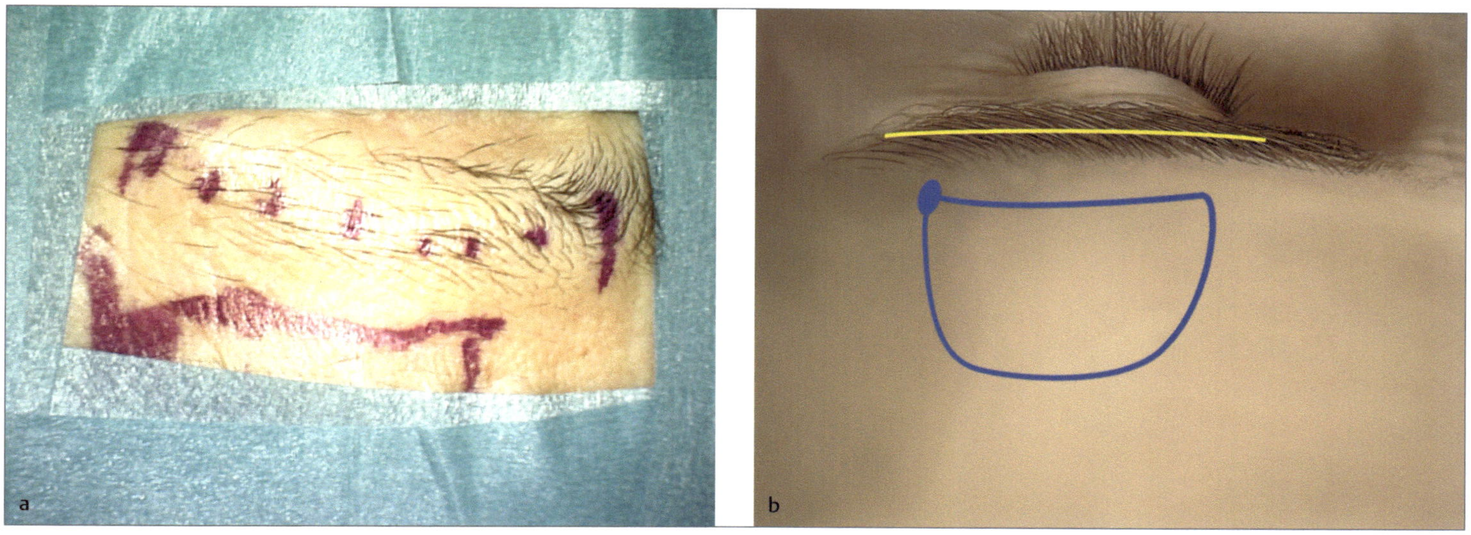

Fig. 5.38 (a, b) Draped position before skin incision. The skin incision should be made within the eyebrow for cosmetic reasons, in particular in patients with thin eyebrows. In patients with no eyebrows, the skin incision may be made in a wrinkle. The length is typically 3 to 4 cm.

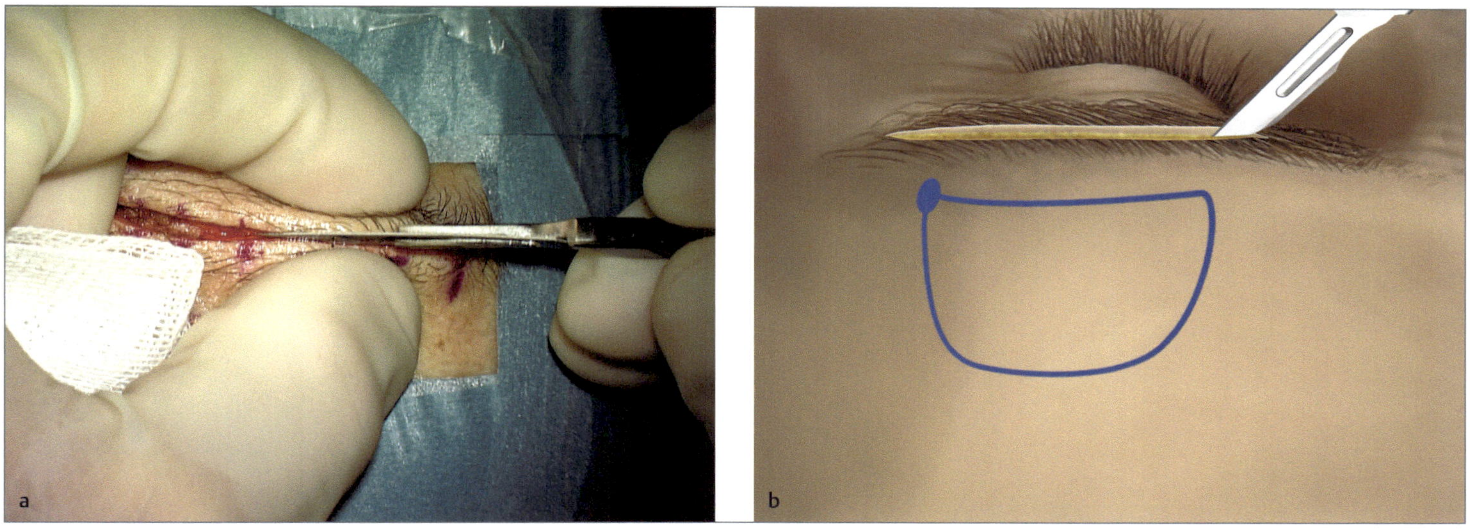

Fig. 5.39 (a, b) Skin incision. The skin incision spares the frontal and orbicularis oculi muscle fascia and is made just lateral to the supraorbital foramen extending to the lateral margin of the eyebrow.

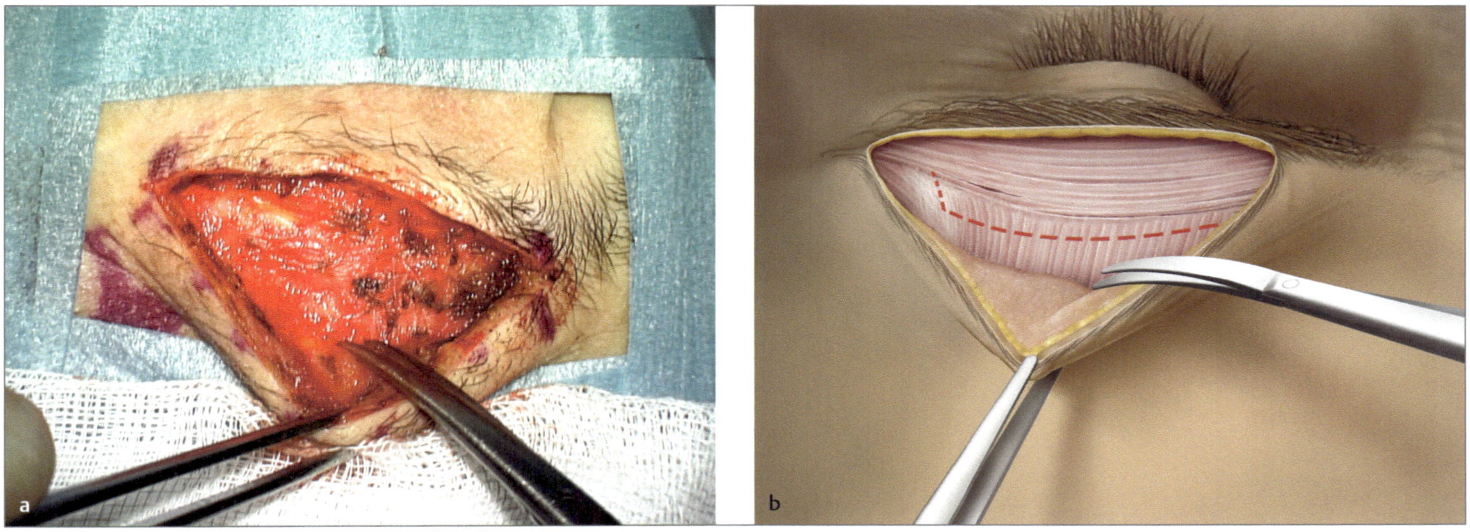

Fig. 5.40 (a, b) Subgaleal flap preparation. The skin flap is dissected between the galea and the frontal muscle fascia only superiorly, since the craniotomy will be located entirely superior to the skin incision. The planned incision is outlined.

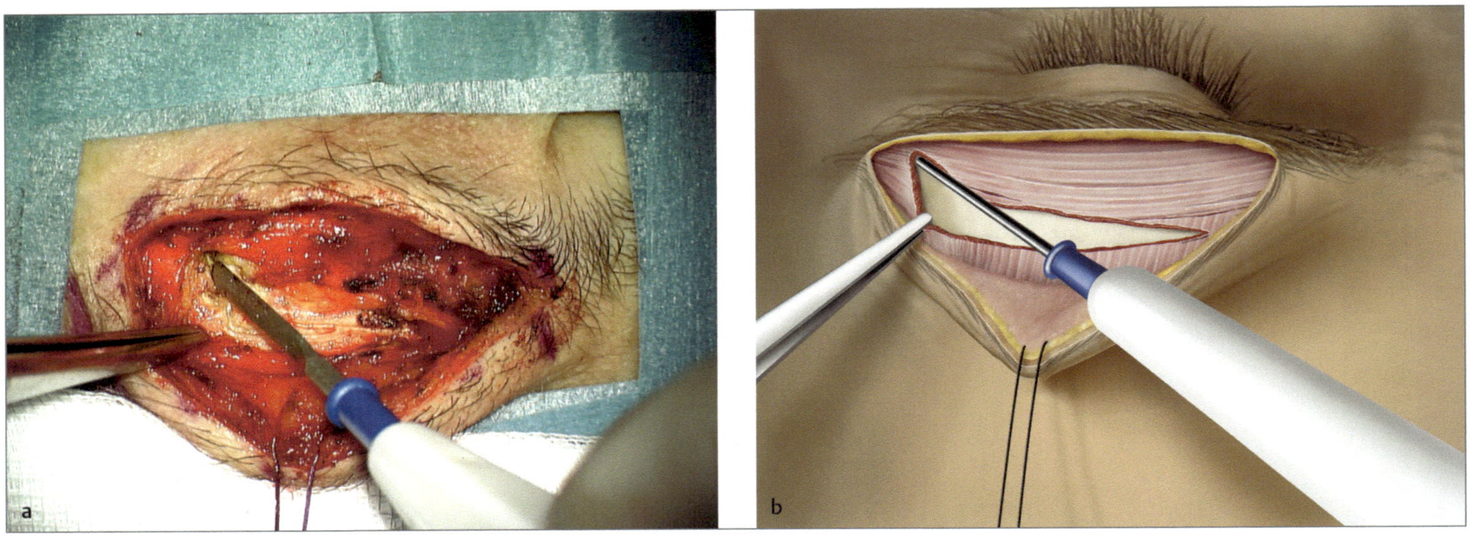

Fig. 5.41 (a, b) Subgaleal flap preparation. The frontal muscle is cut perpendicular to its fibers with a monopolar device, not more than 2 cm superior to the orbital rim and not extending the temporal line laterally, to avoid injury to the facial nerve. Then, the muscle flap is completed by detaching it from the temporal line, cutting in an inferior direction, and pulling it inferiorly with fish hooks or sutures. The temporal muscle is then detached from the temporal line in a very limited area.

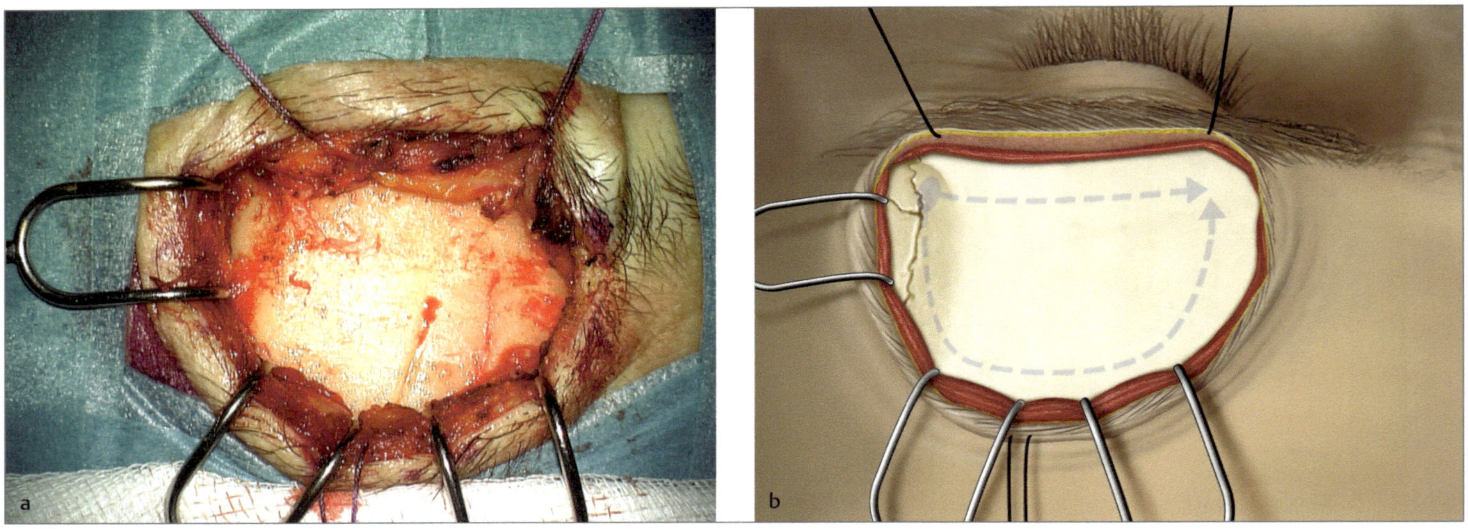

Fig. 5.42 (a, b) Craniotomy planning. Fish hooks or sutures gently pull the detached temporal muscle laterally to keep the anterior superior area of the temporal fossa exposed. The illustration on the right side depicts the planned craniotomy. It must be flush with the floor of the anterior skull base to allow subfrontal access without retraction. The lateral extension is just lateral to the temporal line. The medial extension varies and is typically limited to the level of the supraorbital foramen. Superiorly, it is 1.5–2 cm.

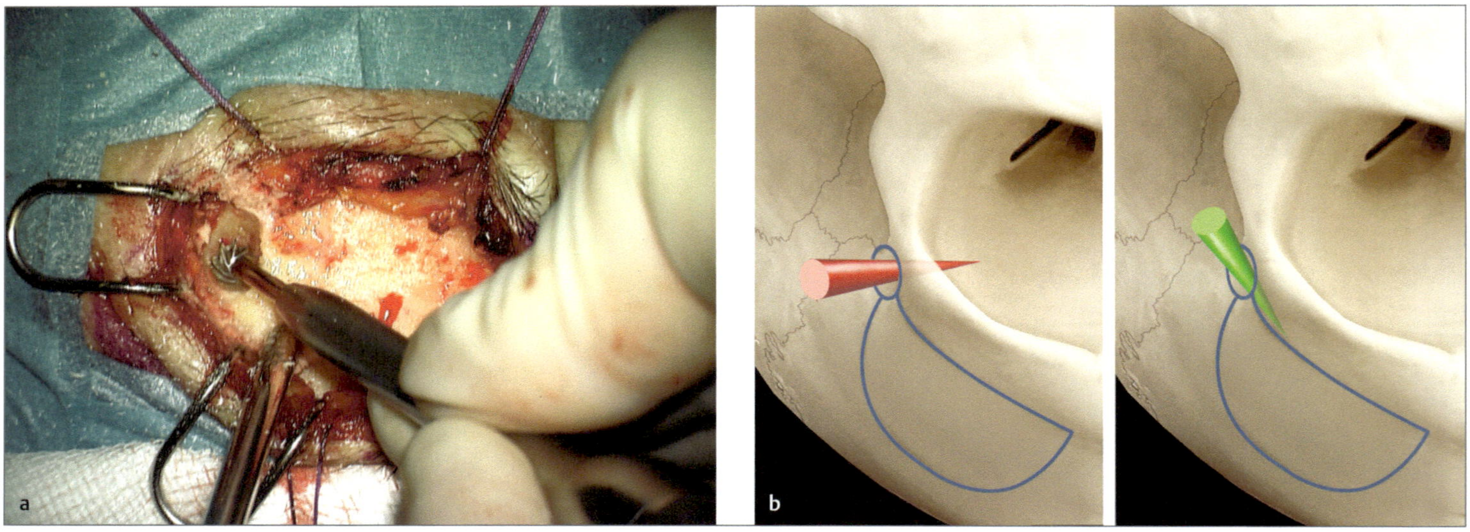

Fig. 5.43 (a, b) Burr hole. The burr hole is made with a cutting or diamond drill. The burr hole is located at the cranial base; therefore, the direction of drilling should be toward the surgeon to avoid entering the orbita. The burr hole should be just big enough to accommodate the craniotome, to achieve a cosmetically acceptable result avoiding sinking of the skin.

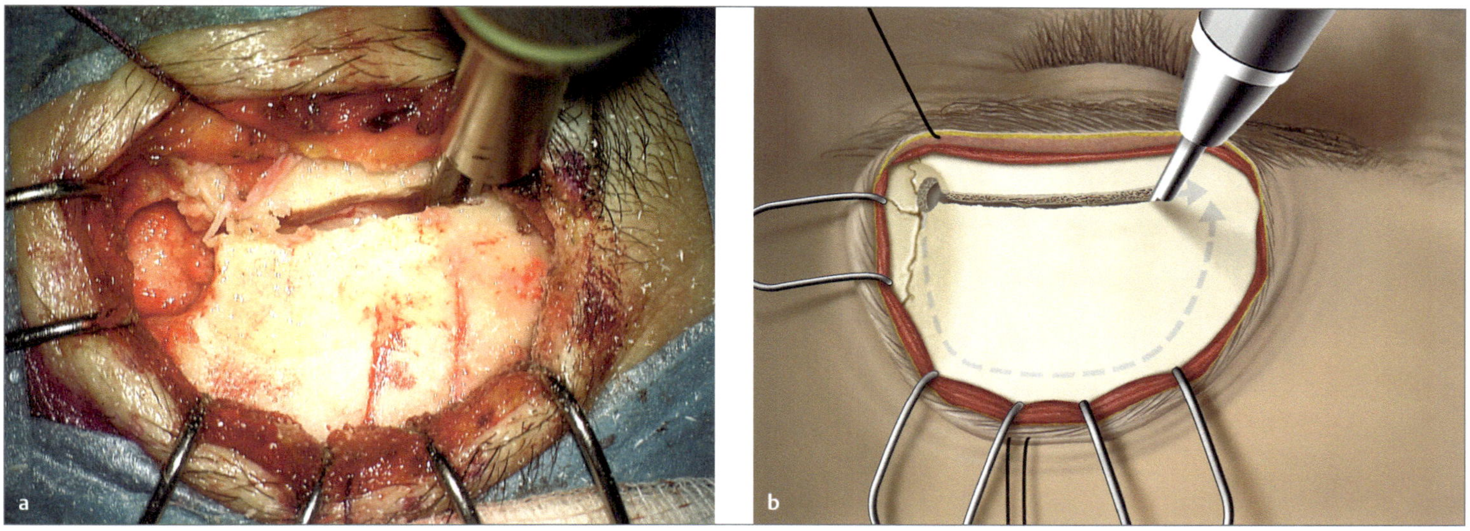

Fig. 5.44 (a, b) Craniotomy. The craniotomy is performed from the burr hole medially and parallel to the frontal skull base. The craniotome should be angled slightly inferiorly to avoid further drilling of the tabula externa.

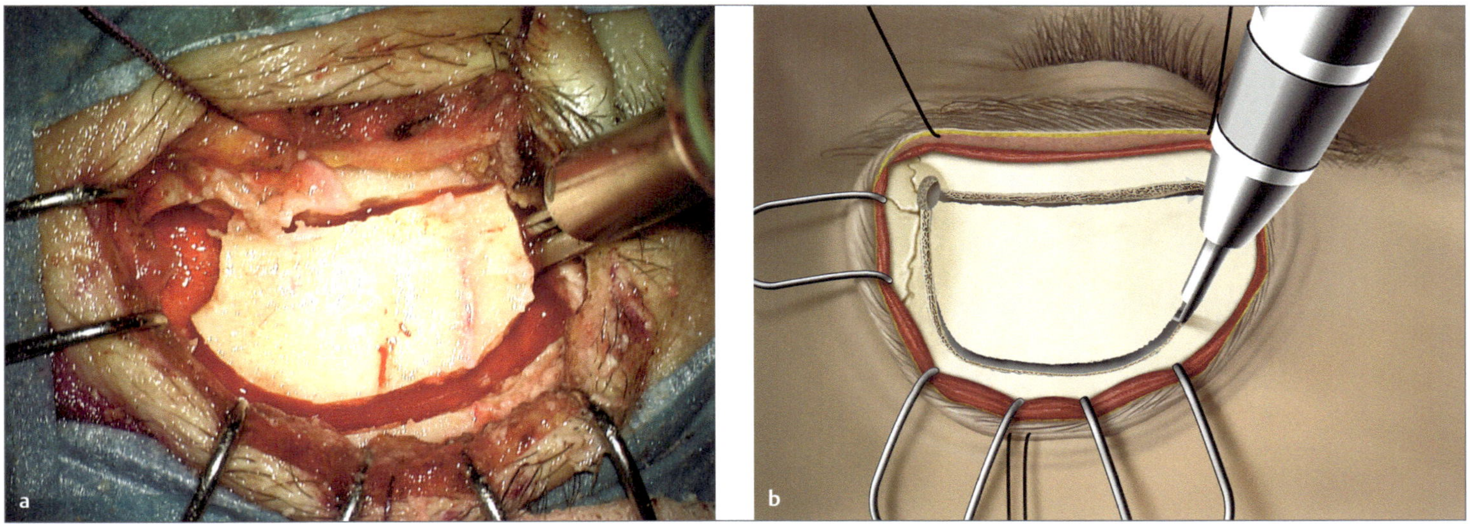

Fig. 5.45 (a, b) Craniotomy. Then, the craniotome is moved back to the burr hole and the craniotomy completed by a C-shaped cut starting from the lateral edge of the burr hole and ending at the medial end of the basal cut. The size of the craniotomy is typically 1.5 × 2.5 cm.

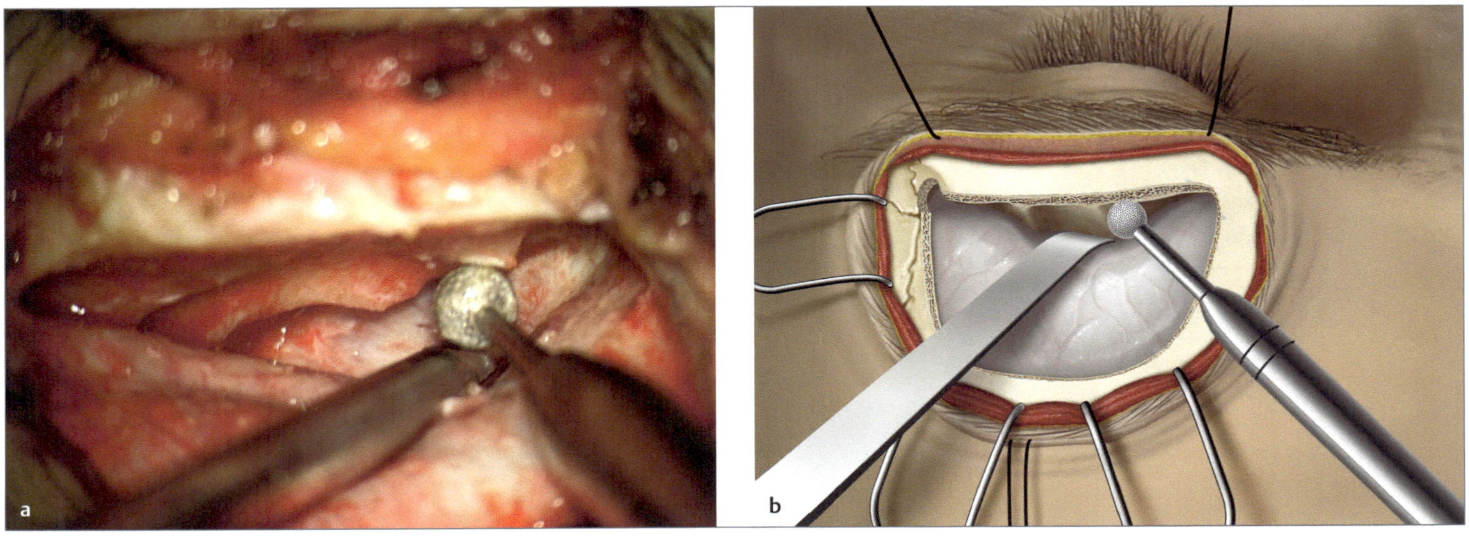

Fig. 5.46 (a, b) Additional bone drilling. After elevation of the bone flap, the inner tabula is drilled with a 4- or 5-mm diamond drill. In so doing, another few millimeters of space is gained to achieve subfrontal access flush with the anterior base to avoid retraction. When completed, the dura should be detached from the base to identify larger bony elevations of the orbital roof, so-called jugae, which may obstruct the view. If present, they should also be flattened with the drill.

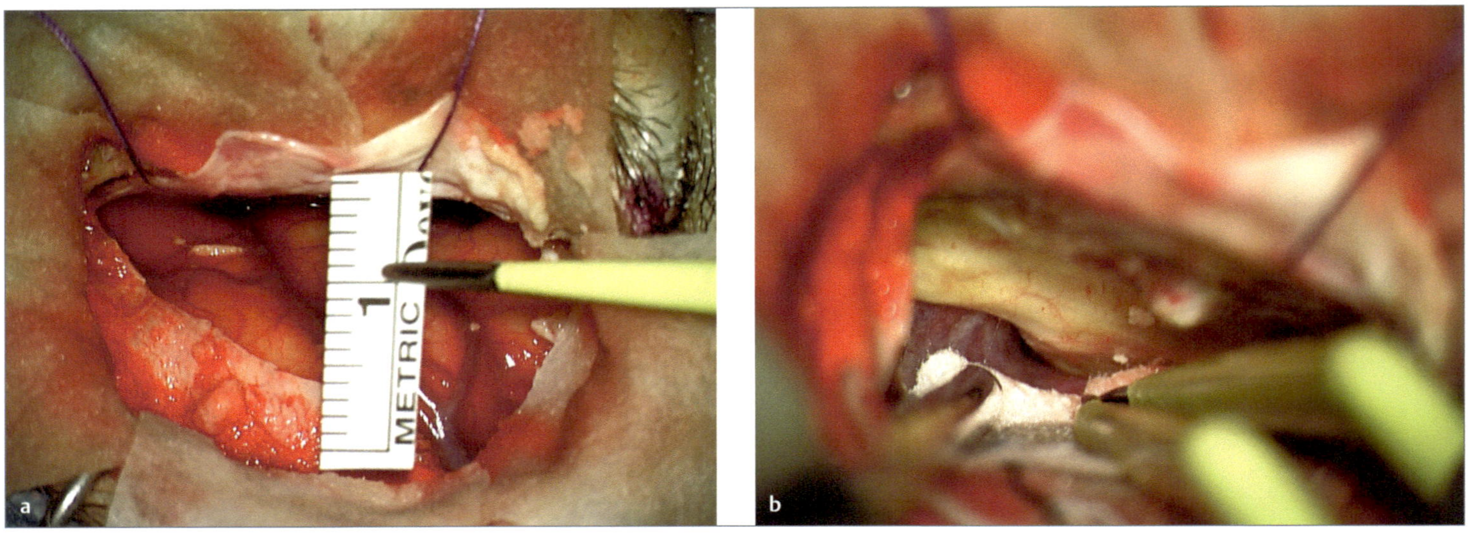

Fig. 5.47 (a, b) **Dura opening.** The dura is opened in a C-shaped manner toward the skull base anteriorly and fixed with tacking sutures. The brain is then covered with wet cottonoids to reduce mechanical damage and avoid exposure to heat from the light source of the microscope or endoscope. The image shows subfrontal access to the anterior cranial base without retraction.

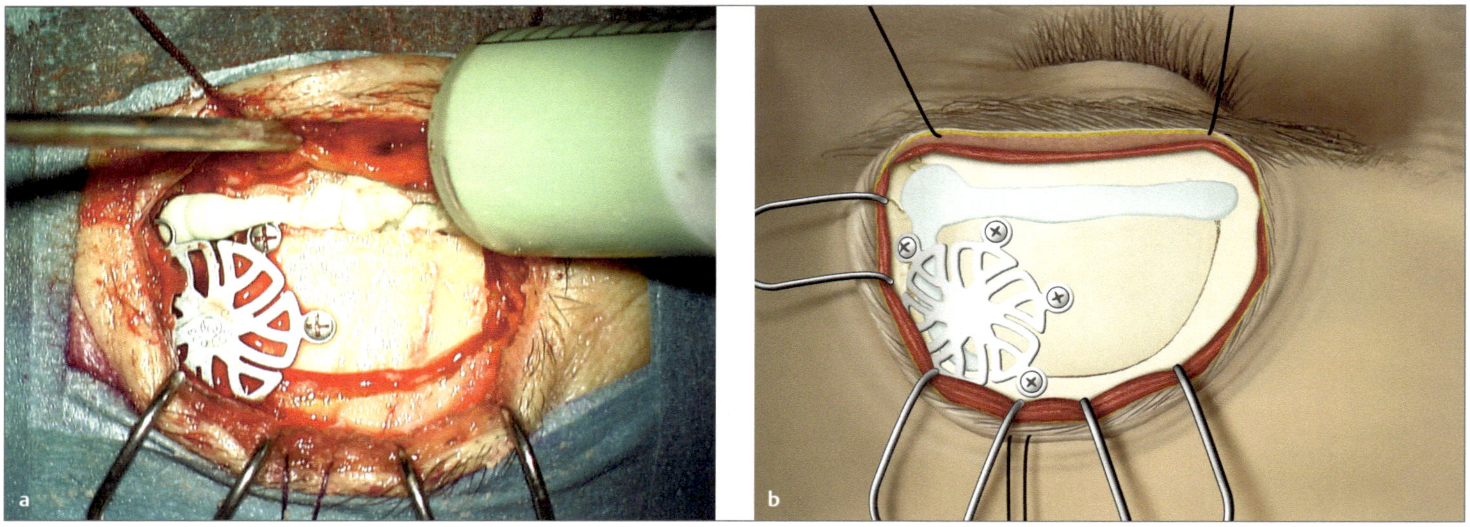

Fig. 5.48 (a, b) **Closure: bone flap.** After closure of the dura, the bone flap is fixed with sutures or a titanium plate as shown on the left image. For cosmesis, the bone flap should be placed superiorly and medially without any gaps. Bone cement, as shown on the image, or other material should be used to fill larger lateral and inferior gaps. Opening the frontal sinus during craniotomy is of less concern but should be avoided if possible.

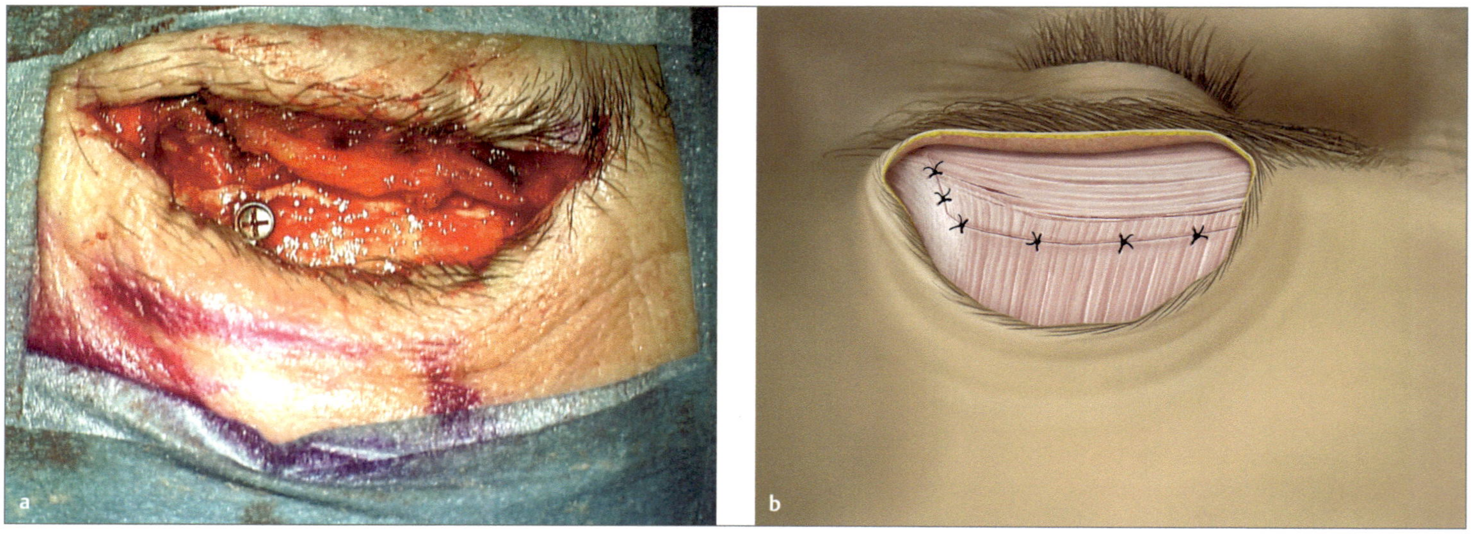

Fig. 5.49 (a, b) **Closure: soft tissue.** The frontal muscle flap is sutured medially and superiorly and to the temporal muscle fascia. Then, the subcutaneous tissue is sutured tightly to achieve a narrow scar.

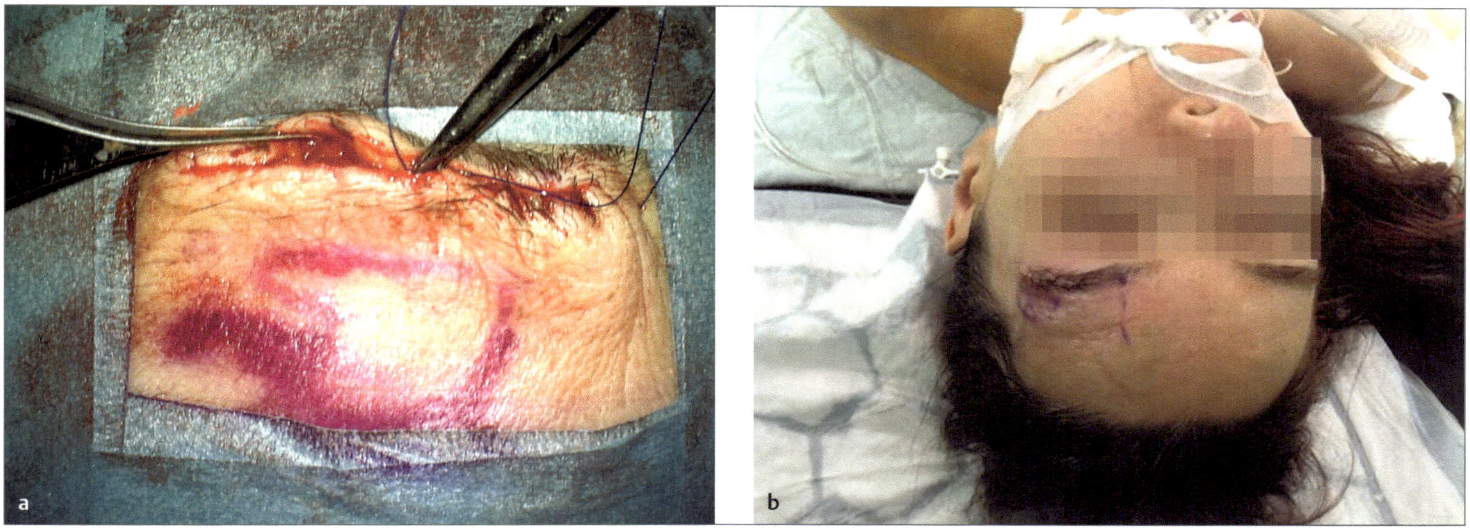

Fig. 5.50 (a, b) Closure: skin. The skin may be closed with an intracutaneous suture as shown in the left image **(a)**. Alternatively, a monofilament running suture **(b)**, sterile strips, or acrylic glue may be used. Surgeons should check cosmesis during follow-up of the patients to obtain feedback on the results of the technique they are using.

Checklist

- Palpate the supraorbital foramen and temporal line and estimate the level of the frontal skull base about 1.5 cm superior to the inner edge of the orbital rim.
- Make the incision within the eyebrow and not above it.
- Mobilize skin only superiorly.
- Use a small drill for the burr hole for cosmetic reasons.
- Direct the burr toward your body when making the burr hole to avoid entering the orbita.
- Angle the craniotome inferiorly during the basal cut of craniotomy.
- Drill the tabula interna for better access to the base while leaving the tabula externa intact.
- Detach the dura mater basally from the orbital roof and check for large jugae that obstruct your view along the anterior skull base.
- Avoid superior and medial bone gaps when placing the bone flap. Cover the burr hole with temporal muscle.

5.2.4 Frontolateral

Andreas Raabe

See ▸Fig. 5.51, ▸Fig. 5.52, ▸Fig. 5.53, ▸Fig. 5.54, ▸Fig. 5.55, ▸Fig. 5.56, ▸Fig. 5.57, ▸Fig. 5.58, ▸Fig. 5.59, ▸Fig. 5.60, ▸Fig. 5.61, ▸Fig. 5.62, ▸Fig. 5.63, ▸Fig. 5.64, ▸Fig. 5.65, ▸Fig. 5.66, and ▸Fig. 5.67.

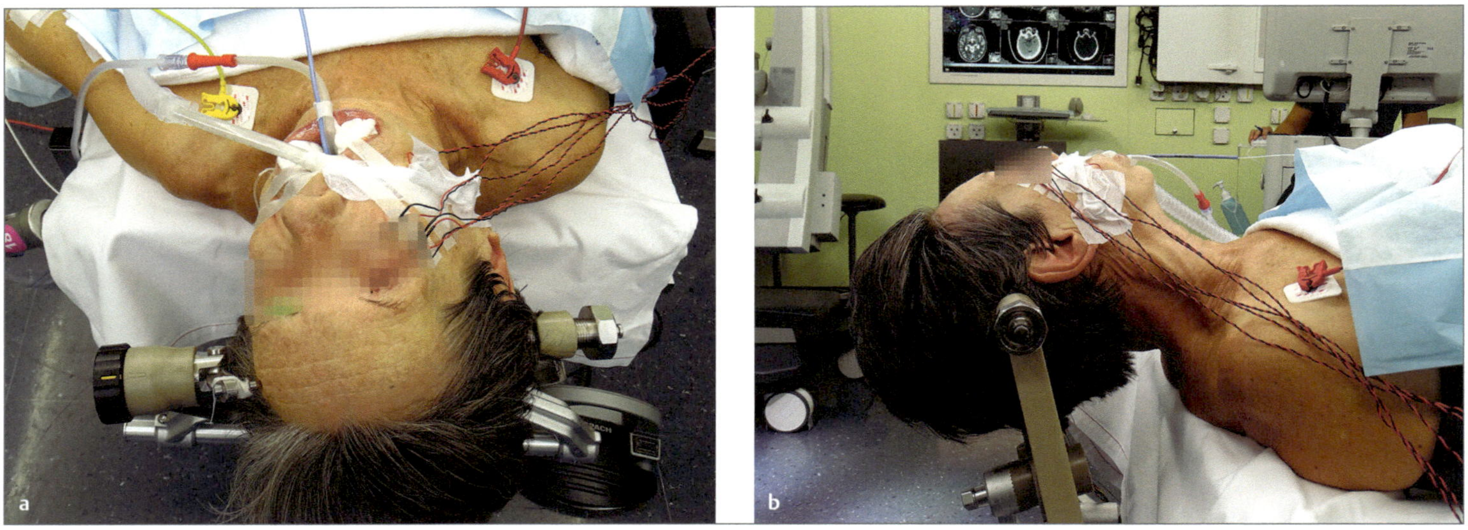

Fig. 5.51 (a, b) Positioning. The frontolateral craniotomy is used for subfrontal, parasellar, tentorial, and midline lesions including the contralateral side and transsylvian approaches. Positioning of the head is similar to that for the pterional approach with the zygoma being the highest point and head rotation to provide a perpendicular line from the craniotomy to the target. The angle of head rotation varies accordingly between 15° and 60° (30° for most cases).

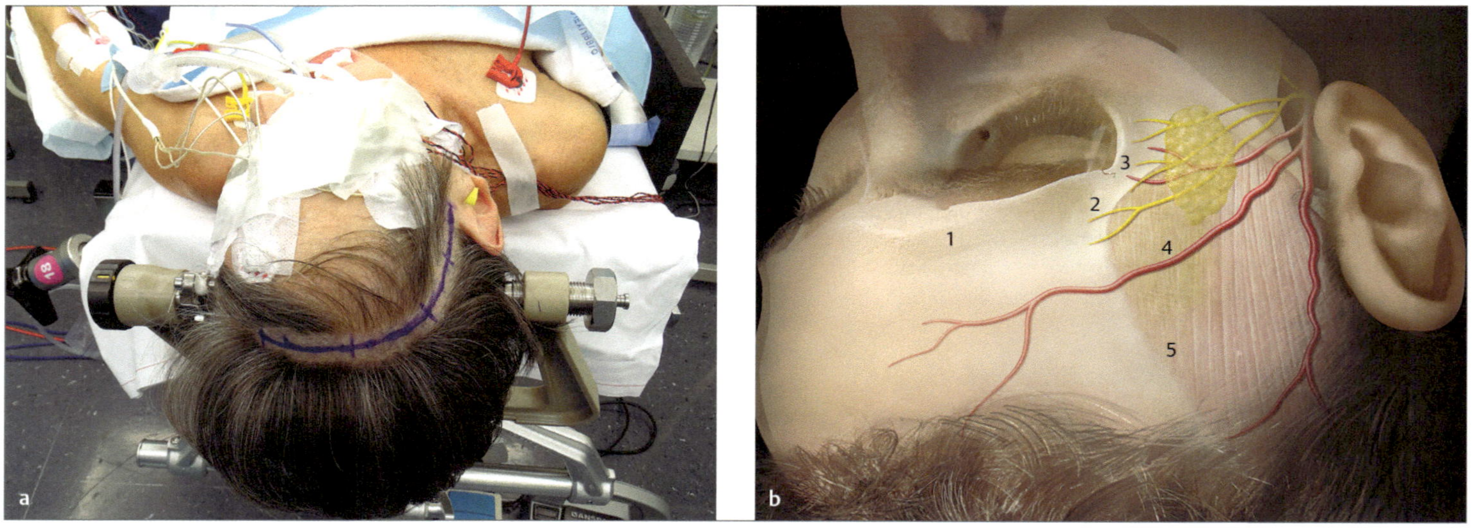

Fig. 5.52 (a, b) Anatomy overview. Important landmarks are (1) the supraorbital foramen, (2) the posterior lateral edge of the zygomatic process of the frontal bone (landmark: frontotemporale) indicating the cranial base, (3) the frontozygomatic suture as a rough landmark for the sphenoid ridge, (4) the frontal branch of the superficial temporal artery, and (5) the fascia of the temporal muscle originating from the superior temporal line. For planning of the length of the skin incision, the frontotemporale (2) should be located by palpation. A common misconception is that a small craniotomy such as the frontolateral craniotomy needs a small skin incision. For cosmetic reasons, the incision should be covered by hair, i.e., it should be behind the hairline, and as large as necessary to gain access to the skull base. Therefore, in patients with more anterior hairlines, the incision will be shorter, and in patients with more posterior hairlines it will be longer.

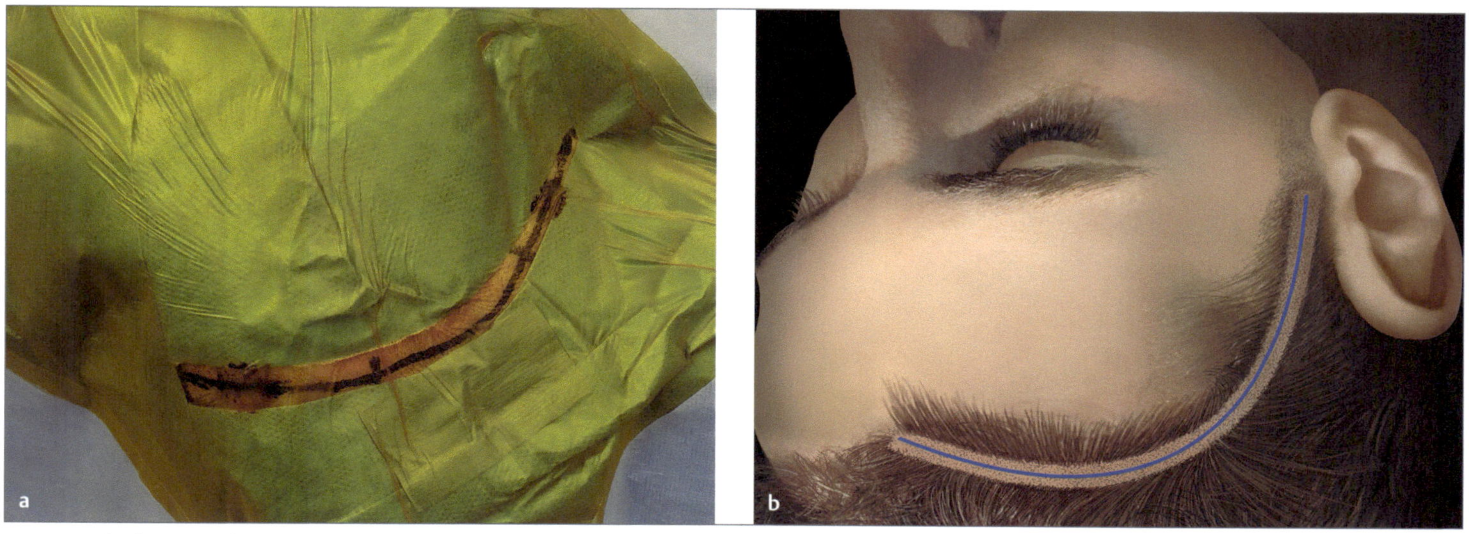

Fig. 5.53 (a, b) Draped position before skin incision. The skin incision is similar to that for the pterional approach, but does not extend so far inferior on the temporal side. It should allow visualization and opening of the sylvian fissure. When the frontolateral approach is used, exposure of the temporal lobe is not usually planned. The skin incision should be made behind the hairline for cosmesis. In bald patients, the incision should be made in a wrinkle on the forehead 1–2 cm above the eyebrow, or within the eyebrow when a smaller supraorbital approach is used. The beginning and the end of the planned skin incision should be checked to make sure that the cranial base point will be exposed during craniotomy.

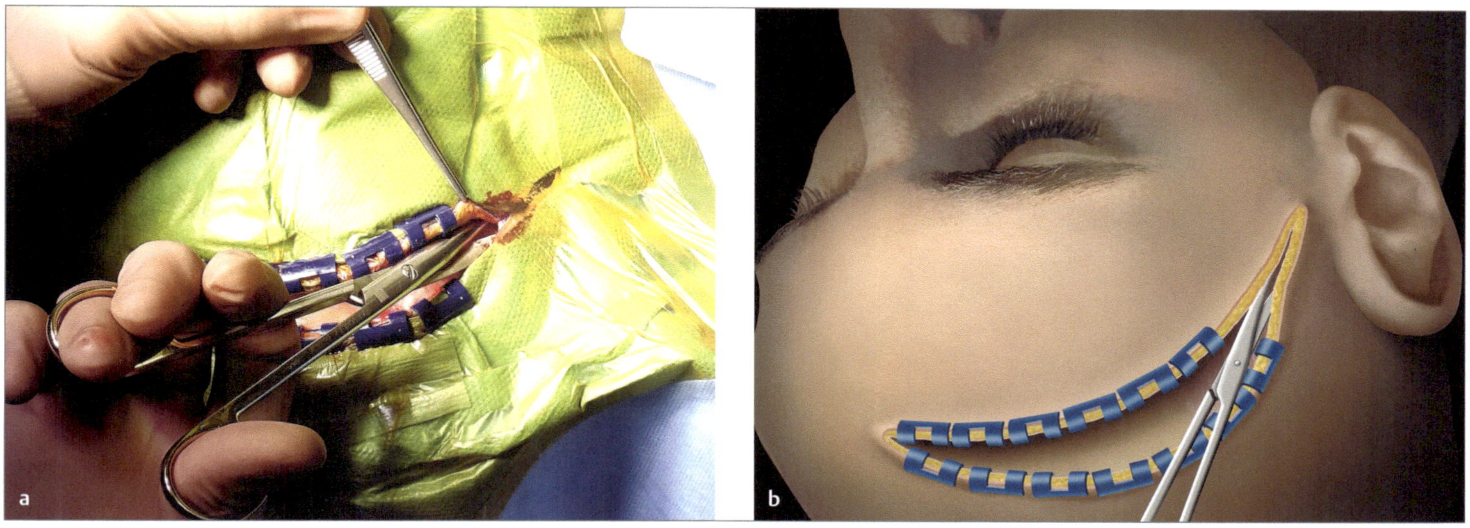

Fig. 5.54 (a, b) Skin incision. The skin incision spares the temporal muscle fascia. Upon reaching the temporal third of the planned incision, care is taken to preserve the superficial temporal artery. Our technique is to dissect the horizontal tissue layers in the skin flap in a subcutaneous and a deep galea layer to end up with two separate layers. The superficial temporal artery can be found on top of the galea in the deep layer.

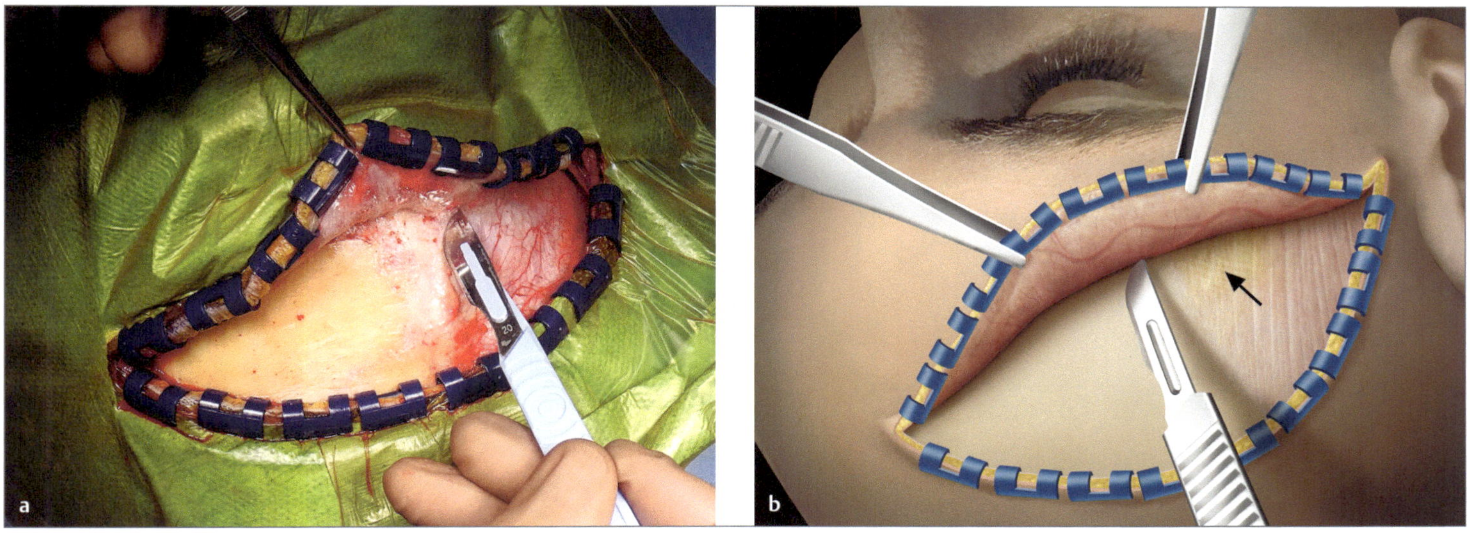

Fig. 5.55 (a, b) Subgaleal flap preparation. The skin flap is dissected between the galea and the temporal muscle fascia anteriorly. Usually, the yellow interfascial fat pad (*black arrow*) becomes visible through the temporalis fascia in the superoanterior part of the temporalis muscle. The temporal muscle fascia attaches to the superior temporal line. Medially (=above) the superior temporal line, the pericranium is detached from the skull in one layer with the galea, using a raspatorium.

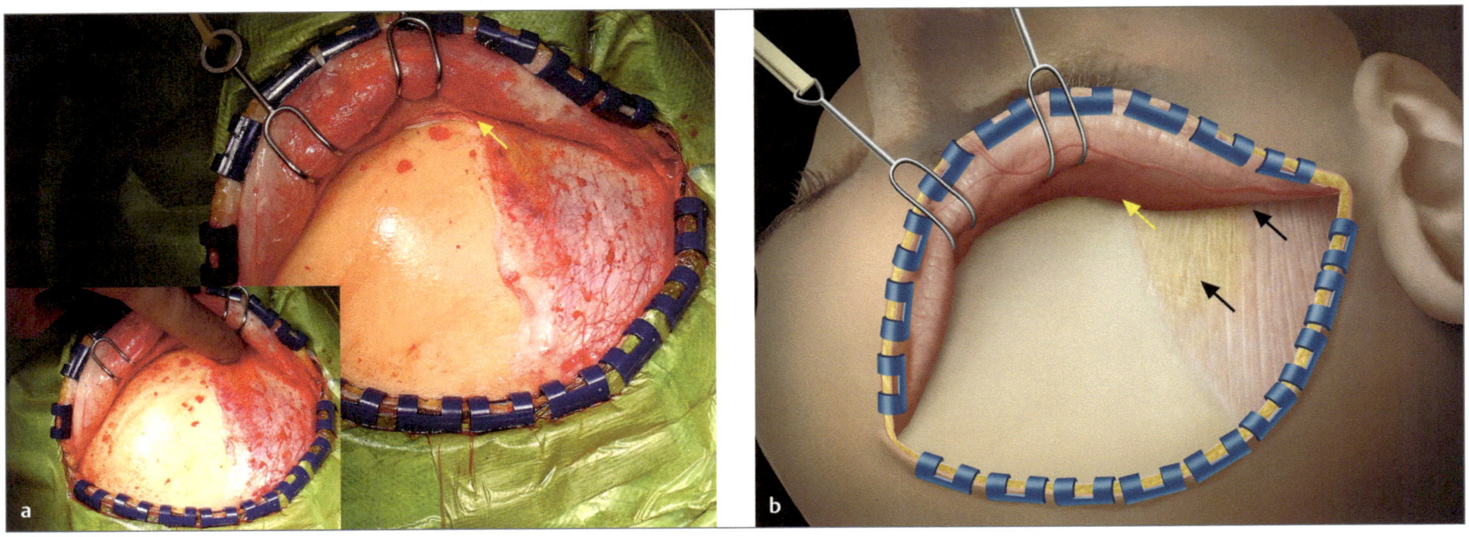

Fig. 5.56 (a, b) Subgaleal flap preparation. When the bony edge of the zygomatic process (= the landmark frontotemporale) (*arrow*) can be palpated with the finger through the galea and intact muscle, the anterior border of the galeal dissection is almost reached. The risk of facial nerve injury is low with this approach, because the facial nerve crosses into the galea in the area of the suprafascial fat pad (*black double arrow*), which is situated below and temporal of the interfascial fat pad (*black arrow*, see also Chapter 5.2.1, Facial Nerve Anatomy and Protection).

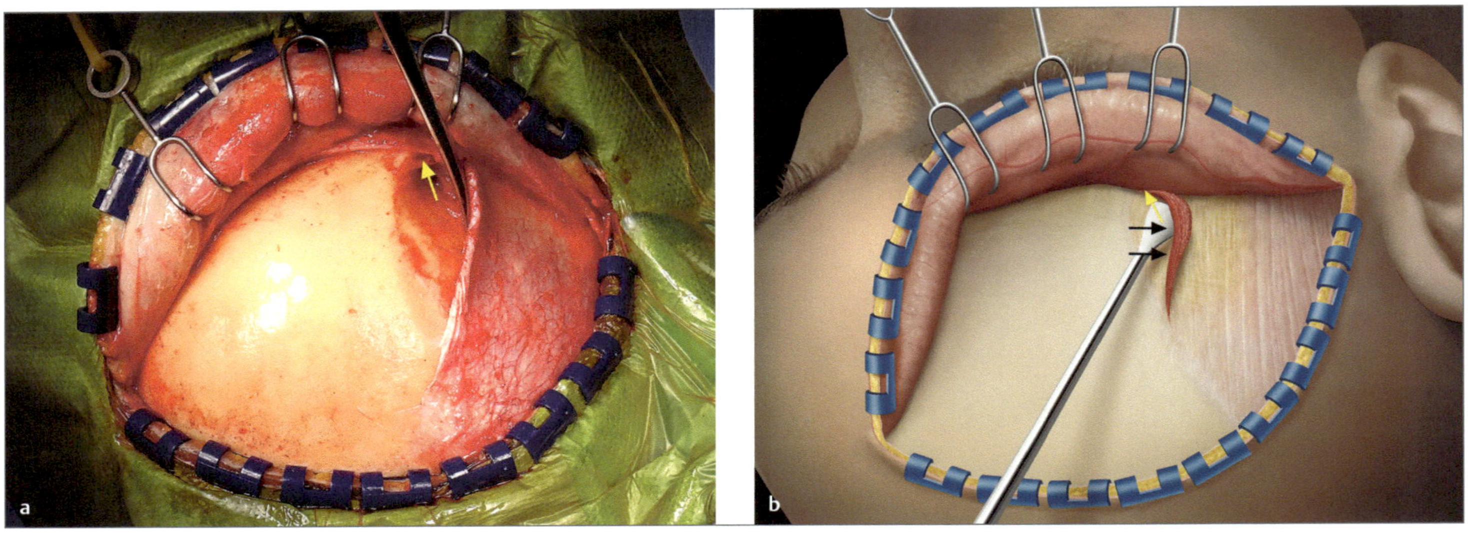

Fig. 5.57 (a, b) Subperiostal elevation of upper anterior temporal muscle. The anterior temporalis muscle is detached subperiostally from the bone to expose the bone below the superior temporal line (*black arrows*). It is elevated, also subperiostally, from the zygomatic process and upper orbital rim (*yellow arrow*). This is required to expose the area for the burr hole and the anteroinferior craniotomy border.

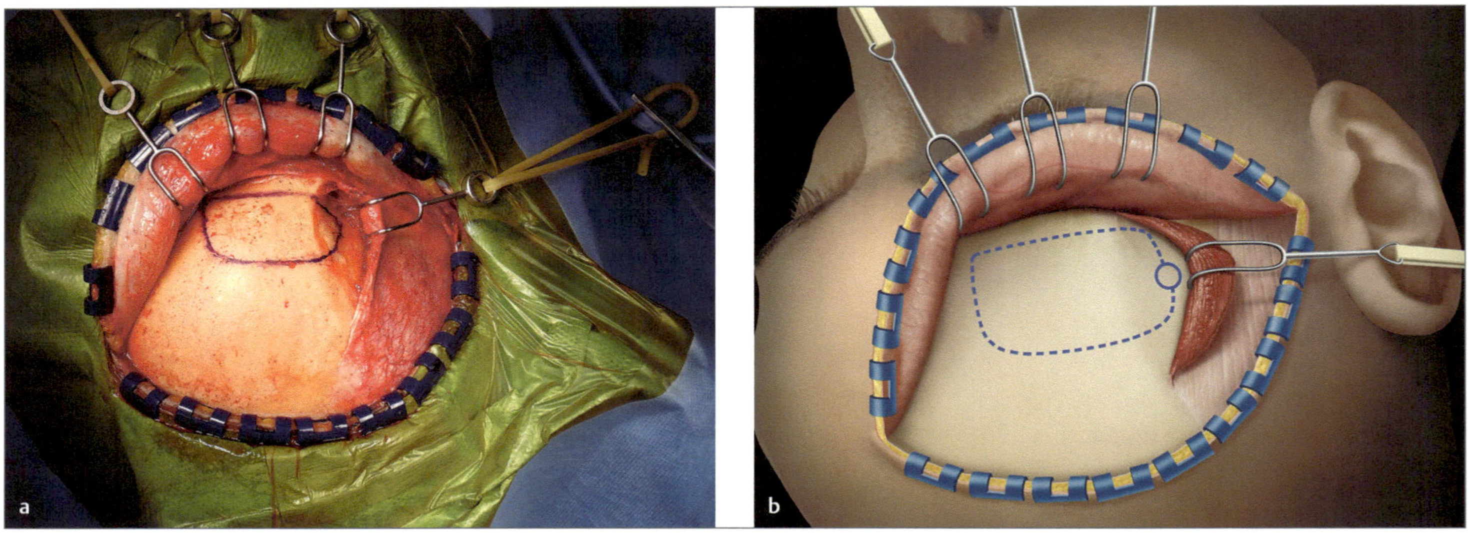

Fig. 5.58 (a, b) Craniotomy planning. A fish hook gently holds the detached muscle inferiorly without pressure, to keep the anterior superior temporal fossa exposed. The outline of the planned craniotomy can be drawn on the bone. It must be flush with the floor of the anterior skull base to allow subfrontal access without retraction. The lateral extension is about 2–3 cm into the temporal muscle fossa close to or connecting with the sphenoid ridge and gives access to the sylvian fissure. The medial extension varies but is typically limited to the midpupillary line or the level of the supraorbital foramen. Superiorly, its size can vary from 2.5 to 5 cm. Usually, the target is at the skull base and not much superior extension is required.

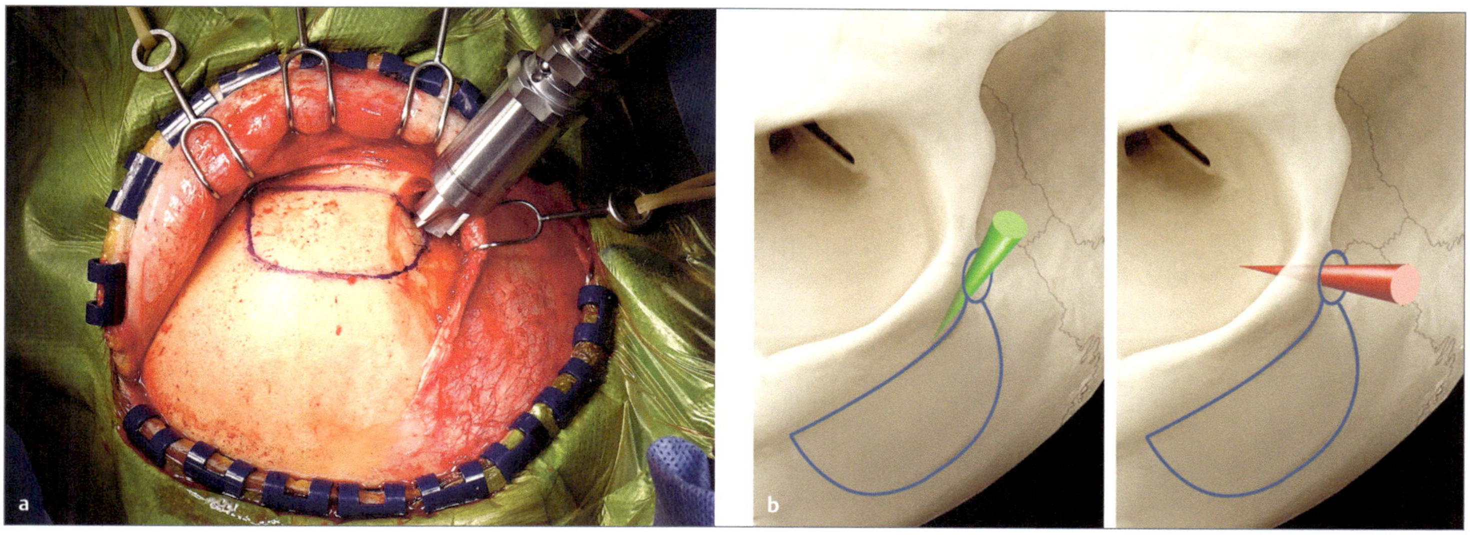

Fig. 5.59 (a, b) Burr hole. For the burr hole, a small trephine or a diamond drill should be used. The burr hole can be placed at the classical MacCarty location (keyhole, left photograph) or on the superior temporal line. For the MacCarty burr hole, the direction of drilling should be toward the surgeon (*green cone*) to avoid entering the orbita (*red cone*). Remember that this is a cosmetically sensitive area where the skin may sink some months after surgery as a result of temporal muscle atrophy or bone defects. Therefore, large burr holes and tension on the retracted temporalis muscle should be avoided.

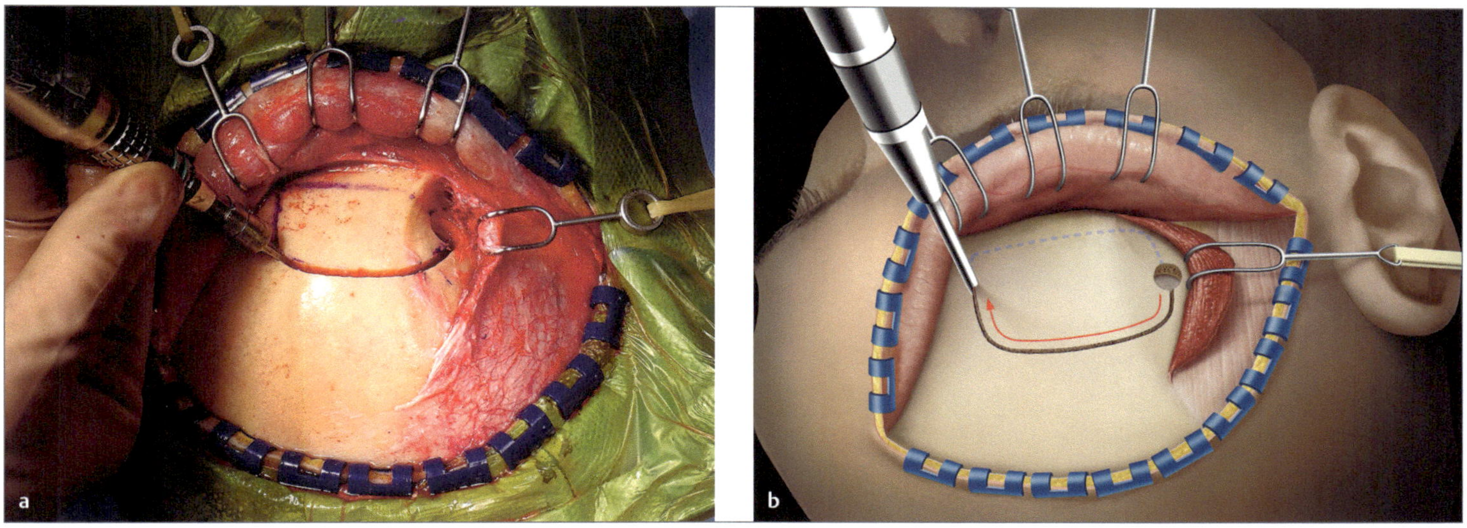

Fig. 5.60 (a, b) Craniotomy. On the left side, the skin flap seems to be too large for the craniotomy. However, this exposure is given by the height of the hairline of the individual patient. The craniotomy starts from the burr hole toward superiorly, crosses the temporal line, curves toward the midline, and then down to the frontal base approximately at the midpupillary line.

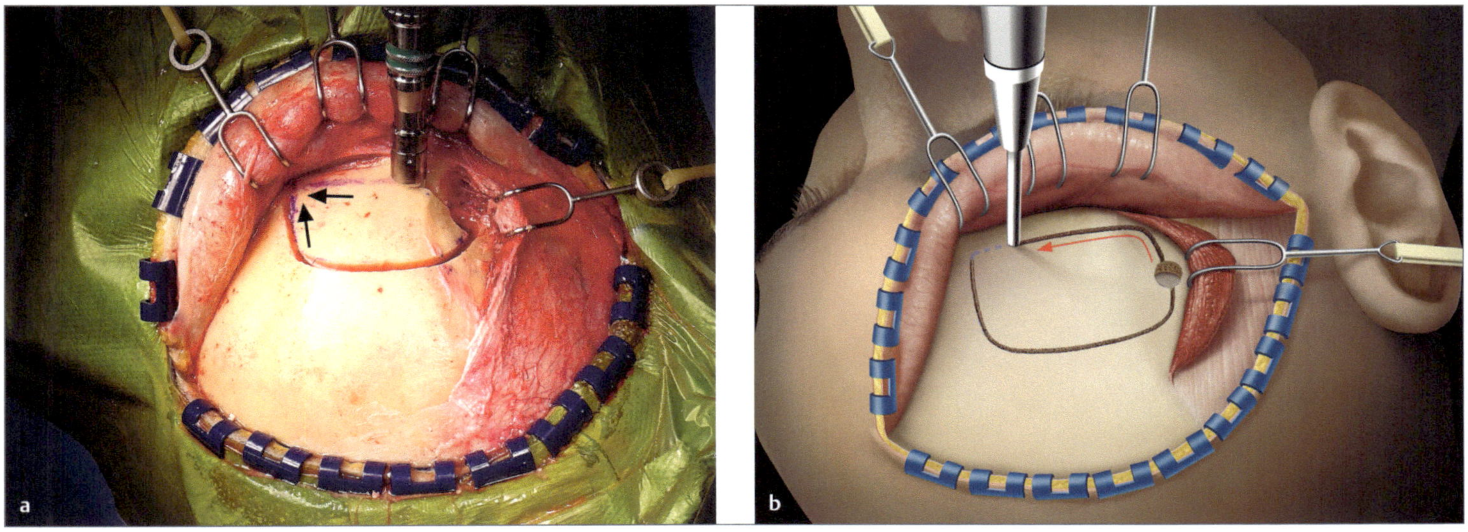

Fig. 5.61 (a, b) Craniotomy. Care should be taken to disconnect the bone from the base with a 90° angle laterally and medially to make sure that the working angle and view to the anterior base is not limited, and retraction is avoided. At the area at the level of the zygomatic process of the frontal bone, the cranial base rises a few millimeters and the craniotome can get blocked. This area corresponds to the frontolaterale, which is a landmark for the anterolateral cranial base.

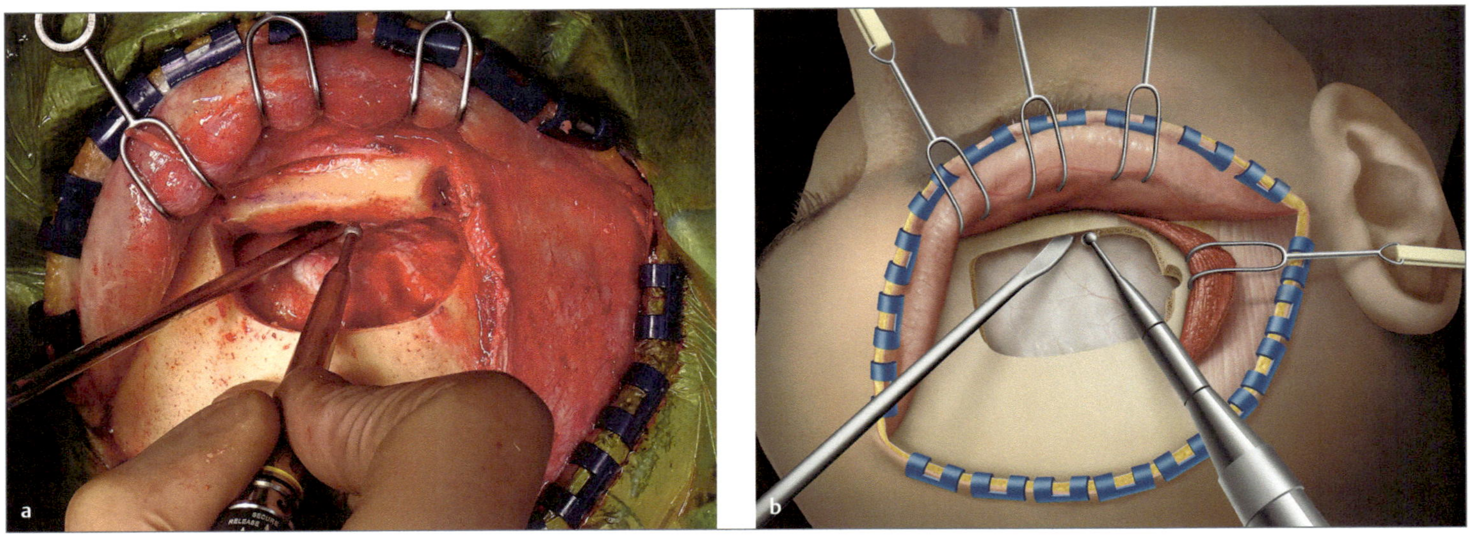

Fig. 5.62 (a, b) **Additional bone drilling.** After elevation of the bone flap, the inner tabula is drilled with a 4–5-mm diamond or cutting drill. In so doing, another 2-mm space is gained to achieve subfrontal access flush with the anterior base and avoid retraction. When completed, the dura should be detached toward the base for 1–2 cm to identify large bony elevations of the orbital roof that may obstruct the view. If present, they should also be flattened with the drill. We prefer to place the dural tacking sutures at this stage to see accidental pial vessel injury and to minimize epidural oozing during surgery.

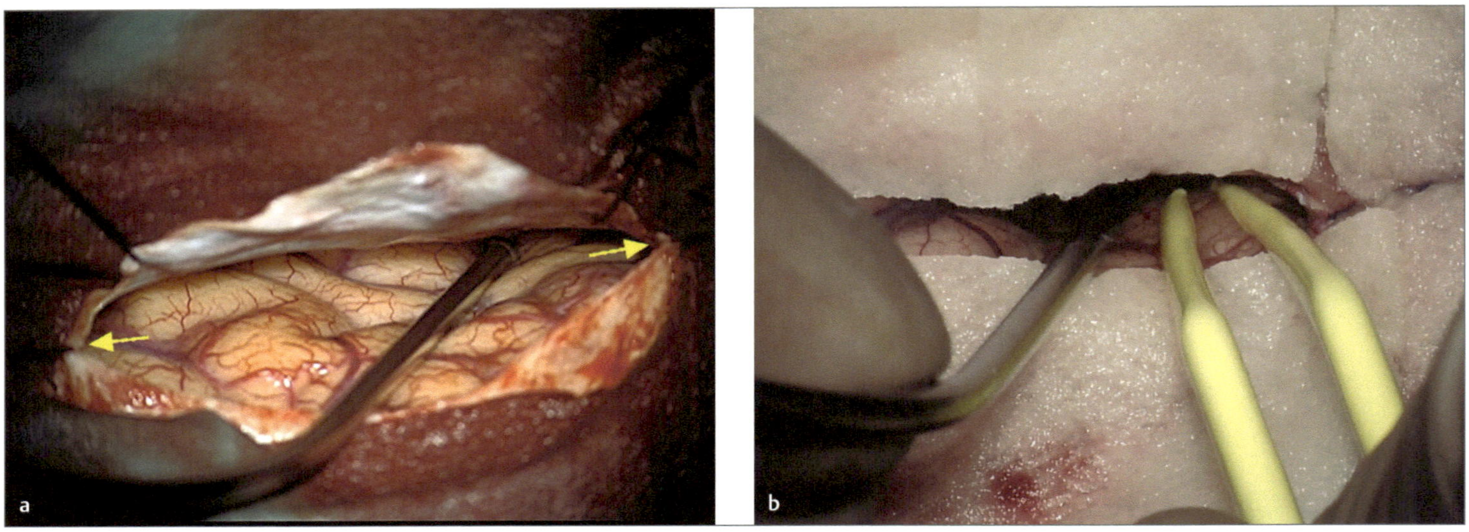

Fig. 5.63 (a, b) **Dura opening.** The dura is opened with the base anteriorly and fixed with tacking sutures. These sutures are also placed at the lateral and medial borders to open the space and allow a better view (see *arrows*). The dura and the brain are then covered with wet cottonoids to avoid exposure to heat from the light source of the microscope. The right image shows subfrontal access to the anterior cranial base without retraction.

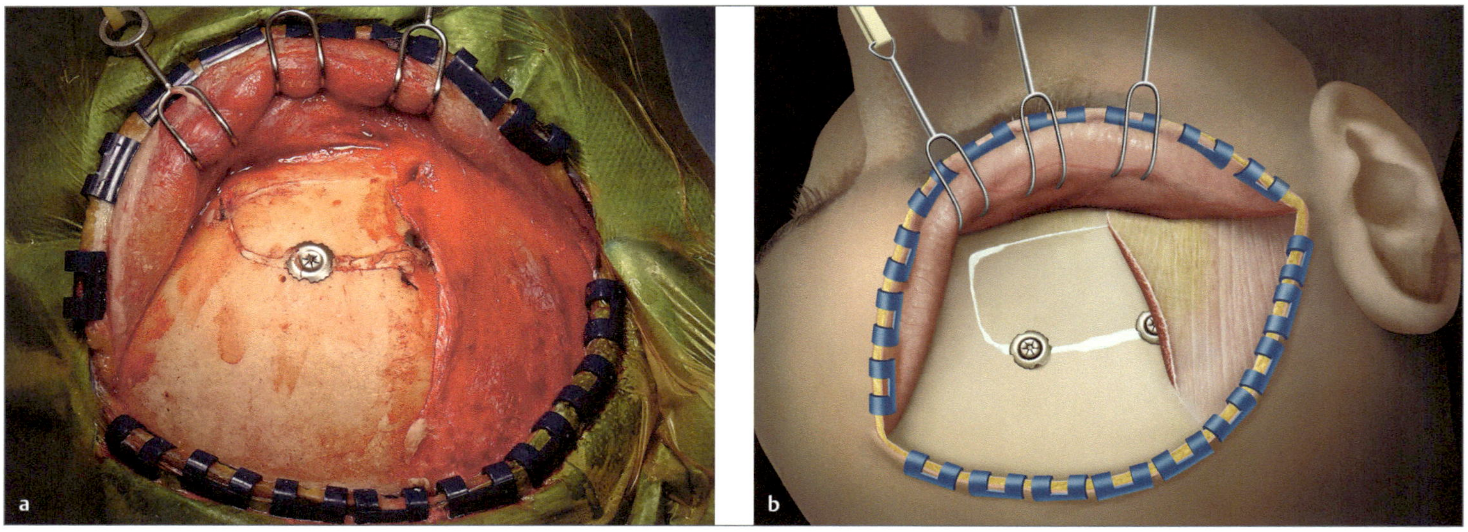

Fig. 5.64 (a, b) **Closure: bone flap refixation and filling gaps with bone cement.** After closure of the dura, the bone flap is fixed. For cosmesis, care should be taken to fix the bone basally and medially without leaving any gaps and to use bone cement or other material to fill larger lateral and superior gaps. Entering the frontal sinus during craniotomy is of less concern as our goal is to gain access flush to the base. However, before replacing the flap in cases of frontal sinus opening some rules should be followed (see Chapter 1.9, Frontal Sinus Breach and Repair).

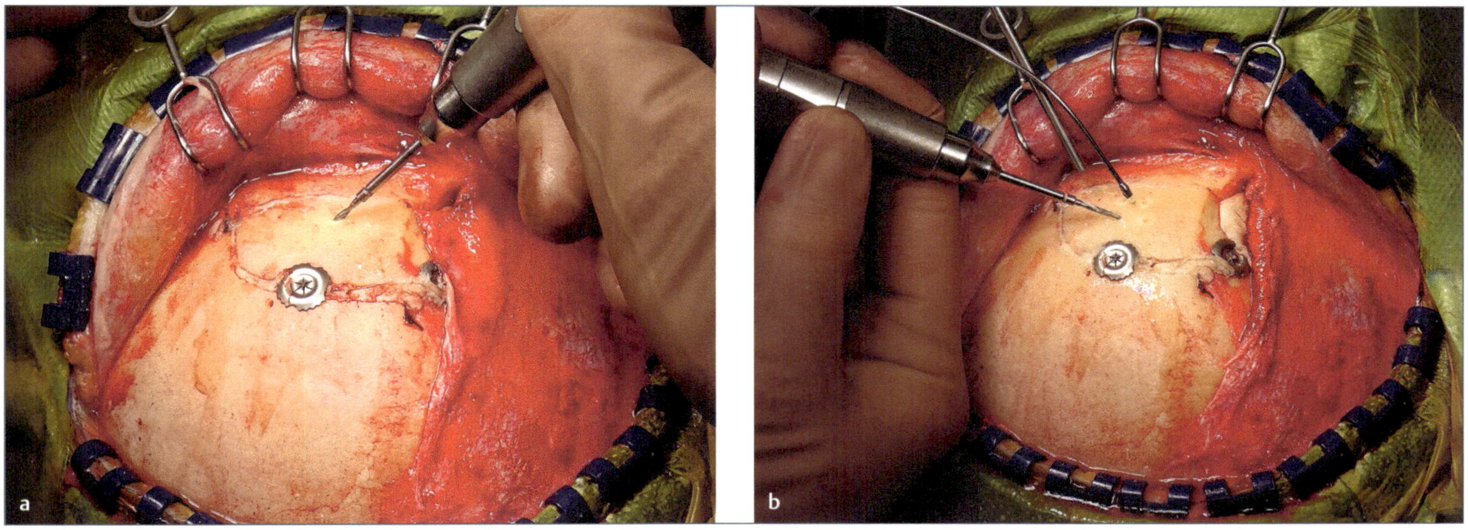

Fig. 5.65 (a, b) Closure: fixation of the temporalis muscle fascia. V-shaped holes may be drilled for sutures to reattach the elevated temporal muscle. The drill is angulated to create two shallow canals that allow a needle to pass through the surface of the bone as an anchor to elevate and fix the fascia of the temporalis muscle.

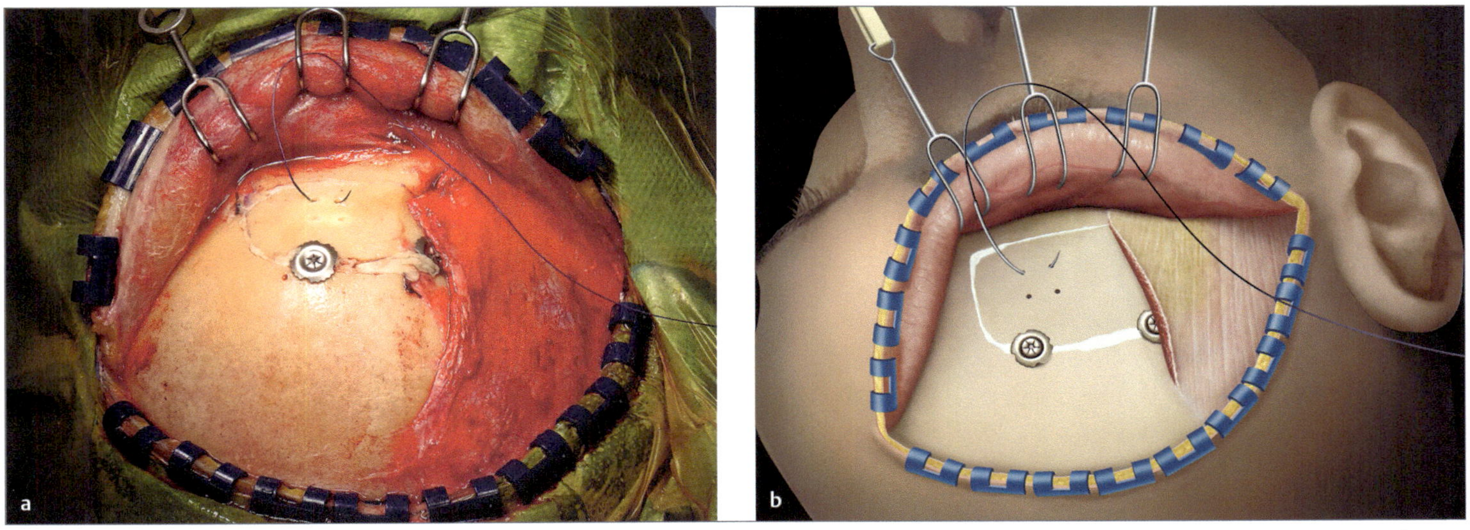

Fig. 5.66 (a, b) Closure: fixation of the temporalis muscle fascia. The temporal fascia is sutured. The edge of the temporal fascia/muscle may be pulled upward and fixed using the V-shaped drill holes and sutures.

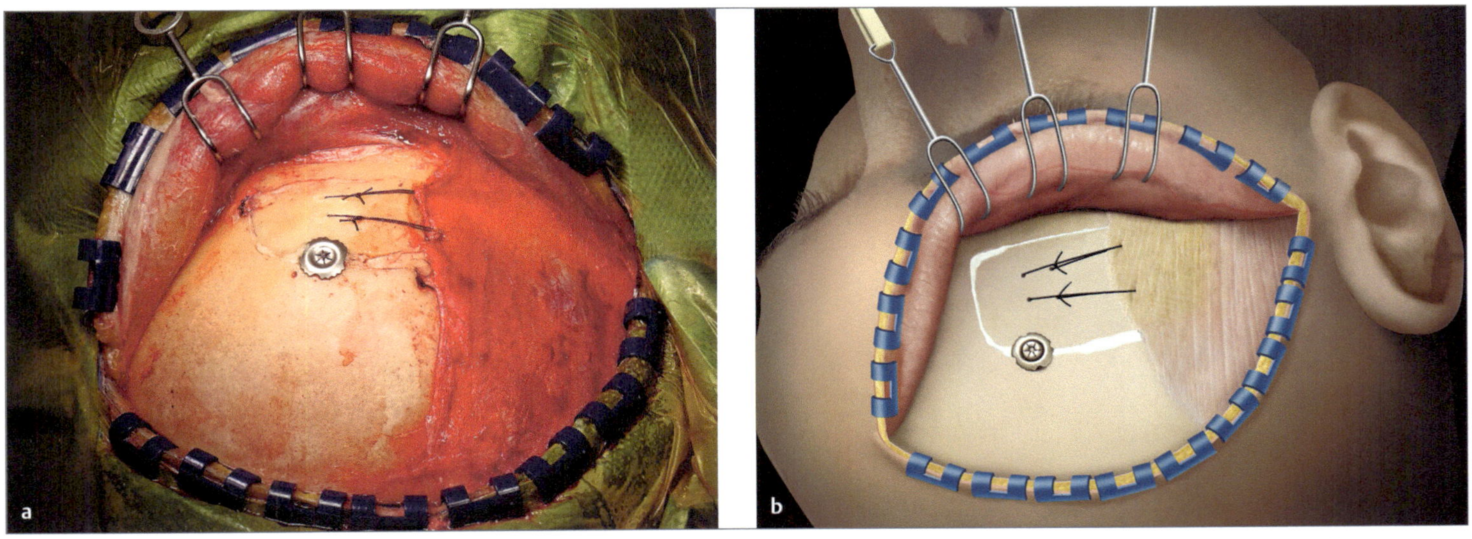

Fig. 5.67 (a, b) Closure: fixation of the temporalis muscle fascia. Careful handling of the temporal muscle in this area provides an excellent cosmetic result and symmetrical appearance of the visible skin. Surgeons should check cosmesis during follow-up of these patients to obtain feedback on the results of the technique they are using.

Checklist

- Palpate the bony edge formed by the orbital rim (the posterior lateral zygomatic process of the frontal bone = frontolaterale) = cranial base point.
- Incision line allows mobilization of the skin flap down to the cranial base point.
- Mobilize skin downward until the frontolaterale can be palpated.
- Use a small craniotome or diamond drill for the burr hole; avoid large burr holes for cosmetic reasons.
- Direct burr toward your body when drilling the burr hole.
- Make sure to have a 90° angle laterally and medially at the base of the craniotomy.
- Drill the tabula interna for better access to the base while leaving the tabula externa intact for cosmesis.
- Dissect the dura mater 1 to 2 cm basally from the bone and check for large bony elevations of the orbital roof that might obstruct the view to the anterior skull base.
- During closure, take care to avoid bony defects. Cover the burr hole and place the temporal muscle above it.

5.2.5 Helsinki Lateral Supraorbital

Juha Hernesniemi and Hugo Andrade-Barazarte

Introduction

The lateral supraorbital approach (LSO) is a simpler, faster, and less invasive modification of the pterional approach popularized by Gazi Yaşargil. The LSO allows excellent exposure of anterior fossa lesions, sellar and suprasellar areas, most anterior circulation aneurysms, and some basilar tip aneurysms (see ▶ Fig. 5.68, ▶ Fig. 5.69, ▶ Fig. 5.70, ▶ Fig. 5.71, ▶ Fig. 5.72, ▶ Fig. 5.73, ▶ Fig. 5.74, ▶ Fig. 5.75, ▶ Fig. 5.76, ▶ Fig. 5.77, ▶ Fig. 5.78, ▶ Fig. 5.79, ▶ Fig. 5.80, ▶ Fig. 5.81, ▶ Fig. 5.82, ▶ Fig. 5.83, and ▶ Fig. 5.84).

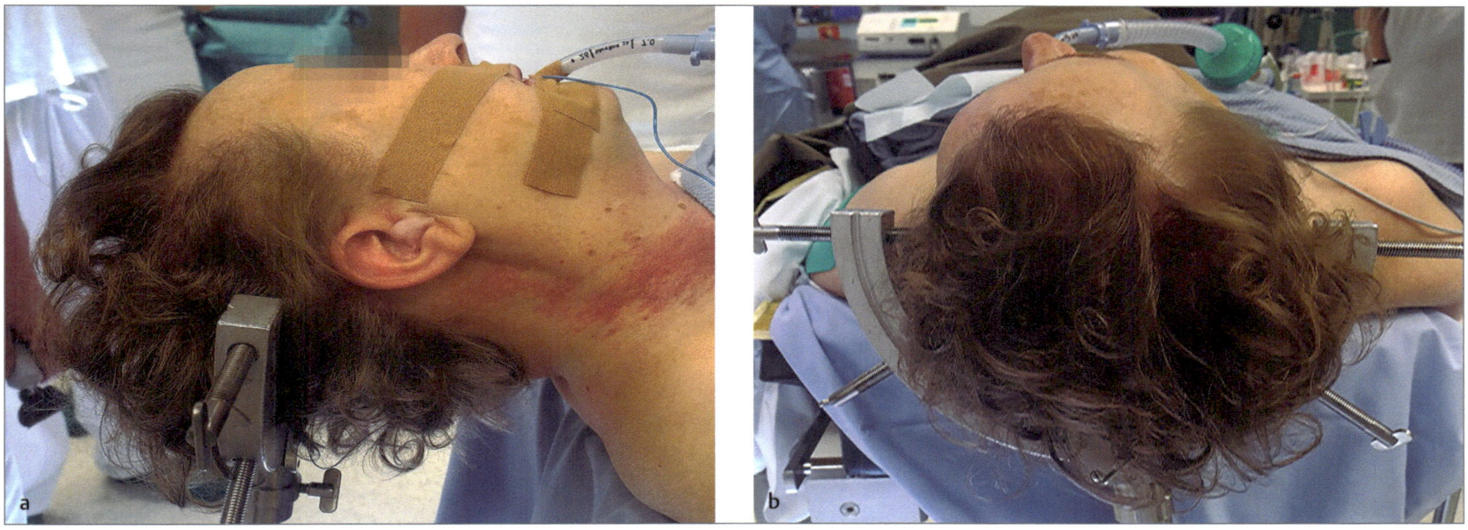

Fig. 5.68 (a, b) Positioning. The patient is placed in the supine position, with the head and shoulders elevated above the heart level to reduce bleeding. The head is fixed with three or four pins to the Sugita or Mayfield frame. The rotation of the head varies from 15° to 30° toward the opposite side, depending on the lesion to be treated. Additionally, the head is tilted slightly laterally toward the opposite shoulder to orientate the sylvian fissure vertically. The degree of lateral tilt depends on the pathology, skull base relationship, and surgical trajectory. For patients with middle cerebral artery aneurysms, the head is rotated approximately 15° toward the contralateral side, avoiding more extensive rotation of the head to prevent the temporal lobe obstructing the sylvian fissure. The LSO represents a tailored craniotomy; the degree of head rotation depends on the target projection, but as a general rule the head is rotated approximately 20° to 30° toward the contralateral side. Again, an important consideration during the positioning for aneurysms of the anterior communicating artery (AcoA) is the lateral flexion of the head, allowing a horizontal surgical trajectory to the AcoA complex.

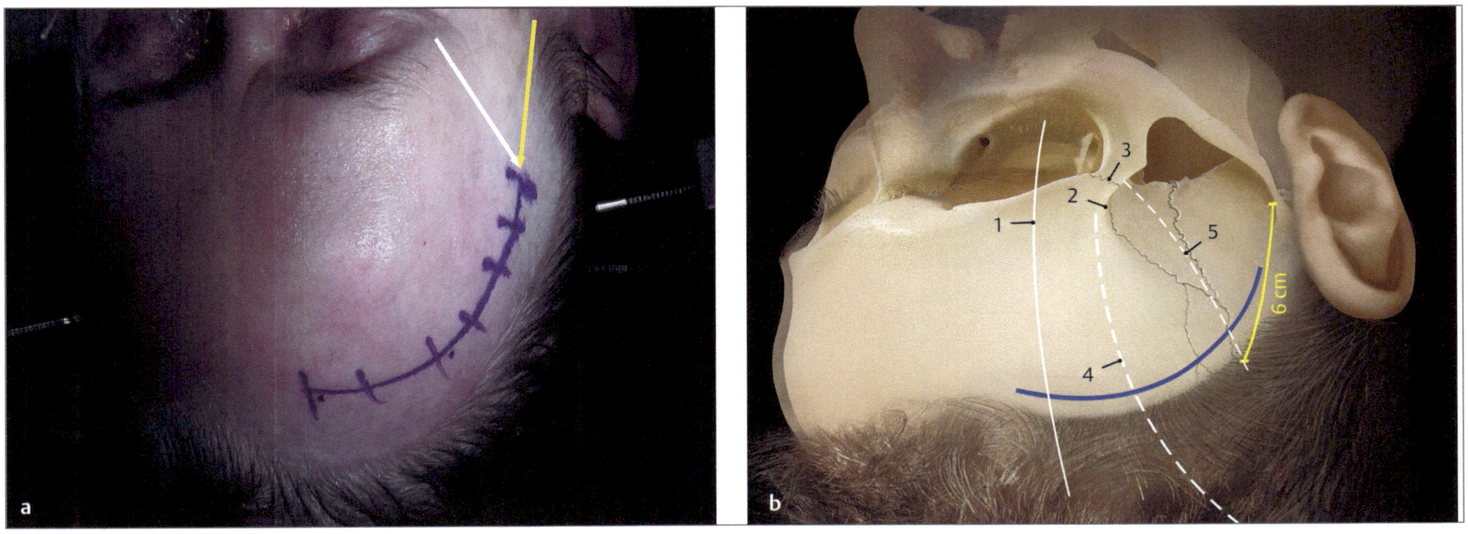

Fig. 5.69 (a, b) Anatomy overview. Important landmarks are: (1) ipsilateral midpupillary line, (2) zygomatic process of the frontal bone, (3) frontozygomatic suture, (4) superior temporal line, and (5) projection of the sylvian fissure over the skin. *White line*: a horizontal line from the external orbital wall (lateral canthus intersecting a *yellow vertical line* projected 6 cm above the tragus).

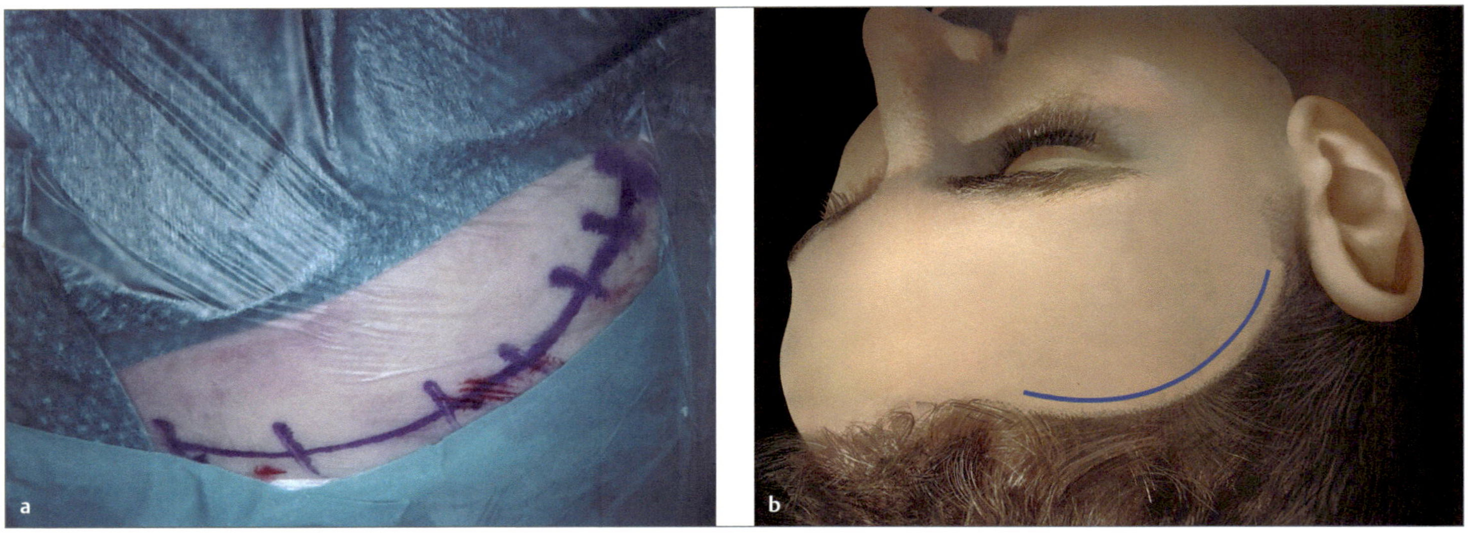

Fig. 5.70 (a, b) Draped position before skin incision. After minimal shaving, a frontotemporal curved skin incision is made at the hairline. It starts approximately 5 cm above the zygoma and is directed in a curvilinear fashion to the ipsilateral midpupillary line ending 2 cm medial of it. The incision does not extend to the midline or contralateral side. In balding patients, the skin incision may be made in a wrinkle to provide better cosmetic results. The LSO is intended to be a tailored craniotomy. Furthermore, the place of the skin incision varies according to the hairline of the patient. Some patients have a lower hairline allowing for placement of the skin incision closer to the important landmarks.

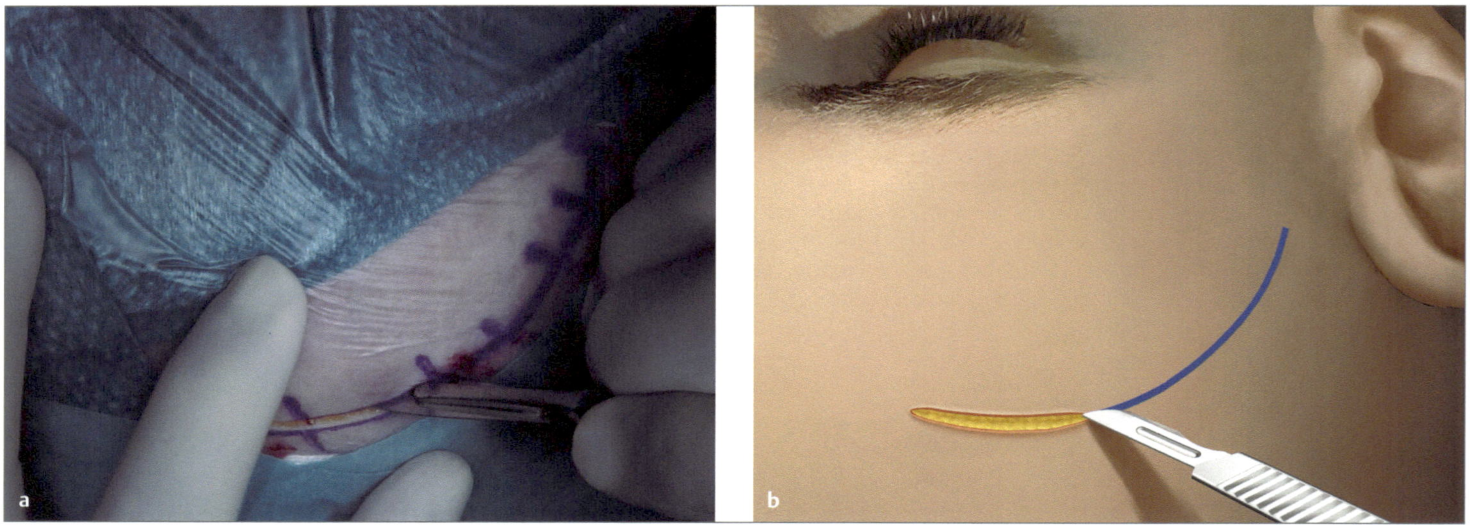

Fig. 5.71 (a, b) Skin incision. The skin–galea and the temporalis muscle are cut in a single layer.

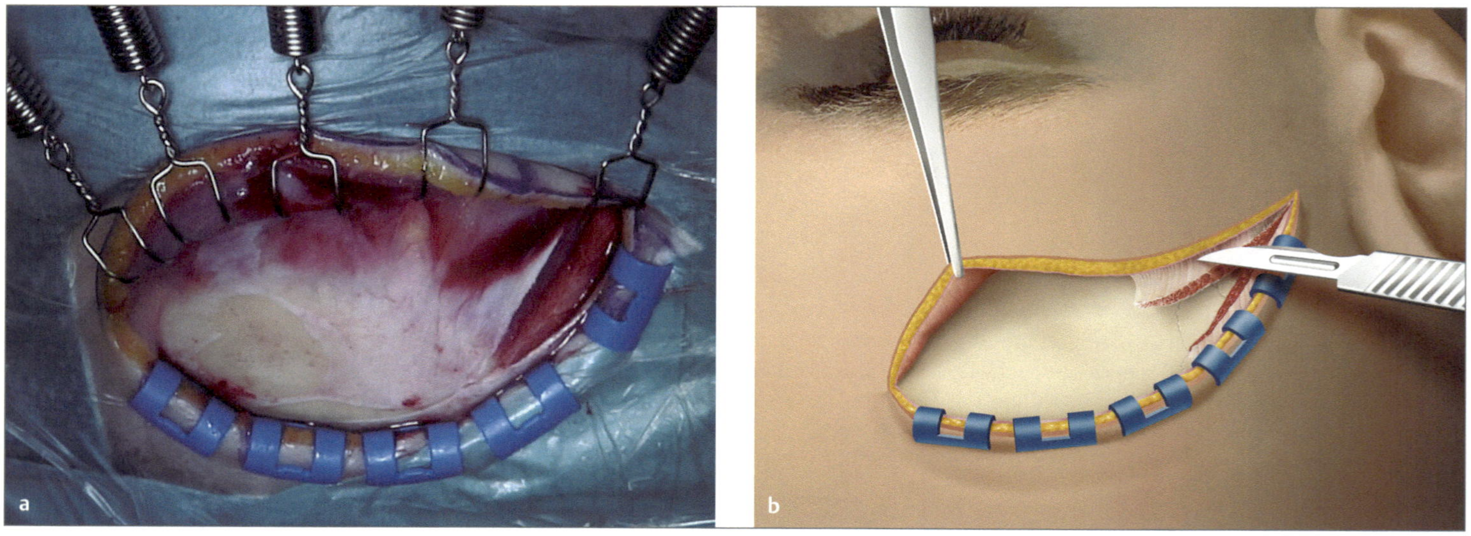

Fig. 5.72 (a, b) Flap preparation. Only the superior part of the temporal muscle is exposed. Multiple spring hooks are placed over the skin–galea flap, starting at the posterior temporal side and directed progressively anterior. This is done to retract the flap anteriorly and to provide hemostasis. Multiple Raney clips are placed on the posterior margin of the skin incision to stop the bleeding as well.

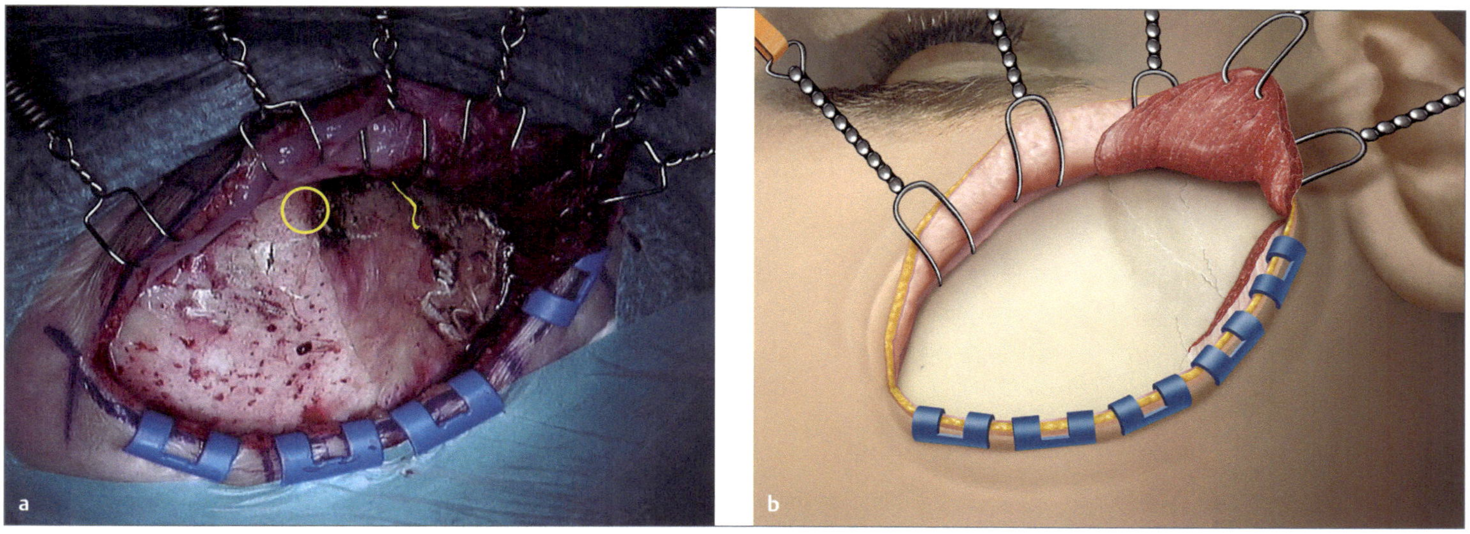

Fig. 5.73 (a, b) **Detaching temporal muscle.** This step represents one of the main tricks of the LSO. Once the most superior part of the temporal muscle is detached, a spring hook is placed underneath to retract this segment laterally and the remaining superior insertion of the temporal muscle is detached until the bony landmarks are exposed. Additionally, all the spring hooks are repositioned to mobilize the flap anteriorly and to expose the zygomatic process of the frontal bone (*yellow circle*) and the frontozygomatic suture (*yellow line*).

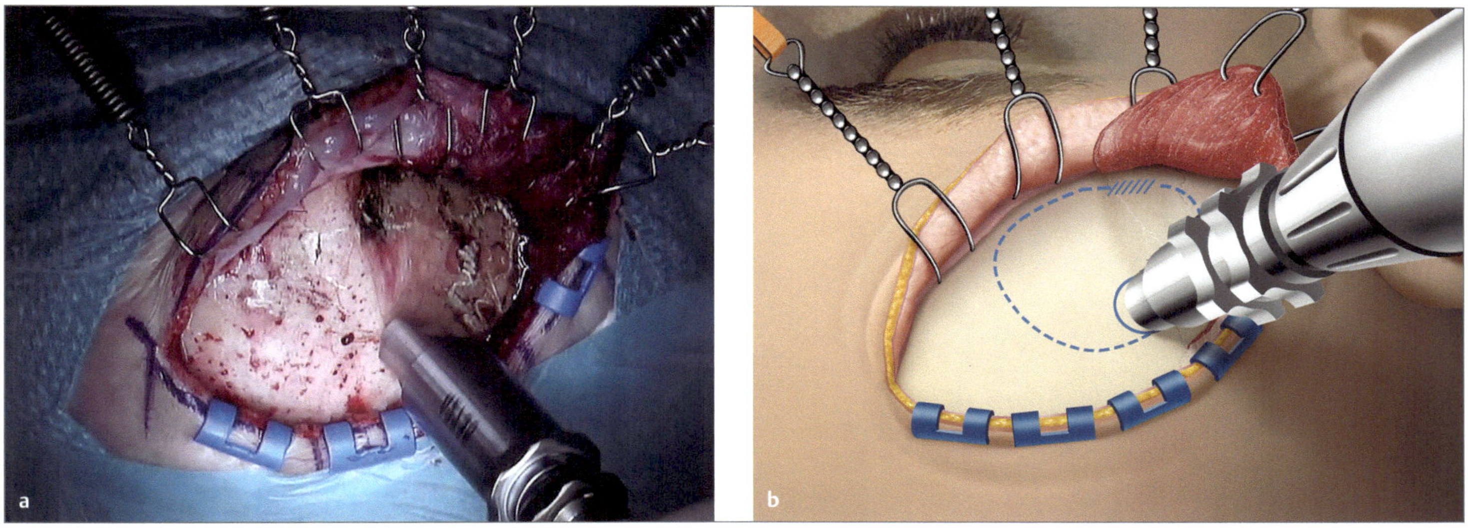

Fig. 5.74 (a, b) **Burr hole.** A single burr hole is made at the superior temporal line. This is done to enable the dura to be detached easily and to avoid tearing of the dura during the craniotomy. In elderly patients with a strongly attached dura, an extra burr hole may be made.

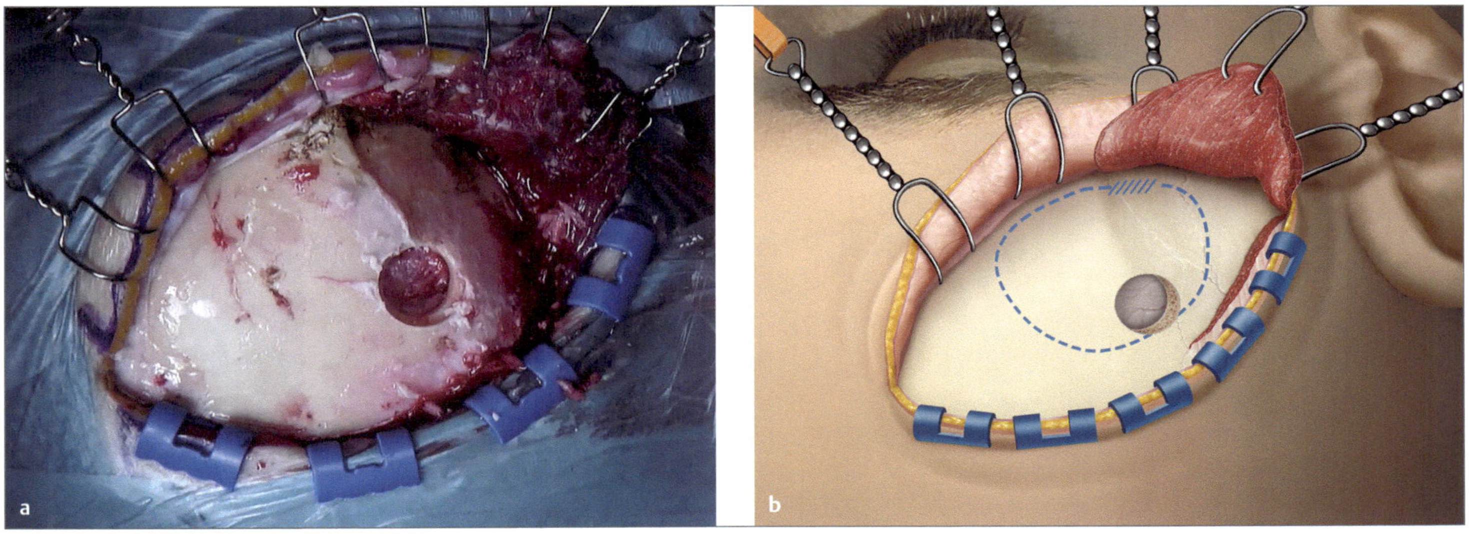

Fig. 5.75 (a, b) **Detaching the dura.** A stout, curved dissector is used to detach the dura from the inner table, beginning with the frontal region and then proceeding to the temporal region.

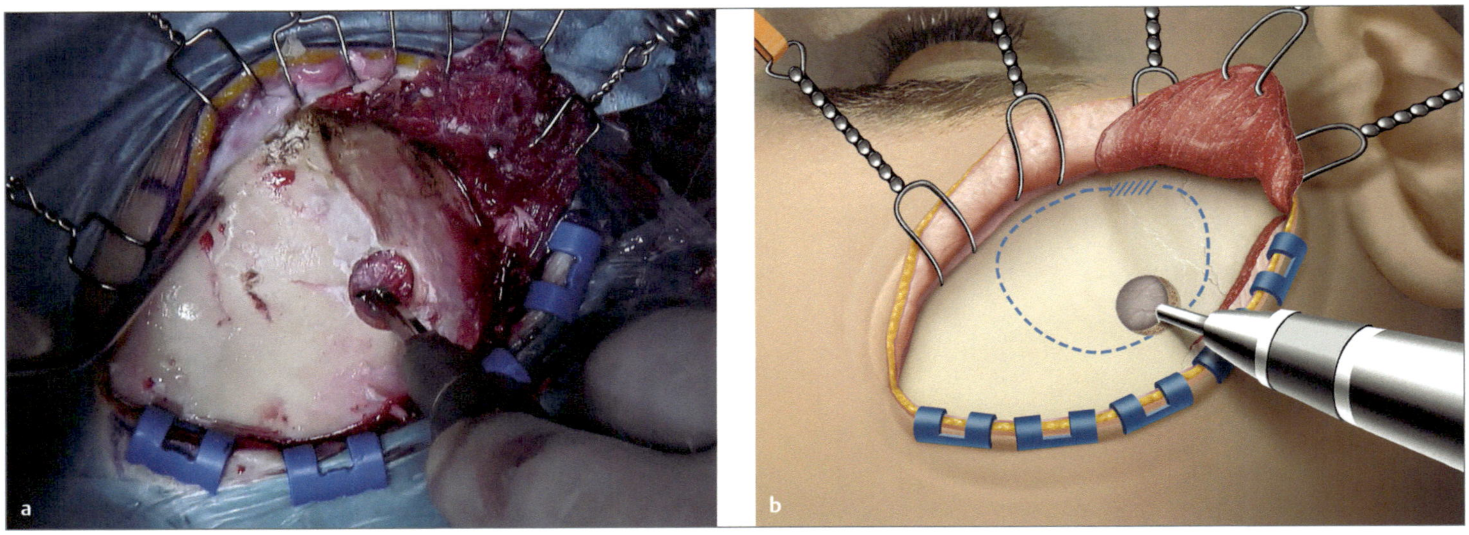

Fig. 5.76 (a, b) **Craniotomy.** Two cuts are made using the side-cutting burr with footplate protection.

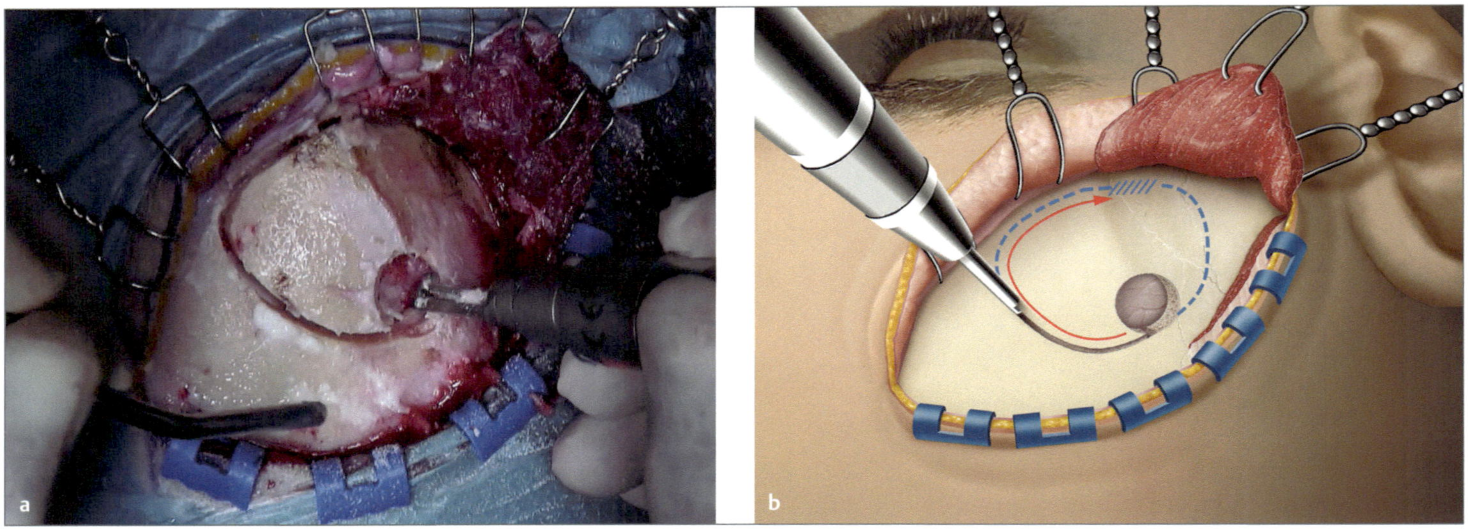

Fig. 5.77 (a, b) **Craniotomy: frontal cut.** The first cut starts from the burr hole extending toward the frontal region in a curvilinear fashion passing over the zygomatic process of the frontal bone.

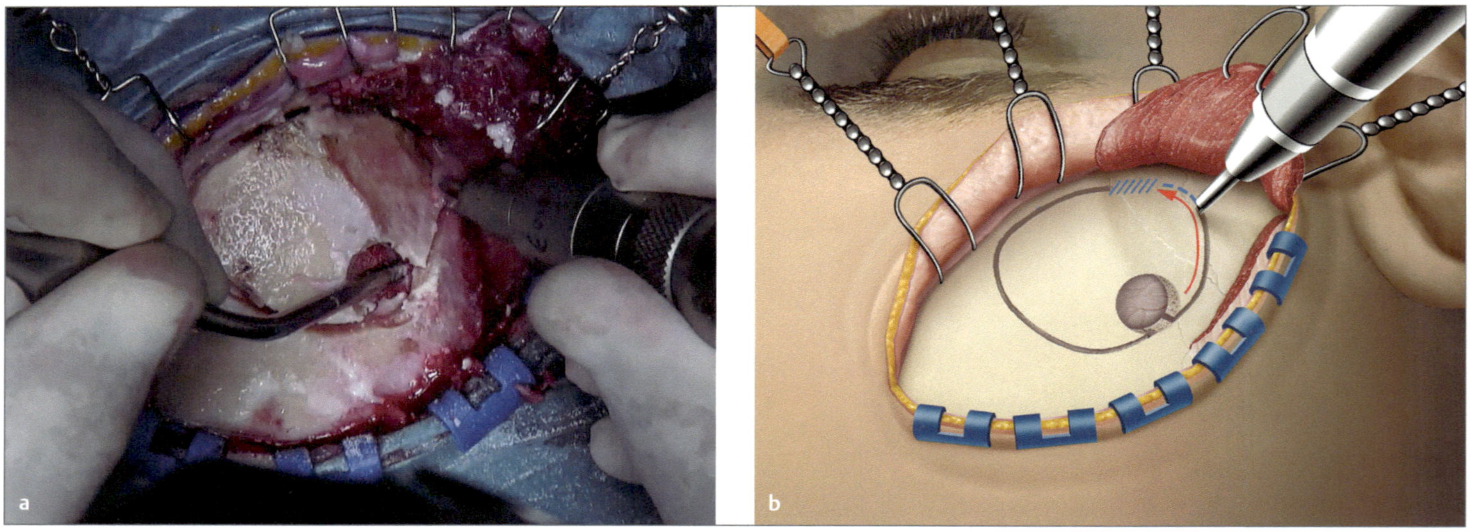

Fig. 5.78 (a, b) **Craniotomy: temporal cut.** The second cut starts from the burr hole extending toward the temporal bone, almost in a straight line, leaving the sphenoid ridge between these two cuts.

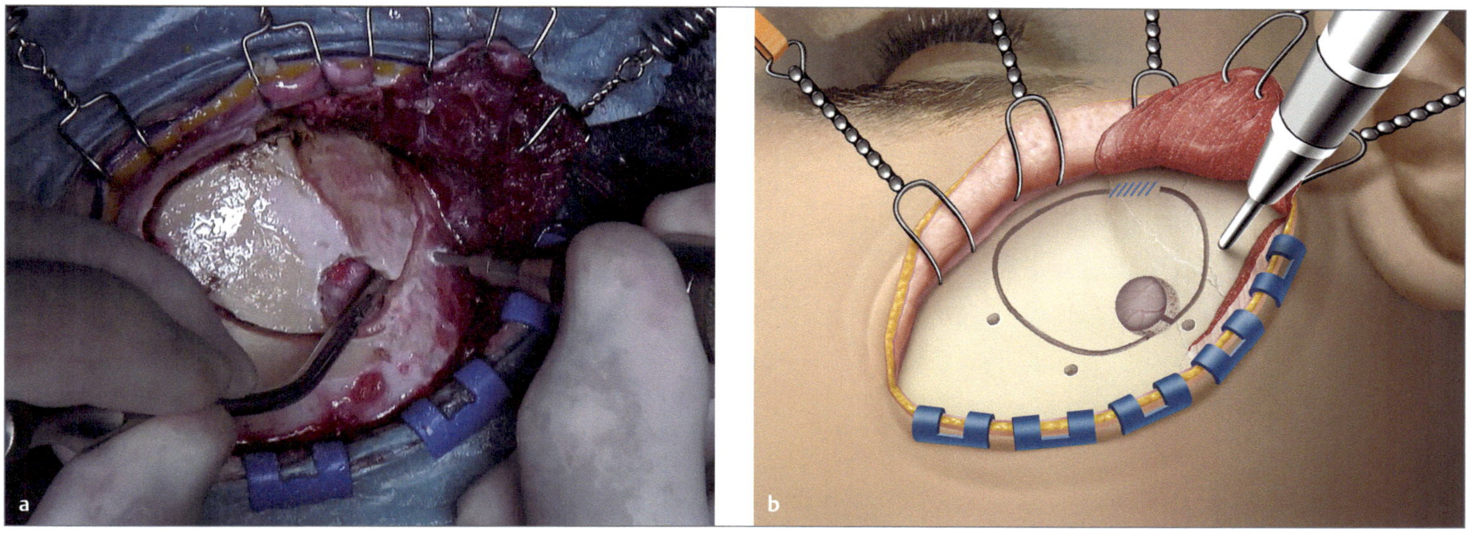

Fig. 5.79 **(a, b) Placing burr holes for tack-up sutures.** The side-cutting craniotome without footplate is used to drill small holes around the edges of the craniotomy in preparation for later placement of tack-up sutures.

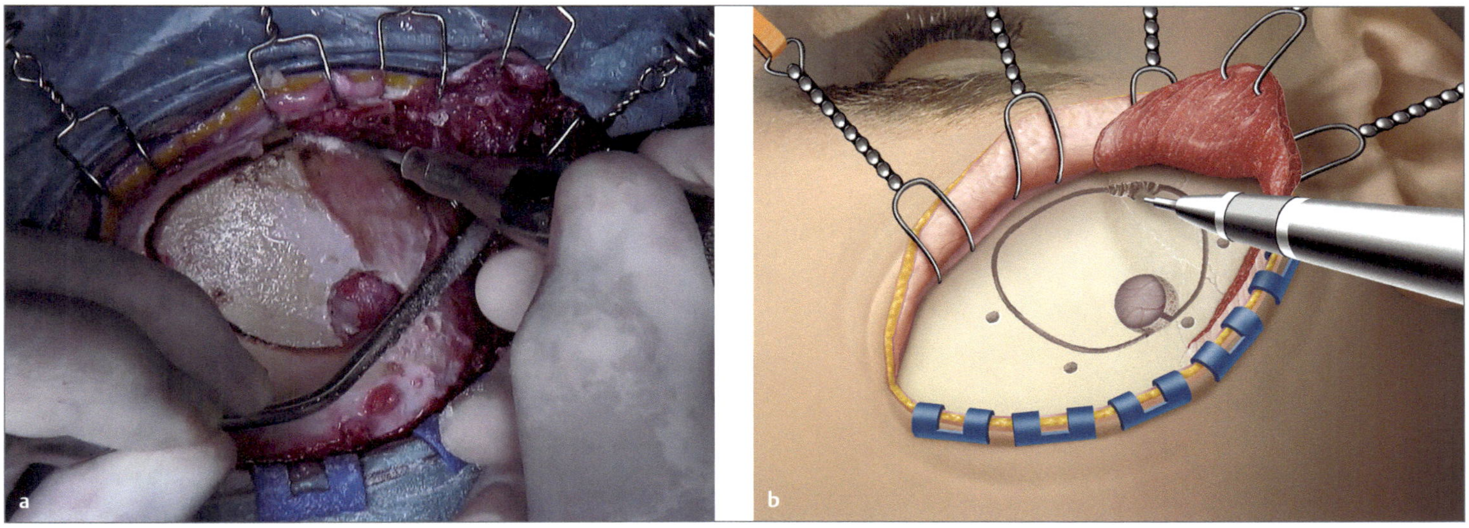

Fig. 5.80 **(a, b) Thinning off sphenoid ridge bone attachment.** The remaining frontal bone and sphenoid ridge are thinned off using the side-cutting drill without footplate. The bone flap is then elevated from its posterior segment directed anteriorly and cracked along the drilled line over the frontal bone and the sphenoid ridge.

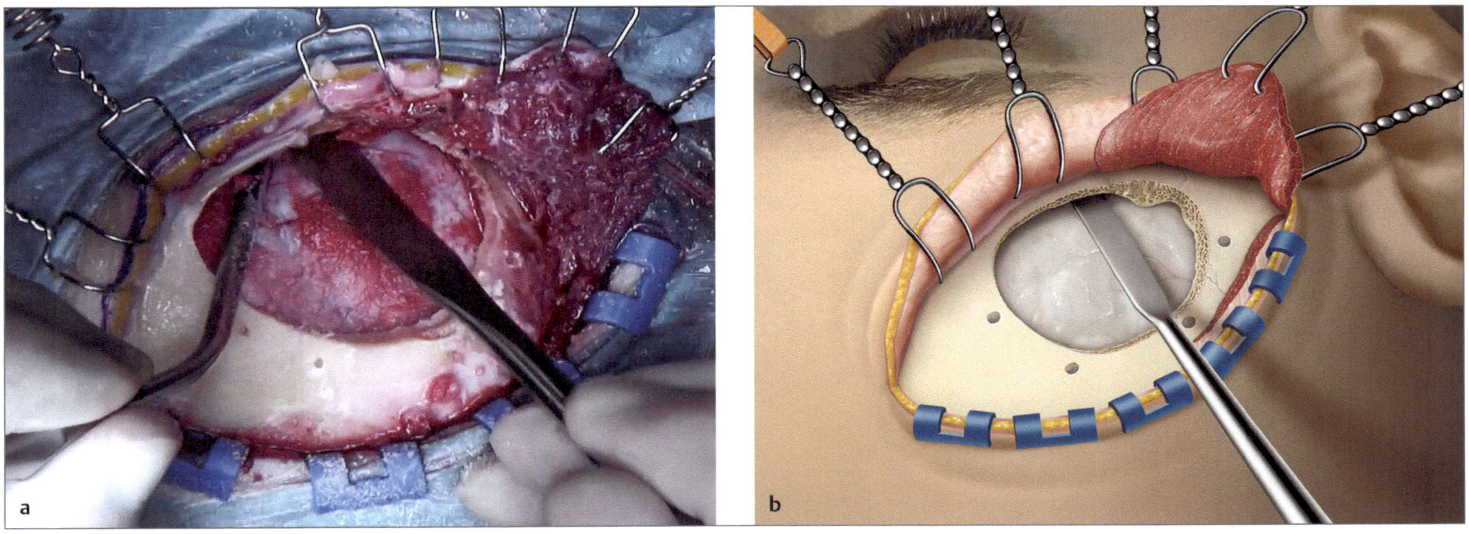

Fig. 5.81 **(a, b) Detaching the dura to prepare for additional bone drilling.** After removal of the bone flap, a dissector is used to detach the dura from the posterior and lateral aspect of the orbit.

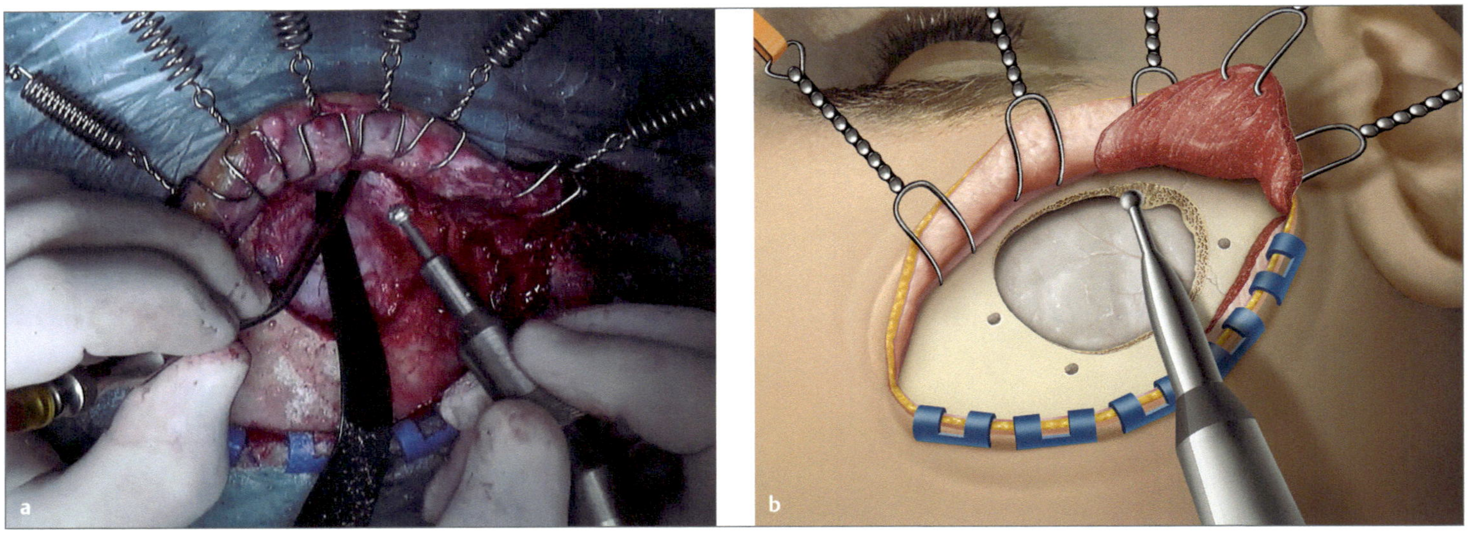

Fig. 5.82 (a, b) Additional bone drilling. The remaining sphenoid ridge is drilled off using a high-speed drill with cutting burr, starting from the lateral aspect of the orbit to the lesser sphenoid wing. The drilling is then continued with a diamond burr without irrigation to smooth the surface and stop bone bleeding ("hot drilling technique"). This technique offers excellent hemostasis while finishing the bone removal.

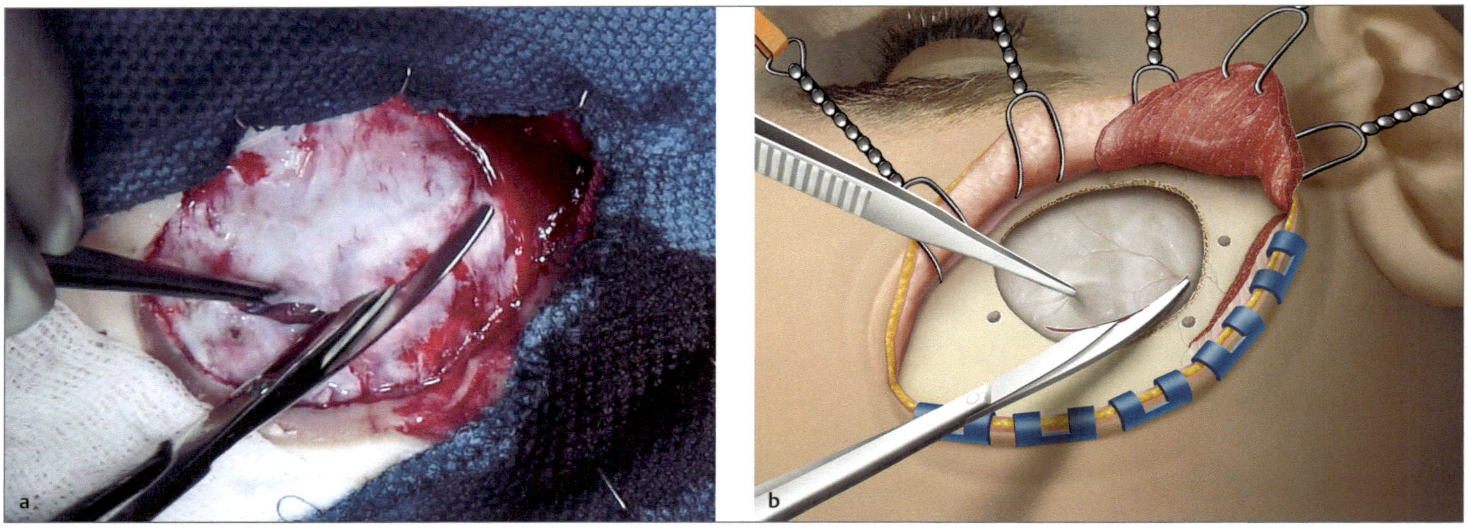

Fig. 5.83 (a, b) Dura opening. Before opening the dura, the area surrounding the craniotomy is covered with three towels soaked with hydrogen peroxide for antimicrobial effect. Then a dry green cloth is attached with staples to the anterior and inferior limit of the craniotomy to decrease the color imbalance in the operative field.

The dura is opened in a curvilinear fashion, starting at the superoposterior margin and directed inferiorly and anteriorly. Multiple tack-up sutures are placed over the dural edges, to retract the dura over the craniotomy margins and prevent bleeding from the epidural space. Before beginning the intracranial work, meticulous care should be taken to achieve hemostasis and ensure a clear surgical field.

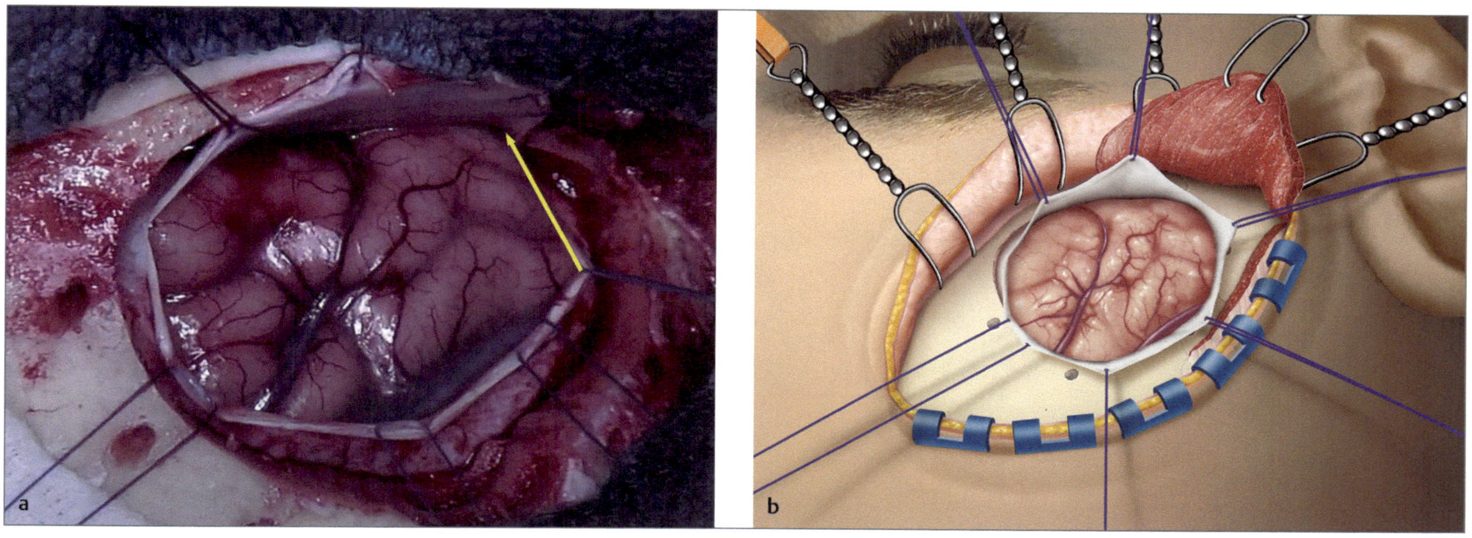

Fig. 5.84 (a, b) Dura opening. The sylvian fissure (yellow line) represents the inferior border of the craniotomy. The intracranial work starts along the frontobasal surface of the frontal lobe, slightly medial and proximal to the sylvian fissure. The goal of this stage is to reach the basal cisterns and/or the lamina terminals to release cerebrospinal fluid and further relax the brain.

Checklist

- Slight rotation toward the contralateral side (15–30°).
- Curvilinear skin incision at the hairline.
- Skin incision and flap preparation.
- Superior portion of temporal muscle split.
- Zygomatic process of the frontal bone and superior temporal line exposed.
- One single burr hole over the superior temporal line.
- Craniotomy.
- Multiple small holes for tack-up sutures.
- Dura opening in a curvilinear fashion.
- Meticulous attention to achieving hemostasis before intracranial work.

5.2.6 Pterional

Peter Vajkoczy and Andreas Raabe

See ▶Fig. 5.85, ▶Fig. 5.86, ▶Fig. 5.87, ▶Fig. 5.88, ▶Fig. 5.89, ▶Fig. 5.90, ▶Fig. 5.91, ▶Fig. 5.92, ▶Fig. 5.93, ▶Fig. 5.94, ▶Fig. 5.95, ▶Fig. 5.96, ▶Fig. 5.97, ▶Fig. 5.98, ▶Fig. 5.99, ▶Fig. 5.100, ▶Fig. 5.101, ▶Fig. 5.102, ▶Fig. 5.103, ▶Fig. 5.104, and ▶Fig. 5.105.

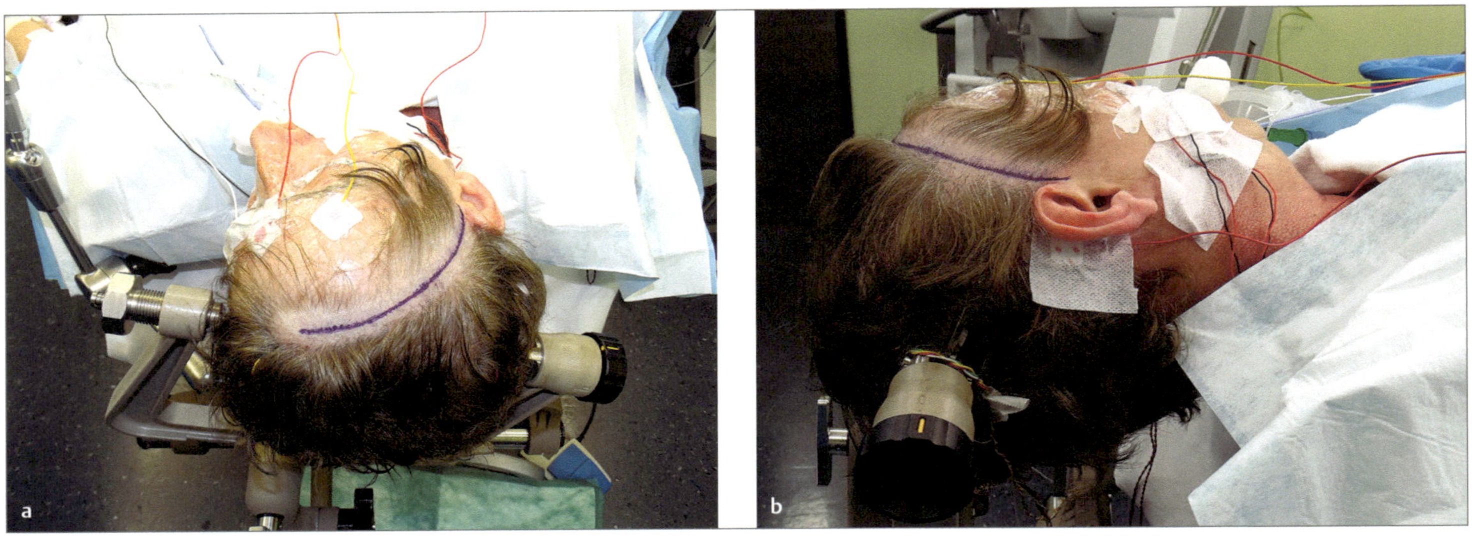

Fig. 5.85 (a, b) Positioning. The pterional approach is used for subfrontal, temporal, parasellar, tentorial, and midline lesions including the contralateral side. The head is rotated between 30° and 60° depending on the surgical target and is slightly extended so that the zygoma reaches the highest point. The amount of extension also depends on the surgical target and the preferred position of the surgeon. Tilting the head 10° to 20° to the contralateral side places the sylvian fissure in a vertical position and may facilitate its opening.

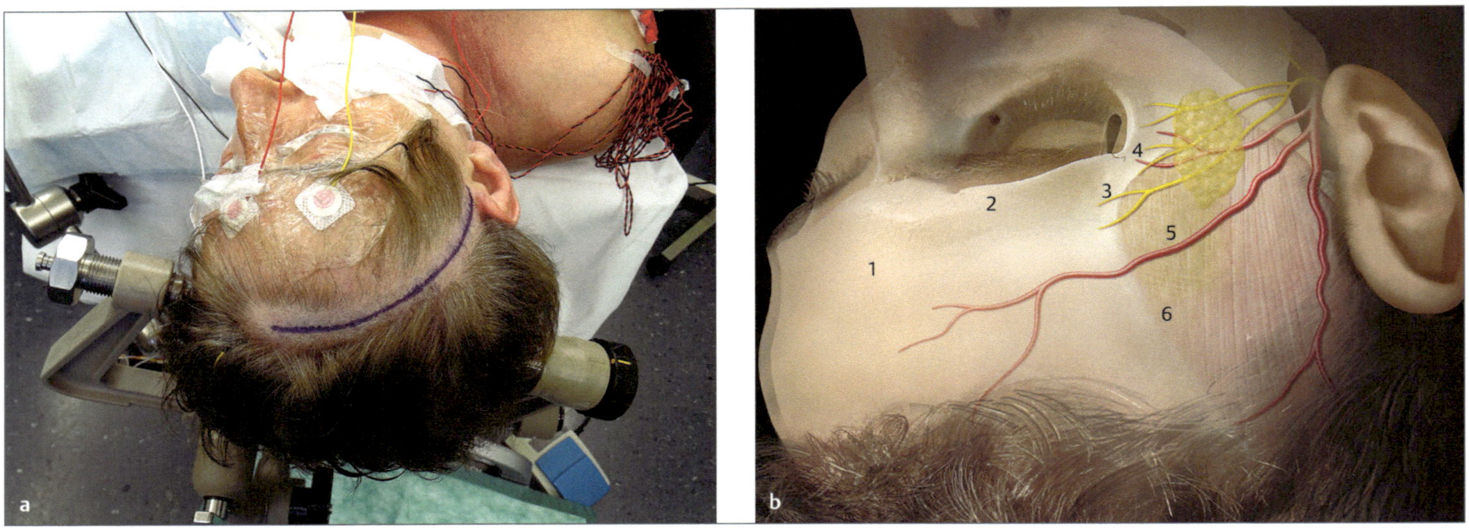

Fig. 5.86 (a, b) Anatomy overview. Important landmarks are (1) the midline, (2) the midpupillary line as the medial limit of the craniotomy, (3) the posterior edge of the zygomatic process of the frontal bone (landmark frontotemporale) indicating the cranial base, (4) the most lateral part of the orbit, corresponding to the frontozygomatic suture as a rough landmark for the sphenoid ridge, (5) the frontal branch of the superficial temporal artery, and (6) the fascia of the temporal muscle originating from the superior temporal line.

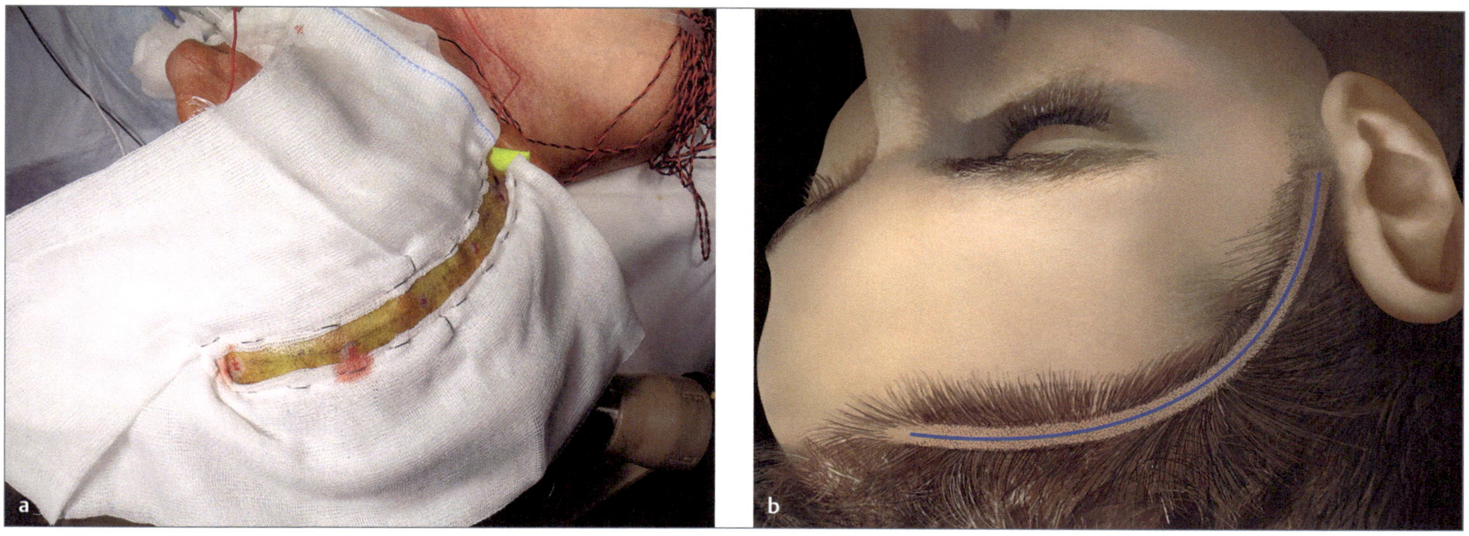

Fig. 5.87 (a, b) Draped position before skin incision. The length of the skin incision depends on the hairline of the patient and the size of the pterional craniotomy. On the temporal side, it stops 0–10 mm above the zygomatic arch. Frontally, the incision should be planned as far toward (or even crossing) the midline as necessary to make sure that the frontotemporale (see chapter 2.2 Craniocerebral Topography), which indicates the skull base is reached and can be exposed. The incision is marked with a pen and the hair is shaved 0.5–1 cm on each side of the planned incision. We prefer to spare 1 cm hair anteriorly to the incision for immediate postoperative cosmesis. In bald patients, the incision can be made in a wrinkle > 3 cm above the eyebrow or within the eyebrow when a smaller supraorbital approach is feasible (see chapter 1.6 Esthetic Considerations in Neurosurgical Procedures).

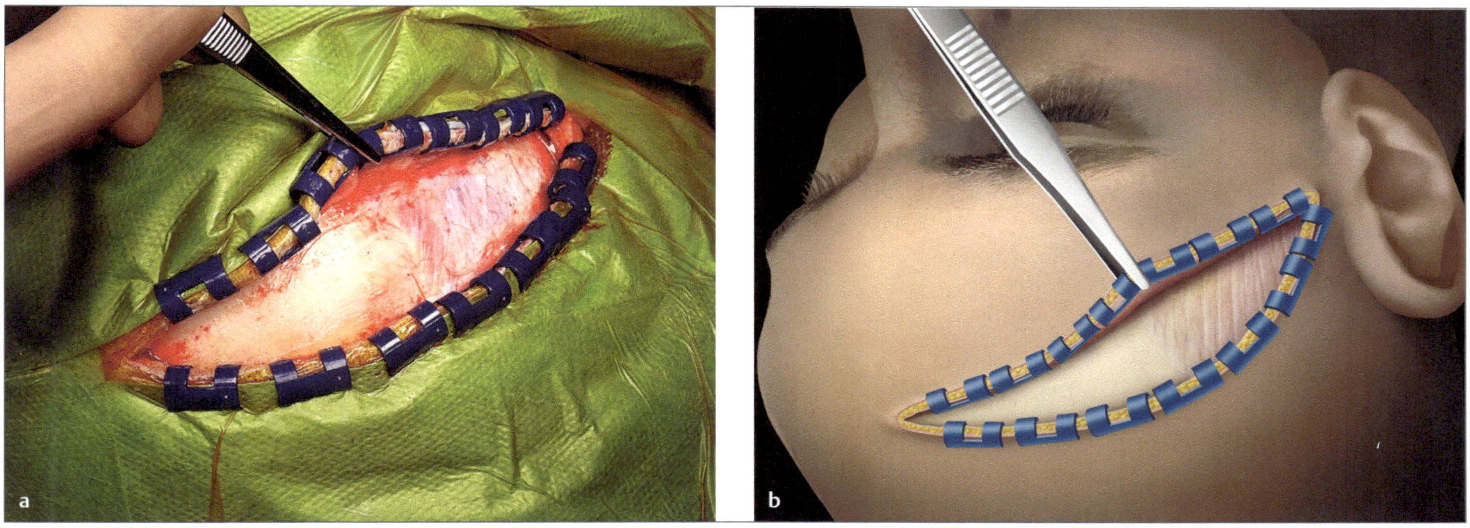

Fig. 5.88 (a, b) Skin incision. The skin incision spares the temporal muscle fascia. When reaching the temporal third of the planned incision, care should be taken to preserve the superficial temporal artery. Our technique is to dissect the horizontal tissue layers in the skin flap in a subcutaneous and a deep galea layer. The superficial temporal artery can be found on top of the galea in the deep layer (see Chapter 5.2.2 Superficial Temporal Artery Preservation during Frontolateral Approaches).

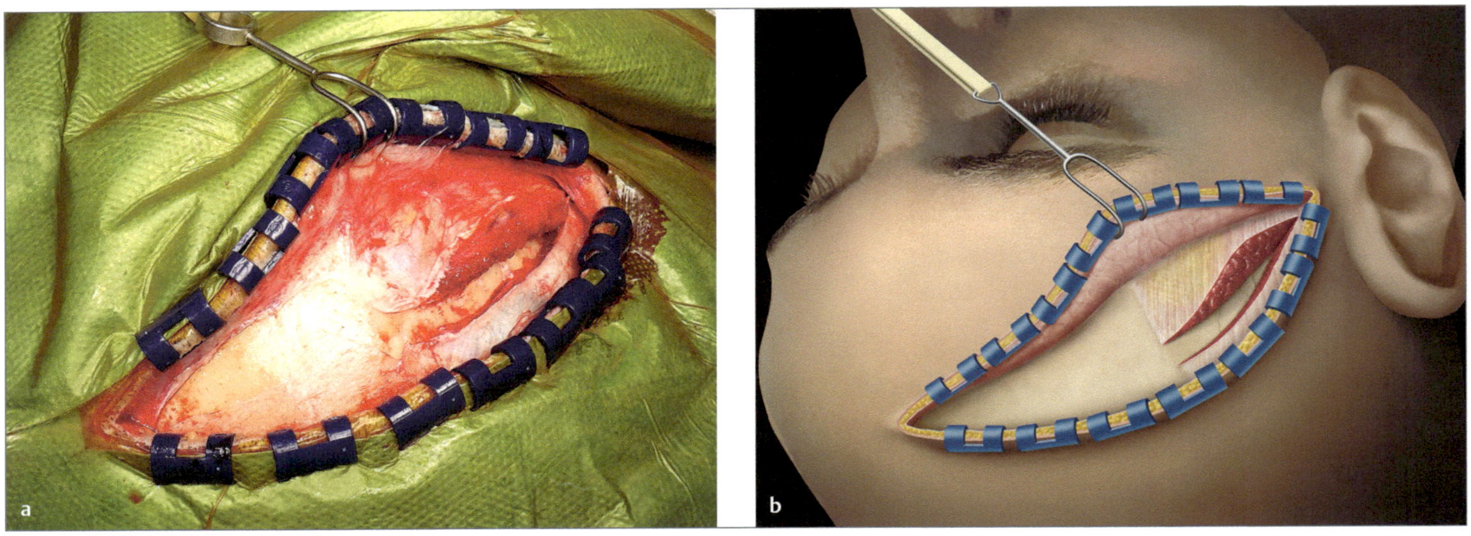

Fig. 5.89 (a, b) Combined skin–galea–muscle flap. For pterional craniotomy, a single-layer, skin–galea–muscle (=musculocutaneous), flap can be used in most cases. The temporalis muscle and skin–galea remain as one layer that will not be separated. The temporalis muscle is incised down to the bone. Venous bleeding may occur close to the zygoma and hemostasis is performed.

The combined musculocutaneous flap is quick and easy, prevents displacement and atrophy of the temporalis muscle, and achieves excellent cosmesis.

For pterional craniotomy, many textbooks still describe interfascial or subfascial dissection to separate the skin–galea from the muscle, and to turn the skin anteriorly but the muscle inferiorly (see Chapter 5.2.1, Facial Nerve Anatomy and Protection). In our opinion, this is only required if the lateral orbital rim has to be exposed, or in rare cases where the surgeon anticipates that the line of sight to the surgical target is likely to be obstructed by the temporal muscle.

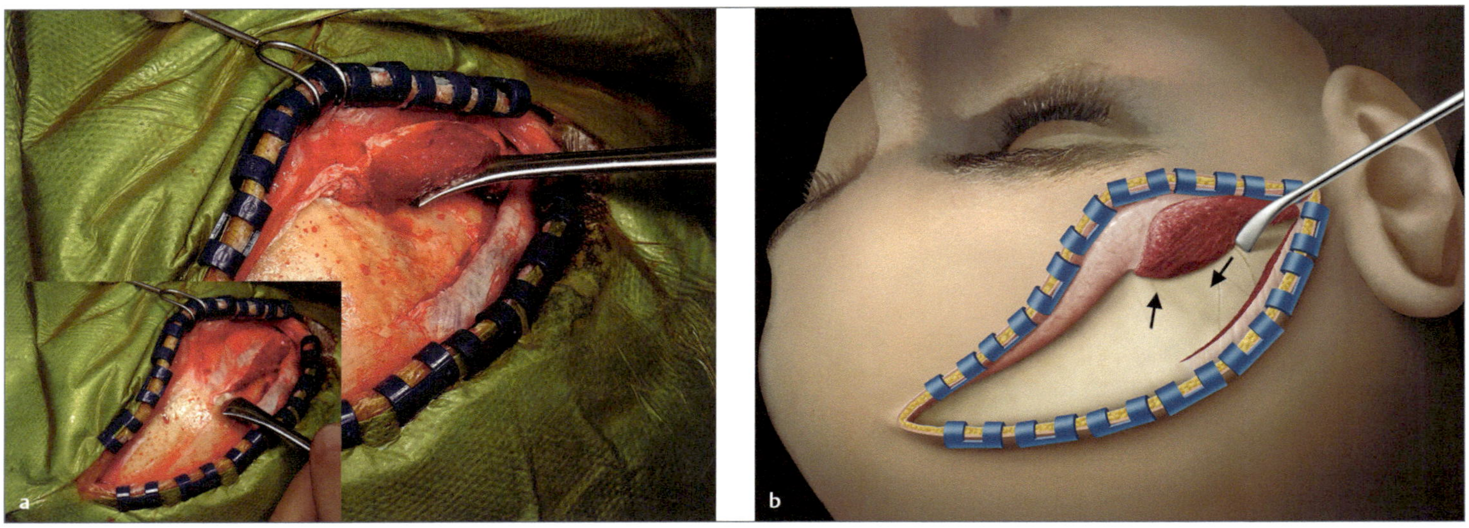

Fig. 5.90 (a, b) Temporalis muscle detachment and lifting the combined flap. The flap is now lifted in one layer by detaching the temporalis muscle from the bone and the fascia from the superior temporal line. Because of the direction in which the temporalis muscle fibers attach to the bone, the sharp rasp is moved subperiostally in an inferior-to-superior direction. This prevents injury of the muscle by slipping above the muscle fibers when detaching it in a superior-to-inferior direction. This, together with avoiding extensive monopolar dissection, prevents injury of the blood vessels, shrinkage, and atrophy of the muscle.

We do not leave a muscle cuff at the superior temporal line for the combined musculocutaneous flap, unless this is necessary when a subfascial or interfascial dissection is performed.

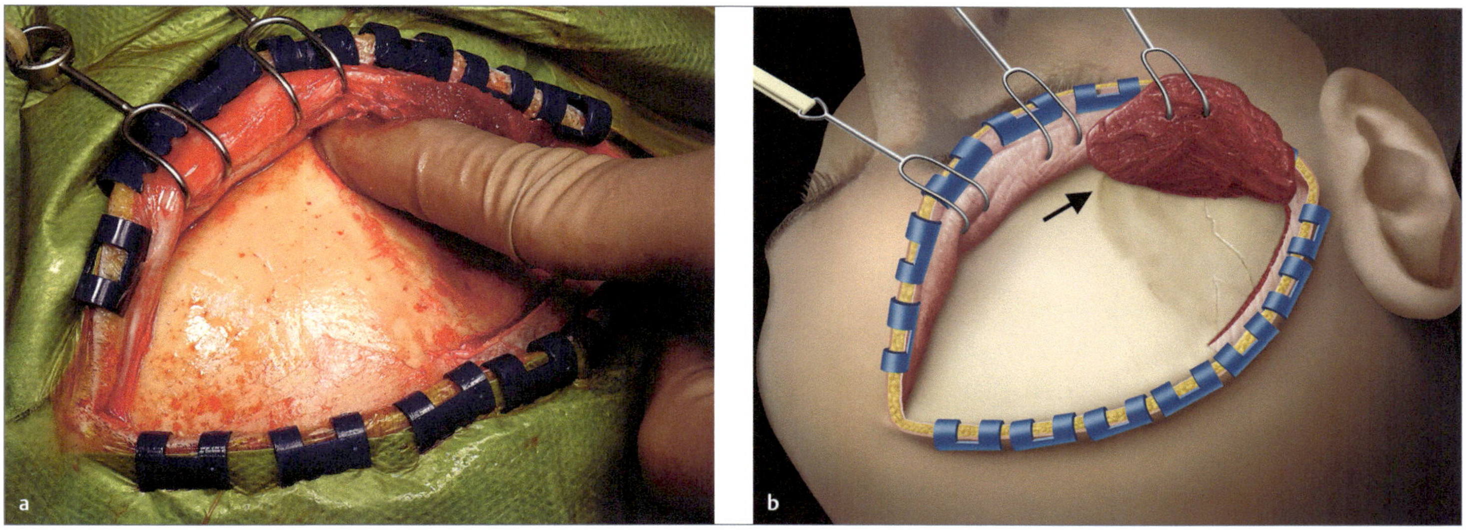

Fig. 5.91 (a, b) Exposing the frontotemporale. When the bony edge of the zygomatic process and its connection to the lateral orbital rim (the landmark frontotemporale indicating the frontal cranial base) can be palpated with the finger, the anterior = basal border of exposure is reached. There is no risk of injury to the facial nerve, because the flap is lifted in a single layer and the facial nerve remains embedded in its natural course and is safe as long as a single-layer musculocutaneous flap is preserved (see Chapter 5.2.1 Facial Nerve Anatomy and Protection).

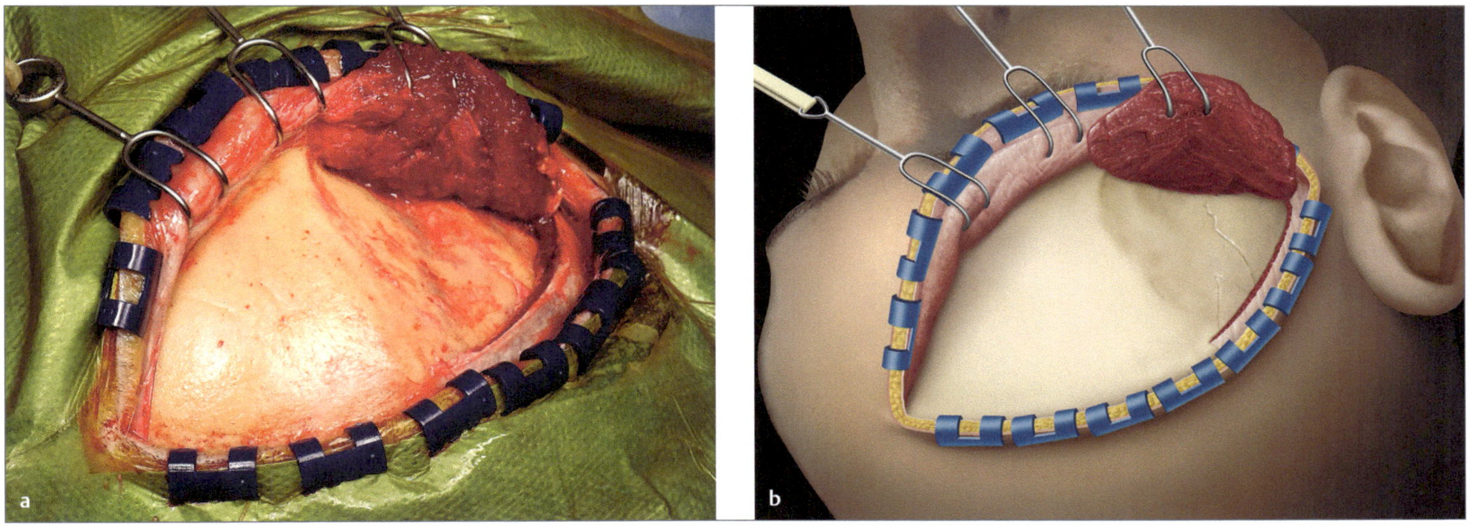

Fig. 5.92 (a, b) Bony exposure. The muscle is held with fish hooks. Often only minimal tension is required to keep the temporalis muscle in place. While the skin–galea may be retracted with more tension, the muscle should be handled more carefully to prevent pressure- or tension-induced damage and atrophy. The position of the pterion can be used as a landmark for further planning to tailor the size and position of the bone flap.

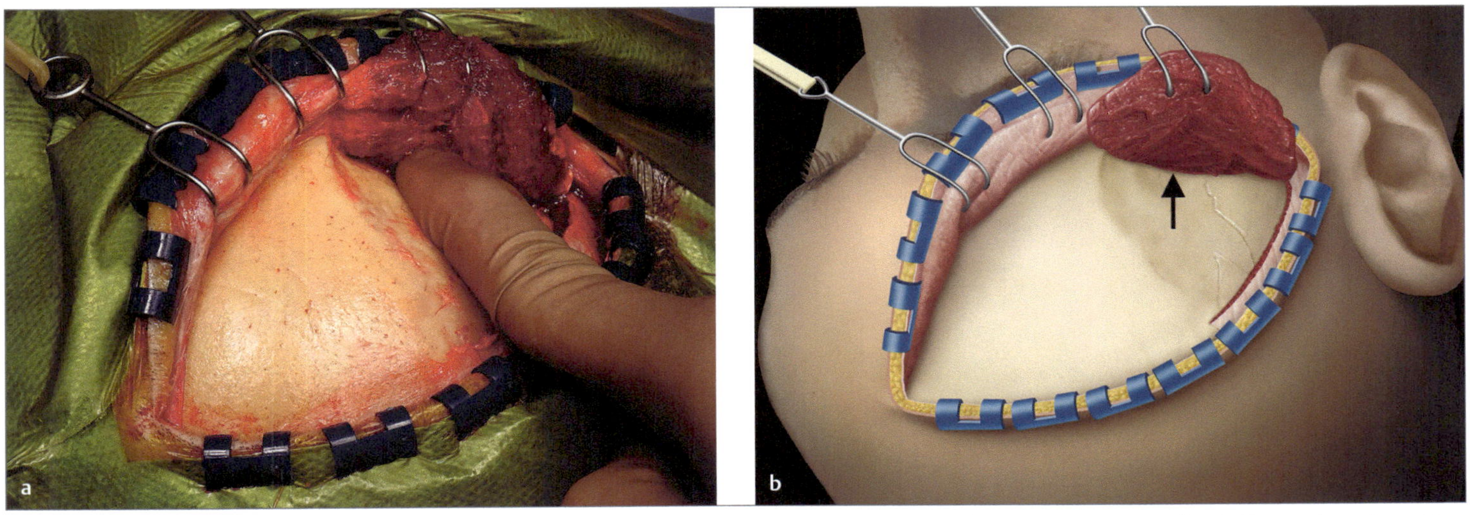

Fig. 5.93 (a, b) Determining the position of the sphenoid ridge. Another landmark is the shallow but constant groove that indicates the sphenoid ridge and the course of the sylvian fissure. When using a finger to palpate the bone in the direction of the sylvian fissure, the finger slips into the groove indicating the sphenoid ridge. The area felt by the fingertip indicates where the craniotome will be blocked by the sphenoid ridge, and a drill is used to complete the craniotomy in most cases.

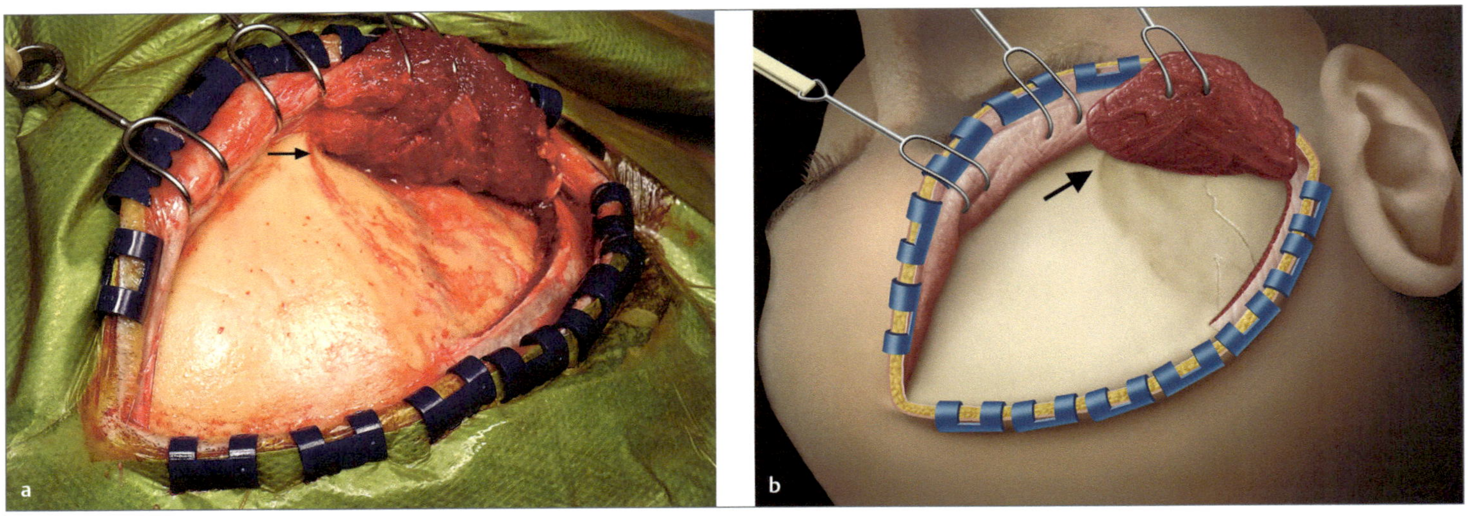

Fig. 5.94 (a, b) Craniotomy planning. As previously described, the pterional craniotomy typically extends two-thirds frontally and one-third temporally. Because it is a skull base approach that should provide access below the frontal lobe and along the sylvian fissure without brain retraction, it has to be flush with the anterior skull base at the basal extension of the frontal part of the craniotomy. A landmark for the anterior cranial skull base is the frontotemporale (*arrow*), which corresponds to the base of the zygomatic process of the frontal bone forming the upper lateral border of the orbital rim.

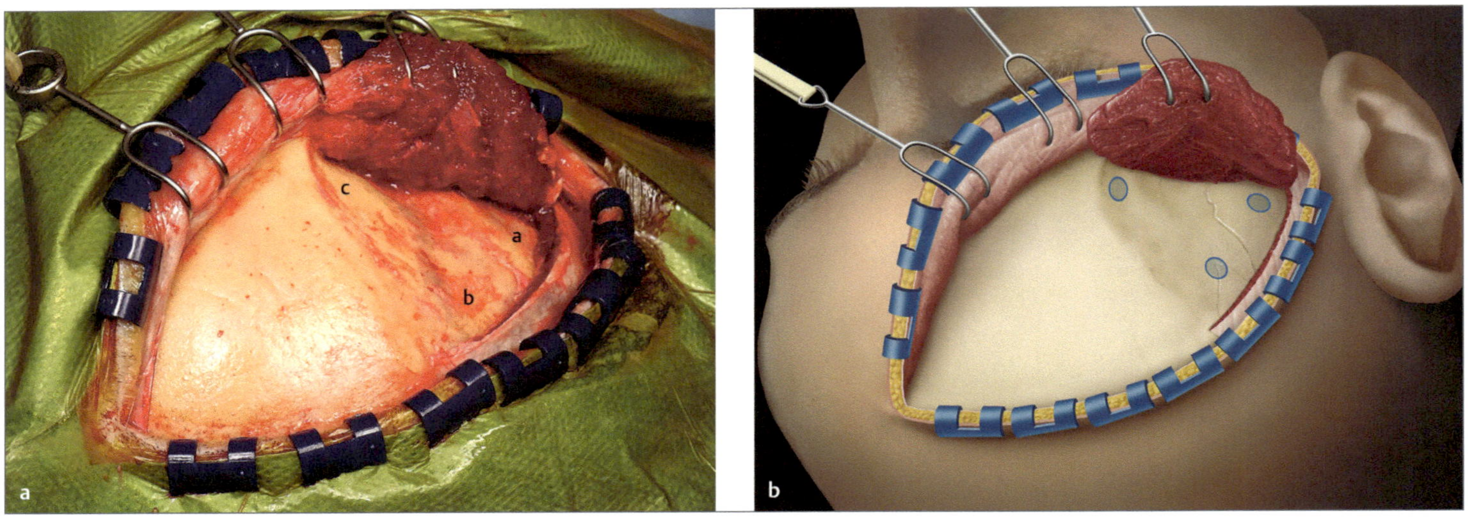

Fig. 5.95 (a, b) Burr hole. There are three typical locations for the burr hole: (a) at the lowest temporal extension of the planned craniotomy; (b) at the posterior level of the sphenoid ridge. Usually, the dura mater is more fixed at this point, and starting from here gives a good plane in the frontal and temporal direction. Both the temporal and sphenoid ridge burr holes are later covered by the temporal muscle. The third site for a burr hole (c), the so-called MacCarty keyhole, is 5–10 mm below the superior temporal line at the most basal-anterior position, but no closer than 5 mm posterior to the frontozygomatic suture. It gives worse cosmetic results than a and b. It was initially intended to open both the orbit and the frontal fossa with the same burr hole. For pterional craniotomy this is not needed, and the frontotemporale can be used instead as a reliable marker to gain access flush with the anterolateral skull base.

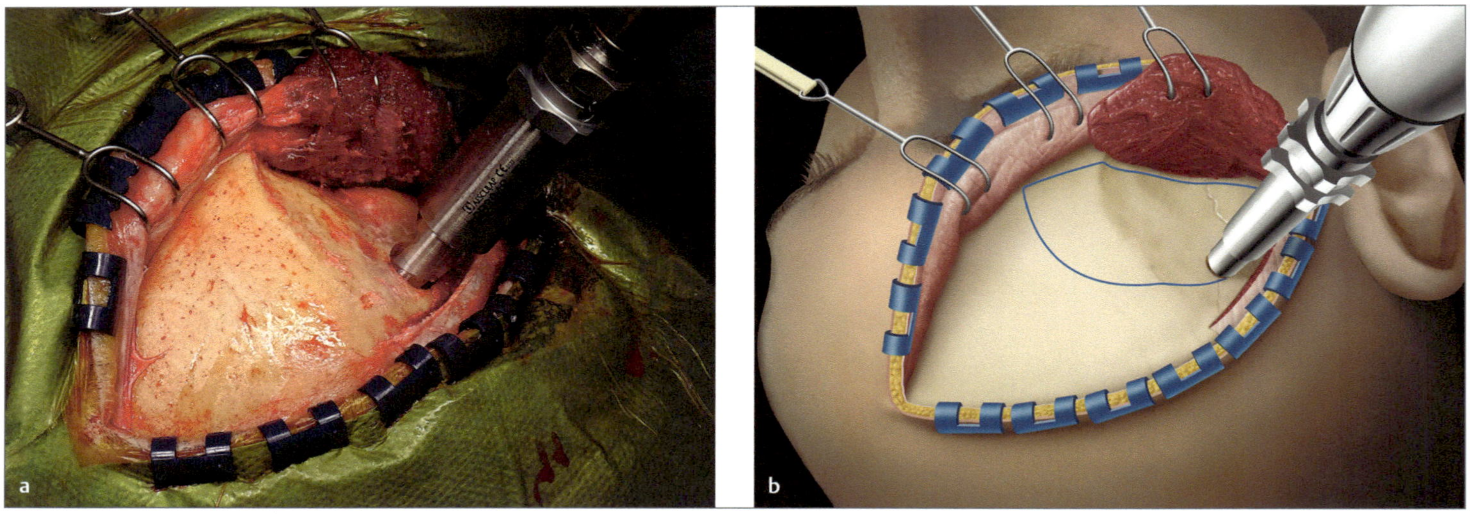

Fig. 5.96 (a, b) Burr hole. A burr hole is made at the distal sphenoid ridge. With the help of modern craniotomy instruments, we try to use only one burr hole. However, when we feel, during advancement of the craniotomy, that the dura is adherent or lacerated, additional burr hole(s) are made. There is a direct relationship between long-term postoperative cosmesis and the location (MacCarty burr hole should be avoided), the size, and the number of burr holes, even when they are covered with titanium plates. We use medium-sized burrs (6–9 mm) rather than large ones (14–16 mm).

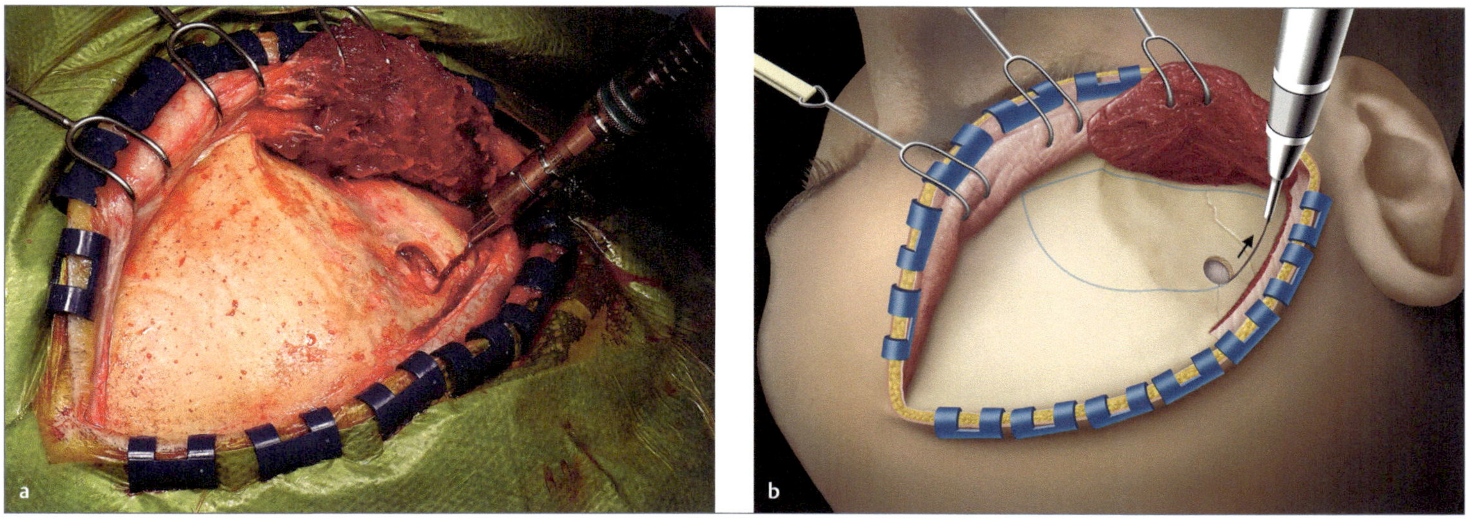

Fig. 5.97 (a, b) Craniotomy. In this example, the craniotomy is started from the posterior rim of the burr hole toward the temporal base and then goes upward, parallel to the temporal muscle, toward the sphenoid ridge. When the resistance of the sphenoid ridge is felt, the craniotome is moved back to the burr hole and the frontal craniotomy is performed. Arterial bleeding may occur from the middle meningeal artery, which should be stopped using bone wax. Therefore, some groups recommend performing the temporal cut at the end of the craniotomy immediately before lifting the flap.

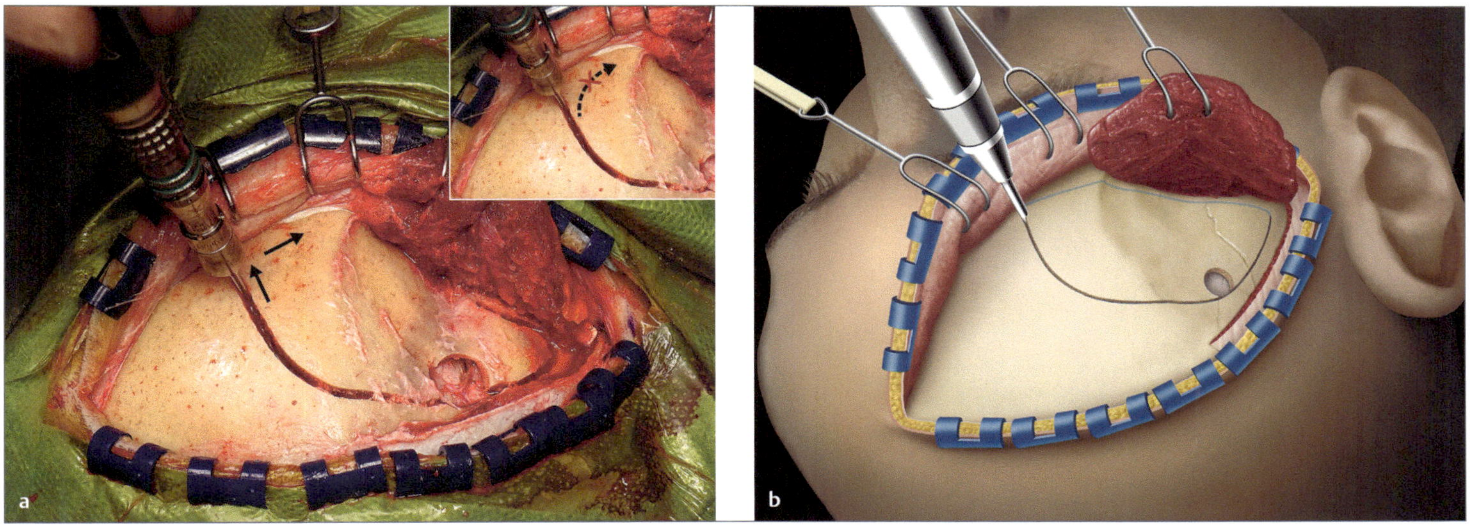

Fig. 5.98 (a, b) Craniotomy. Frontally, the craniotomy line should be straight down to the base rather than being curved. It should be continued all the way down until it hits the frontal base. Note that the craniotome has to be advanced slightly into the depth to reach the true base. Using the 90° dura dissector ensures that the base is reached and the dura is detached from the bone (see Chapter 1.7, Protection of the Dura Mater). Violation of the frontal sinus may occur, but access flush to the cranial base is a higher priority than sparing the frontal sinus. Limiting the medial border of the craniotomy to the midpupillary line helps to avoid the frontal sinus in most cases.

Now the blade of the craniotome is turned 90° and then follows the anterior base toward the frontozygomatic process. The cranial base rises a few millimeters laterally and the craniotome can get blocked at the frontozygomatic process, which is proof that the basal exposure is adequate. Care should be taken to cut the bone at the base at a 90° angle instead of in a curve to ensure that the view to the anterior base is not limited by incomplete bone removal

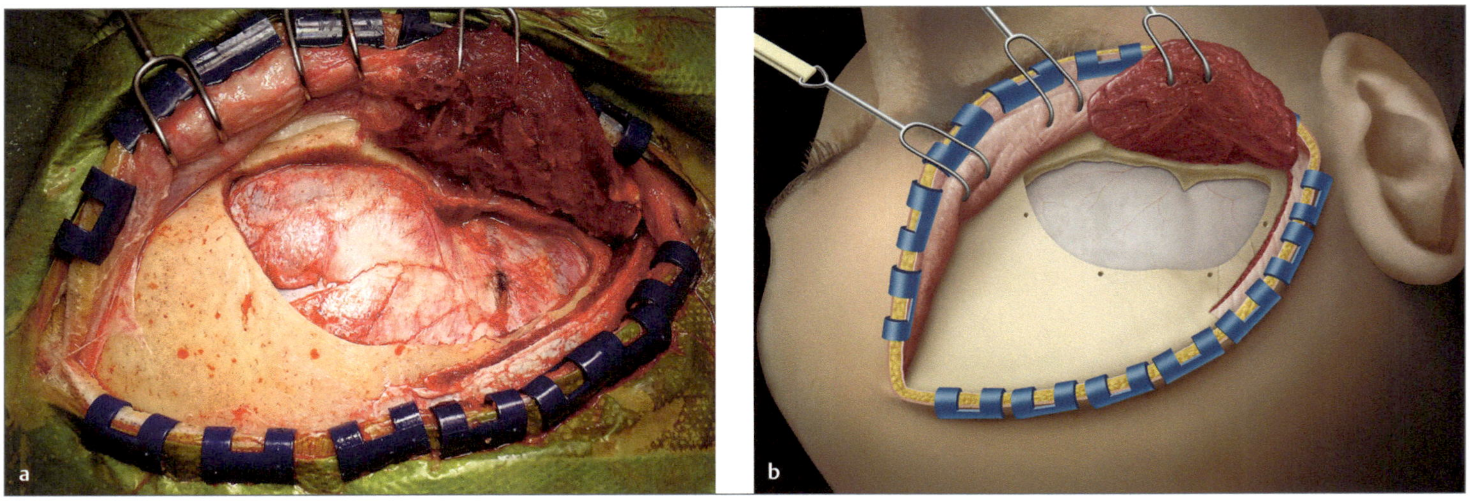

Fig. 5.99 (a, b) **Bone flap and tacking sutures.** After completing the craniotomy, the bone flap is elevated. In the case of a more solid sphenoid wing, additional drilling with the craniotomy blade or a 3–5 mm burr is required above the remaining attachment between the frontal and temporal basal cuts. We prefer to place two to five dural tacking sutures at the time of opening instead of at closure to enable the detection of rare accidental injury to the pial vessel by the tacking suture, and to minimize epidural oozing during surgery. These sutures are temporary and are released when closing the dura and tied afterward.

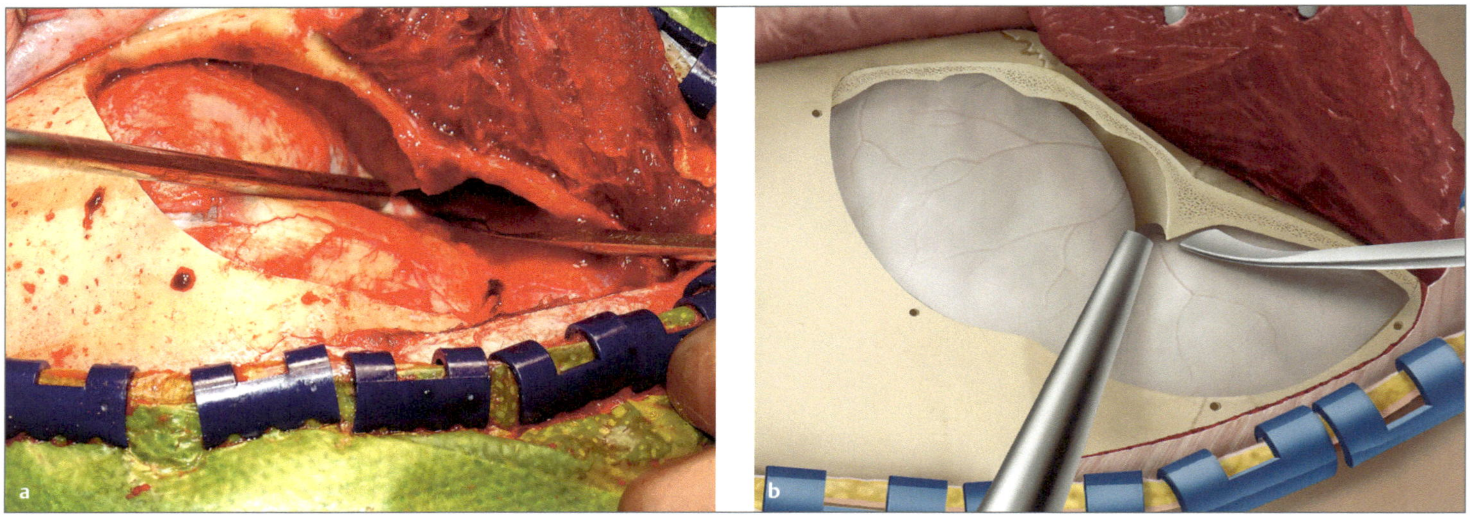

Fig. 5.100 (a, b) **Detaching the dura mater from the frontal and temporal bone.** Now the dura is detached 1–2 cm frontally and temporally, around the sphenoid wing. The next landmark is the meningo-orbital ligament, which indicates the superior orbital fissure and the proximal end for the drilling of the sphenoid wing. It is easily identified by (1) its position at the temporal side of the sphenoid wing and (2) unlike the frontal and temporal dura, it cannot be detached from the bone; instead, it connects the temporal dura with the periorbita.

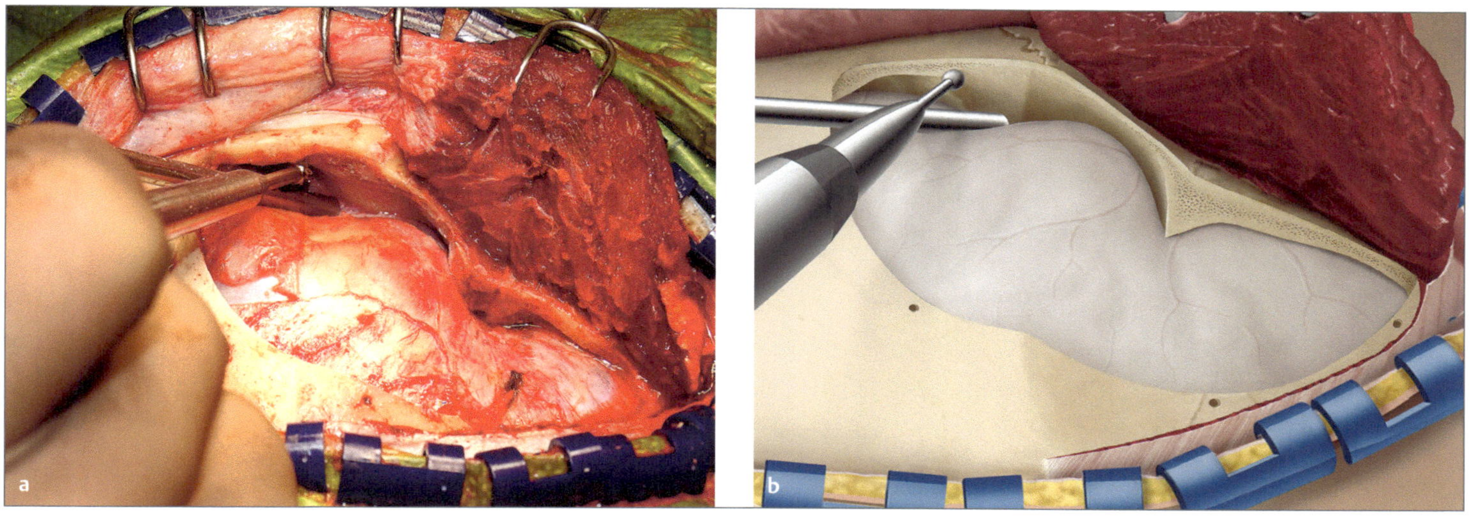

Fig. 5.101 (a, b) **Additional drilling of frontal and temporal bone.** The inner tabula is thinned with a 4–5-mm diamond or cutting drill. In so doing, another 2-mm space is gained to achieve subfrontal access flush with the anterior base. Care should be taken not to touch the frontal external tabula, for cosmetic reasons. When detaching the dura toward the frontal base, large bony elevations of the orbital roof should also be flattened with the drill, because they may obstruct the view. If needed, additional bone removal can also be performed at the temporal base using the drill or a rongeur.

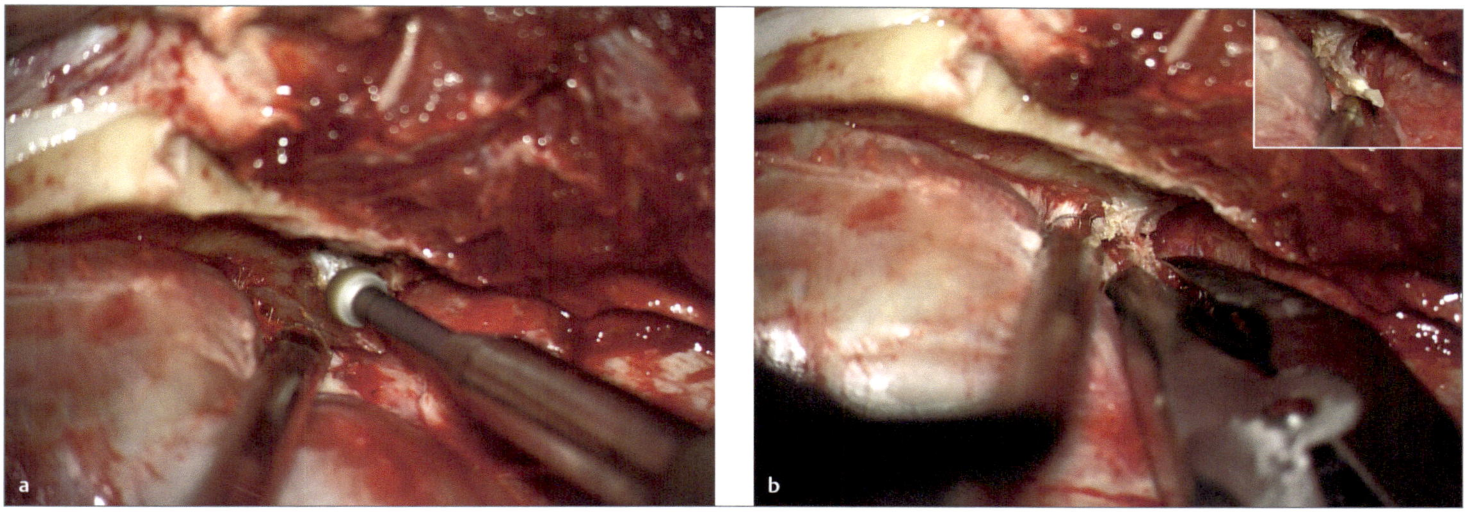

Fig. 5.102 (a, b) **Flattening of the sphenoid ridge.** After detaching the dura from the frontal and temporal bone, the sphenoid wing is drilled down to the meningo-orbital ligament using a 4–5-mm diamond or cutting drill (left) or a rongeur (right). Care should be taken to protect the dura mater from injury. The sphenoid wing obstructs a line of sight parallel to the skull base at the level of the sylvian fissure. To gain access to the optic nerve, internal carotid artery, the parasellar, the temporal, or tentorial region via a pterional approach, either retraction of the brain or removal of the bone is required to visualize these regions. The rule "remove bone, save brain" is the principle of skull base exposures.

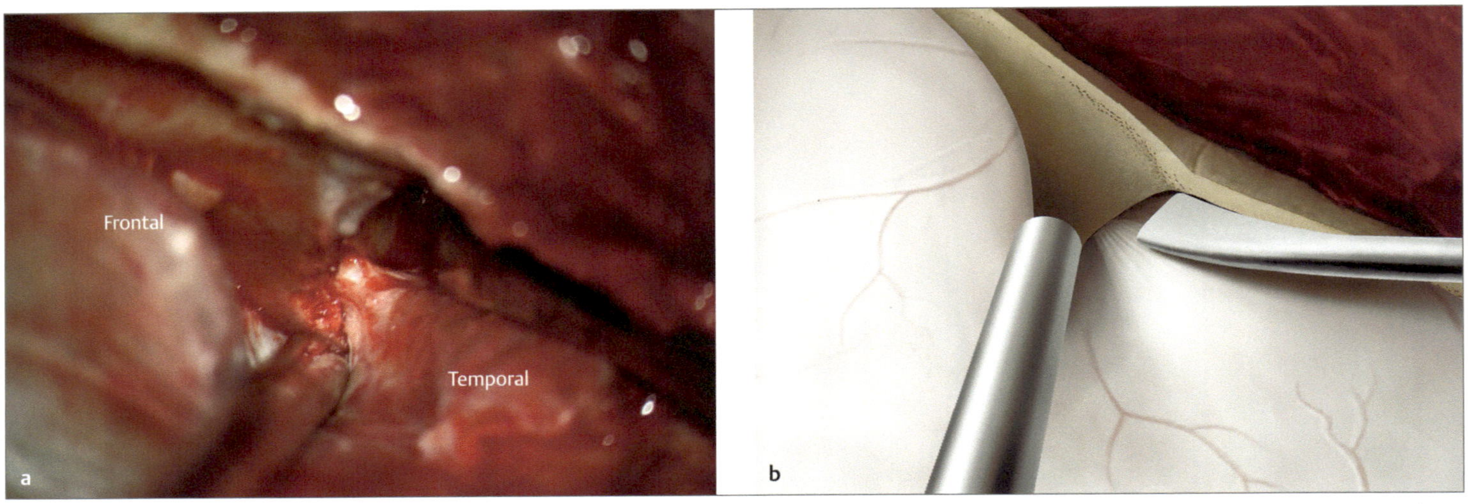

Fig. 5.103 (a, b) The meningo-orbital ligament. The meningo-orbital ligament connects the dura of the temporal side of the sphenoid wing with the periorbita. It is identifiable because it remains adherent to the dura when the frontal and temporal dura is detached from the bone. It marks the most superior part of the superior orbital fissure. It can be cut when the dura needs to be detached more widely, as for extradural clinoidectomy or a transcavernous approach, because this part of the superior orbital fissure does not contain nerves.

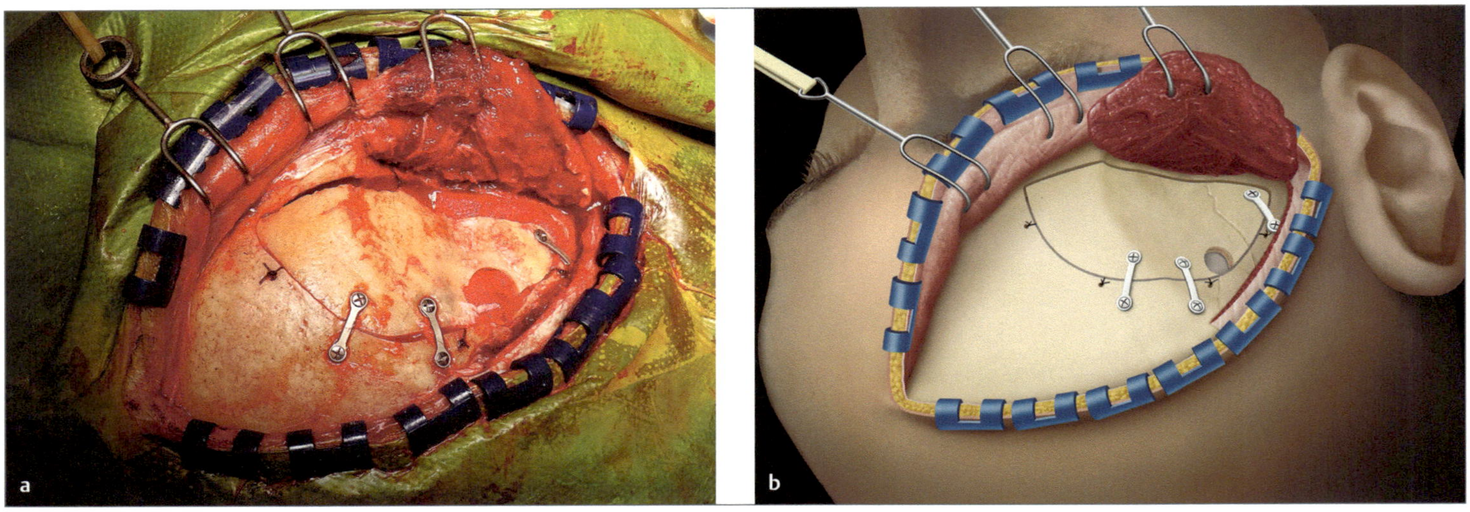

Fig. 5.104 (a, b) Closure: bone flap fixation. After closure of the dura, the bone flap is fixed with mini-plates or CranioFix. For cosmesis, care should be taken to fix the bone frontally without any gaps. Small temporal or dorsal gaps will be covered by the temporal muscle. Bone cement or titanium mesh should be used to fill larger gaps. As already mentioned, entering the frontal sinus during craniotomy is of less concern than the need to gain access flush to the base. However, before replacing the flap, any frontal sinus opening should be closed (see Chapter 1.9, Frontal Sinus Breach and Repair). For more information about cosmesis, see Chapter 1.6, Esthetic Considerations in Neurosurgical Procedures.

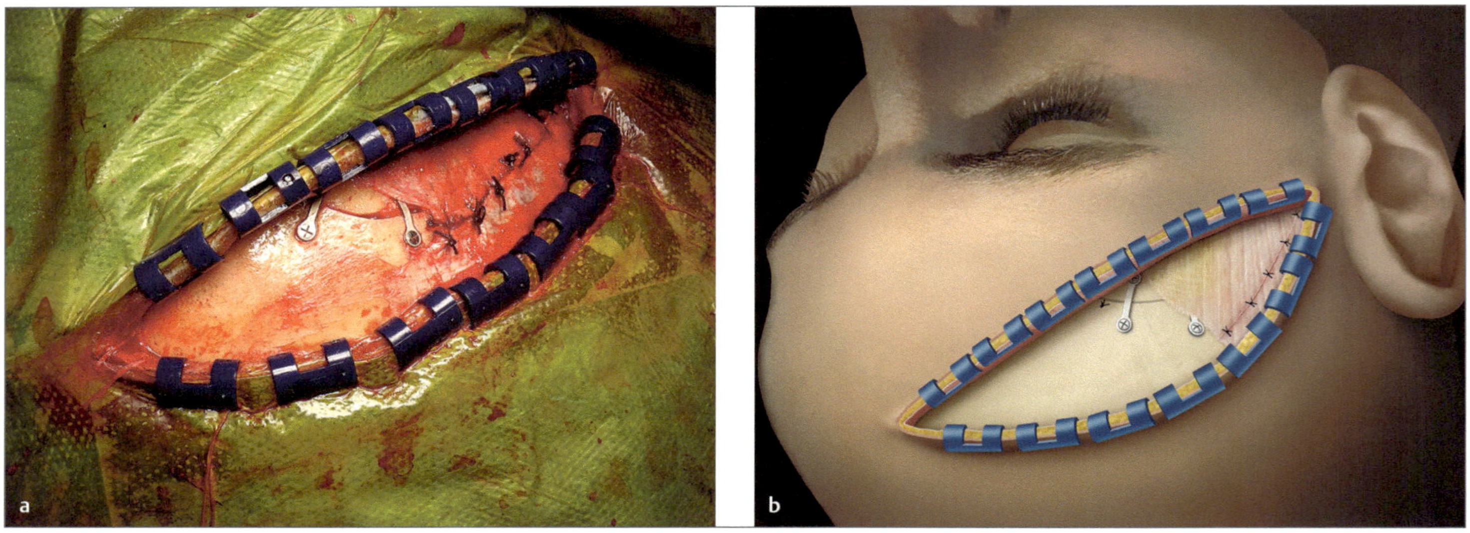

Fig. 5.105 (a, b) Closure: temporalis muscle. The temporal muscle fascia is sutured. Care is taken to lift the fascia rather than to sew it downward, i.e., the suture hole should be a few millimeters higher on the posterior part of the temporalis muscle fascia. This assures an upward tightening and correct replacement of the muscle with excellent cosmetic results.

Checklist

- Before skin incision, check that the skin incision is > 1 cm behind the hairline and is sufficiently large to reach the base of the zygomatic process of the frontal bone (landmark frontotemporale).
- Elevate a combined musculocutaneous flap without separating the muscle from the galea.
- Detach the muscle fibers in an inferior-to-superior direction rather than a superior-to-inferior direction.
- Expose the frontotemporale which is a landmark for the anterior skull base, i.e., sufficient basal exposure.
- Avoid the MacCarty burr hole for cosmetic reasons.
- Use medium-sized or small burrs rather than large ones.
- Make sure that the direction of the craniotome is perpendicular to the frontal skull base; use the 90° dura dissector to detach the dura and to make sure that the exposure is basal enough.
- Turn the craniotome 90° and follow the most basal part to achieve a craniotomy that is flush with the skull base.
- Incidental dural laceration most often occurs between the zygomatic process and the sphenoid ridge; make sure to detach the dura with the 90° dissector along the craniotomy line and 1 cm beyond toward the intended craniotomy line and take care to handle the craniotome very gently.
- Drill the tabula interna for better access to the base while leaving the tabula externa intact for cosmesis.
- Dissect the dura mater about 2 cm frontally, temporally, and around the sphenoid ridge, with the goal of visualizing the meningo-orbital band.
- Drill down the sphenoid ridge to the level of the meningo-orbital band.
- Insert the dural tacking sutures at the beginning of the surgery before dural opening rather than at the end after closure.
- When closing, take care to avoid bony defects anteriorly and medially where no temporal muscle is covering them. Use bone cement or titanium mesh or plates to cover large bony defects and larger or multiple burr holes.

5.3 Temporal Craniotomies

5.3.1 Temporobasal Craniotomy

Bernhard Meyer

Introduction

The temporobasal craniotomy is one of the so-called workhorses of standard craniotomies for basal access and should therefore be mastered early on in training, at least conceptually. As opposed to the other two options (pterional/frontolateral and lateral suboccipital), this craniotomy is seemingly easier, but access to the basal target area (i.e., the tentorial edge) is more difficult due to the concavity of the temporal base.

The classic target area is the tentorial edge and everything in its proximity, i.e., the tip of the pyramid, upper clivus/posterior clinoid, cavernous sinus, Meckel's cave, lateral brainstem (pons), tip of the basilar artery, and P1/P2 segment of the posterior cerebellar artery. The mesial structures of the temporal lobe itself (hippocampus and parahippocampal gyrus) can also be reached. While the "standard" temporobasal craniotomy is centered on the outer auditory canal, it can be shifted anteriorly or posteriorly according to the desired angle of access, thus allowing visualization of structures in front of or behind the brainstem. Incising the tentorium from medially (its edge) to laterally behind the tip of the pyramid makes further visualization and access to the posterior fossa possible. If the tip of the pyramid is drilled away too (the so-called Kawase approach), additional access of approximately 10 mm into the posterior fossa is gained. In the author's experience, however, this is very rarely necessary. With these extensions, the cranial nerves III–VI and partly VII and VIII can be seen, as well as the upper surface of the cerebellum, the superior cerebellar artery, the middle clivus, and Dorello's canal.

The limits cranially are clearly determined by the restricted possibility of retracting the temporal lobe, which is the key drawback of the subtemporal route. Due to the above-mentioned concavity of the temporal base and the temporobasal draining veins, a safe retraction beyond 15 mm mesially is rarely possible, even after drainage of large quantities of cerebrospinal fluid (CSF) from the ambient cistern.

The spectrum of pathologies amenable to subtemporal access via a temporobasal craniotomy ranges from hippocampal tumors, tentorial edge or upper clival meningiomas, brainstem cavernomas, basilar tip or P1/P2 aneurysms, schwannomas of the trigeminal nerve, to tumors of the pyramidal tip.

With these prerequisites in mind, it becomes clear that the key feature of this craniotomy is its placement as basally as possible. A lateral entrance flush with the temporal base is essential (▶Fig. 5.106, ▶Fig. 5.107, ▶Fig. 5.108, ▶Fig. 5.109, ▶Fig. 5.110, ▶Fig. 5.111, ▶Fig. 5.112, ▶Fig. 5.113, ▶Fig. 5.114, ▶Fig. 5.115, and ▶Fig. 5.116).

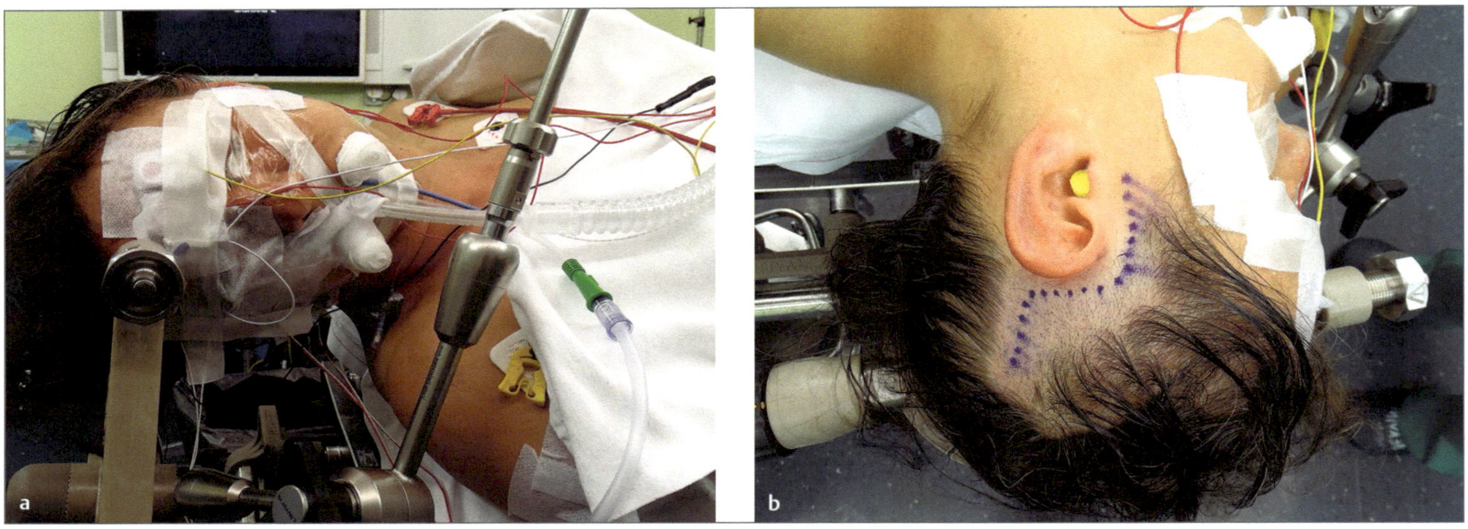

Fig. 5.106 (a, b) Positioning. Patient positioning for a left-sided approach. Patient is prone and the head is turned 90° toward the contralateral (right) side. Some support under the ipsilateral (left) shoulder is recommended. The head is flexed only slightly downward to facilitate temporal lobe retraction by gravity. To avoid distortion of the neck and venous outflow constriction, excessive flexion should be avoided. If necessary, the table can be tilted in the direction of the surgeon's lap, once CSF has been released from the ambient cistern.

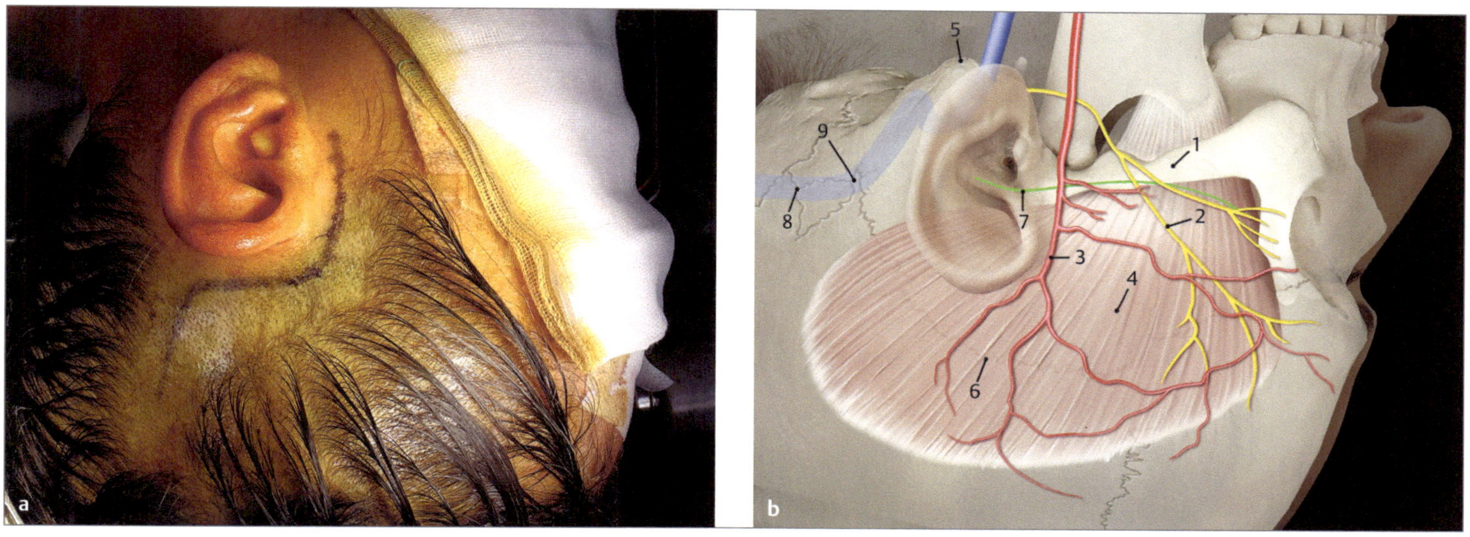

Fig. 5.107 (a, b) Anatomy overview. Important landmarks or structures are (1) zygomatic arch, (2) facial nerve, (3) superficial temporal artery, (4) temporal muscle, (5) mastoid process, (6) sutura temporalis (squamosa), (7) floor of the middle fossa, (8) asterion, and (9) the sinus knee (transition zone of transverse-to-sigmoid sinus).

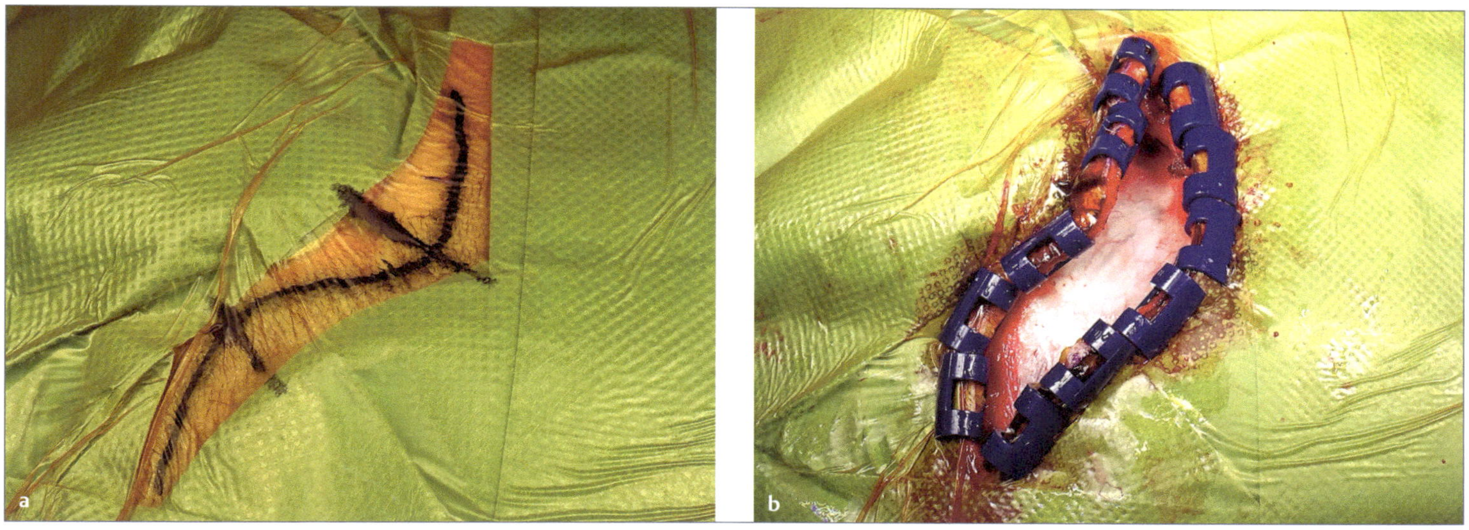

Fig. 5.108 (a, b) Skin incision. (a) Outline of the skin incision after draping, **(b)** a "lazy-Z" type skin incision starting 1 cm below the zygoma, turning backward immediately above the ear and then extending 4–5 cm upward. Care should be taken not to incise the fascia of the temporal muscle.

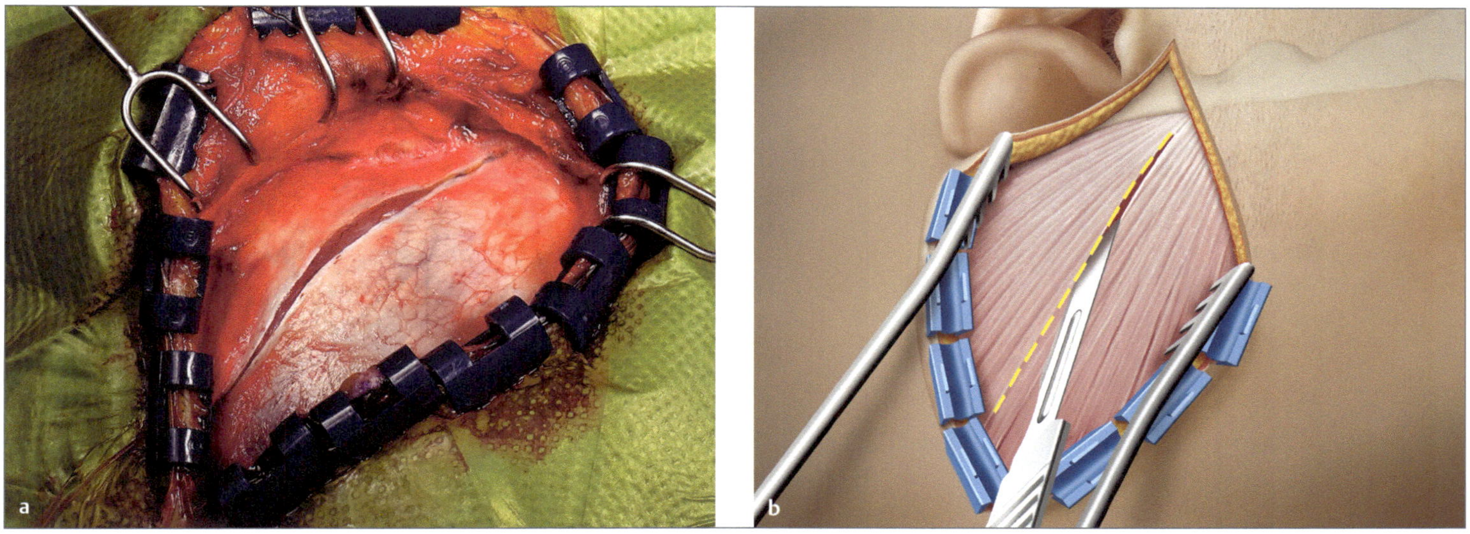

Fig. 5.109 (a, b) Incision and detachment of temporalis muscle. The fascia of the temporal muscle is incised separately. It is not incised with the skin in order to avoid cutting muscle fibers instead of separating them bluntly. The fibers of the temporalis muscles run in a superoposterior direction that is different from the lazy-Z skin incision. The temporalis muscle is bluntly separated in an inferior-to-superior direction. The use of monopolar coagulation is avoided to preserve the vascular supply and minimize postoperative atrophy. Fish hooks or a blunt retractor is used to keep the temporalis muscle aside.

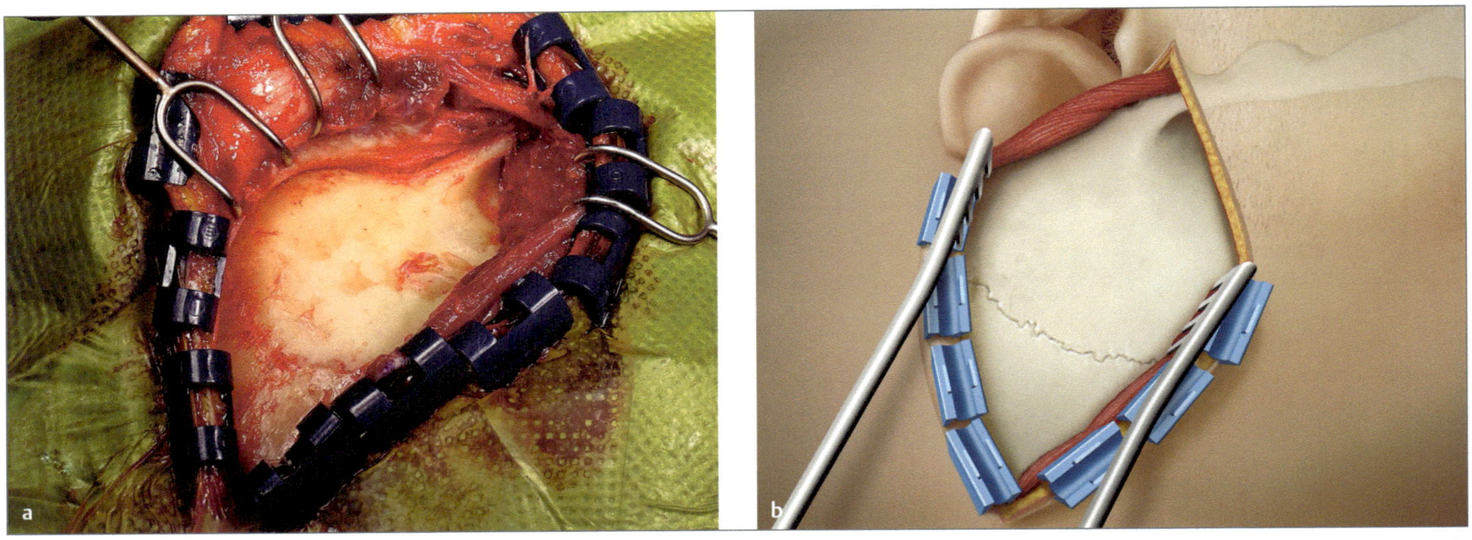

Fig. 5.110 (a, b) Exposure of bony landmarks. Exposure of the three essential bony landmarks before craniotomy: the sutura squamosa, the base of the zygoma, and the groove indicating the upper rim of the meatus acusticus externus. It is important to be able to see all three landmarks to plan and place the craniotomy properly, i.e., basal enough. The most common mistake made by beginners is not to visualize the landmarks, which usually results in a craniotomy being placed too cranially.

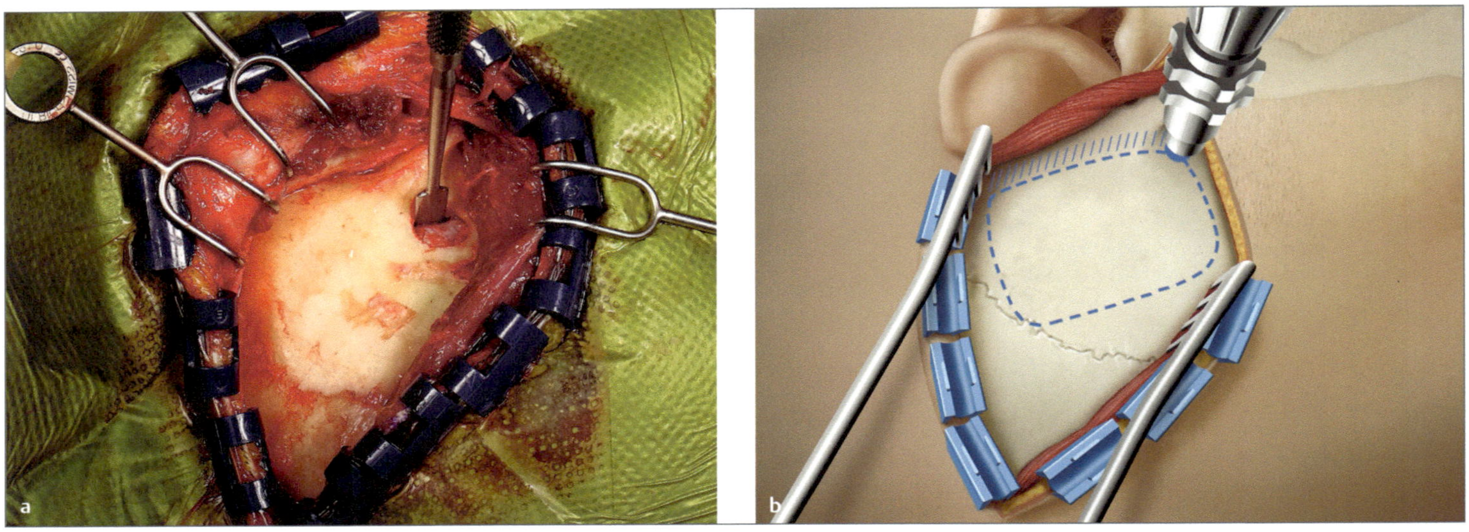

Fig. 5.111 (a, b) Craniotomy planning. The craniotomy is planned to gain access flush with the base of the middle fossa. It is advisable to draw the outline of the craniotomy onto the temporal bone with these landmarks visible. Necessary measurements can be referenced to the temporal base and the auditory canal. The landmark for the temporal base is the line of insertion of the zygomatic arch (Fig. 5.107). The dimension of the craniotomy (including the osteoclastic basal part) should be 3 cm in height as measured from the base. The anteroposterior dimension normally does not exceed 3.5 cm. Because this craniotomy is typically used for a subtemporal intradural approach, therefore there is no need for a longer extension in a superior direction.

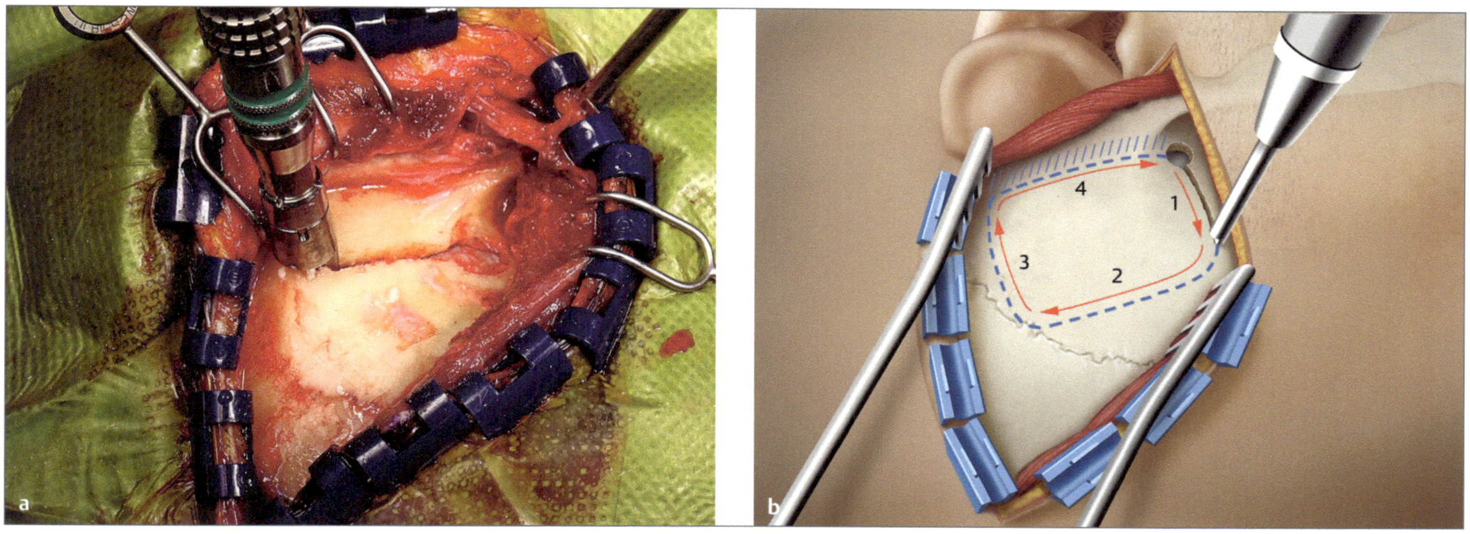

Fig. 5.112 (a, b) Burr hole. A single burr hole is drilled with a 6-mm drill immediately above the zygoma. This is usually the most anterior inferior part of the exposure and marks the lowest point of the middle fossa floor. The temporal base is not horizontally orientated but runs in a posterosuperior oblique direction. The burr hole can also be made at the posterosuperior edge of the craniotomy.The craniotomy should be performed first toward the anterior superior direction (1), then superiorly (2), posterior inferiorly (3), and finally the basal part (4) connecting to the burr hole (clockwise on the left side, counterclockwise on the right side). Moving the craniotome toward the base (3) helps to achieve the most basal craniotomy, instead of performing the basal horizontal cut at the beginning (left image).

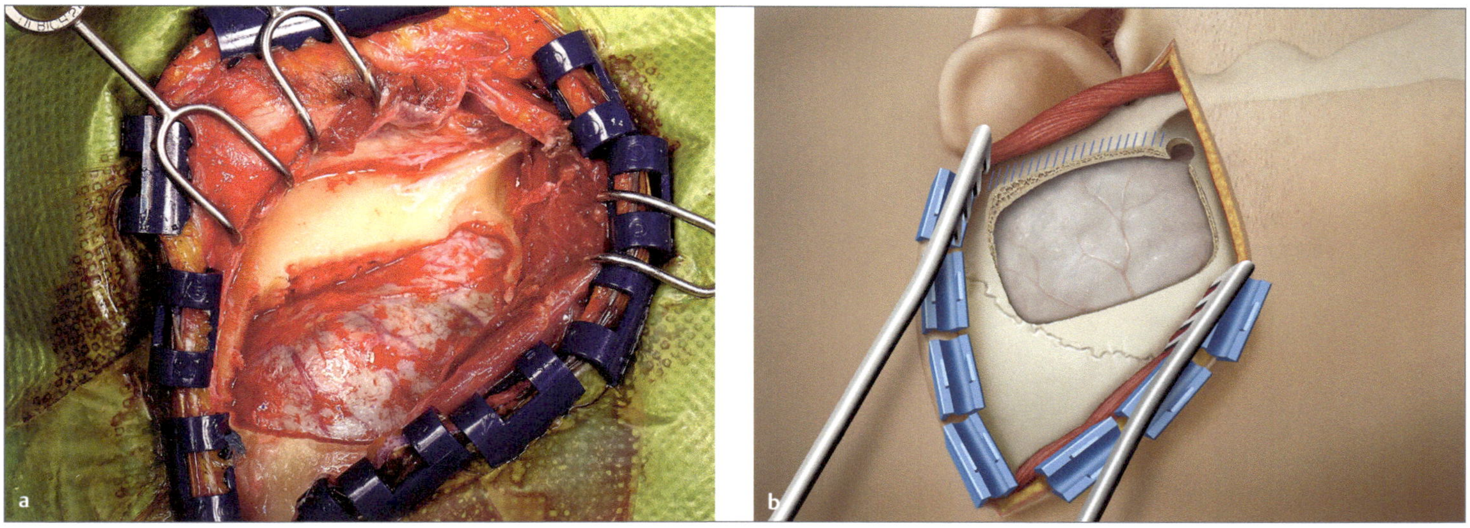

Fig. 5.113 (a, b) Craniotomy. Because of the position of the mastoid cells and the os petrosum, the most basal part of the craniotomy (hatched area) is not amenable to osteoplastic craniotomy; it must be drilled away to gain access flush to the skull base. The dura is gently deflected to visualize the location of the floor of the middle fossa and the amount of drilling.

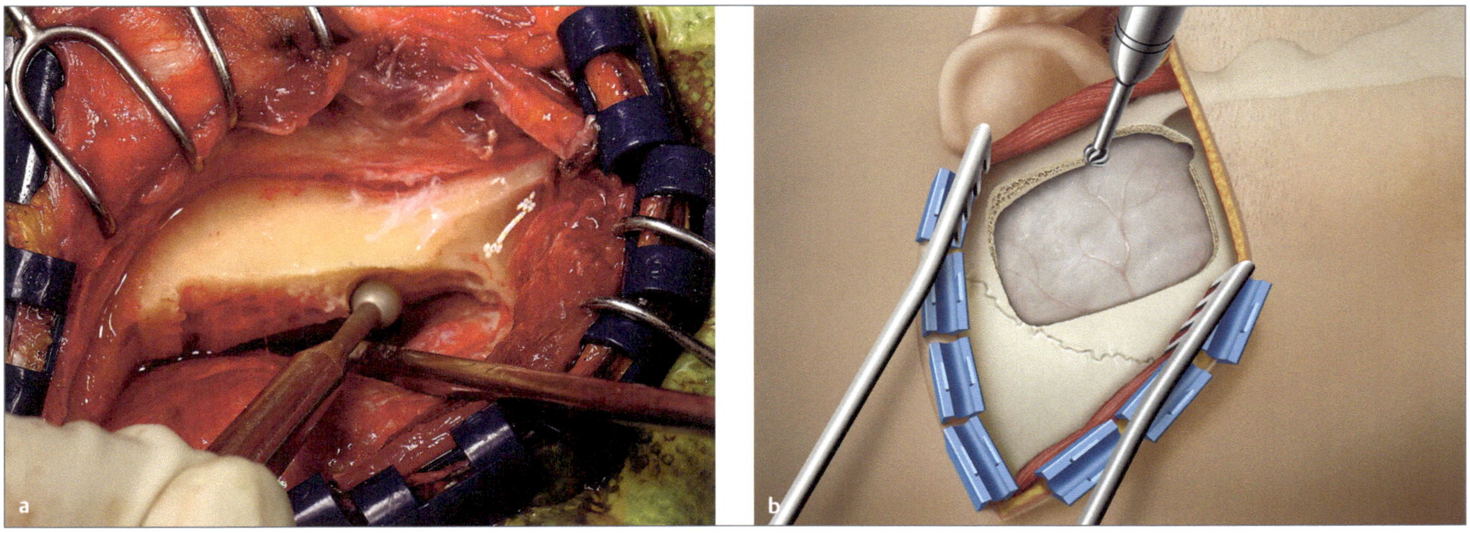

Fig. 5.114 (a, b) Basal drilling. Once the osteoplastic part of the craniotomy has been accomplished, the mastoid air cells are usually already open. A drill now needs to be used to finish the exposure. The final inferior 5 mm of the bone have to be drilled down until it is flush with the temporal base. In the left image, a diamond drill is used; in the right image, a cutting burr is used, with the sharp equator toward the bone to be drilled and the blunter tip (south pole) of the burr toward the dura mater.

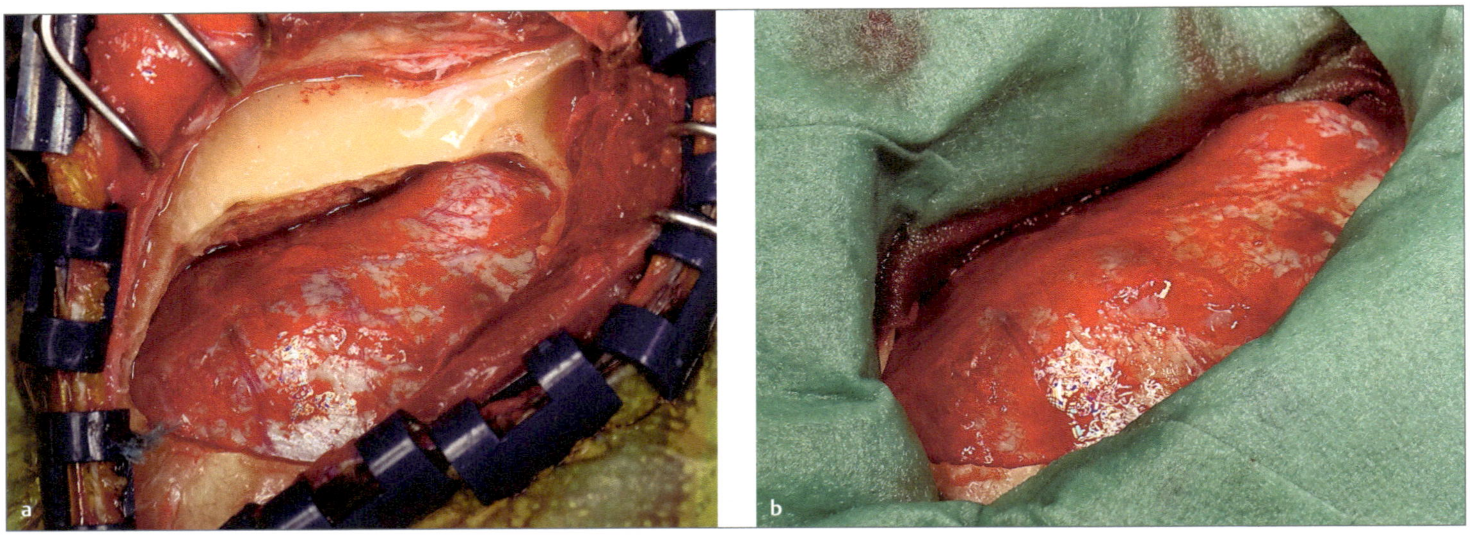

Fig. 5.115 (a, b) Flush access to the middle fossa. After drilling of the basal bone is complete, the mastoid air cells are usually wide open and should be sealed with bone wax. It is essential at this stage to elevate the basal dura in order to check that the lateral remaining bone is indeed flush with the temporal base. If not, it will result in an unnecessary retraction of the temporal lobe during the intradural subtemporal approach. The bone is covered with cottonoids. The dura is opened in a curvilinear fashion, and tacking sutures are placed. After performing the craniotomy as described, the inferior temporal gyrus should be easily visible. Subtemporal access is thus provided by a temporobasal craniotomy.

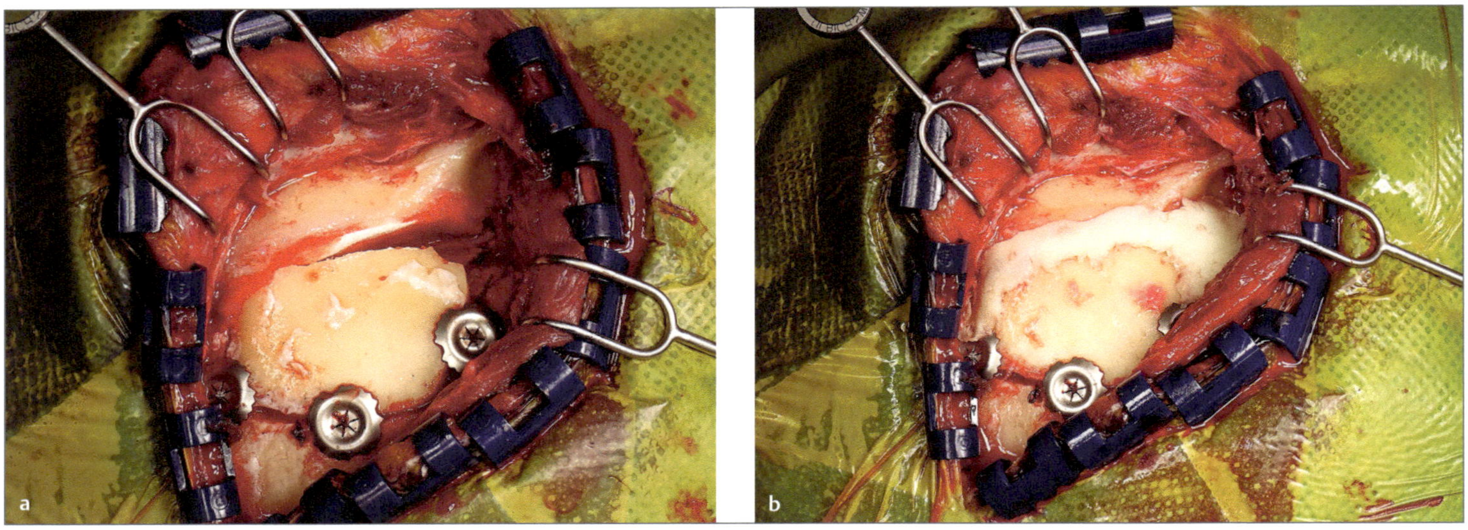

Fig. 5.116 (a, b) Closure. Before the bone flap is replaced, the surface of the osteoclastic part should be carefully inspected to make sure that all air cells are obliterated with bone wax. Alternatively, Gelfoam, fibrin glue, or pieces of muscle can be used. The bone flap is fixed in close contact with the superior edge of the craniotomy with mini-plates or CranioFix. If large defects are present, bone cement can also be used to ensure closure and cosmesis. No routine drainage is used. The fascia of the temporalis muscle is approximated, without suturing.

Checklist

- Position the head horizontally in the two axes: frontal-occipitally and craniocaudally.
- Palpate the base of the zygomatic arch, which is an important landmark.
- Adjust the position of the flap in relation to the external auditory canal.
- Remember that the access will be at the base of the middle fossa, at the inferior border of the craniotomy, only a short distance superior to the external auditory canal.
- Make sure that this position of the flap is reached using a lazy-Z or U-incision.
- Firstly, incise only skin and galea.
- Then incise the fascia of the temporalis muscle along the course of the fibers.
- Split the fibers and retract the muscle.
- Expose the base of the zygomatic arch, make sure you can see the beginning of the groove of the auditory canal and the squamous (temporalis) suture.
- Place a burr hole at the base of the zygomatic arch.
- Perform the craniotomy toward the base to reach it.
- Deflect dura mater after removal of the bone flap to localize the floor of the middle fossa.
- Perform osteoclastic drilling to the floor to ensure a flush access.
- Wax or close the mastoid cells before dura opening.
- After dural closure, inspect mastoid cells again and wax to ensure proper closure.
- Fix flap in contact with the anterior and superior rim of the craniotomy.
- Close gap with bone cement in large gaps.

5.4 Posterior Fossa

5.4.1 Retrosigmoid Craniotomy

Marcos Tatagiba, Florian H. Ebner, and Georgios Naros

See ▶ Fig. 5.117, ▶ Fig. 5.118, ▶ Fig. 5.119, ▶ Fig. 5.120, ▶ Fig. 5.121, ▶ Fig. 5.122, ▶ Fig. 5.123, ▶ Fig. 5.124, ▶ Fig. 5.125, ▶ Fig. 5.126, ▶ Fig. 5.127, ▶ Fig. 5.128, and ▶ Fig. 5.129.

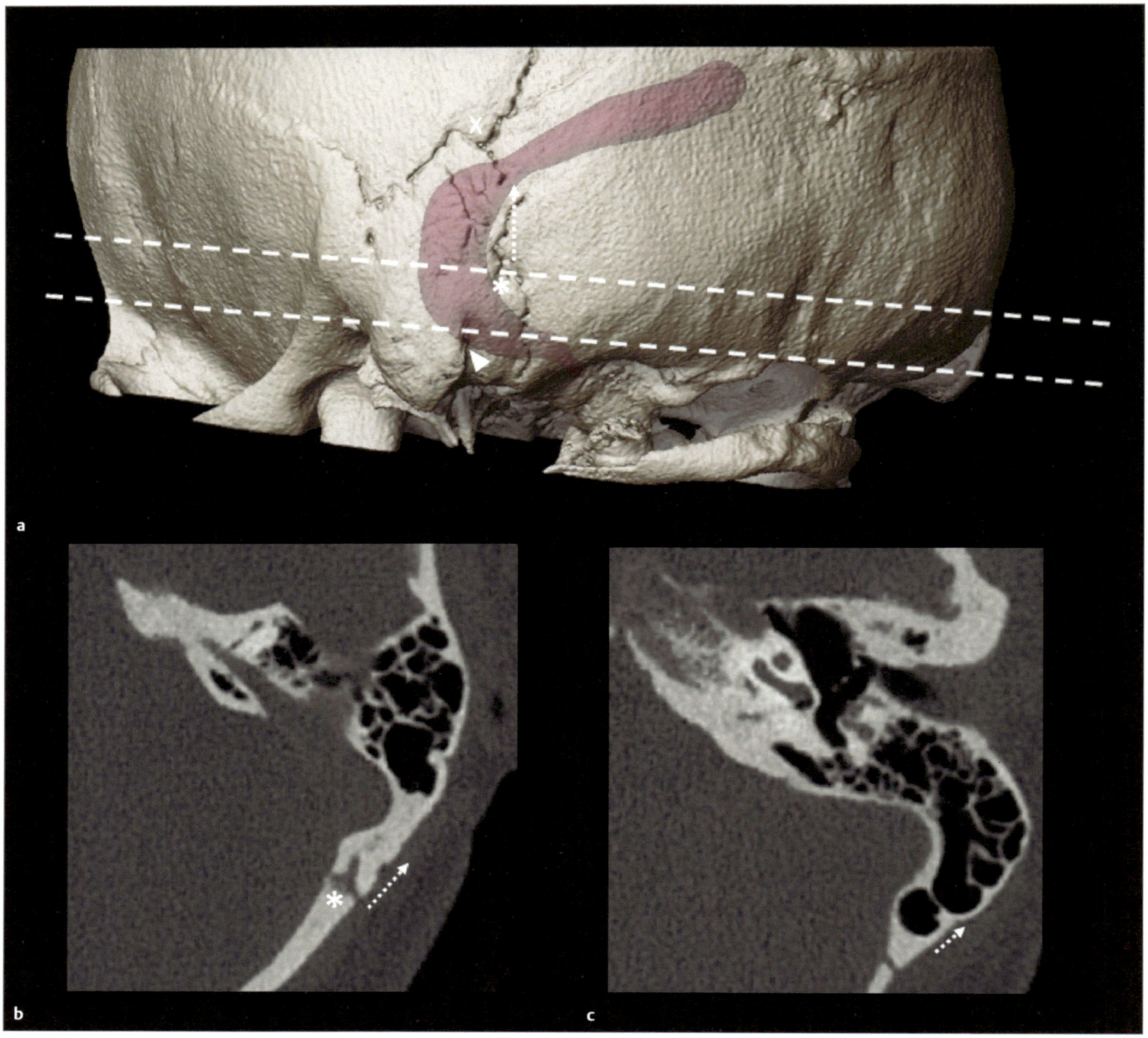

Fig. 5.117 (a–c) Preoperative CT imaging and anatomical considerations. High-resolution CT imaging of the posterior fossa is recommended in all patients scheduled for a retrosigmoid craniotomy. 3D volume rendering (e.g., provided by the BrainLab navigation software) takes only a couple of minutes and provides an excellent visualization of the relevant bony anatomy **(a, top)**. Thus, the asterion (**x**), the mastoid tip with the digastric groove (▲), emissary veins (*), mastoid air cells, and their spatial relationship to the transversal and sigmoidal sinus (→) can be memorized prior to surgery. The asterion is the junction of the lambdoid, parietomastoid, and occipitomastoid sutures. It is considered a key landmark for a retrosigmoid craniotomy, because it usually indicates the sinus knee. However, the case in this figure demonstrates how this landmark could be misleading. In contrast, emissary veins **(b, bottom left)** and mastoid air cells **(c, bottom right)** as seen in the preoperative high-resolution CT scan can be used as reliable anatomical landmarks for the transversal and sigmoidal sinus. Note the course of the sigmoid sinus inside the mastoid bone necessitating a partial mastoidectomy for its exposure.

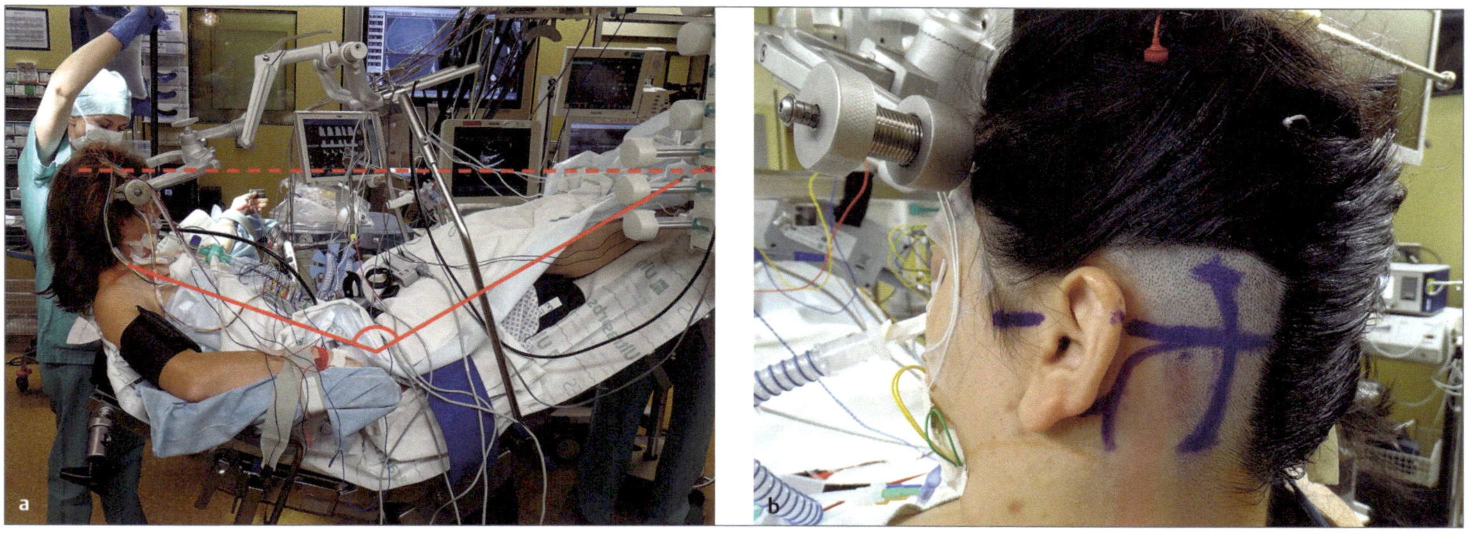

Fig. 5.118 (a, b) Positioning. (a) For large lesions (e.g., T2–T4 vestibular schwannomas), the semisitting position is recommended. For this position, the table is flexed so that the patient's legs are at the level of the head to facilitate venous return while reducing the risk of venous embolism. Note that anesthesiologic monitoring with transesophageal echocardiography should be used to enable immediate detection of air embolism.
(b) The Mayfield skull clamp is positioned with the single pin on the side of the surgery, anterior to the tip of the ear. The final head position results is achieved in four steps: (1) slight elevation; (2) anteposition (to keep the neck straight and avoid jugular vein compression); (3) inclination with slight tilting toward the sternum; (4) 30° rotation toward the side of the tumor. This procedure is carried out under continuous neuromonitoring of the somatosensory-evoked potentials. The lateral neck must be accessible to the anesthesiologist on both sides to allow jugular vein compression when needed during surgery. The mastoid tip is palpated and a surgical incision planned two finger widths behind the ear extending from the level of the tip of the ear to 1 cm below the mastoid tip. Important landmarks are: (1) the iniomeatal line (protuberantia occipitalis externa, external acoustic meatus, root of zygoma), which indicates the direction of the transverse sinus; (2) the mastoid tip, which indicates the direction of the sigmoid sinus; and (3) the asterion, which can sometimes be palpated as a flat area behind the ear.

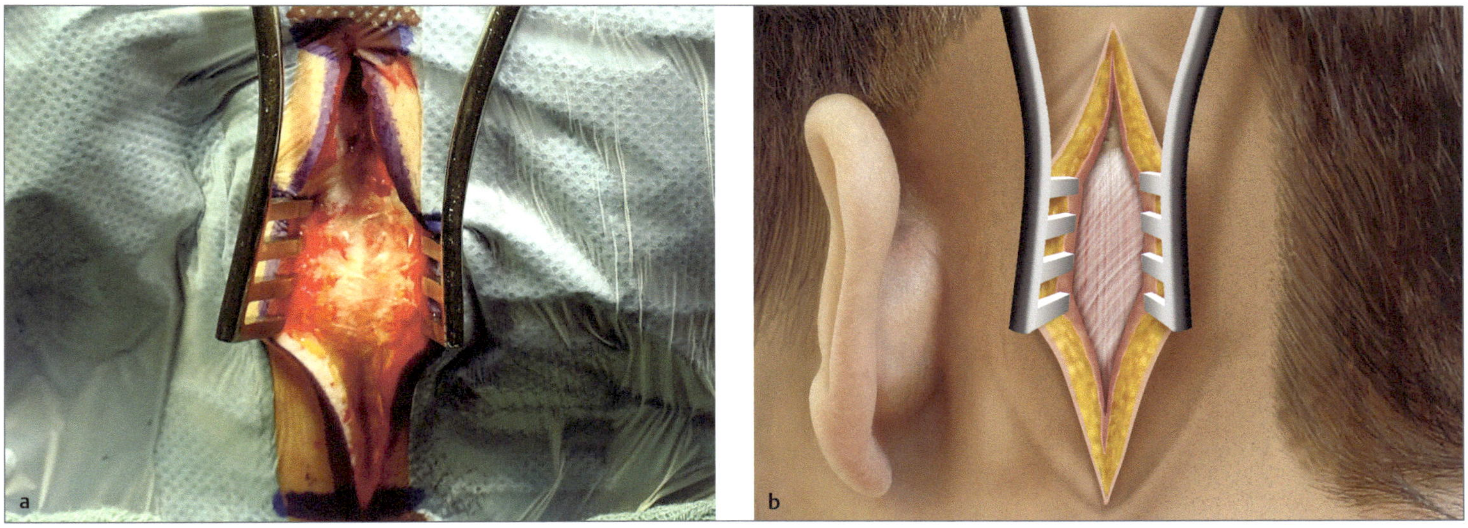

Fig. 5.119 (a, b) Soft tissue dissection. Before the incision, the skin may be infiltrated with Xylocaine/adrenaline (1:200,000) solution to reduce intraoperative bleeding and postoperative pain. However, if there are large emissary veins, great care is advised to prevent intravenous injection.

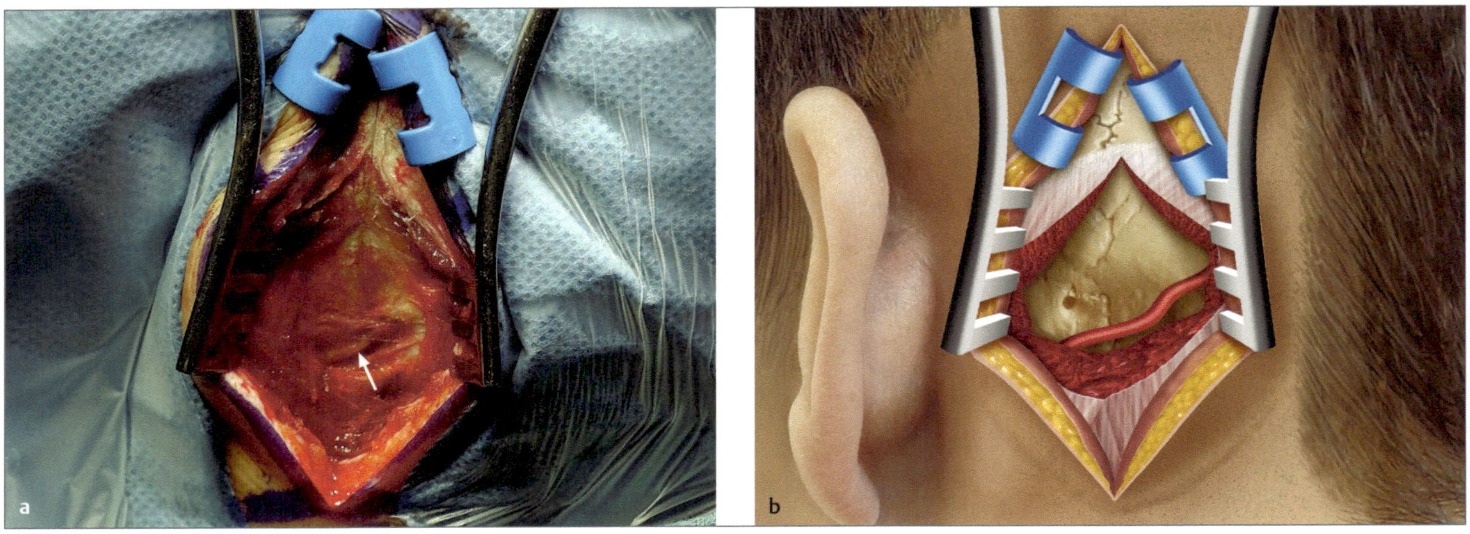

Fig. 5.120 (a, b) Soft tissue dissection. Soft tissue dissection (skin, superficial and deep muscles of the neck) is done in layers, taking care to avoid the lesser and greater occipital nerve, which are usually located medial and lateral to the incision, respectively. However, a large occipital artery (↑) must sometimes be carefully ligated and cut to prevent postoperative bleeding.

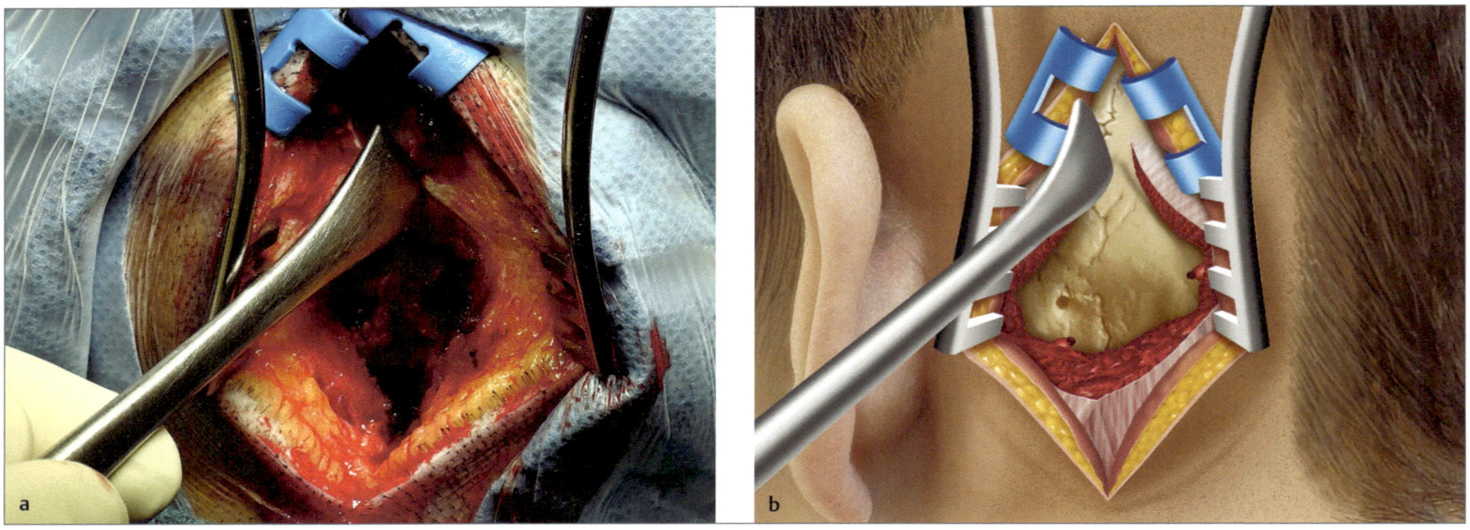

Fig. 5.121 (a, b) Subperiosteal dissection. Once the periosteum has been incised and subperiosteal dissection done (as shown in the figure), bleeding from the mastoid emissary may occur. In this situation, jugular vein compression is carried out by the anesthesiologist and any site of bleeding is closed with bone wax to avoid air embolism. It is recommended to start subperiosteal dissection in a lateral-to-medial direction.

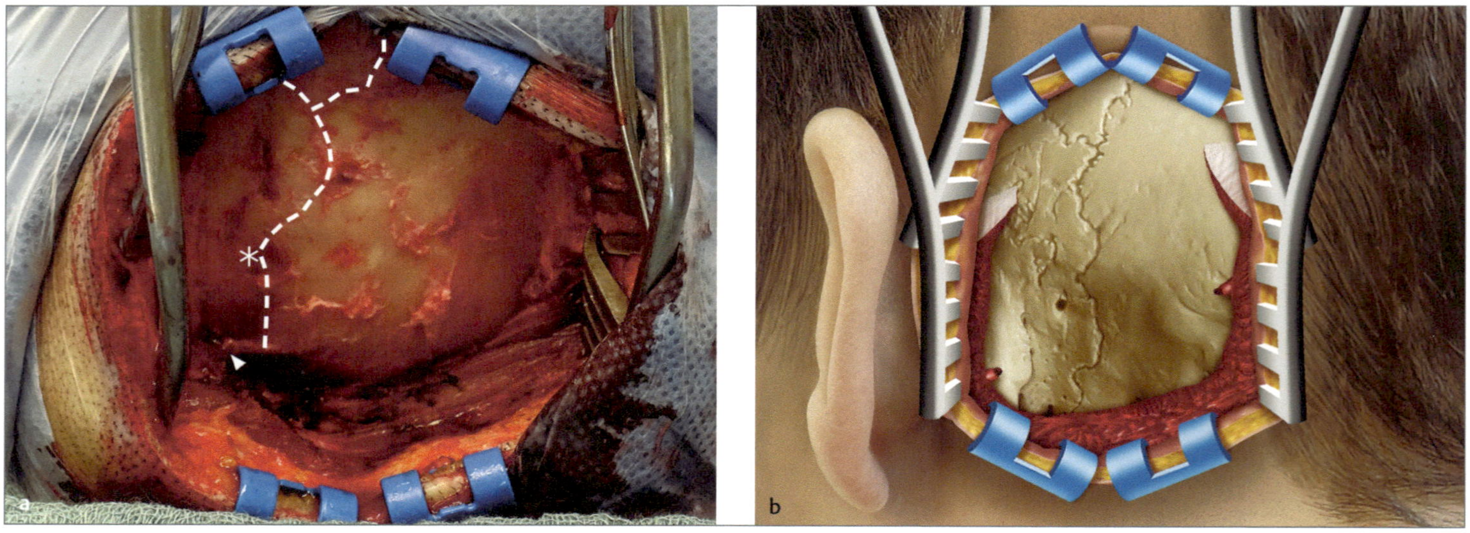

Fig. 5.122 (a, b) Bony landmarks. Once the soft tissue dissection is completed, the bony landmarks should be visible: the asterion at the junction of the lambdoid, parietomastoid, and occipitomastoid sutures; the mastoid tip with the digastric groove (▲); emissary veins (*, note that the emissary vein is closed with bone wax); and the passage from the vertical to the horizontal part of the occipital bone. A curved Apfelbaum retractor is used to increase the exposure.

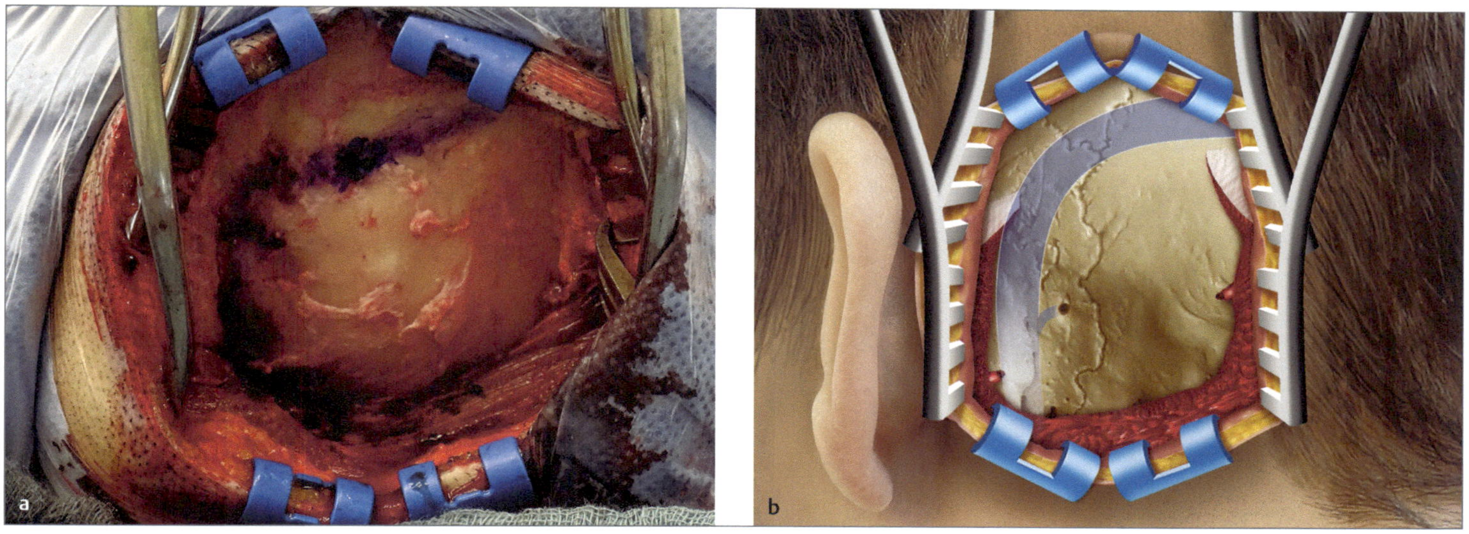

Fig. 5.123 (a, b) Transferring the position of the sinuses. Taking into account the information acquired from the preoperative cCT imaging and the location of the intraoperative bony landmarks, the position of the sigmoid and transverse sinus can usually be determined accurately before craniotomy.

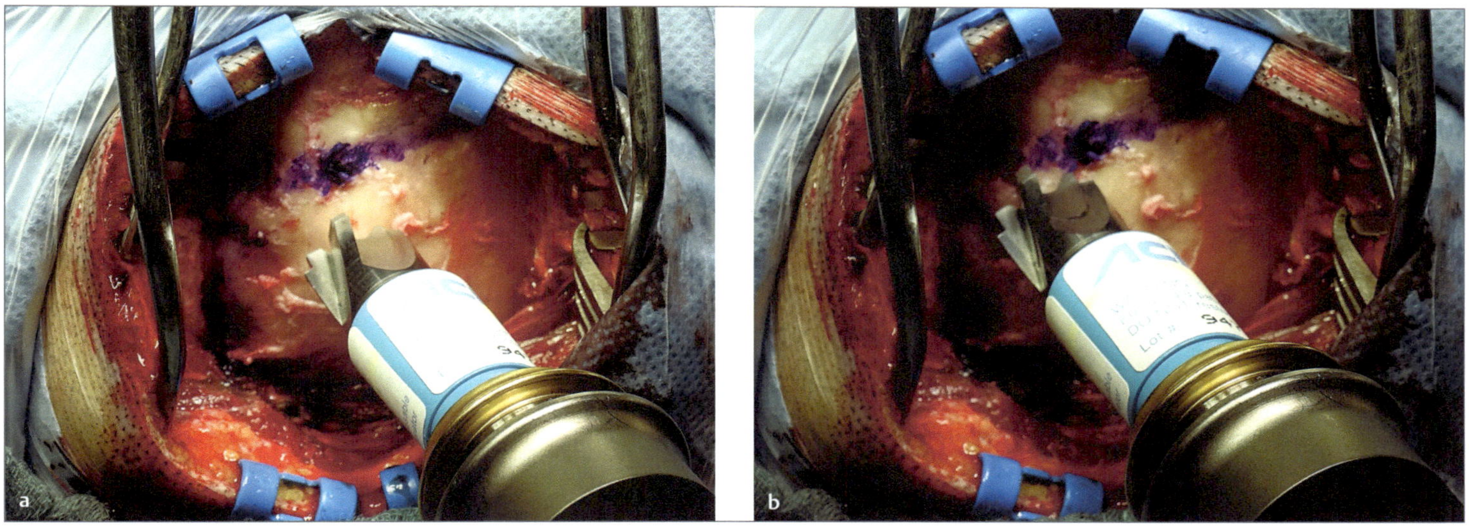

Fig. 5.124 (a, b) Burr hole. If there is any uncertainty about the position, the first burr hole should be made below and medial to the asterion **(a)** and successively enlarged with drills, rongeurs, and/or Kerrison bone punches. In general, this craniectomy is recommended for elderly patients because of the firm attachment of the dura to the bone in older people. If a craniotomy is planned, the burr hole could be positioned close to the expected position of the sinus knee **(b)**.

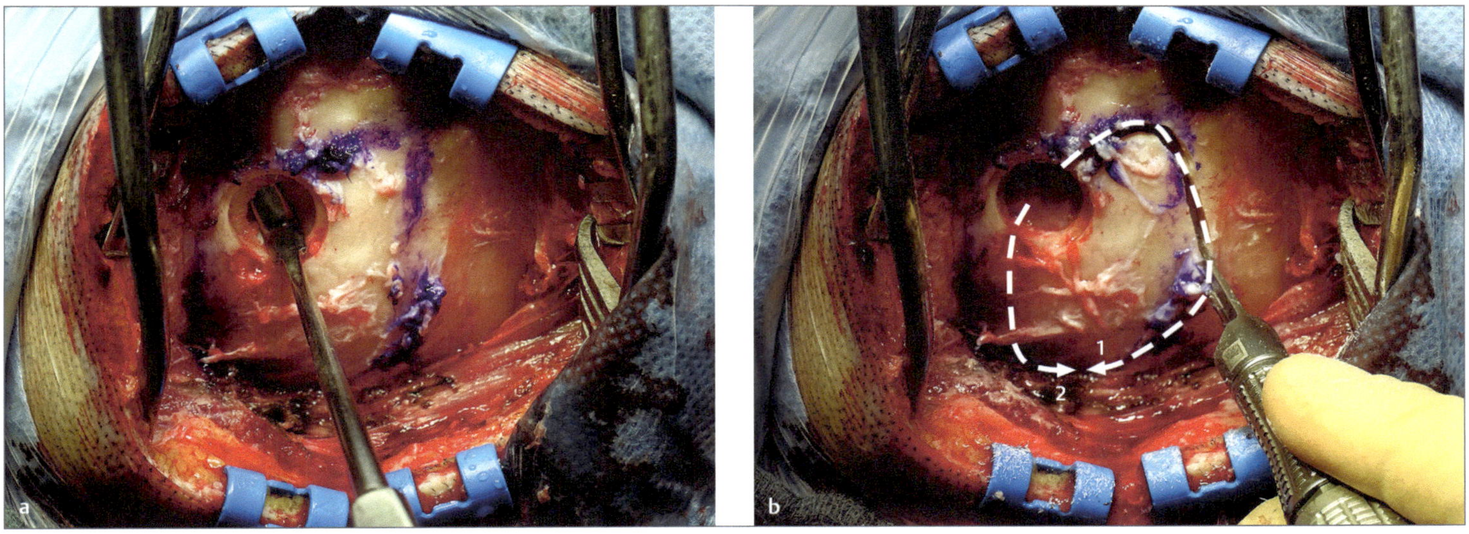

Fig. 5.125 (a, b) Craniotomy. After the burr hole has been made, the distance to the sinus knee and the direction of the transversal and sigmoid sinus is carefully checked using a curved Woodson dissector **(a)**. If the sinus knee has not been reliably identified, the burr hole should be extended with a drill and Kerrison bone punches superiorly lateral toward the sinus knee. The craniotomy is then performed with a high-speed craniotome, first toward the midline and secondly along the sigmoid sinus **(b)**.

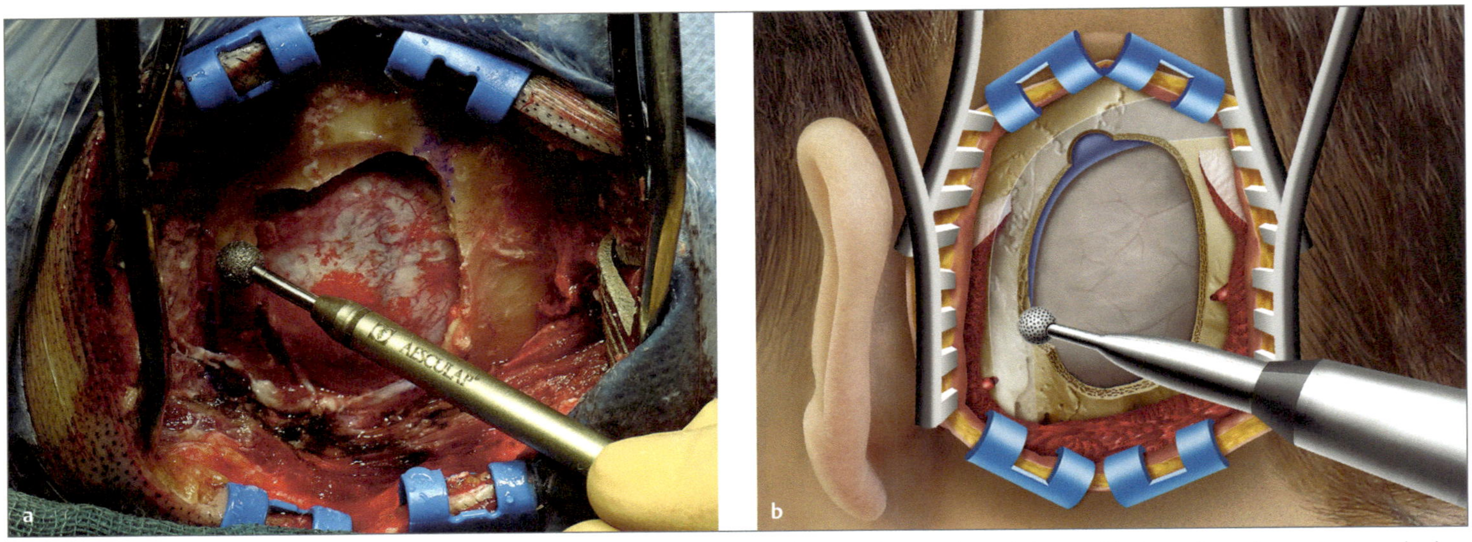

Fig. 5.126 (a, b) Defining the superior and lateral border at the transverse and sigmoid sinus. A partial mastoidectomy is performed using a high-speed drill and Kerrison bone punches, to the medial edge of the sigmoid sinus. The extent of the mastoidectomy (and the pneumatization of the mastoid) that will be necessary can be derived from the preoperative high-resolution cCT scan. Any bleeding from the mastoid emissary vein must be controlled and jugular compression applied to avoid venous air embolism. If the emissary vein is large, a safe way to manage it is to skeletonize the vein with the aid of a high-speed drill and coagulate it under direct view.

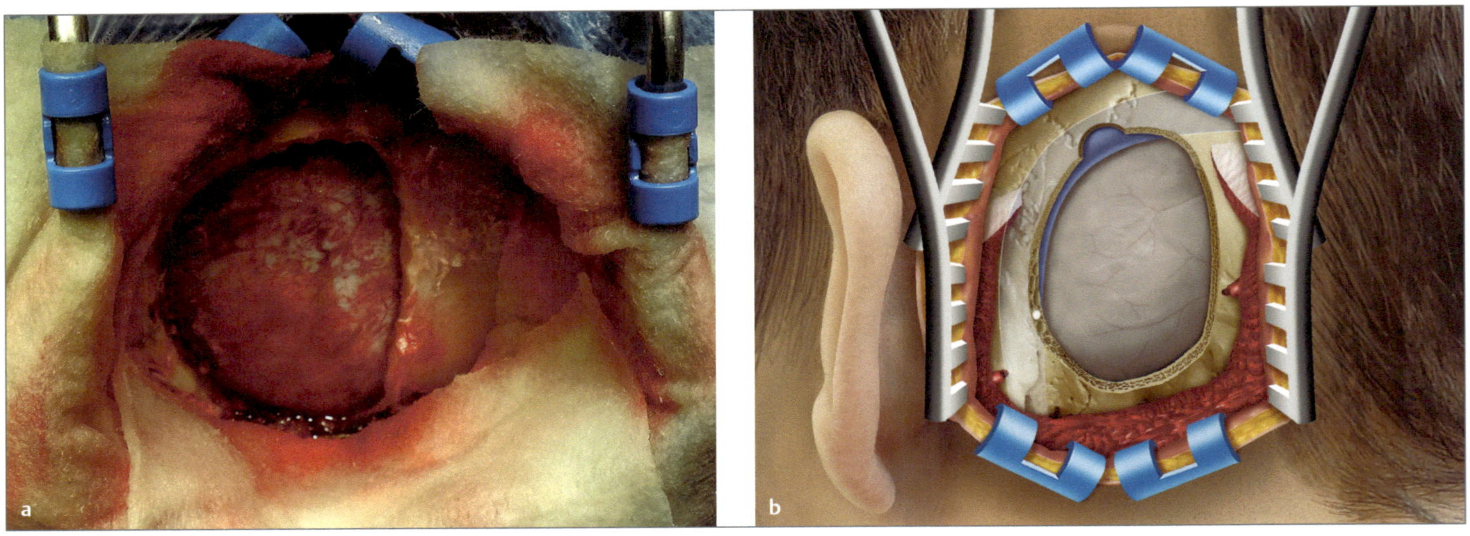

Fig. 5.127 (a, b) Preparation of the operative field for microsurgery. At the end of the craniotomy, the following boundaries should be exposed: superior, the inferior edge of the transverse sinus; superolateral, the transverse-sigmoid sinus junction (sinus knee); lateral, the sigmoid sinus edge; inferior, horizontal part of the posterior cranial fossa; and medial, about 3 cm from the sigmoid sinus edge. The surgical field is covered with wet cotton pads.

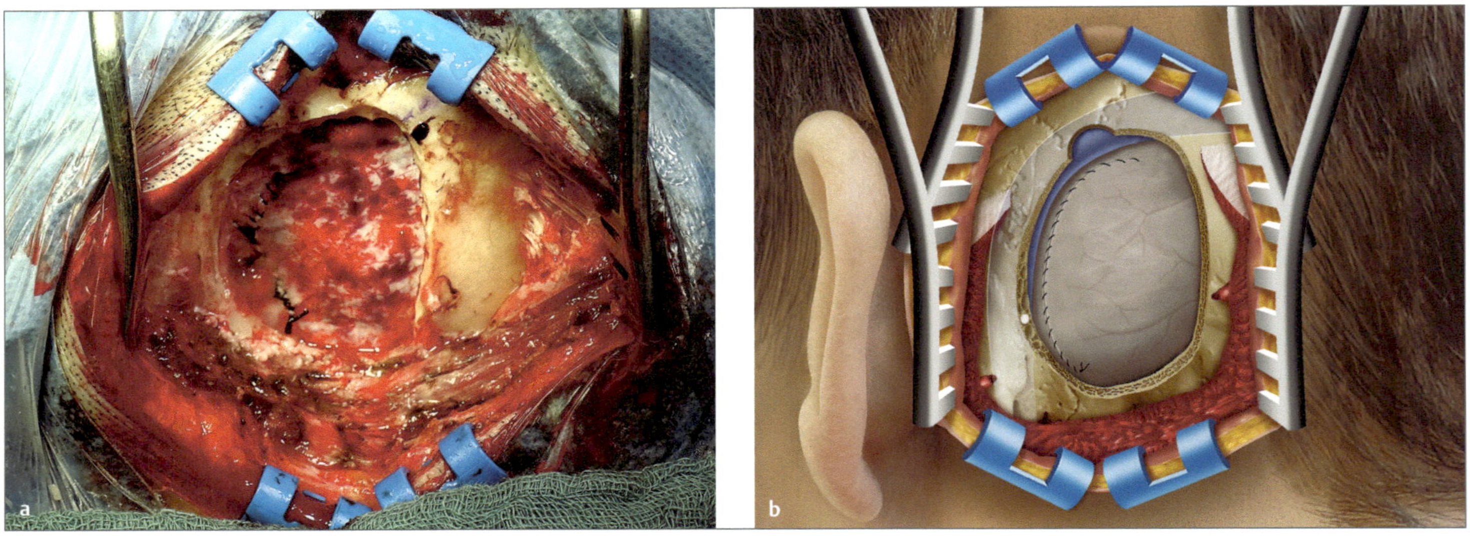

Fig. 5.128 (a, b) Dura closure. The dura is opened under the microscope in semilunar fashion parallel to the course of the sigmoid sinus. Additional cuts are not necessary, which facilitates dura closure. At the end of the surgery, the dura is closed with a continuous running suture. Watertight closure could be ensured by the application of fibrin glue and/or a fibrin sealant patch (e.g., TachoSil).

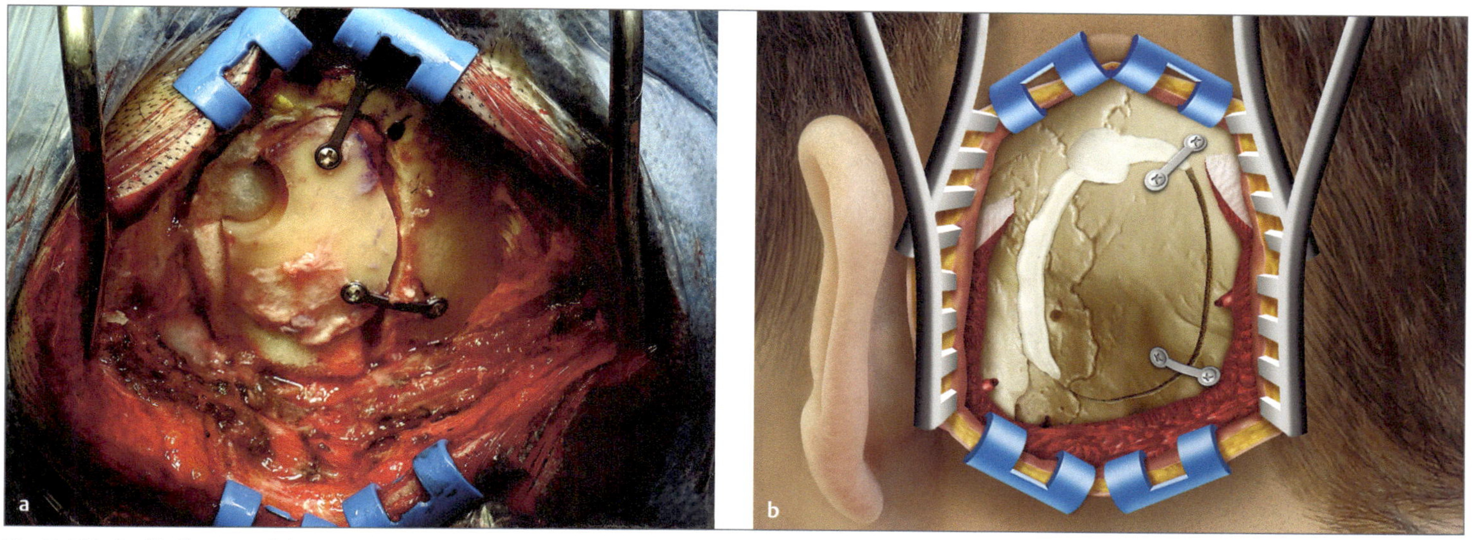

Fig. 5.129 (a, b) Closure of the craniotomy. Finally, opened air cells are closed with muscle and fibrin glue. The dura is covered with a Gelfoam sponge. In the case of a craniotomy, the bone flap is reinserted and fixed with two plates and screws. The bone defect due to a craniectomy is closed with methyl methacrylate plastic. The wound is closed in layers, taking care to achieve a watertight closure of the fascia.

Checklist

- A careful preoperative workup can avoid (or reduce the risk of) intraoperative difficulties. Bone window CT scans (slice thickness 1 mm) are important for evaluation of the pneumatization of the mastoid, the location of the transverse and sigmoid sinus, and the location, position, and size of the emissary veins, which are important for planning the extent of retrosigmoid drilling and determining the safe distance from the sinus.
- Correct positioning of the patient—excessive rotation or flexion of the head has to be avoided, especially in older patients. Close attention to intraoperative neurophysiological monitoring during patient positioning is important to avoid any inadvertent neurological compromise.
- Use of monopolar electrocautery must be avoided at the caudal end of the soft tissue dissection and around C1 (danger of inadvertent injury to the vertebral artery). The course of the vertebral artery at the C1 vertebra can be variable.
- Careful bone removal around major dural sinuses: the dura should be dissected from the bone before using bone punches for bone removal. A diamond drill can be used to thin down the bone, especially the bone close to the sigmoid sinus.
- With the patient in semisitting position, intermittent jugular vein compression by the anesthesiologist (during opening and at the end of the microsurgical work) can prevent venous air embolism.
- Closure of any opened mastoid air cells with muscle and fibrin glue at the end of the surgery is important to prevent postoperative leakage of cerebrospinal fluid.

6 Skull Base Extensions

6.1 Orbitozygomatic Craniotomy

Andreas Raabe

See ▶ Fig. 6.1.

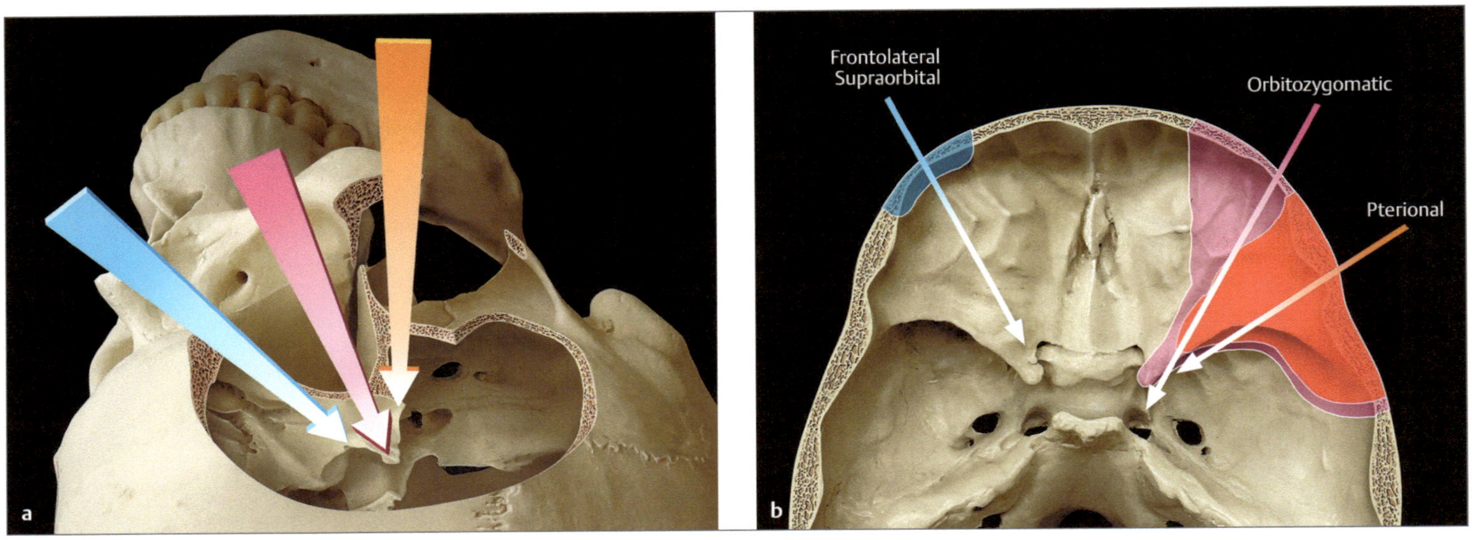

Fig. 6.1 (a, b) Principle of the approach. The orbitozygomatic (OZ) approach is performed when the angle of the surgical corridor toward a deep lesion is higher and/or the lesion is deeper and exposure would require significant brain retraction with a pterional or frontolateral approach. By removing parts of the orbital rim, orbital roof, anterior clinoid process, and/or the zygoma, the entry angle is made shallower and less retraction is necessary for exposure of the target, for example, at the upper clivus, perimesencephalic cisterns, or a high-riding basilar bifurcation.

Orbitozygomatic Craniotomy: One Piece or Two Pieces?

See ▶ Fig. 6.2.

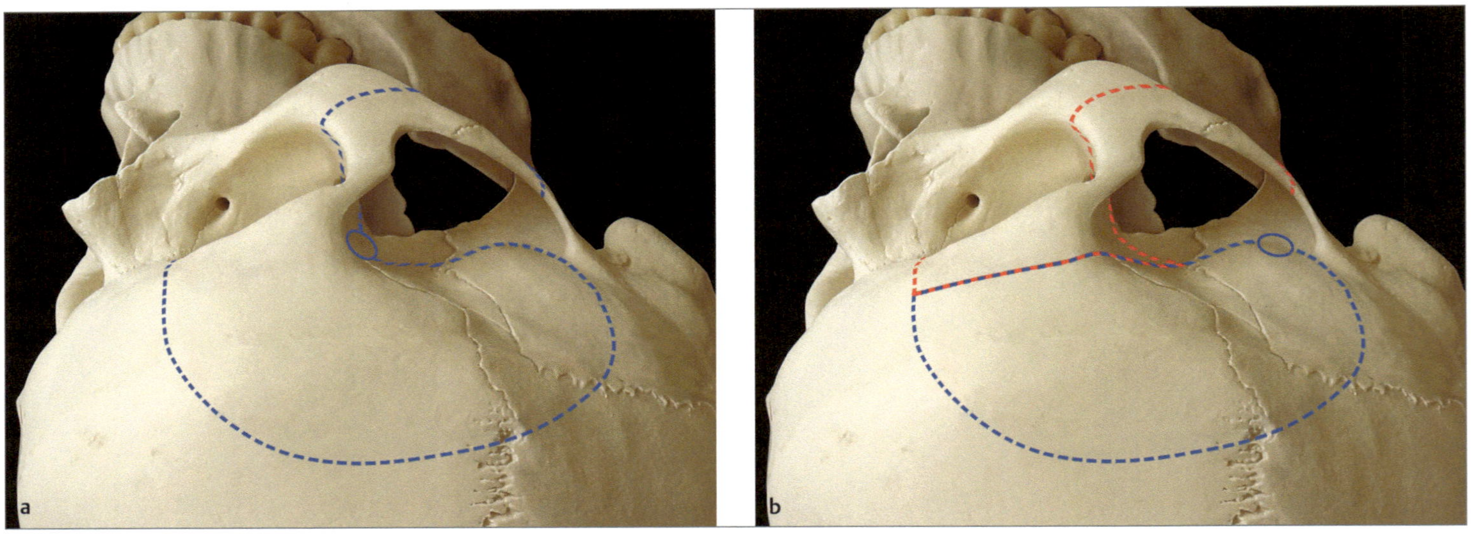

Fig. 6.2 (a, b) One- versus two-piece OZ. The craniotomy can be carried out in one piece **(a)** or in two pieces, when a pterional craniotomy is performed before removal of the orbitozygomatic bar **(b)**. The two-piece OZ gives a better view and is less traumatic, because the dura can be mobilized and the bony cuts can be made under direct visual control.

Full OZ or Partial OZ?

See ▶ Fig. 6.3, ▶ Fig. 6.4, ▶ Fig. 6.5, ▶ Fig. 6.6, ▶ Fig. 6.7, ▶ Fig. 6.8, ▶ Fig. 6.9, and ▶ Fig. 6.10.

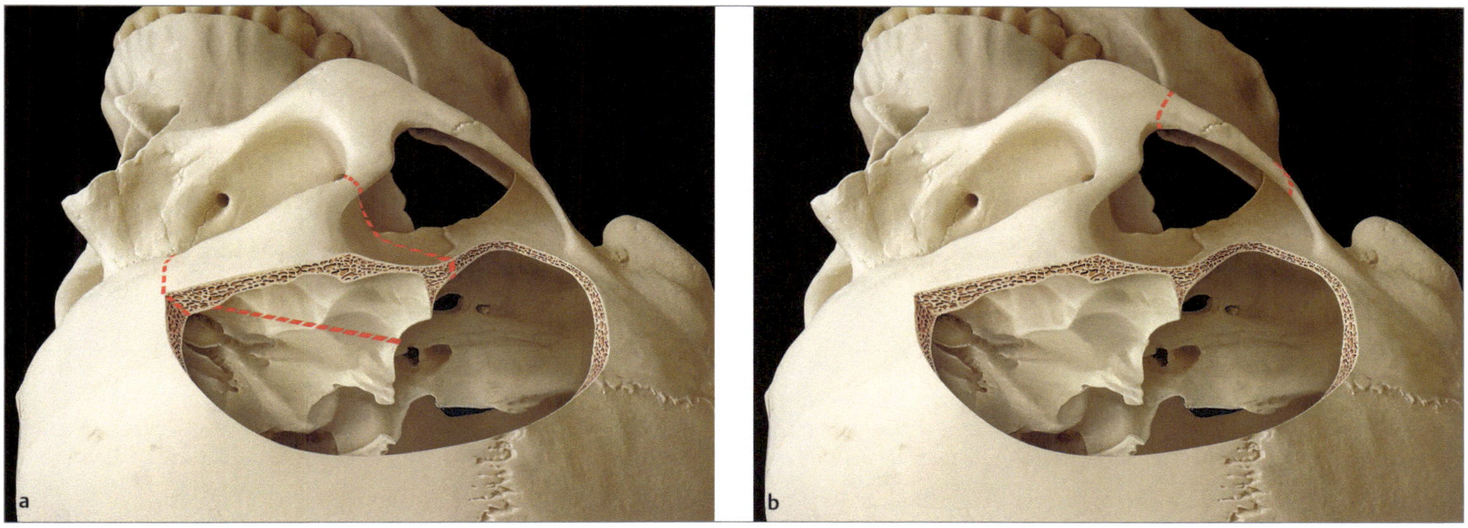

Fig. 6.3 (a, b) Partial OZ. In many cases, a "full" OZ with removal of the orbital and zygomatic bar is not required. A removal limited to either the orbital **(a)** or the zygomatic bar **(b)**, depending on the surgical target, in addition to the pterional craniotomy, may offer the same advantages.

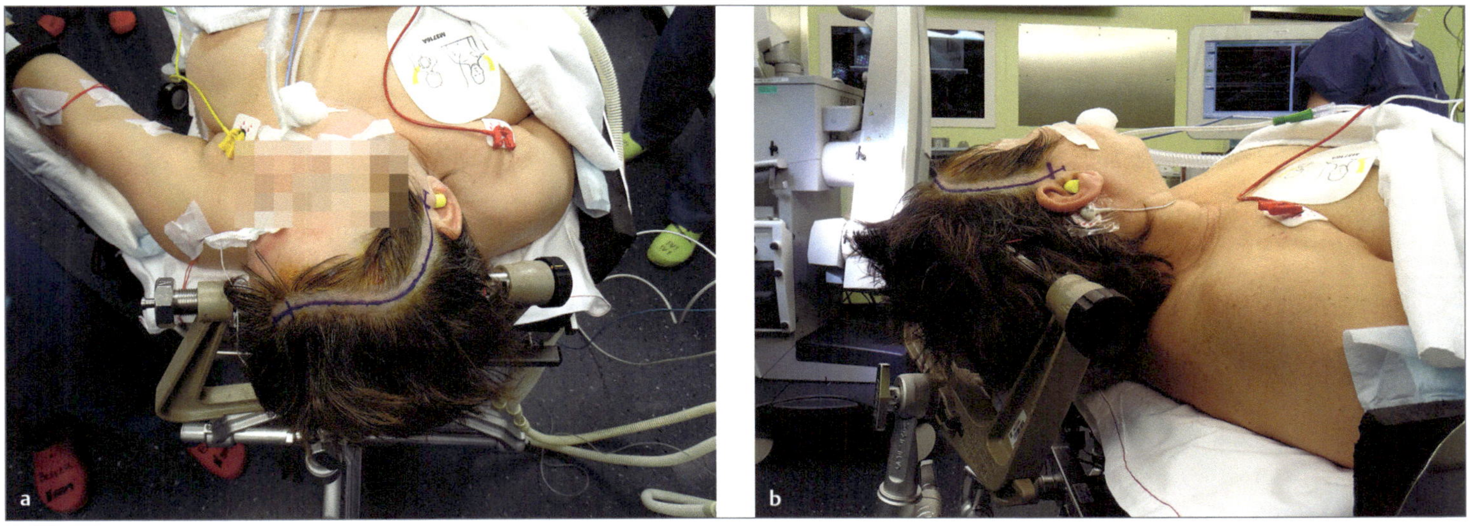

Fig. 6.4 (a, b) The two-piece orbitozygomatic approach. The head is turned 20–60° (most often 30–45°), depending on the surgical target, and tilted toward the floor to place the zygoma at the highest point.

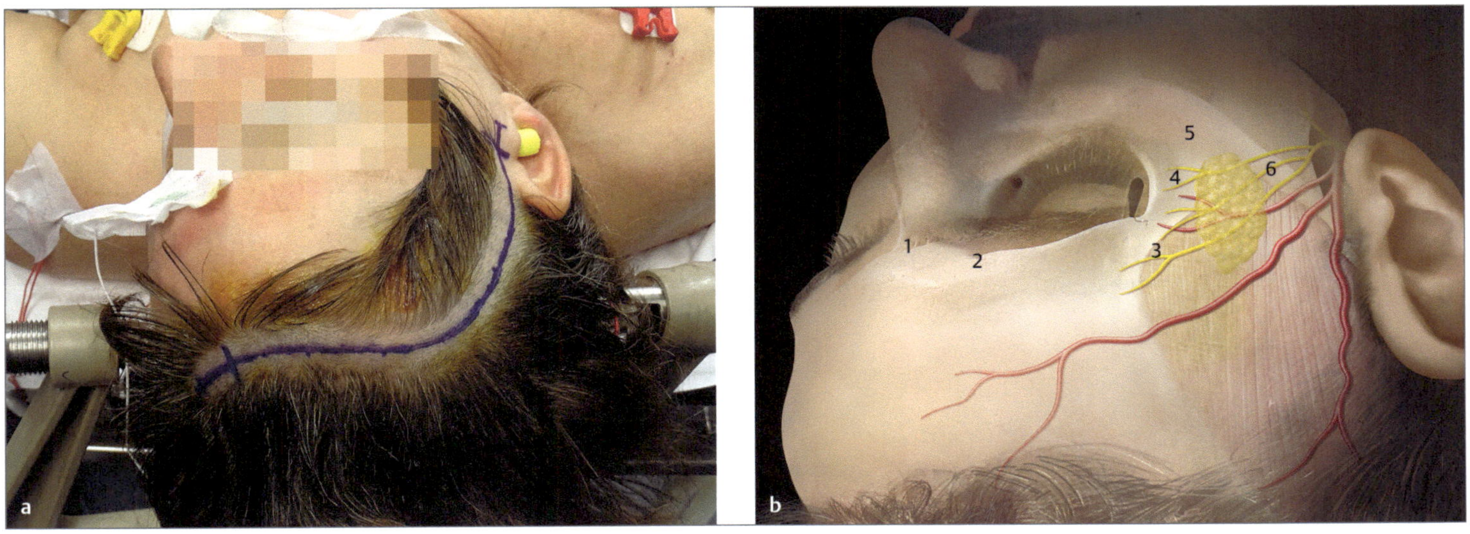

Fig. 6.5 (a, b) Landmarks and skin incision. For sufficient exposure of the orbital rim, the zygoma, and the zygomatic arch, the skin incision has to cross the midline about 2–5 cm and has to extend 1 cm caudal to the zygomatic arch, which is sufficient to expose the arch for the bony cut. The critical distance to the main trunks of the facial nerve is about 1.5 cm, and should be always respected. The following landmarks are useful: nasion (1), supraorbital foramen (2), frontotemporale (3), frontozygomatic suture, which can be palpated (4), zygoma (5), and zygomatic arch (6).

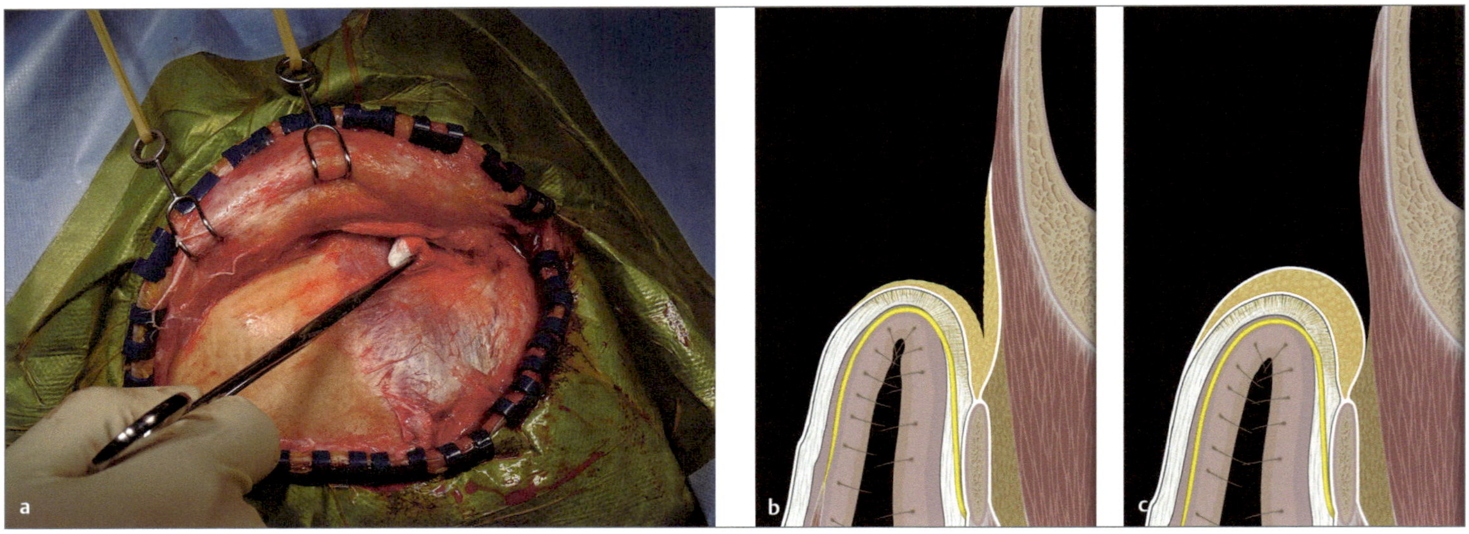

Fig. 6.6 (a–c) **Initial skin flap preparation.** After skin incision and placement of the scalp clips, an interfascial **(b)** or subfascial **(c)** dissection is performed (see Chapter 5.2.1, "Facial Nerve Anatomy and Protection," Fig. 5.19b, c) to remain underneath the branches of the facial nerve. Creating a combined musculocutaneous flap, as with the pterional craniotomy, is not possible because the orbital bar, the zygoma, and the zygomatic arch have to be exposed.

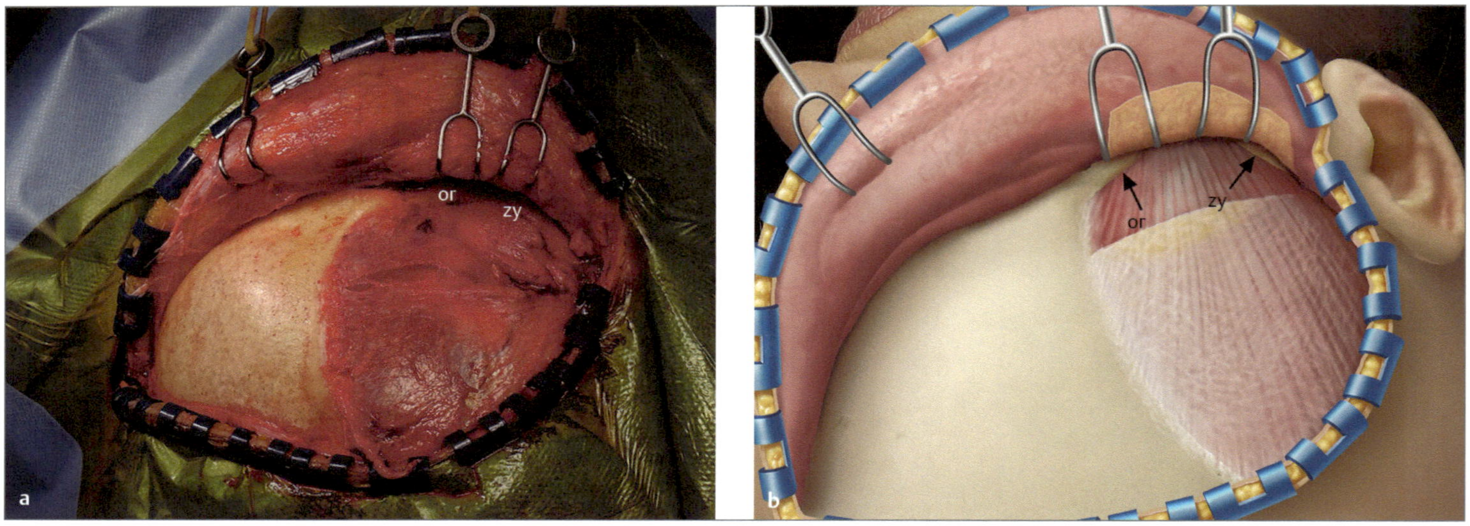

Fig. 6.7 (a, b) **Detachment of the temporalis fascia from the orbital rim and zygoma.** The deep layer of the temporalis fascia is followed to the attachment at the orbital rim and the zygoma. Both the deep and the superficial layer of the temporalis fascia attach to the orbital rim and the zygoma. This attachment is detached and these layers are lifted toward the galea to expose the orbital rim and/or the zygoma (zy) using fish hooks.

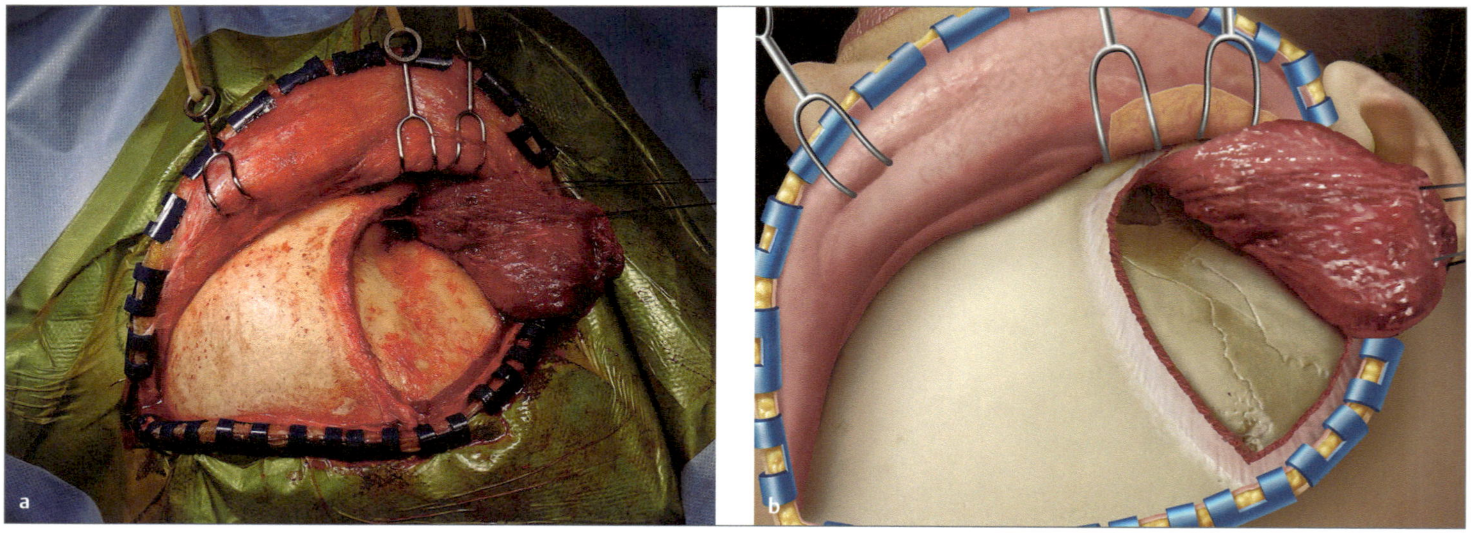

Fig. 6.8 (a, b) **Detachment of the temporalis muscle.** The muscle is cut from the superior temporal line leaving a 1-cm cuff for resuturing the muscle at the end of surgery. This improves cosmesis by preventing the muscle from slipping down or retracting. This maneuver is not necessary when a combined musculocutaneous flap is lifted during a pterional craniotomy. The superficial and the deep temporal fascia are detached from the orbital rim and the zygoma and these structures are exposed.

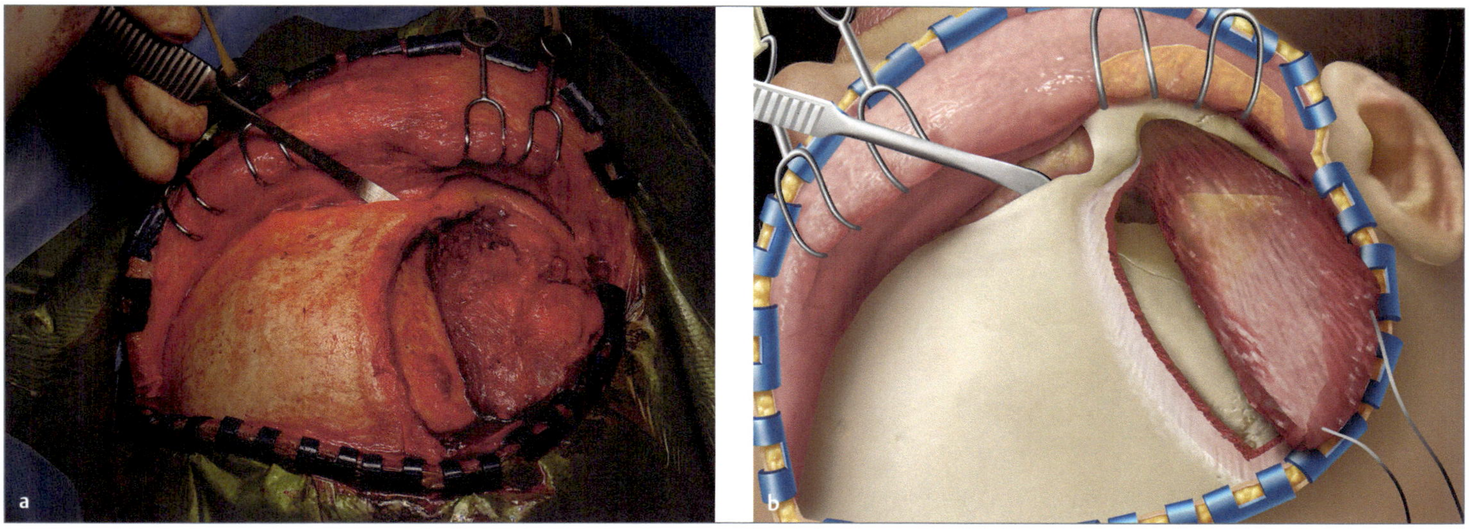

Fig. 6.9 (a, b) Detachment of the periorbita. The periorbita is detached from the intraorbital bone to prepare for the bone cuts. Usually, the detachment extends from the medial edge of the planned craniotomy to the base of the lateral orbital bar, i.e., beyond the frontozygomatic suture until the inferior orbital fissure can be palpated from the inside of the orbit. If the supraorbital nerve is fixed in a supraorbital foramen, the foramen is opened under the microscope using a chisel or a 2–3-mm drill.

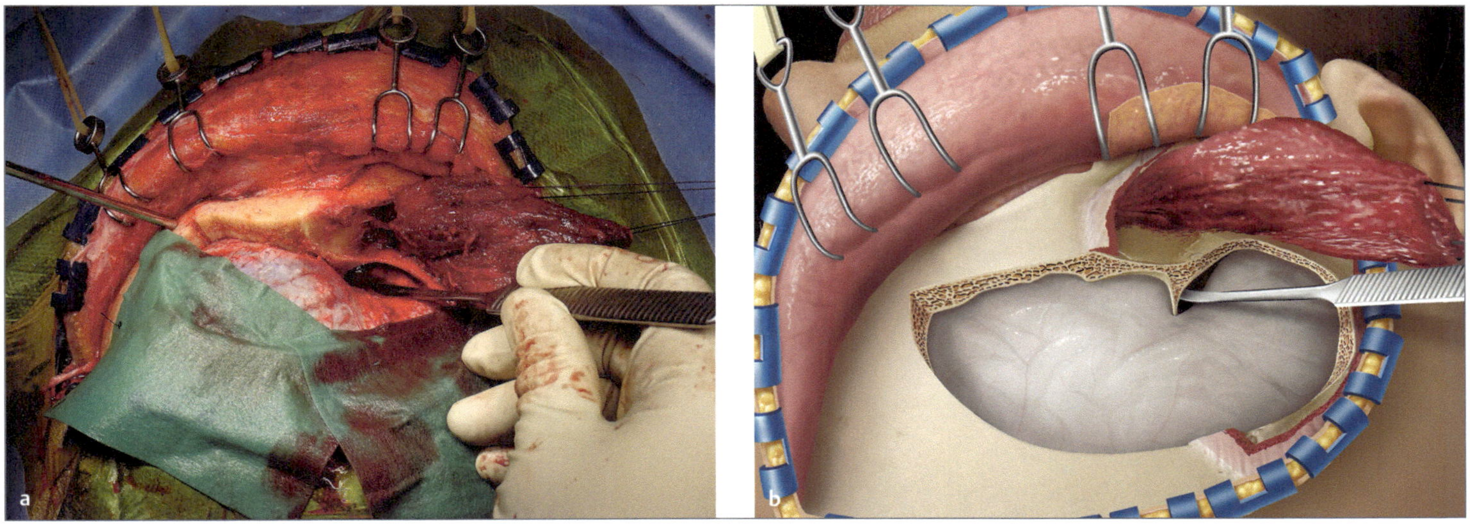

Fig. 6.10 (a, b) Pterional craniotomy and detachment of the dura. A classical pterional craniotomy is performed. The dura is detached frontally and around the sphenoid wing to prepare for the OZ cuts.

Planning of the Orbitozygomatic Bone Cuts

See ▶Fig. 6.11, ▶Fig. 6.12, ▶Fig. 6.13, ▶Fig. 6.14, ▶Fig. 6.15, ▶Fig. 6.16, ▶Fig. 6.17, ▶Fig. 6.18, ▶Fig. 6.19, ▶Fig. 6.20, and ▶Fig. 6.21.

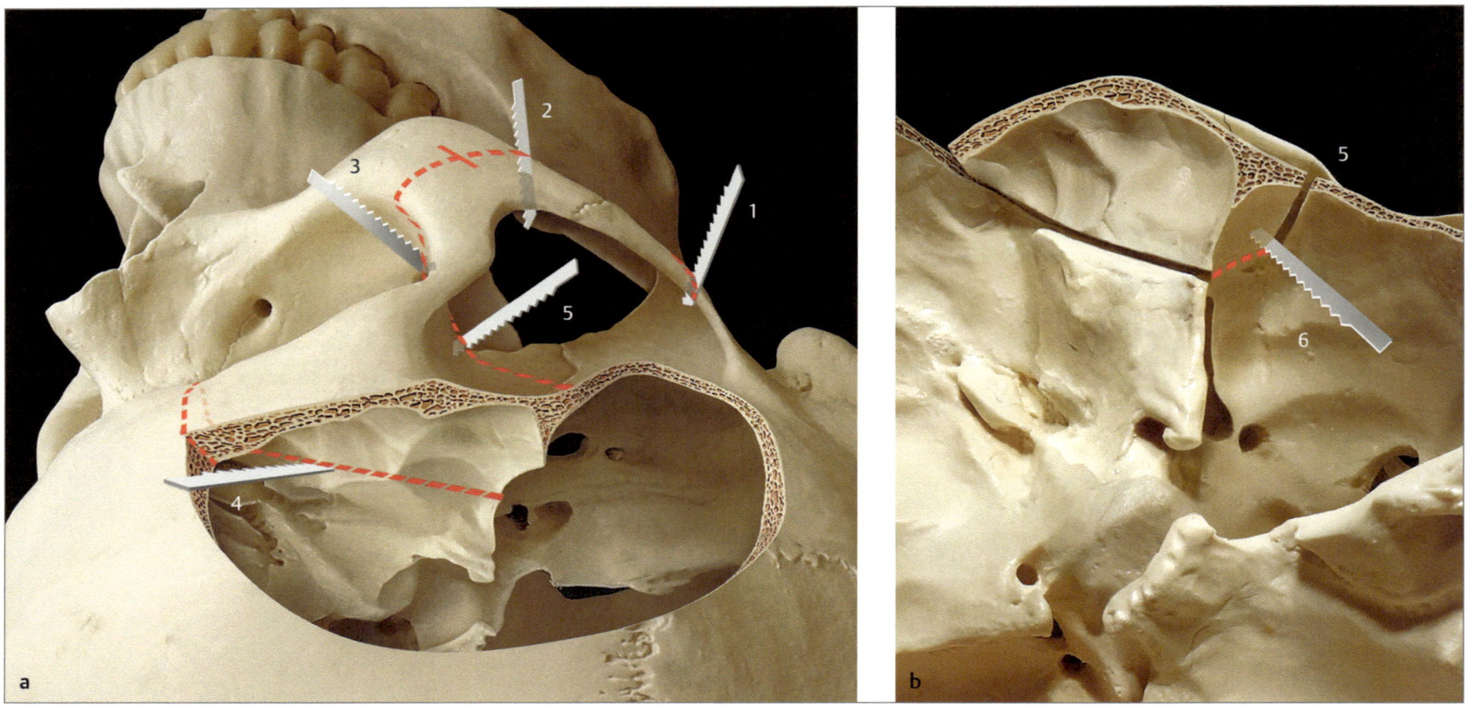

Fig. 6.11 (a, b) Planning of the orbitozygomatic bone cuts. The cuts are performed using an oscillating saw. We prefer to start at the zygomatic arch, but this may be up to the preference of the surgeon.

The cuts will be explained in the following figures (▶Fig. 6.12, ▶Fig. 6.13, ▶Fig. 6.14, ▶Fig. 6.15, ▶Fig. 6.16, and ▶Fig. 6.17).

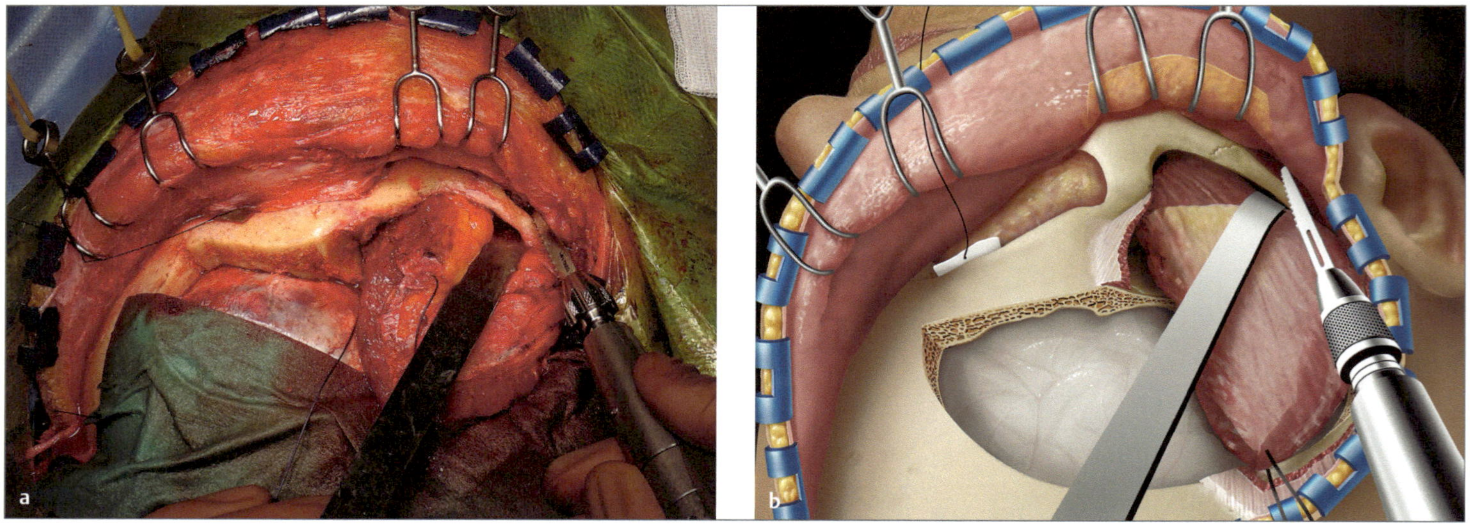

Fig. 6.12 (a, b) Cut 1: zygomatic arch. The masseter muscle is detached from the inferior border of the zygomatic arch. The cut at the zygomatic arch is made at the posterior end in a slightly oblique direction. The idea is to lock the arch into this configuration when the masseter pulls the arch downward after surgery.

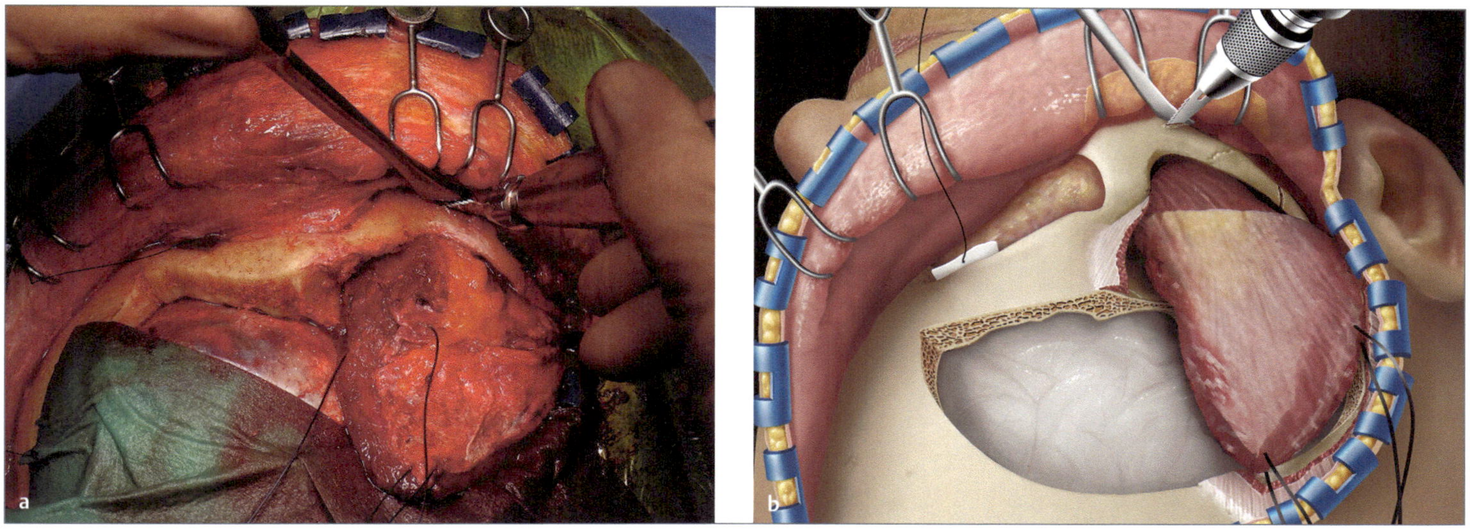

Fig. 6.13 (a, b) Cut 2: the zygoma. The second cut is performed across the zygoma starting at the lateral border below the zygomatic arch and directed toward the inferior orbital fissure, which has already been located by intraorbital palpation. The cut stops in the middle of the zygoma.

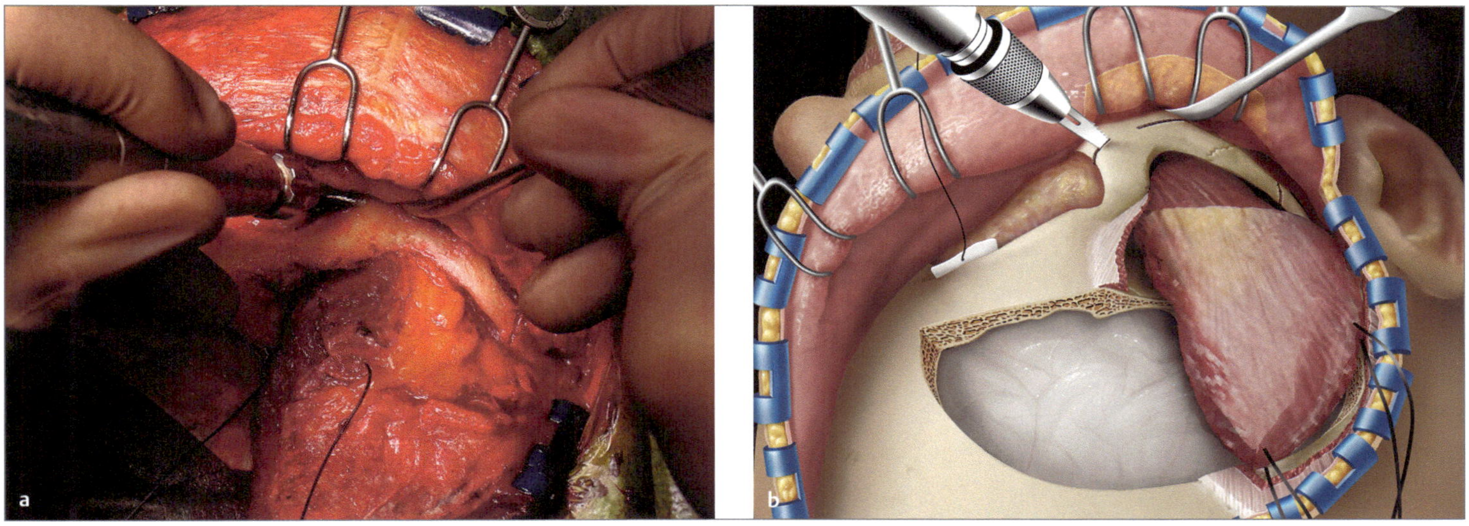

Fig. 6.14 (a, b) Cut 3: completing the cut of the zygoma. The inferior orbital fissure is palpated from intraorbital and the oscillating saw is inserted. The cut of the zygoma is now completed from a medial to lateral direction.

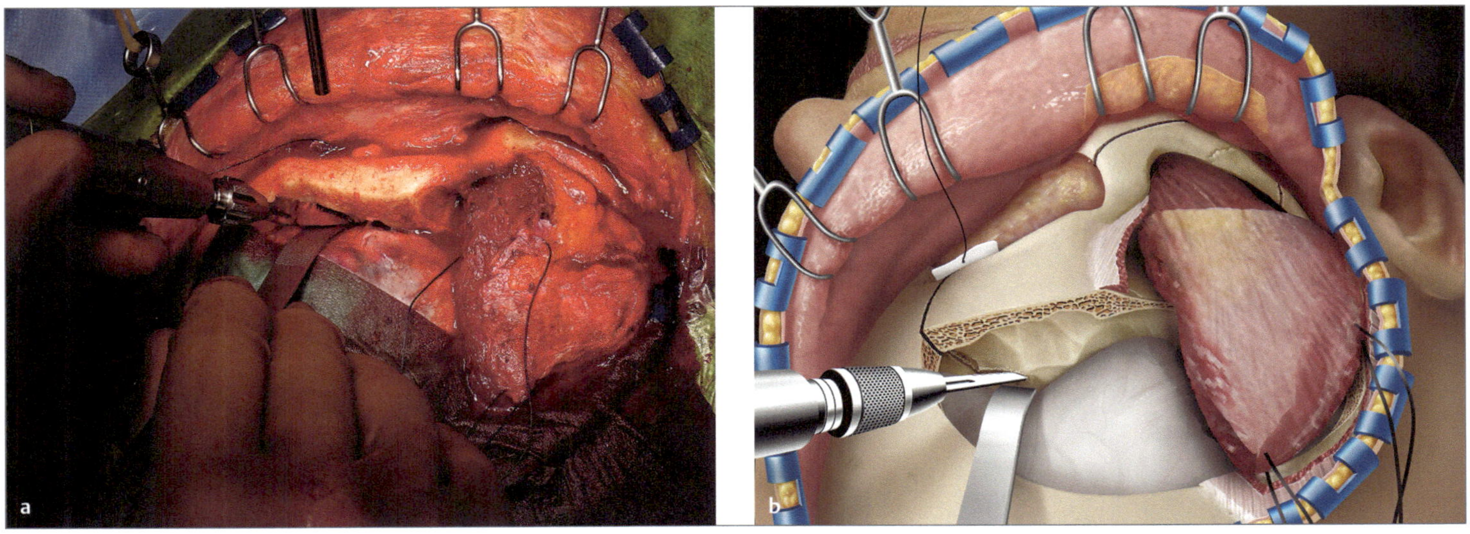

Fig. 6.15 (a, b) Cut 4: orbital roof. The periorbita is detached further toward the upper and lateral edge of the superior orbital fissure. A pad is placed between the periorbita and the bone to protect the periorbita. The dura is also detached and the cut is performed at the medial border of the craniotomy, approximately at the level of the supraorbital foramen toward the upper and lateral edge of the superior orbital fissure.

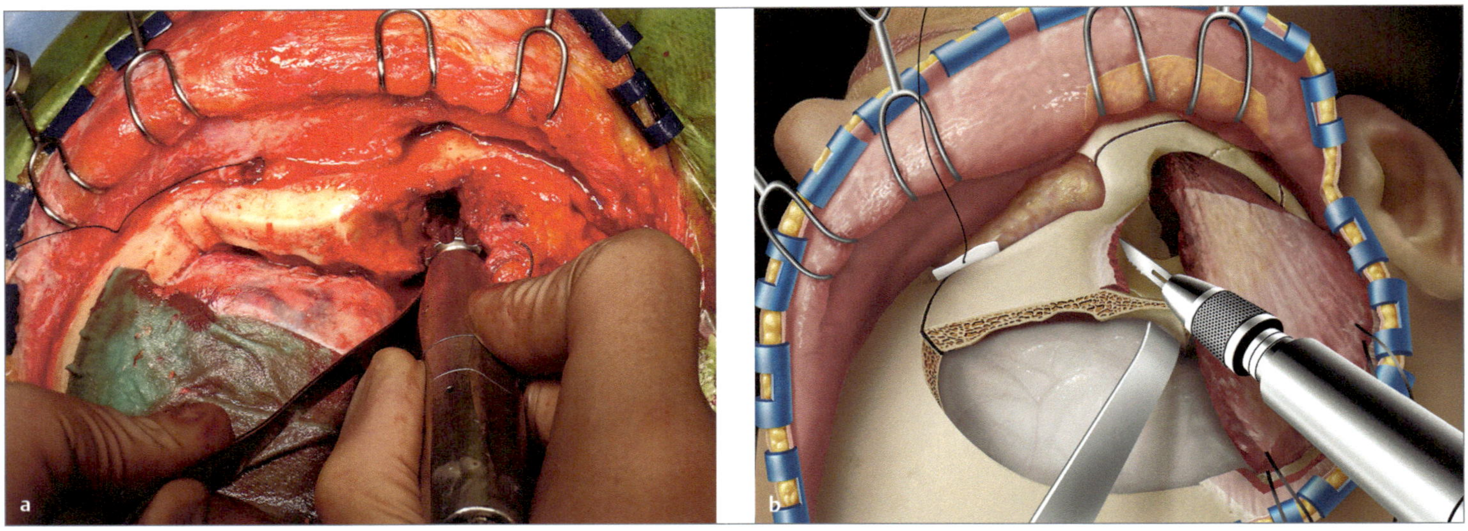

Fig. 6.16 (a, b) Cut 5: inferior sphenoidal cut. The lateral end of the inferior orbital fissure is palpated from outside in the infratemporal fossa and the oscillating saw is inserted. The cut is directed slightly posteriorly to reach the middle fossa approximately 1 cm below the sphenoid ridge. The cut is performed from the outside to the inside. The detached dura is retracted to visualize the entry of the tip of the saw into the middle fossa. It cuts the outer part of the sphenoid in the middle fossa, but not the inner part.

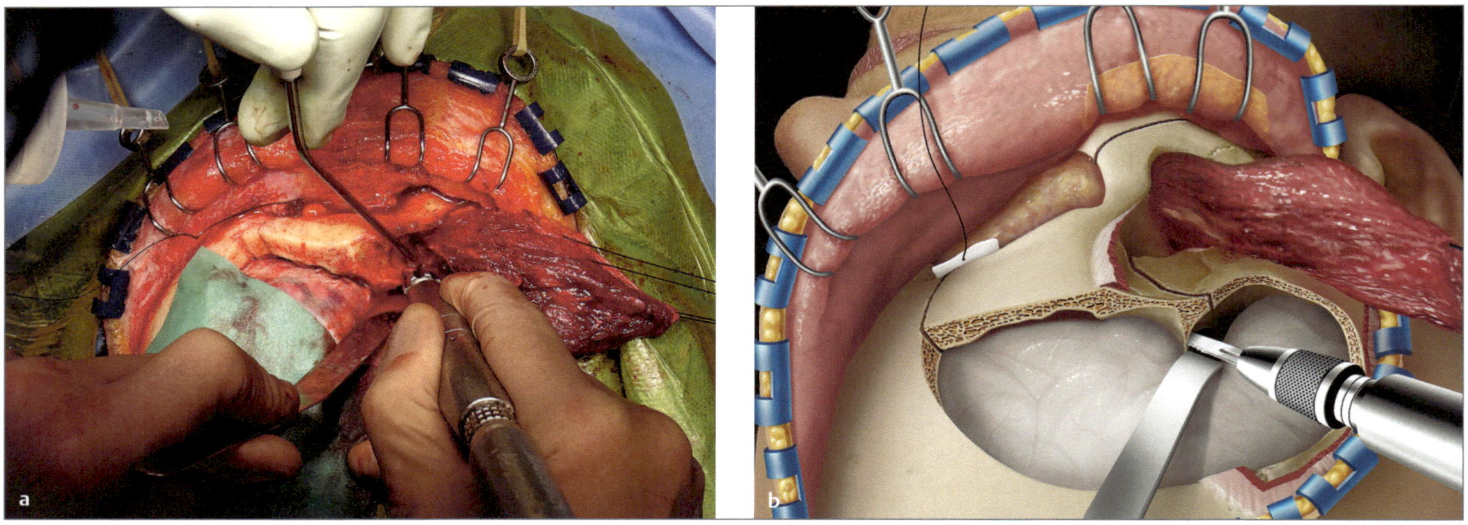

Fig. 6.17 (a, b) Cut 6: superior sphenoidal cut. The final cut divides the inner part of the sphenoid and completes the orbitozygomatic osteotomy. The dura is further detached around the sphenoid wing and the superior lateral edge of the superior orbital fissure is palpated. The line of the previous inferior sphenoidal cut (cut 5) is localized in the middle fossa and the tip of the oscillating saw is inserted. The cut is directed superiorly to the lateral edge of the superior orbital fissure. Care should be taken to use only the tip of the saw to make the cut and to direct it toward the superior and lateral bony end of the fissure, and not into the fissure. The cut connects the osteotomy lines from cut 5 and cut 4 at the lateral edge of the superior orbital fissure or close to it.

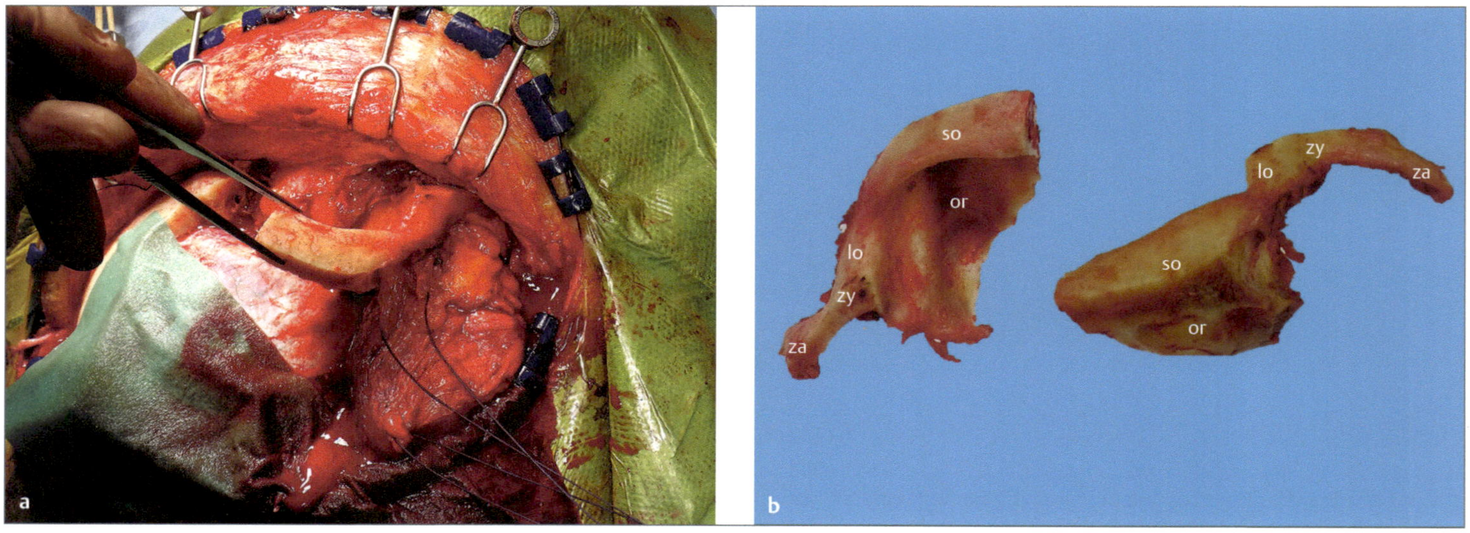

Fig. 6.18 (a, b) Removal of the orbitozygomatic bar. Sometimes the OZ bar is still connected to a small island of bone, but can usually be fractured and then detached from the soft tissue and removed. The view from anterior **(b, left)** and superior **(b, right)**. lo, lateral orbital wall; or, orbital roof; so, superior orbital wall; za, zygomatic arch; zy, zygoma.

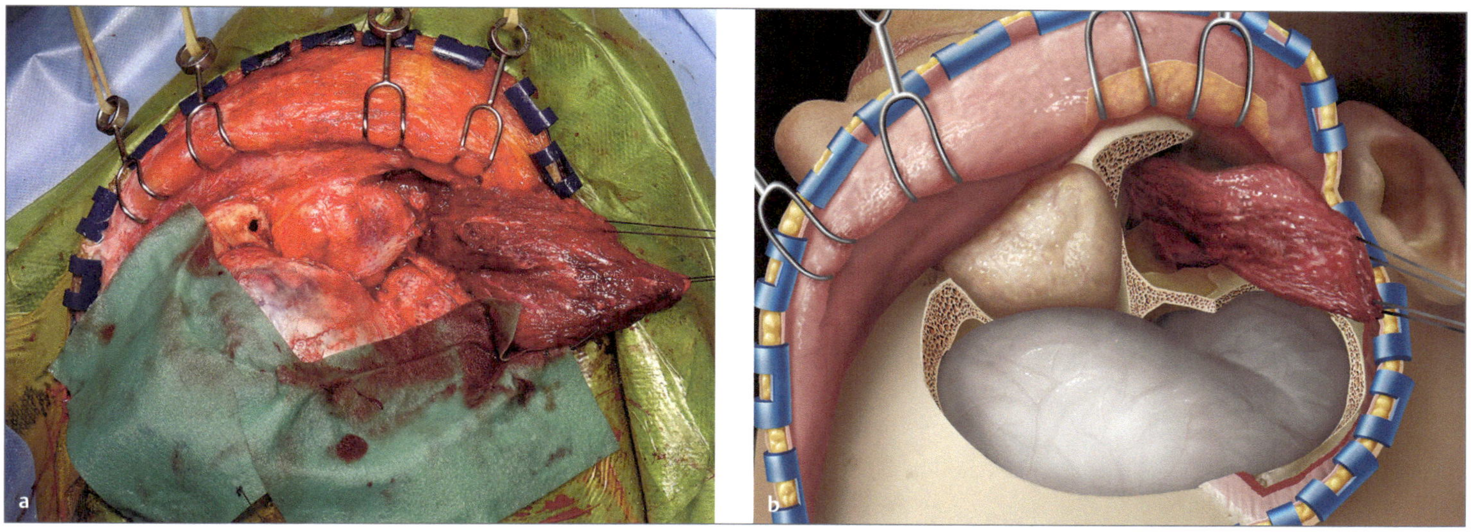

Fig. 6.19 (a, b) Surgical site after orbitozygomatic craniotomy. The angle of the intradural approach is now shallower than with a frontolateral or pterional craniotomy.

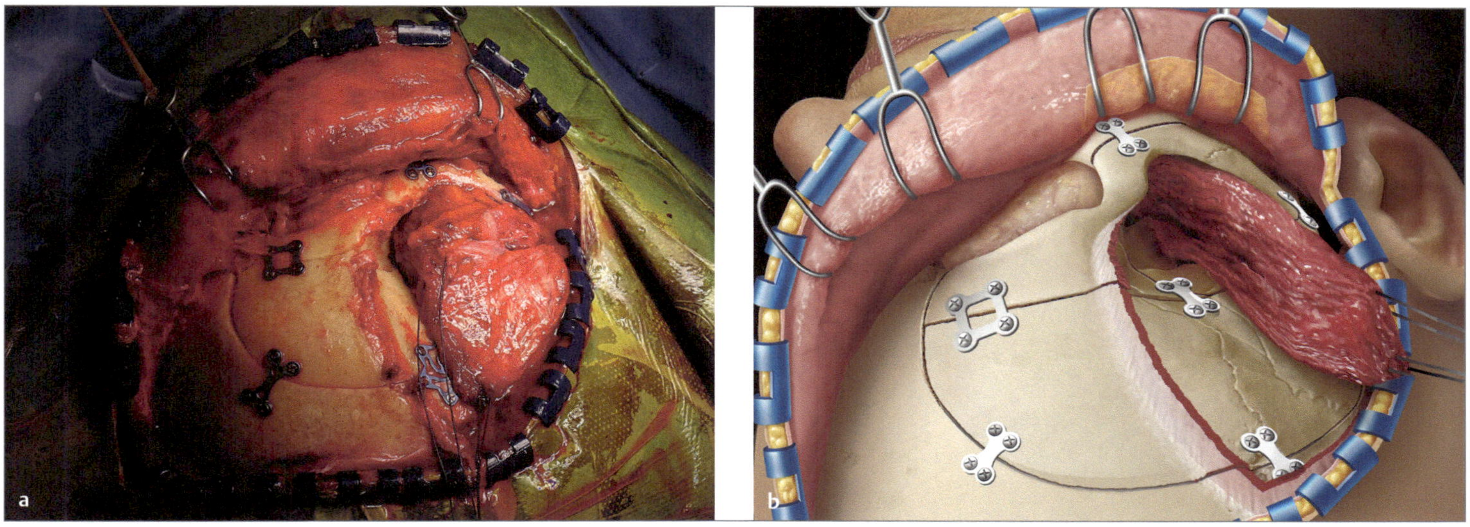

Fig. 6.20 (a, b) Closure and fixation with mini-plates. First, the orbitozygomatic flap is refixed, followed by the pterional flap.

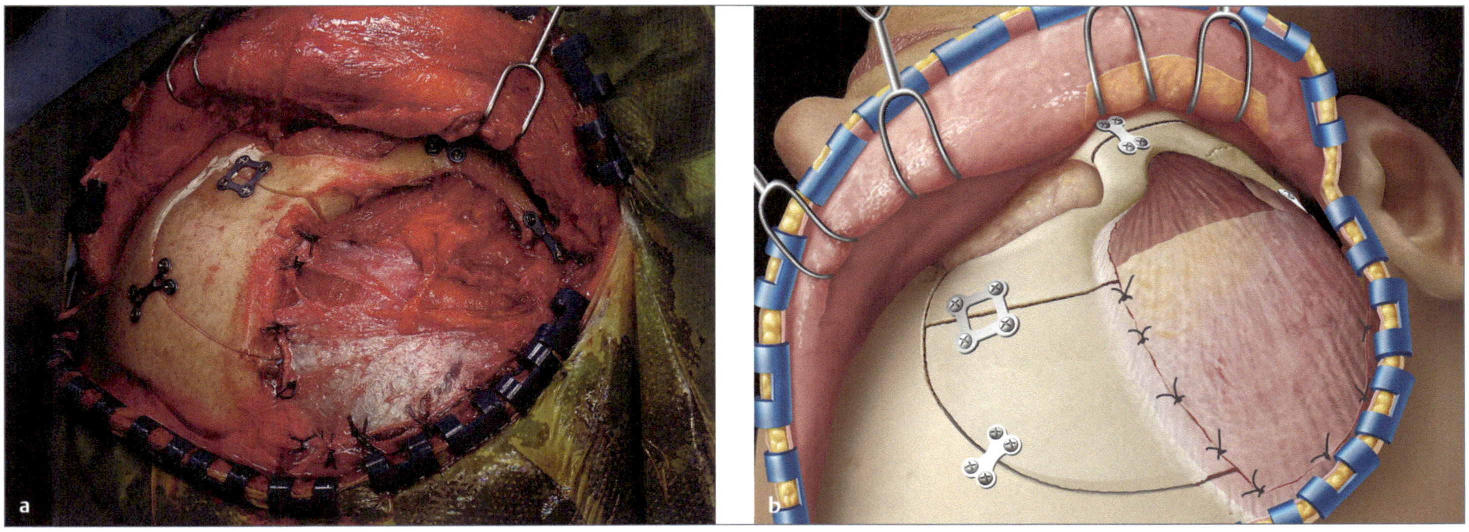

Fig. 6.21 **(a, b)** The muscle is sutured to the cuff at the pterional bone flap and the temporalis fascia posteriorly. The galea and skin are closed in the usual fashion.

Checklist

- Position the head so that the zygoma is the highest point.
- The skin incision must be large enough to expose the zygoma and the zygomatic arch. It has to cross the midline and reach down to 1 cm below the zygomatic arch. Do not go further down; be aware of the facial nerve as it exits the parotid gland.
- Perform interfascial or subfascial dissection of the temporalis muscle.
- Detach the temporalis fascia from the orbital rim and the zygoma and expose the zygoma to see a continuous bony surface from the zygoma to the zygomatic arch.
- Leave a fascia muscle cuff to facilitate refixation of the temporalis muscle.
- Carefully detach the periorbita.
- Perform the cuts as described.
- Place a cotton pad between the periorbita and the orbital roof before performing cut 4.
- Despite cut 6, the bone fragment may still not be entirely mobile. However, slight elevation should crack the final bony bridge. There may still be soft tissue attaching to the bone fragment, which should be detached carefully.

Further Readings

Lemole GM Jr, Henn JS, Zabramski JM, Spetzler RF. Modifications to the orbitozygomatic approach. Technical note. J Neurosurg 2003;99(5):924–930

Youssef AS, Willard L, Downes A, et al. The frontotemporal-orbitozygomatic approach: reconstructive technique and outcome. Acta Neurochir (Wien) 2012;154(7):1275–1283

Zabramski JM, Kiriş T, Sankhla SK, Cabiol J, Spetzler RF. Orbitozygomatic craniotomy. Technical note. J Neurosurg 1998;89(2):336–341

6.2 Orbitocraniotomy

Daniel Hänggi

See ▶Fig. 6.22, ▶Fig. 6.23, ▶Fig. 6.24, ▶Fig. 6.25, ▶Fig. 6.26, ▶Fig. 6.27, ▶Fig. 6.28, ▶Fig. 6.29, and ▶Fig. 6.30.

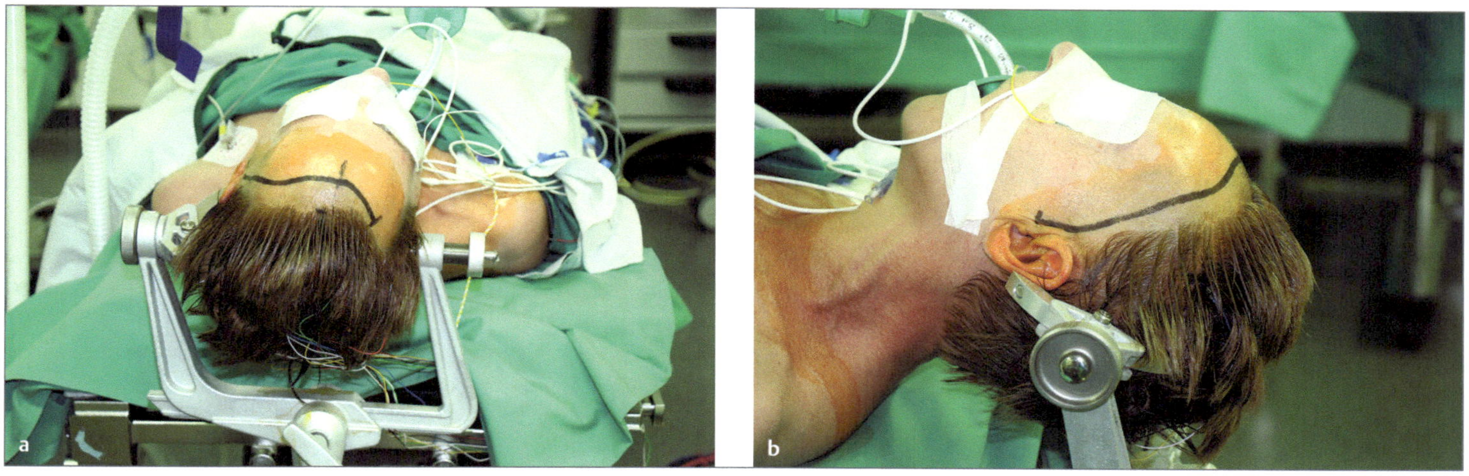

Fig. 6.22 (a, b) Positioning. The transorbital approach is used for midline and parasellar lesions including aneurysms of the anterior communicating artery complex. The head is positioned at an angle of 30–45° toward the contralateral side and hyperextension of 15°. The lateral aspect of the orbital rim is considered as the highest point.

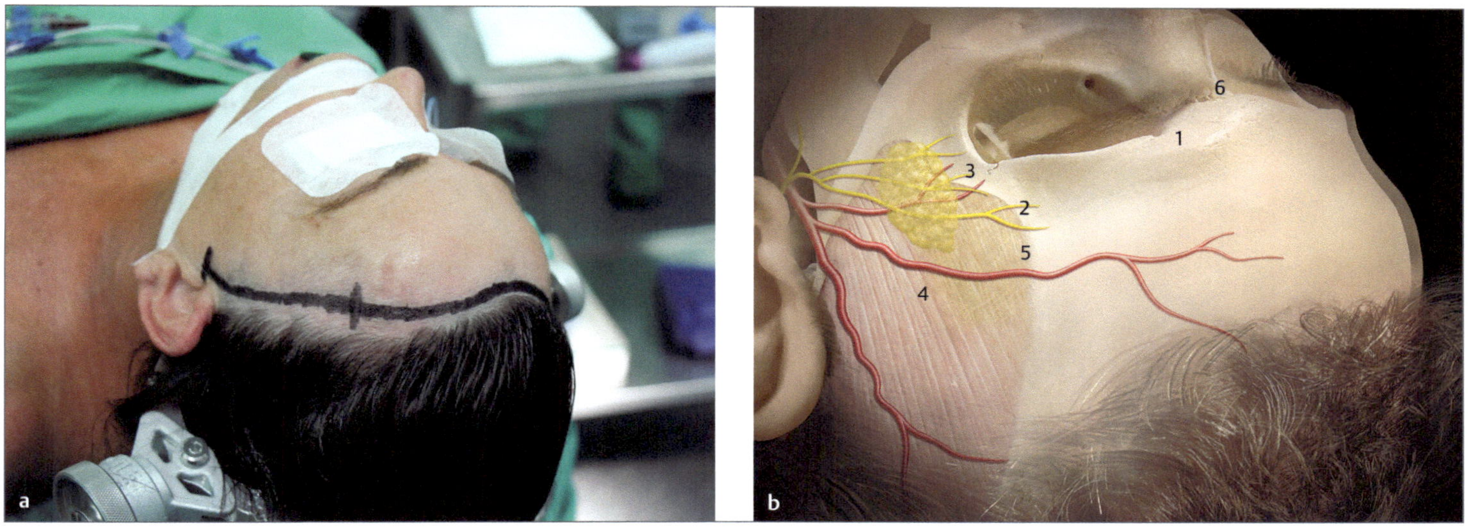

Fig. 6.23 (a, b) Anatomy overview. The left image shows the planned skin incision. The hair has been shaved and the incision is located behind the hairline. Important landmarks are: (1) the supraorbital foramen, (2) the posterior lateral edge of the zygomatic process of the frontal bone indicating the cranial base, (3) the frontozygomatic suture as the landmark for the sphenoid ridge, (4) the frontal branch of the superficial temporal artery, (5) the fascia of the temporal muscle connecting to the superior temporal line, and the nasion (6). For planning the length of the skin incision, the upper part of the zygomatic process and the nasion to determine the midline should be located by palpation.

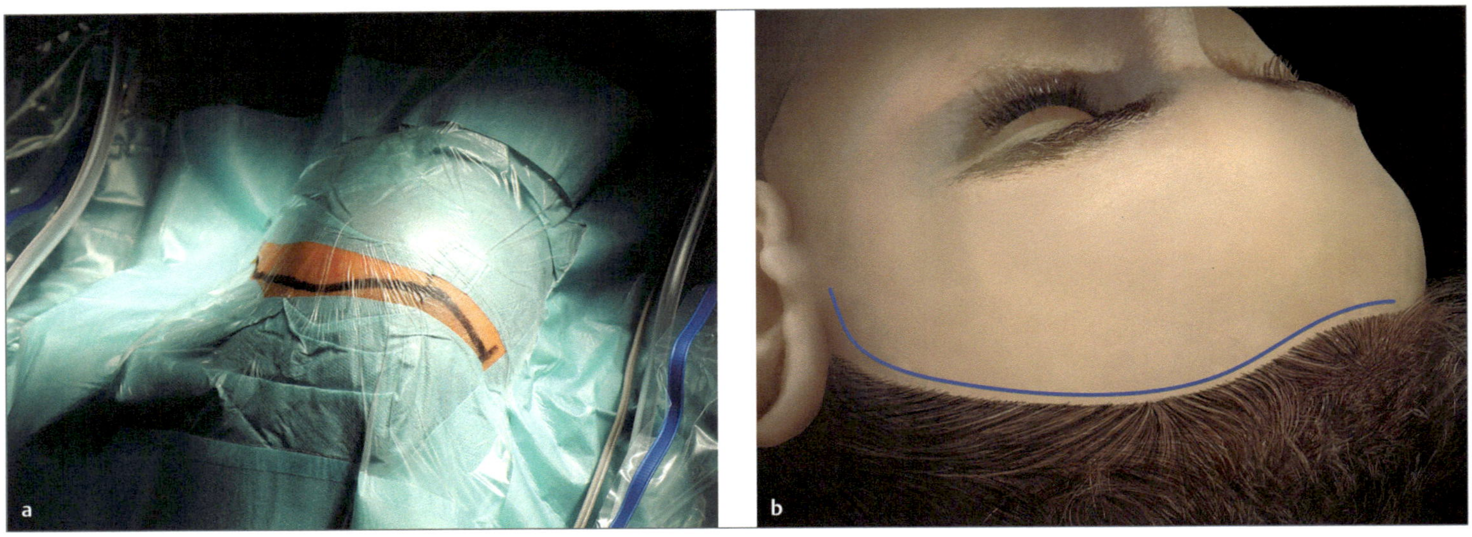

Fig. 6.24 (a, b) Draped position before skin incision. The skin incision is similar to the pterional approach, but, first, it does not extend as far inferior on the temporal side and, second, it should extend beyond the midline to facilitate exposure of the supraorbital foramen, which serves as the landmark for the medial burr hole. Later, it also facilitates intraorbital preparation. The skin incision should be made behind the hairline for cosmesis. We still prefer a frontotemporal hairline incision, although the eyebrow incision may be an acceptable alternative for bald patients.

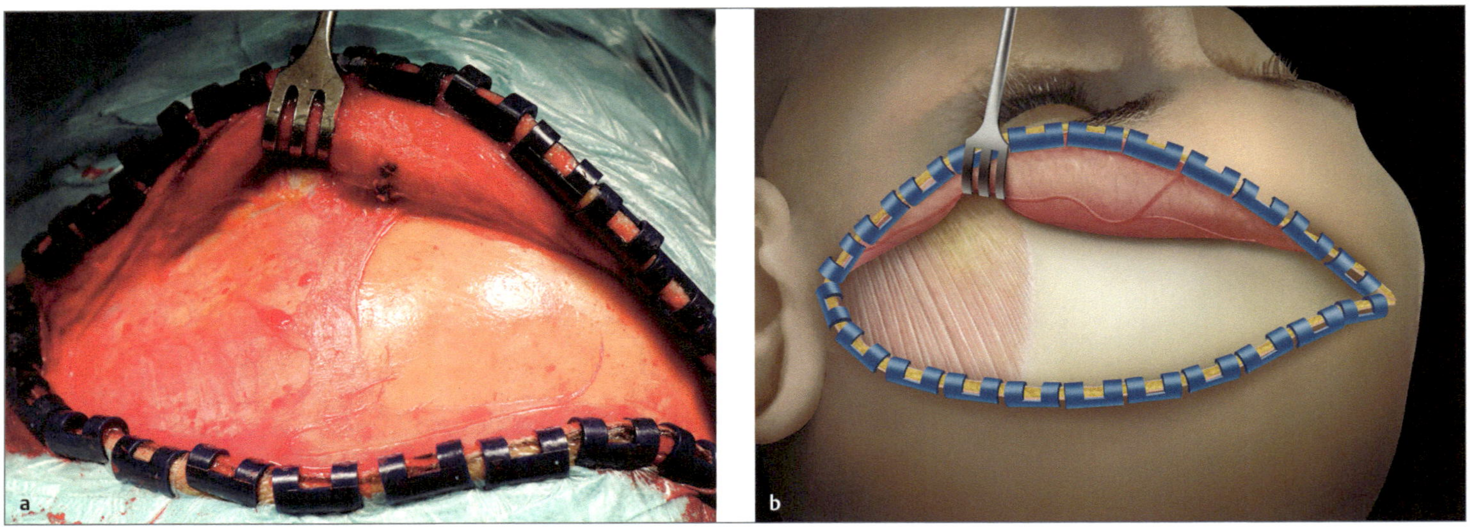

Fig. 6.25 (a, b) Flap preparation. After a cautious incision of the skin and the galea, the superficial temporal artery is identified within the temporal fascia. The frontal or parietal branch of the artery is divided if necessary (see Chapter 6.1.2, Full OZ or Partial OZ). In the case of arterial injury, a small hemoclip is recommended to secure the proximal stump to prevent rebleeding. The temporalis muscle is left intact. The flap is developed anteriorly until the yellow fat pad of the temporal muscle becomes visible.

This yellow appearance of the temporal muscle fascia is caused by the interfascial temporal fat pad that contains the frontal branch of the facial nerve. After reaching the yellow fat pad, the temporal fascia is incised and dissection is continued anteriorly in the interfascial or subfascial plane (see Chapter 6.1.2, Full OZ or Partial OZ). This step protects the frontal branch of the facial nerve from stretching or injury. The superior temporal line is identified by the attachment of the temporal muscle fascia. The interfascial fat pad must be left at and mobilized together with the scalp flap to prevent injury to the frontal branch of the facial nerve. The scalp flap is retracted basally with the help of galea hooks. Because of the danger of traction to the frontal branch of the facial nerve, it is important to avoid deep insertion of galea hooks on the temporal side.

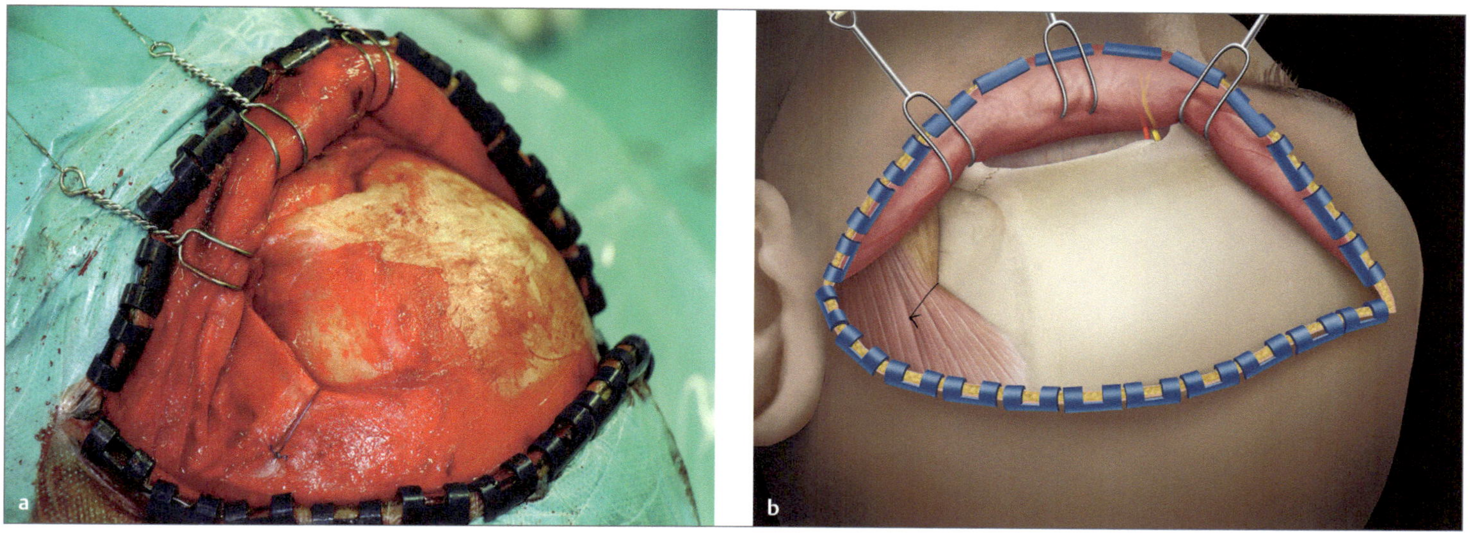

Fig. 6.26 (a, b) Subperiosteal elevation of the anterior part of the temporalis muscle and dissection of the periorbita. The anterior attachment of the temporal muscle at the orbital pillar and the anterior aspect of the linea temporalis are incised sharply. The temporal muscle is then dissected from the underlying bone and pulled back with the help of a galea hook. The temporal muscle should not be mobilized more than necessary for the limited craniotomy. The lateral and superior orbital rims are then dissected from the periorbita using a blunt curved dissector. At this stage, attention should be paid to the frontal nerve as it turns around the orbital rim at the medial aspect of the planned craniotomy. Occasionally, it may be necessary to mobilize the frontal nerve out of its bony groove or tunnel. Three fishhooks are used to gently pull the detached flap inferiorly; a suture retracts the anterior temporal muscle laterally and downward for positioning the keyhole burr hole.

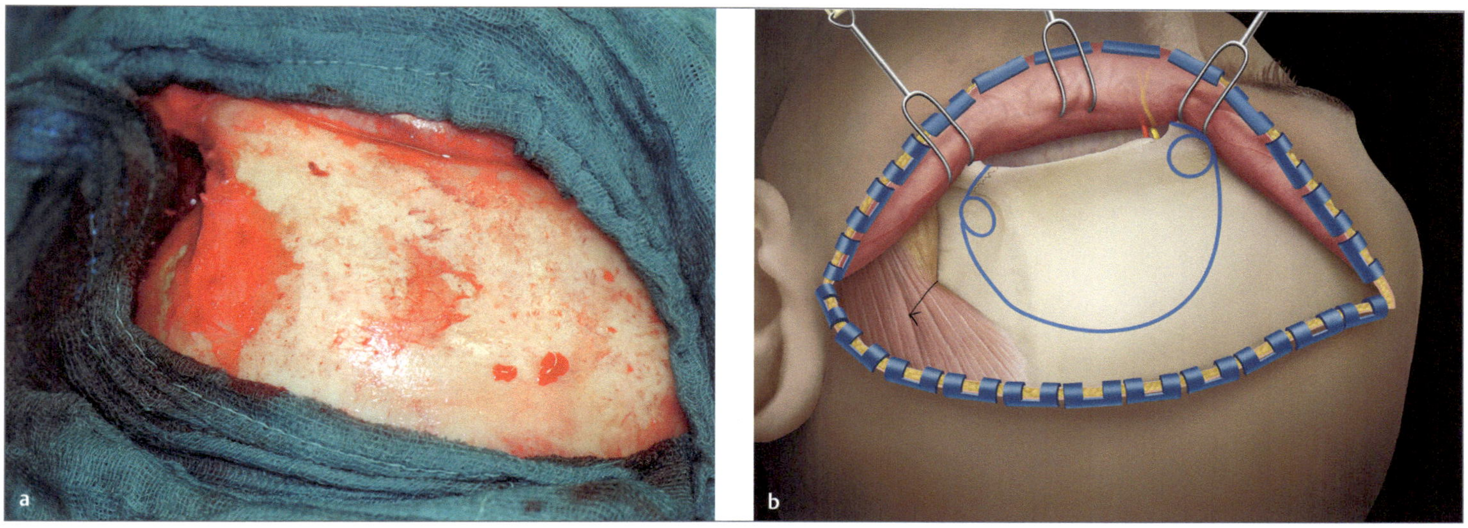

Fig. 6.27 (a, b) Craniotomy planning. A drawing anticipates the planned craniotomy. The lateral extension is toward the sphenoid ridge (i.e., the sylvian fissure); medially the extension should end above the trigeminal nerve root. We recommend two burr holes for the craniotomy. The initial burr hole corresponds to the keyhole of the pterional craniotomy placed at the frontozygomatic suture. The direction of drilling, however, aims more toward the orbit so that the orbit and the anterior cranial fossa are opened simultaneously. If some bone remains on the frontal or the orbital side, use of a diamond drill may become necessary. The second burr hole is made at the medial aspect of the planned craniotomy, immediately above the orbital rim. The dura is separated from the convexity and from the orbital roof through these burr holes using a blunt dissector.

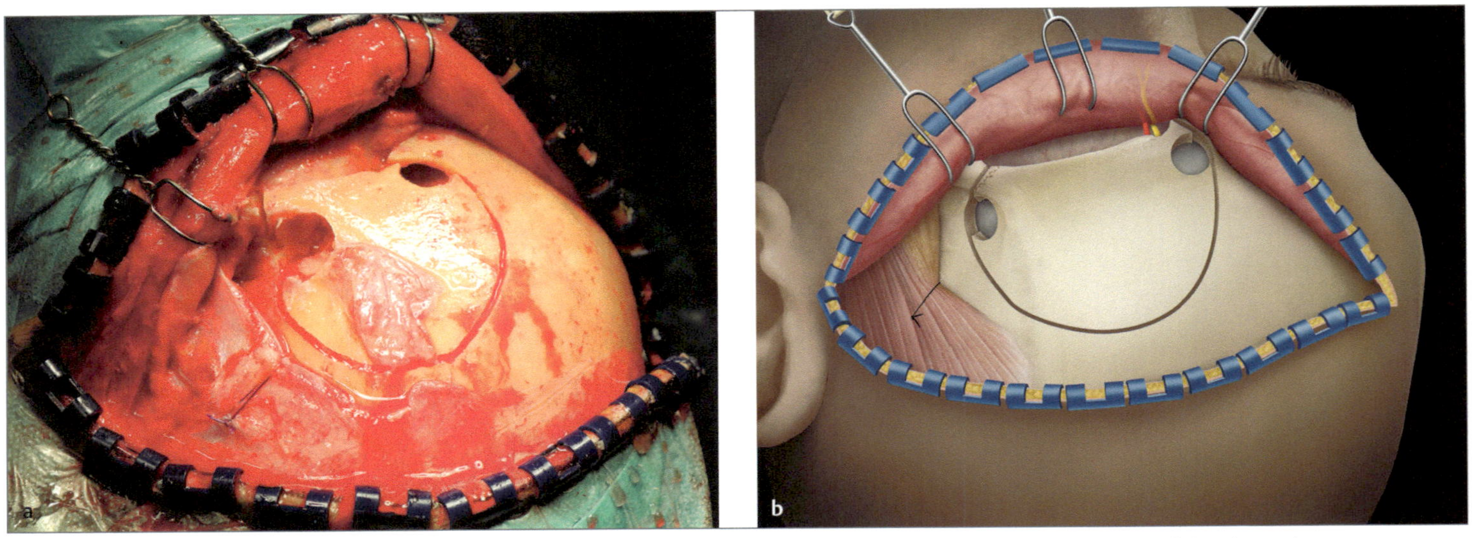

Fig. 6.28 (a, b) Craniotomy. The two burr holes are then connected with the craniotome along the upper delineation of the planned opening. Note that there is no craniotomy planned between the burr holes at the level of the orbit, i.e., the basal part. The superior and lateral orbital rims are best cut using a small bone saw or the craniotome. The dura and the periorbita must be protected with a small spatula. The bone cut in the lateral orbital rim is extended down to the lateral burr hole. With a small punch, starting from the lateral burr hole, the orbital roof is divided along the pterion to a depth of 3 to 4 cm. The anterior aspect of the medial orbital roof is divided through the medial burr hole, again using a small punch or a diamond drill.

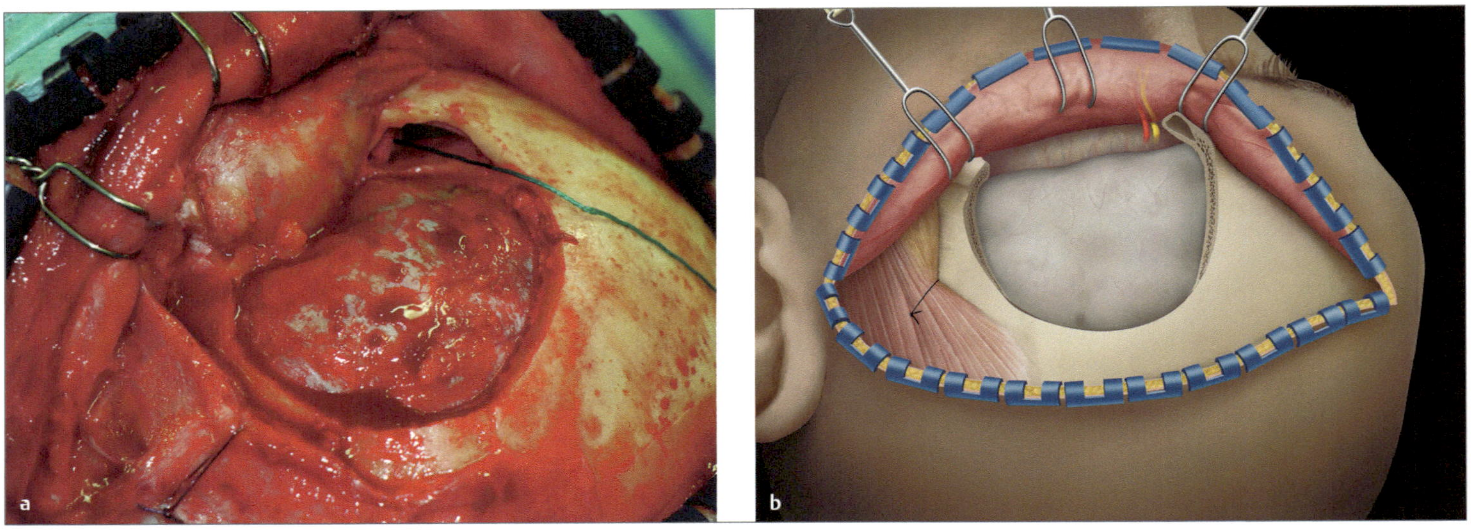

Fig. 6.29 (a, b) One-piece orbitocraniotomy with fracturing of the orbital roof. The bone flap is then elevated and the posterior orbital roof is fractured between the lateral and medial orbital roof incision. Care should be taken to fracture the orbital roof as far back as possible. We do not advocate removal of residual orbital roof in an osteoclastic manner. If this is done, the orbital roof must be reconstructed later with foreign material to prevent orbital roof instability with enophthalmos or pulsating exophthalmos. The dura is opened in a basally pediculated curvilinear fashion. The dural opening does not cross the sylvian fissure.

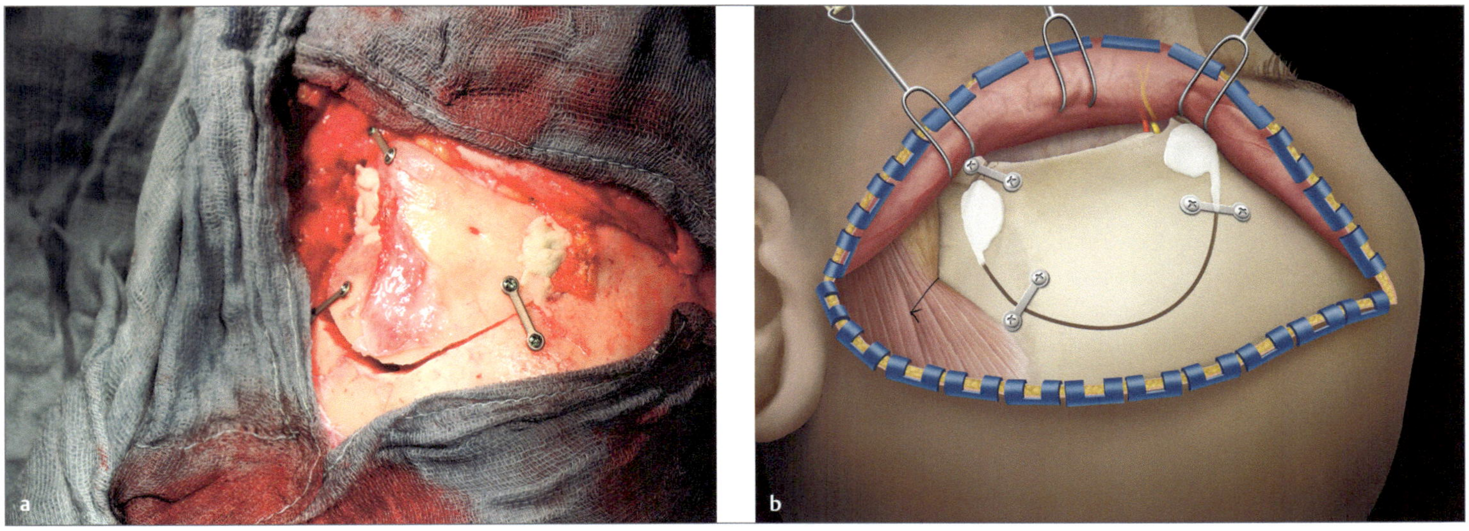

Fig. 6.30 (a, b) Dura closure and bone refixation. The dura is closed so that it is watertight. The periorbita is sometimes injured during dissection from the orbital roof. To prevent protrusion of the orbital fat, periorbital tears should be repaired immediately with a suture. If the frontal sinus has been opened at the medial aspect of the orbitocraniotomy, the defect is plugged with a muscle graft taken from the temporal muscle. We do not recommend a pediculated pericranium flap in this location, because of the risk that it may interfere with eyebrow motility. The bone flap is replaced and attached with rivets or microplates. Burr holes can be closed using Palacos bone cement, miniplates, or titanium mesh. The anterior aspect of the temporalis muscle is reattached at the linea temporalis and the skin flap is closed stepwise.

Checklist

- The head is positioned to have the lateral aspect of the orbital rim as the highest point.
- The upper part of the zygomatic process and the nasion to determine the midline should be located by palpation for later skin incision.
- The temporal fascia is incised and dissection is continued anteriorly in the interfascial or subfascial plane.
- The lateral extension of preparation is the sphenoid ridge, and the medial extension is the supraorbital foramen.
- The initial burr hole corresponds to the keyhole; the second burr hole is made above the orbital rim and then connected with the craniotome along the upper delineation.
- The superior and lateral orbital rims are cut, and the bone cut in the lateral orbital rim is extended.
- The bone flap is then elevated and the posterior orbital roof is fractured between the lateral and medial orbital roof incision.
- The dura is opened in a basally pediculated curvilinear fashion.
- Meticulous closure of bone, muscle, and skin is necessary.

6.3 Intradural Anterior Clinoidectomy

Andreas Raabe and Karl Schaller

The anterior clinoid process (ACP) covers the proximal portion of the internal carotid artery (ICA). Anterior clinoidectomy may be performed when proximal control of ICA aneurysms is required or when a tumor such as a clinoidal or spheno-orbital meningioma needs to be removed.

ACP resection can be done either with a small (i.e., 2–3 mm) diamond drill or by ultrasonic bone aspiration. Care must be taken not to run medially into the optic canal along the optic strut, thereby damaging the optic nerve, or mediobasally into the ICA. There is a choice of several strategies for drilling of the ACP, ranging from "en-bloc nondrilling" to the "eggshell technique" whereby a thin bony membrane is retained, thus providing further protection for the surrounding soft tissue structures.

In this chapter, we present a combination of these techniques (see ▶Fig. 6.31, ▶Fig. 6.32, ▶Fig. 6.33, ▶Fig. 6.34, ▶Fig. 6.35, ▶Fig. 6.36, ▶Fig. 6.37, ▶Fig. 6.38, ▶Fig. 6.39, ▶Fig. 6.40, ▶Fig. 6.41, ▶Fig. 6.42, ▶Fig. 6.43, ▶Fig. 6.44, ▶Fig. 6.45, ▶Fig. 6.46, ▶Fig. 6.47, ▶Fig. 6.48, and ▶Fig. 6.49).

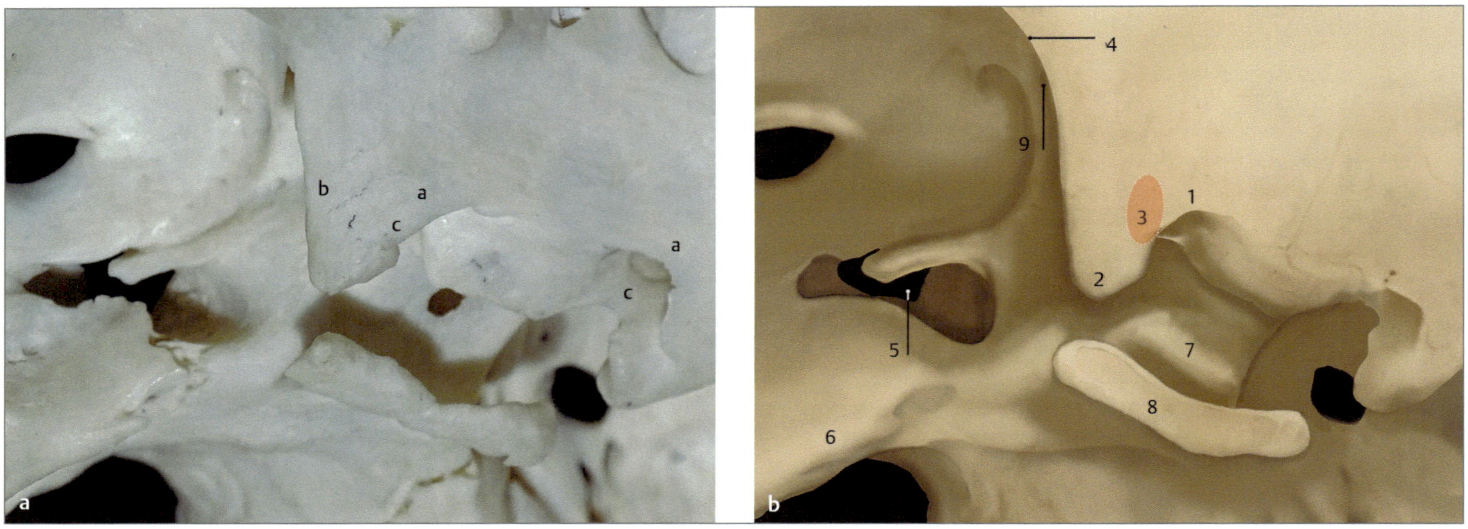

Fig. 6.31 (a, b) Bony anatomy overview. The ACP is attached to the skull base at three points. It is attached (a) medially to the lateral edge of the optic canal, (b) laterally to the sphenoid bridge, and (c) inferiorly to the optic strut. These attachments must be drilled down to mobilize the ACP. (1) Optic canal, (2) ACP, (3) area of optic strut underneath the ACP, (4) sphenoid ridge, (5) foramen lacerum, (6) petrous bone, (7) sella, (8) posterior clinoid process, (9) superior lateral extension of the superior orbital fissure underneath the sphenoid ridge.

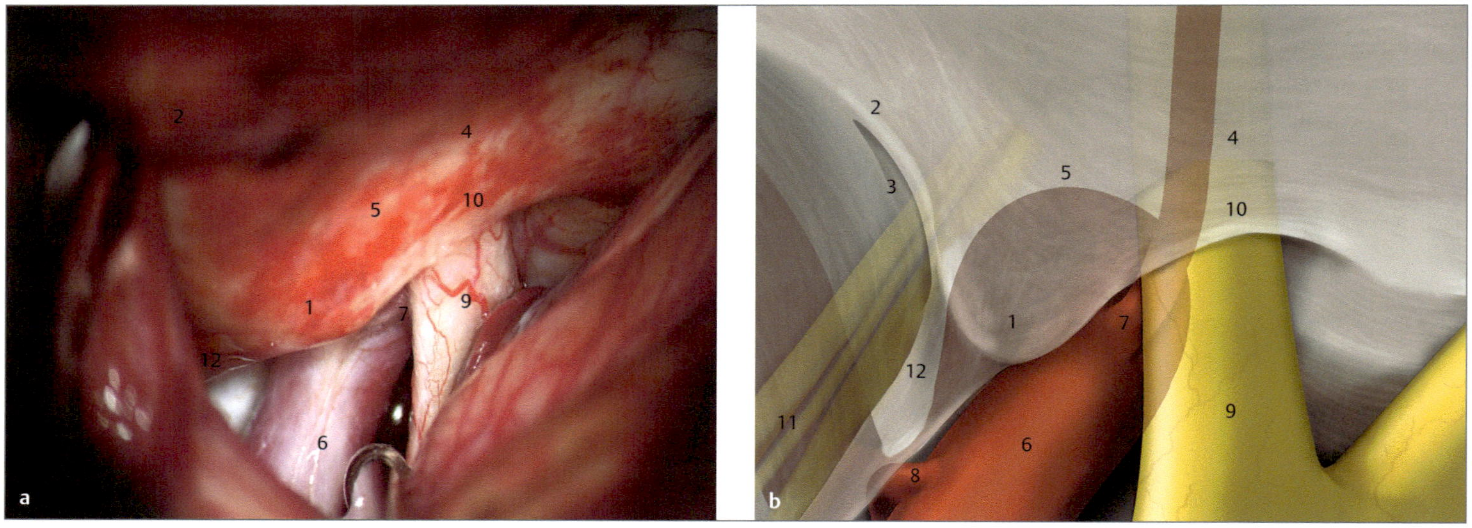

Fig. 6.32 (a, b) Intradural anatomy overview. View following standard pterional or frontolateral craniotomy. Anatomical landmarks are: (1) ACP, (2) lesser sphenoid wing (lateral root of ACP), (3) superior orbital fissure, (4) bony roof of optic canal (medial root of ACP), (5) optic strut (forming the inferior root of the ACP and the base of the optic canal), (6) ICA, (7) ophthalmic artery (ophA), (8) posterior communicating artery (pcomA), (9) optic nerve (CN II), (10) falciform ligament, (11) oculomotor, ophthalmic, trochlear, and abducens nerve, (12) anterior petroclinoid fold.

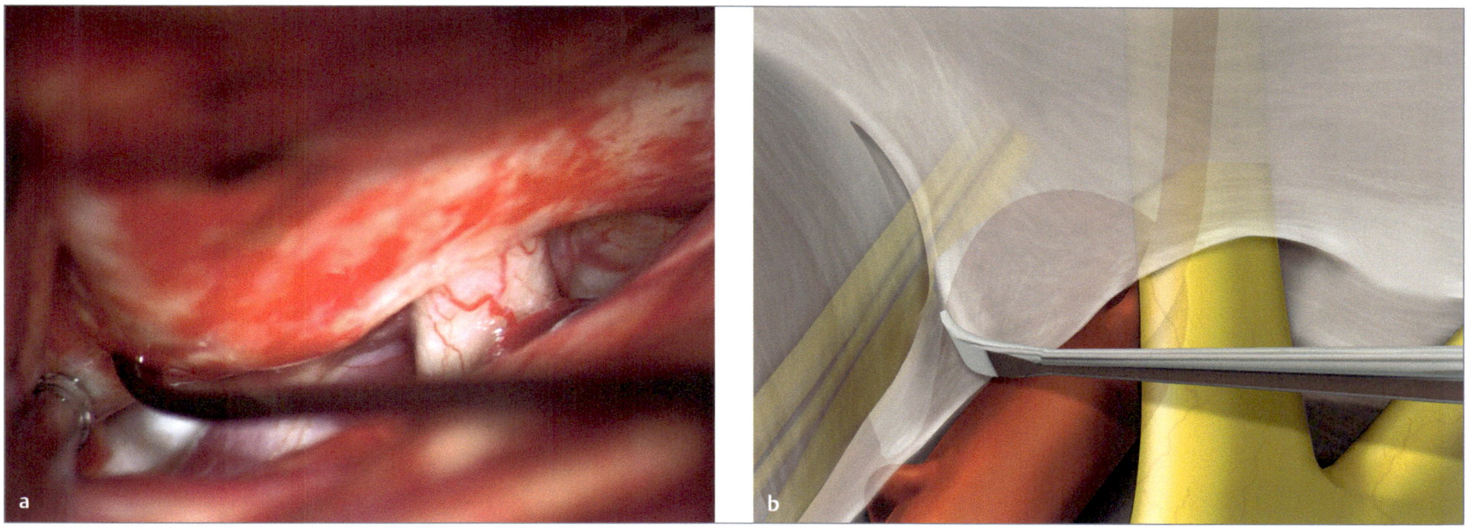

Fig. 6.33 (a, b) **Palpation of ACP.** The ACP can be palpated with a dissector to delineate the borders and gain a better understanding of the anatomy.

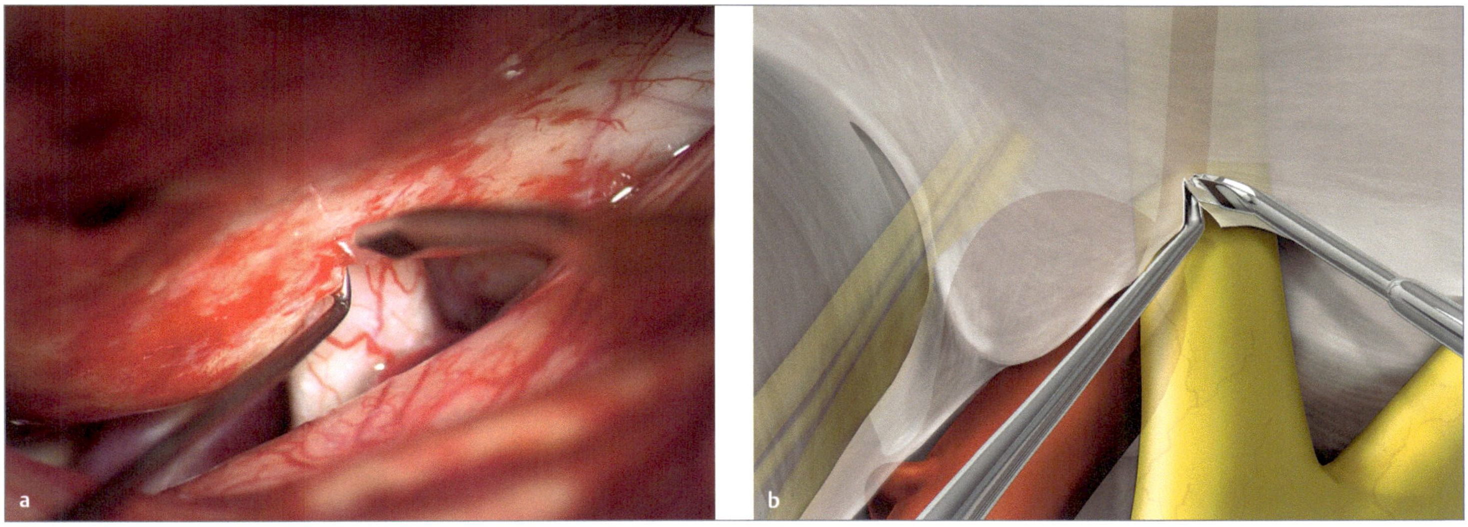

Fig. 6.34 (a, b) **Opening of the falciform ligament.** The optic nerve is tethered by the falciform ligament proximal to the entrance into the optic canal. This ligament is opened using a 90° diamond knife or a dissector elevating the dura and a straight knife. This step helps to identify the bony entrance into the optic canal.

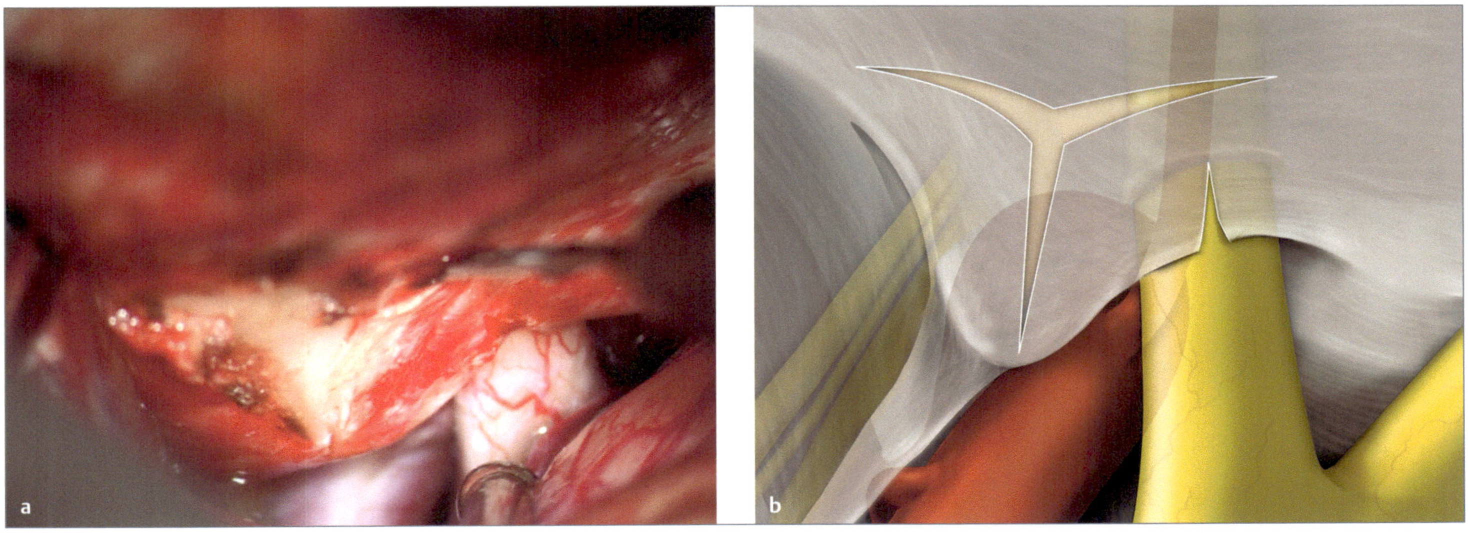

Fig. 6.35 (a, b) **Dural incision on the ACP.** After coagulation of the dura, the dura mater is incised in a **Y**-shape starting at the tip of the clinoid and then going laterally. The second incision completes the **Y**-shape, going medially and crossing the bony roof of the optic canal approximately 5 mm anterior/rostral to the entrance of the optic nerve into the optic canal.

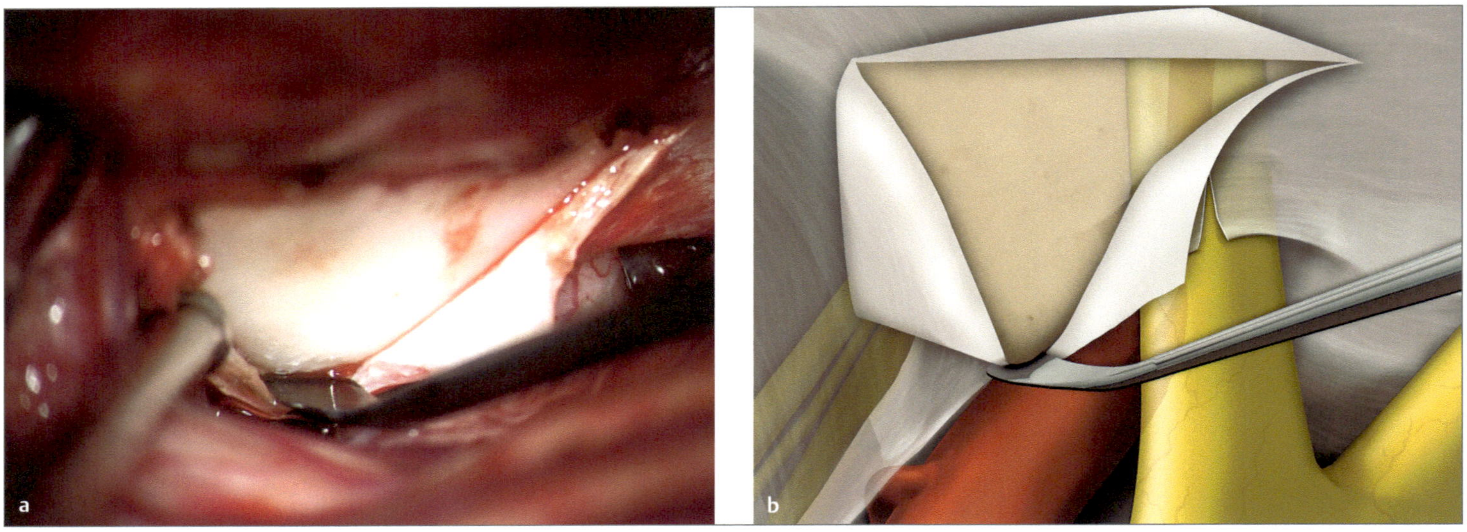

Fig. 6.36 (a, b) Exposing the ACP. The dura mater is peeled away from the bone toward the lateral and medial side. Care has to be taken to extend the cuts to the projected medial side of the optic nerve. Finally, the full bony contour of the ACP and the roof of the optic canal is exposed.

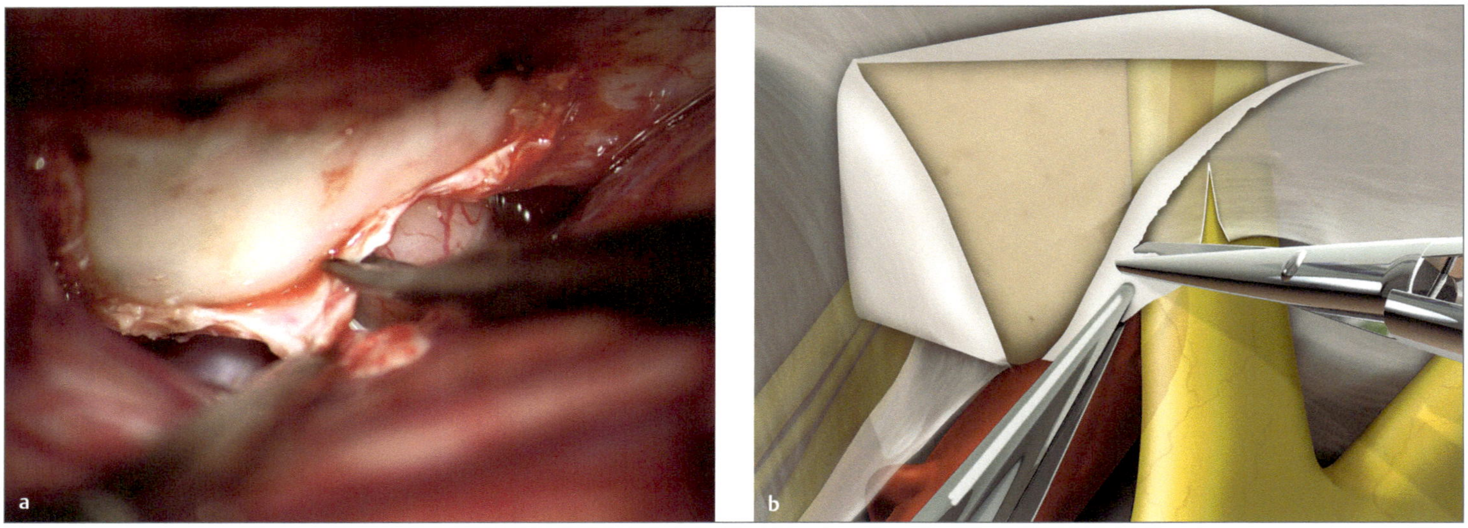

Fig. 6.37 (a, b) Trimming the dura. Here, some neurosurgeons trim the loose dura to prevent the ends being drawn into the drill. Others keep the dura in place as a protective sleeve during ensuing drilling and ACP resection.

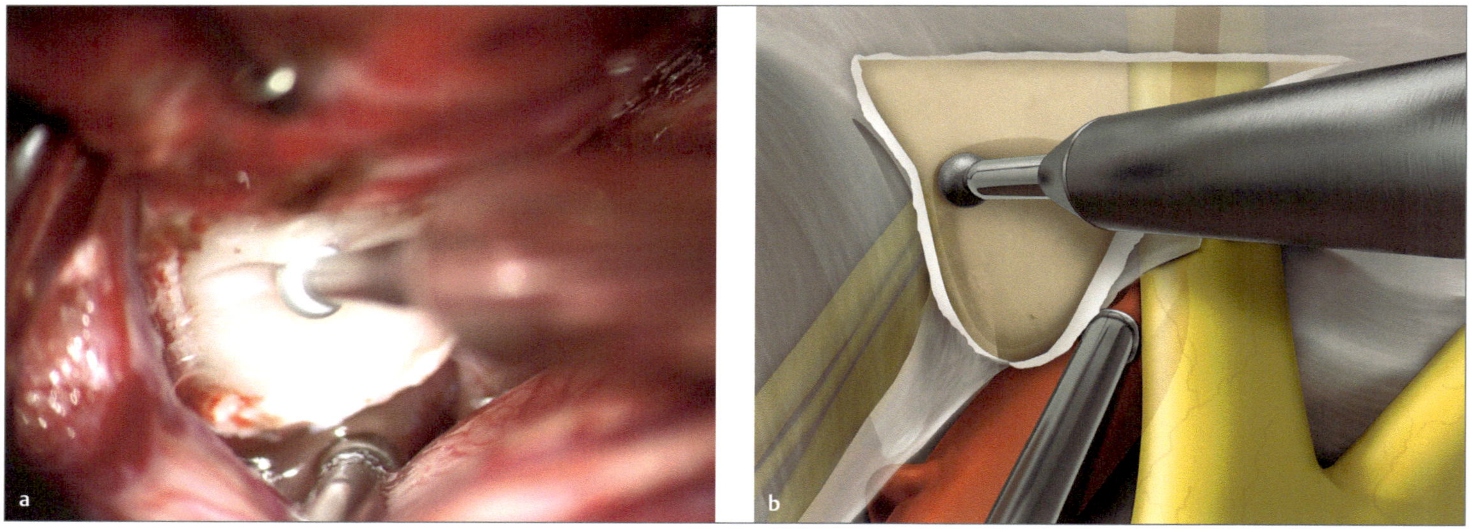

Fig. 6.38 (a, b) Initial drilling. Drilling is started with a 2-mm diamond drill bit at the center of the anterior border in a horizontal direction either toward the lateral or the medial direction. Drilling is also performed toward the inner bone to hollow the clinoid.

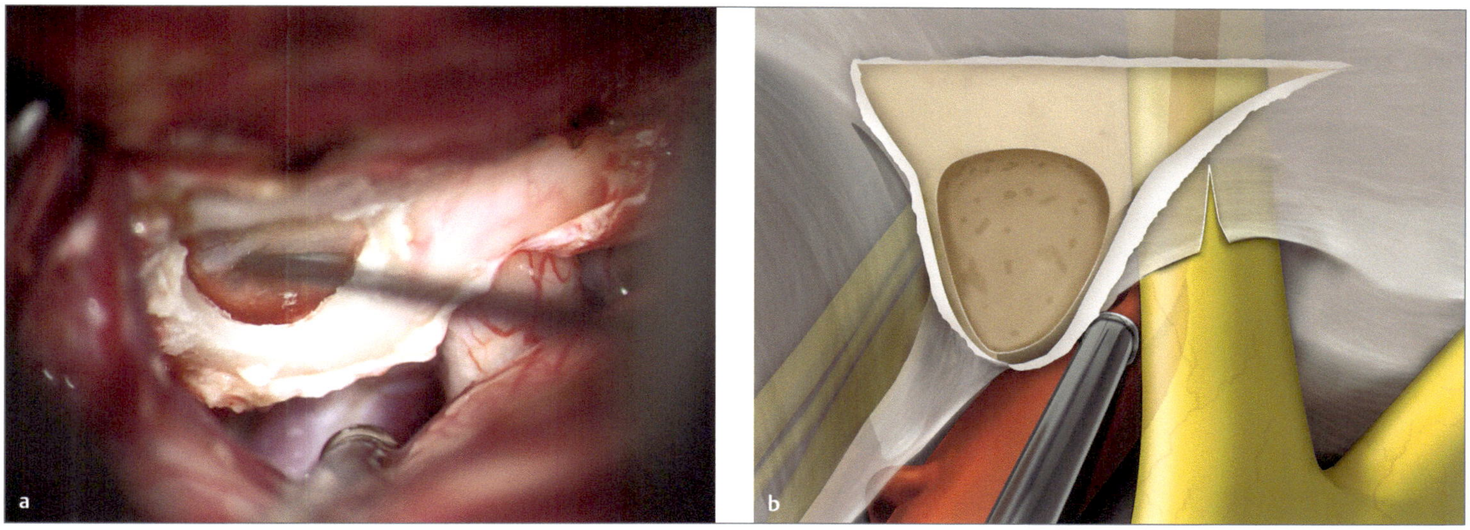

Fig. 6.39 (a, b) Pneumatized ACP. In this patient, the ACP was pneumatized. The intact mucosa is visible. It is mobilized and gently pushed to the inside using a small piece of Gelfoam. Normally, the ACP is solid, as seen in this illustration. In cases of pneumatized ACP, there is a considerable risk of CSF leakage and closure must be performed using a muscle plug or another suitable technique (see Lawton's yoyo technique).

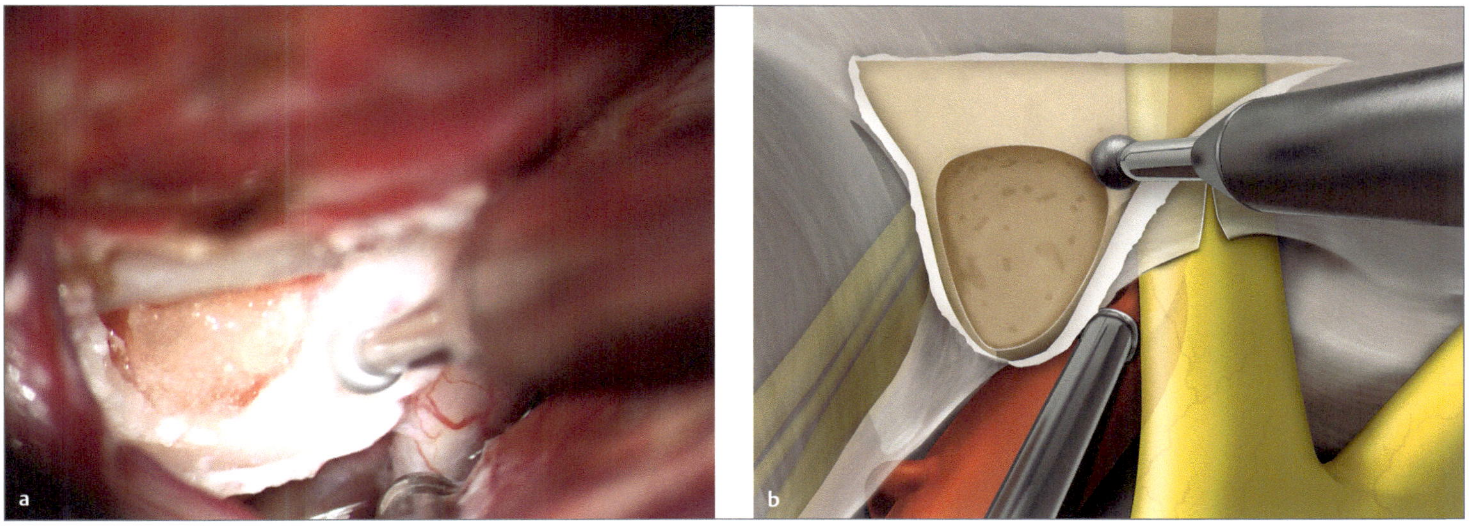

Fig. 6.40 (a, b) Drilling continued. The next drilling step is performed at the medial edge of the clinoid, but laterally to the optic nerve. A virtual line of continuation of the optic nerve can serve as a guide for drilling. Drilling should proceed cautiously and with continuous irrigation.

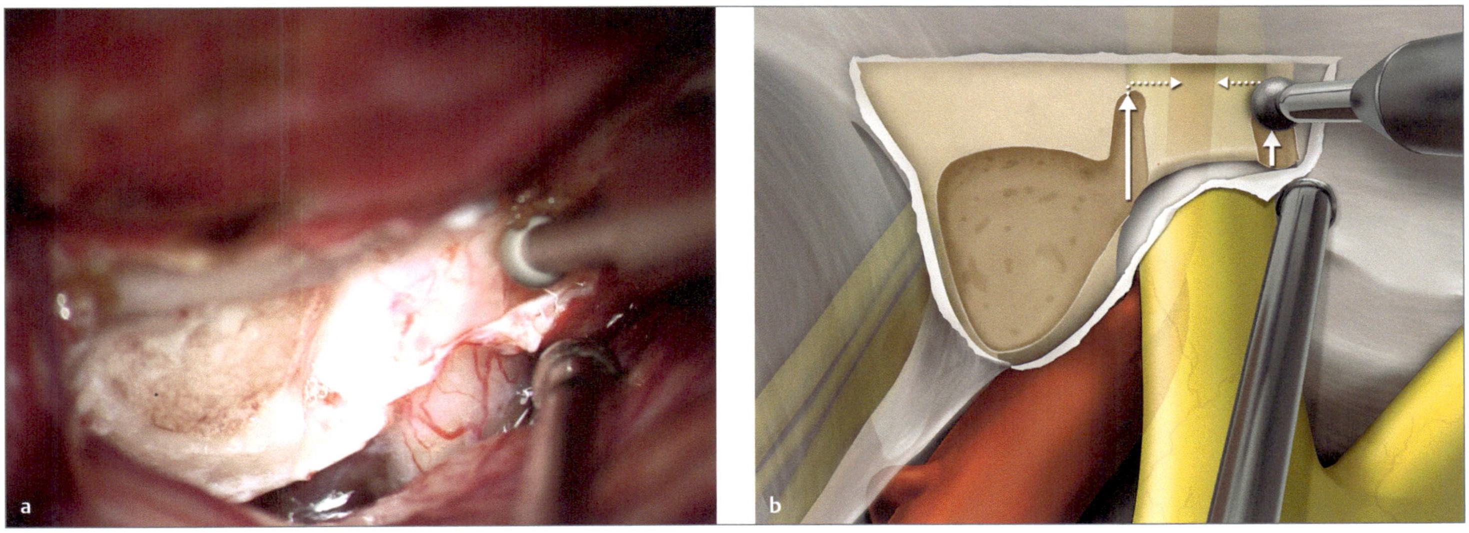

Fig. 6.41 (a, b) Unroofing the optic canal. Then, drilling is performed to unroof the optic canal. This should be performed with a 2-mm diamond drill with almost no pressure and under continuous irrigation. The lateral border of the optic nerve can serve as a landmark for the lateral border of the optic canal. A fine dissector or nerve hook can be used to repeatedly test whether the bone is thinned sufficiently to crack it.

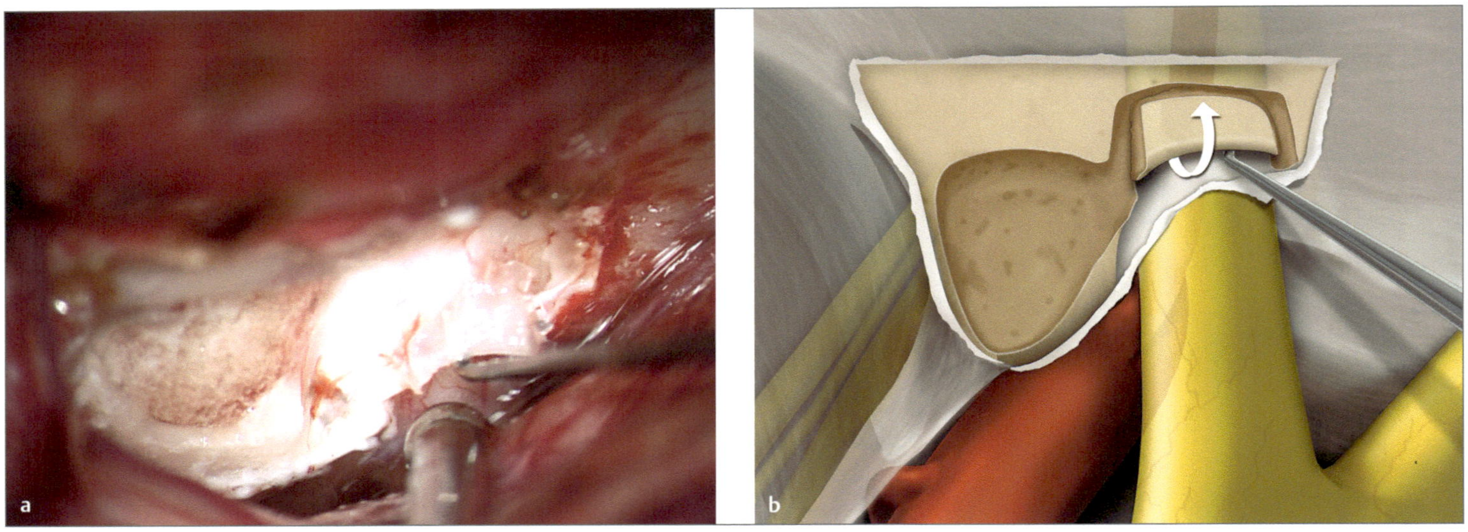

Fig. 6.42 (a, b) Opening of the optic canal. Unroofing the canal can be performed (1) by thinning the whole roof and then elevating it using the "eggshell" technique (= fracturing it upward away from the nerve) or (2) by thinning the bone at the medial and lateral border of the nerve and finally at 90° to the distal border using the same technique and then lifting the bone covering the optic canal or (3) a combination of both techniques. This step is performed to free the optic nerve from its ligamentous and bony fixation so that the nerve can be shifted to one side during the subsequent surgical steps, e.g., of aneurysm clipping, instead of being compressed. In addition, it helps to define the medial attachment of the ACP.

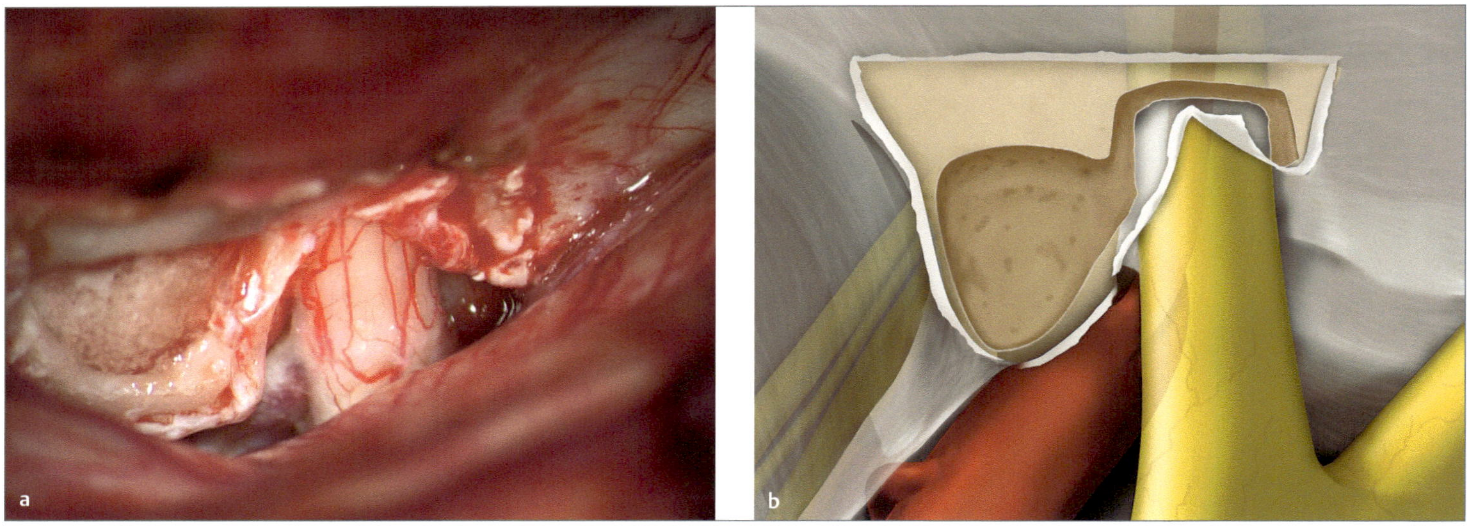

Fig. 6.43 (a, b) Further opening of the falciform ligament. Unroofing of the optic canal is finished. The falciform ligament is further opened. This allows mobilization of the nerve, if required, e.g., for the clipping of paraclinoid aneurysms.

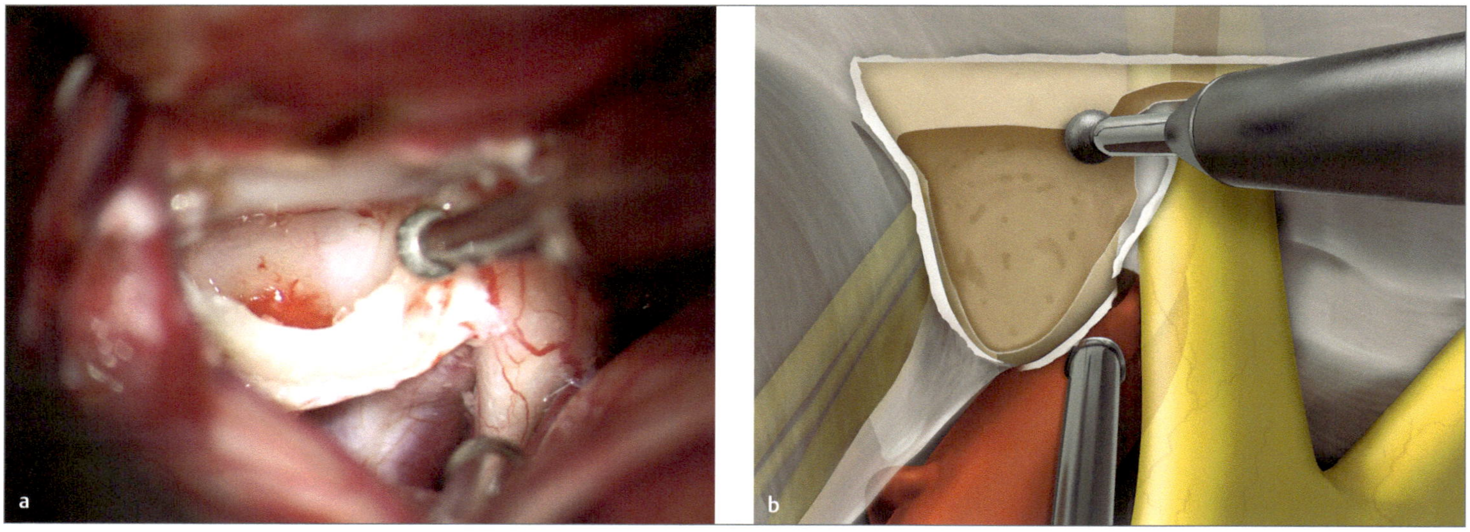

Fig. 6.44 (a, b) Disconnecting the ACP by further drilling. After unroofing the optic canal, hollowing of the ACP is continued. In addition, disconnection of the medial attachment of the ACP is finished by slowly and carefully drilling the remaining bone at the lateral wall of the optic canal. If necessary, drilling returns to the more lateral and central portions to disconnect the ACP laterally. This step is not required when the lateral and medial disconnection has already been achieved. Then, drilling is again focused on hollowing out the ACP and the final attachment of the ACP, which is represented by the optic strut. The landmark for localizing the optic strut is the line between the ACP and the optic canal parallel to the optic nerve.

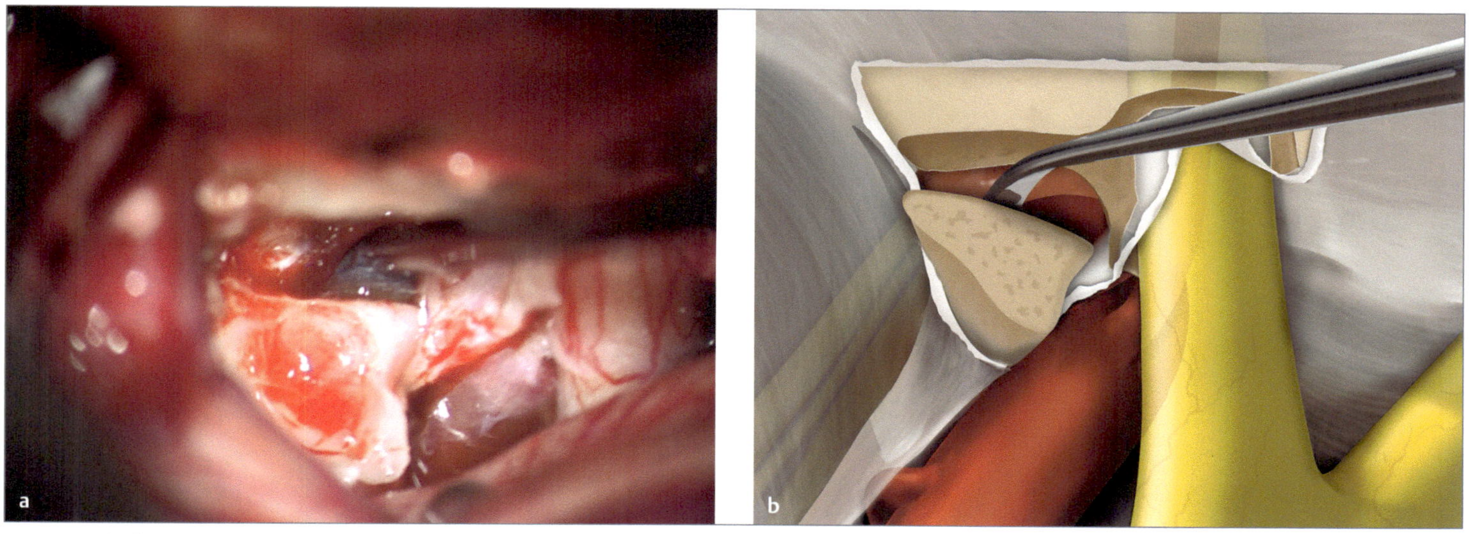

Fig. 6.45 (a, b) **Removing the final piece of ACP.** The apex of the ACP now becomes mobile, usually in one piece, but there may be fragments that are still adherent to the dura mater posterior or laterally. Using a dissector, these bone chips including a larger chip containing the apex of the ACP can be freed and removed.

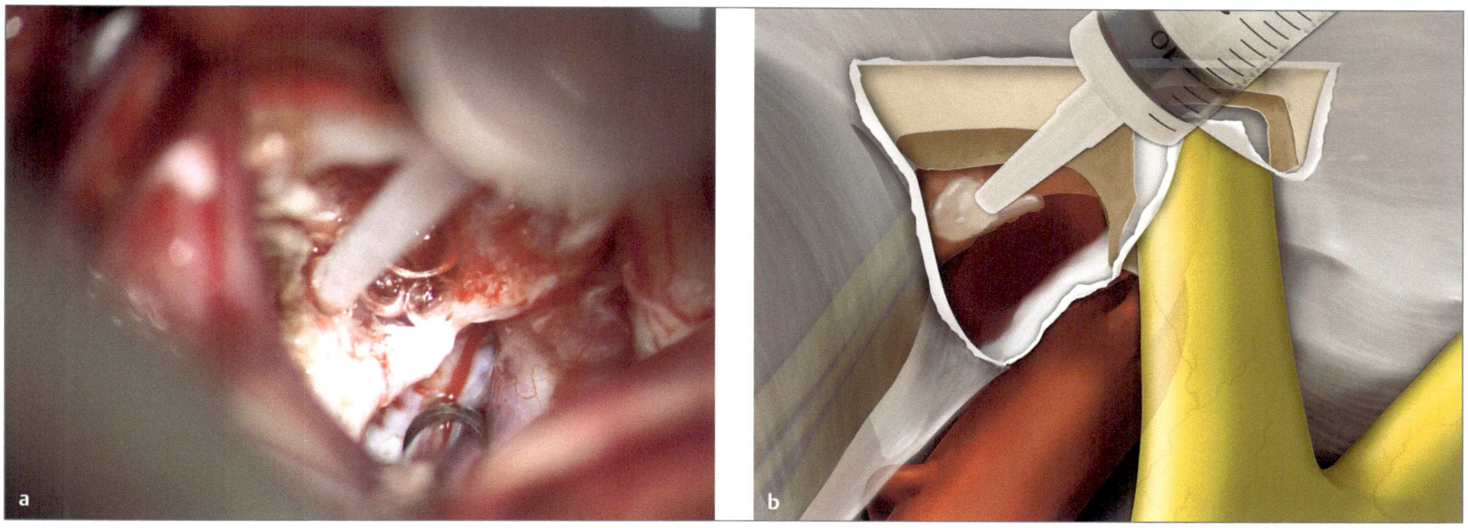

Fig. 6.46 (a, b) **Hemostasis.** Typically, there is venous bleeding from the cavernous sinus that is stopped by injecting fibrin glue into the cavernous sinus.

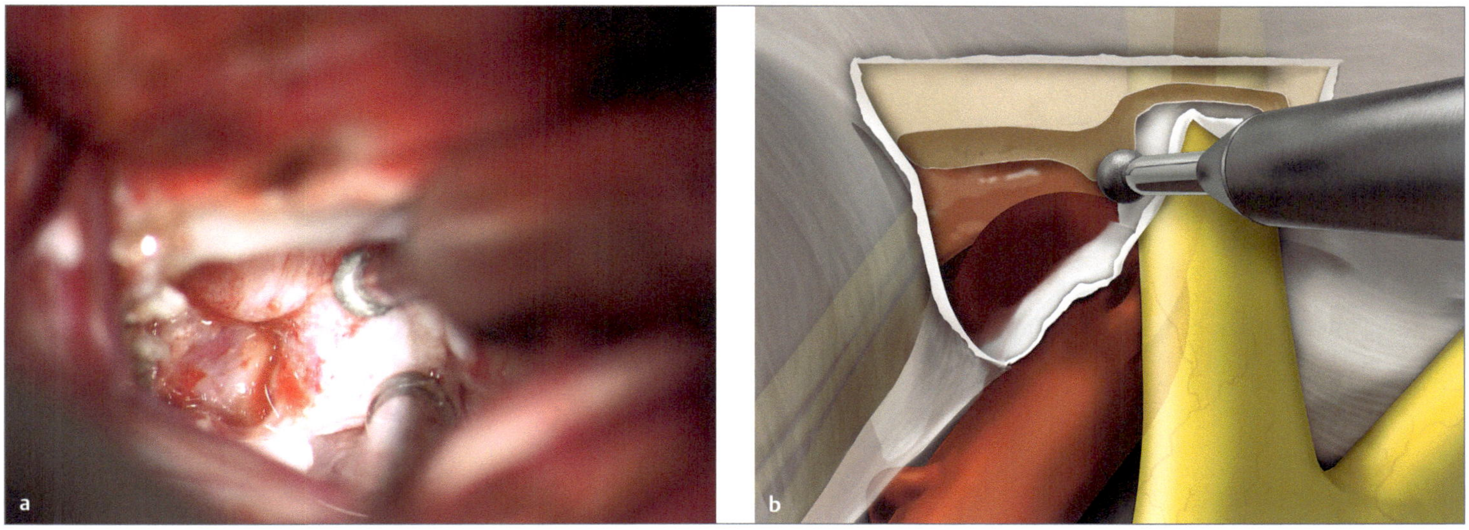

Fig. 6.47 (a, b) **Drilling the optic strut.** The remaining optic strut is now drilled down to gain access to the distal dural ring.

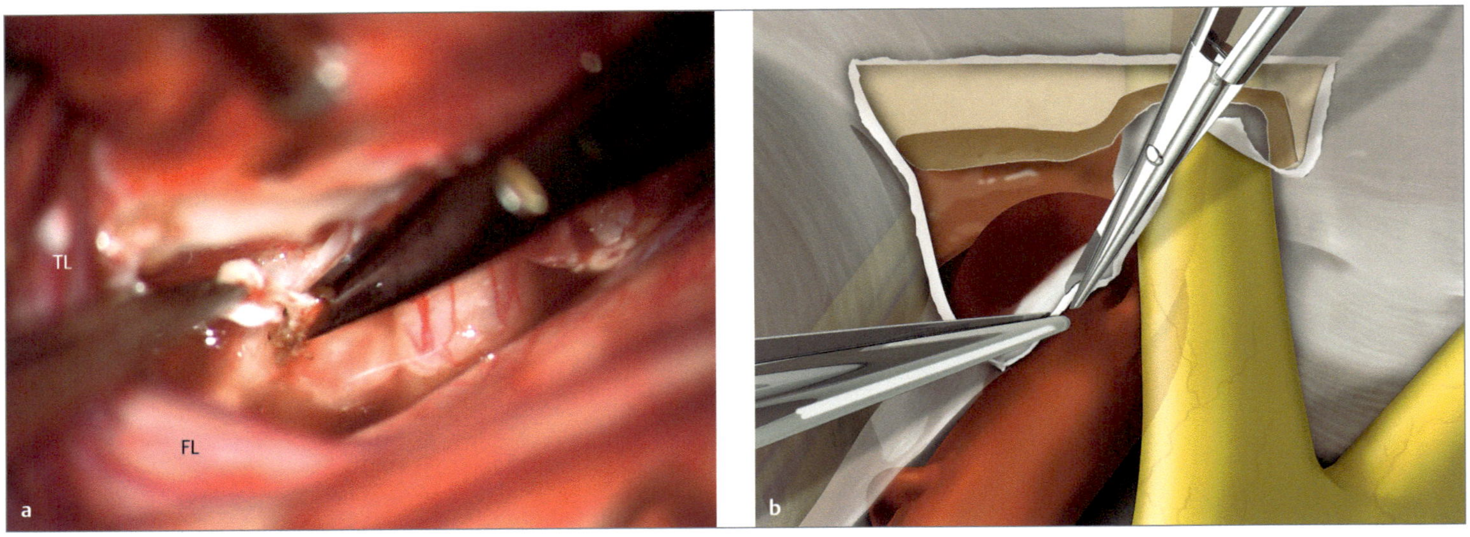

Fig. 6.48 (a, b) Trimming the dura at the distal ring. The lateral part of the optic nerve sheath fades into the distal dural ring. Therefore, the lateral optic nerve sheath is used as a landmark leading toward the distal dural ring. It is cut and followed downward and anteriorly until it fuses with the distal dural ring. The ICA is then identified proximal and distal to the distal dural ring. Then, the loose edges of the dura mater are trimmed to the distal dural ring, i.e., the carotid wall (FL = frontal lobe, TL= temporal lobe).

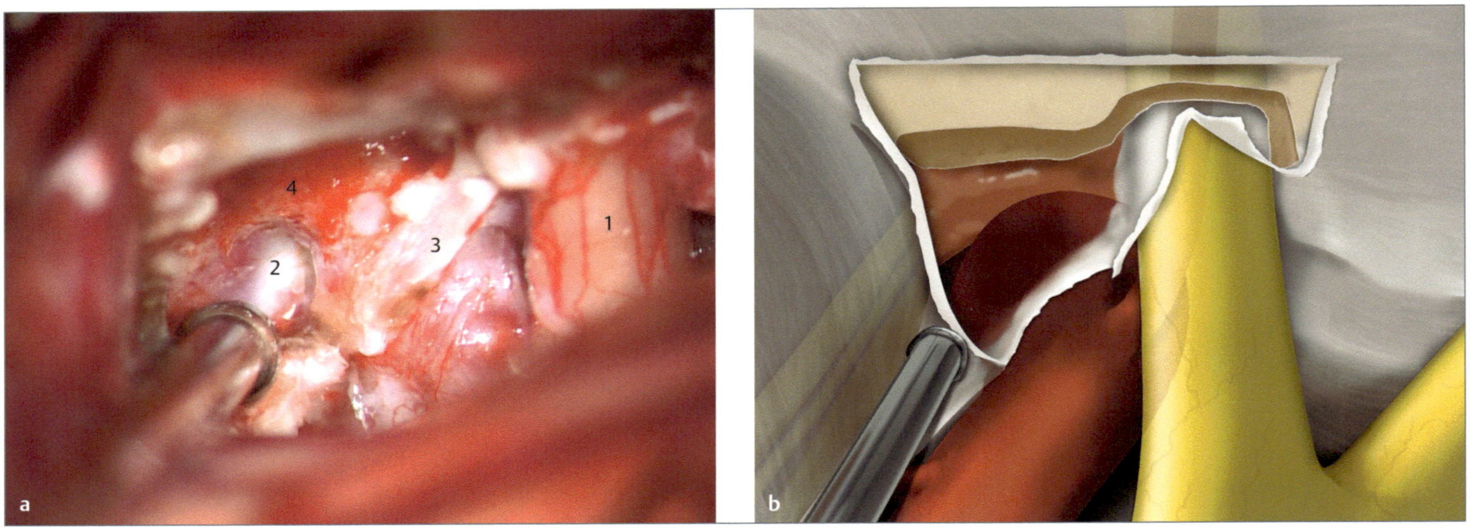

Fig. 6.49 (a, b) Final anatomic view. The dura along the distal dural ring is rather thick laterally but thins out toward the optic nerve. Finally, the following structures are exposed: (1) intracanalicular optic nerve, (2) extradural ICA, (3) dural ring, and (4) cavernous sinus. As already mentioned, meticulous closure of any pneumatized ACP is mandatory to prevent CSF leakage. We recommend using Lawton's yoyo technique (Chi JH, Sughrue M, Kunwar S, Lawton MT. The "yo-yo" technique to prevent cerebrospinal fluid rhinorrhea after anterior clinoidectomy for proximal internal carotid artery aneurysms. Neurosurgery 2006; 59 (Suppl 1):ONS-101–ONS-107).

Checklist

- Palpate clinoid process.
- Open falciform ligament to untether the optic nerve and to localize the bony roof of optic nerve.
- Make a Y-shaped opening of the dura.
- Dissect dura from the clinoid and the roof of the optic canal.
- Drill clinoid and unroof optic canal. The upper drilling border is identical; therefore, these two steps are related. Finish unroofing the optic canal before completing the clinoidectomy.
- Finish disconnecting the clinoid tip, and mobilize it. The dura must be completely detached, before the clinoid tip can be removed. Roll away from the optic nerve, but beware of the carotid artery laterally.
- Use fibrin glue to stop bleeding at the cavernous sinus.
- Drill down optic strut, but protect the optic nerve.
- Cut the dura from the dural ring.

6.4 Far (Enough) Lateral Approach

Andreas Raabe, Johannes Goldberg, and David Bervini

The far-lateral approach originated when skull base surgery was at its height, and was refined with numerous extensions and corresponding terms, such as the lateral, the condylar fossa, transcondylar, juxtacondylar, transjugular, and extreme lateral approach.

Today, for most indications (>90%), the far-lateral approach can be regarded as an extension of a lateral suboccipital approach with opening of the foramen magnum. This approach is used for lesions of the anterior or anterolateral aspect of the clivus, the brainstem, or the craniovertebral junction. It includes additional bone removal at the condylar fossa, the occipital condyle, and/or the jugular tubercle, but only as much as required. We therefore like to call it the "far *enough* lateral approach," a term coined by the Helsinki group, because the amount of drilling is tailored to the needs and anatomy of the individual patient, just enough to reach the lesion (see ▶ Fig. 6.50, ▶ Fig. 6.51, ▶ Fig. 6.52, ▶ Fig. 6.53, ▶ Fig. 6.54, ▶ Fig. 6.55, ▶ Fig. 6.56, ▶ Fig. 6.57, ▶ Fig. 6.58, ▶ Fig. 6.59, ▶ Fig. 6.60, ▶ Fig. 6.61, ▶ Fig. 6.62, ▶ Fig. 6.63, ▶ Fig. 6.64, ▶ Fig. 6.65, ▶ Fig. 6.66, ▶ Fig. 6.67, ▶ Fig. 6.68, ▶ Fig. 6.69, ▶ Fig. 6.70, ▶ Fig. 6.71, and ▶ Fig. 6.72).

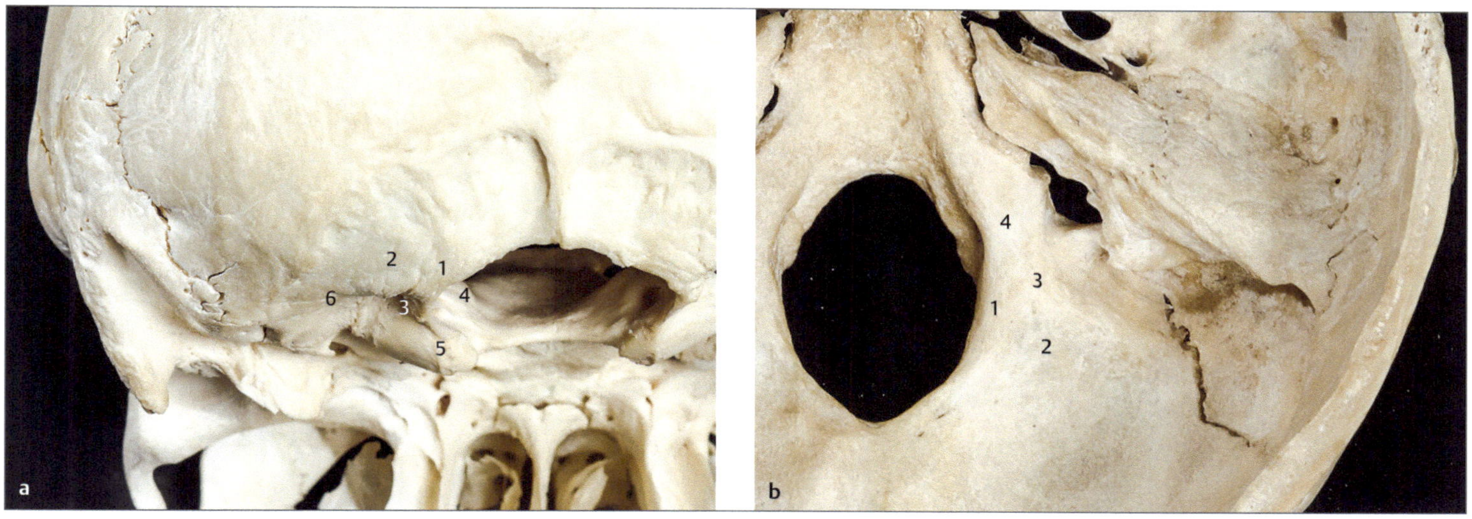

Fig. 6.50 (a, b) Anatomy. Intra- and extracranial view. The idea behind the far-lateral approach is to reach medial targets more easily. The same principle applies as for the orbitozygomatic approach, where in order to look more superior and to retract less, we need to come from more inferior. For the far-lateral approach, to look more medial and anterior to the brainstem, we need to come more from lateral.There are five bony structures that may obstruct the view to the anterolateral clivus and brainstem: (1) posterolateral foramen magnum, (2) suboccipital bone, (3) bone of the condylar fossa, (4) jugular tubercle, and (5) occipital condyle. In more extensive approaches, the bone lateral to these structures may also be drilled (6).

A prominent jugular tubercle can be drilled extradurally or intradurally. The intradural option allows more tailoring, but in the far-lateral approach once the dura is opened, it can be reflected easily back and forth and the required drilling can be completed according to the desired angle of the approach. For most intracranial anteromedial targets, a supracondylar and partial transcondylar approach with resection of the superomedial condyle will be sufficient. The biomechanical stability of the atlanto-occipital joint is directly related to the amount of condylar resection. As a rule of thumb, >50% resection requires C0–C1 fixation and 30 to 50% resection should be followed by imaging and clinical examination. As there is no reliable landmark for the amount of resection, imaging is usually required for quantification.

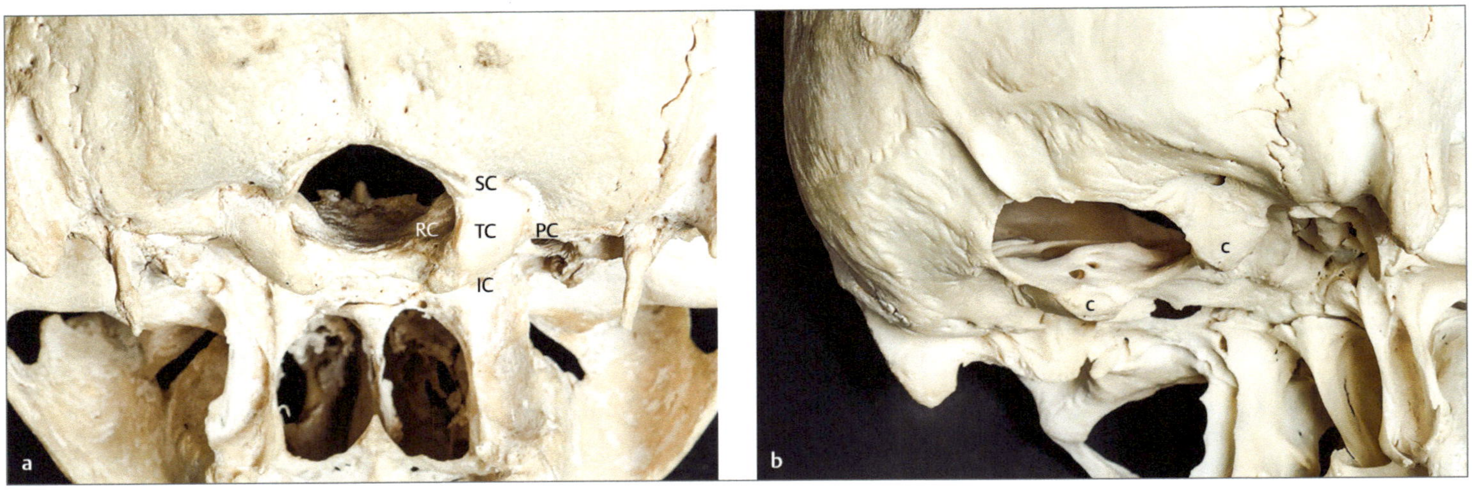

Fig. 6.51 (a, b) The occipital condyle and the terminology of the variants of the far-lateral approach. The occipital condyle (c) is a central landmark for the far-lateral approach. The variants of the far-lateral approach work around or through the occipital condyle. For intracranial targets, only the condyle needs to be dealt with, but for targets below the hypoglossal canal, the entire atlanto-occipital joint—of which the condyle is only the superior part—is involved. *Retrocondylar (RC)*: the access is medial to the condyle (comparable to "retro"sigmoid).*Supracondylar (SC)*: above the condyle. *Paracondylar (PC)*: lateral to the condyle. *Infracondylar (IC)*: below, for spinal tumors. *Complete transcondylar (TC)*: the condyle is removed to gain access, but this is very rarely required; these cases often have a pathology involving the condyle itself. *Partially transcondylar*: an oblique plane either from posterolateral to anteromedial (more correctly: posteroinferolateral to anterosuperomedial) is drilled to gain more laterality.

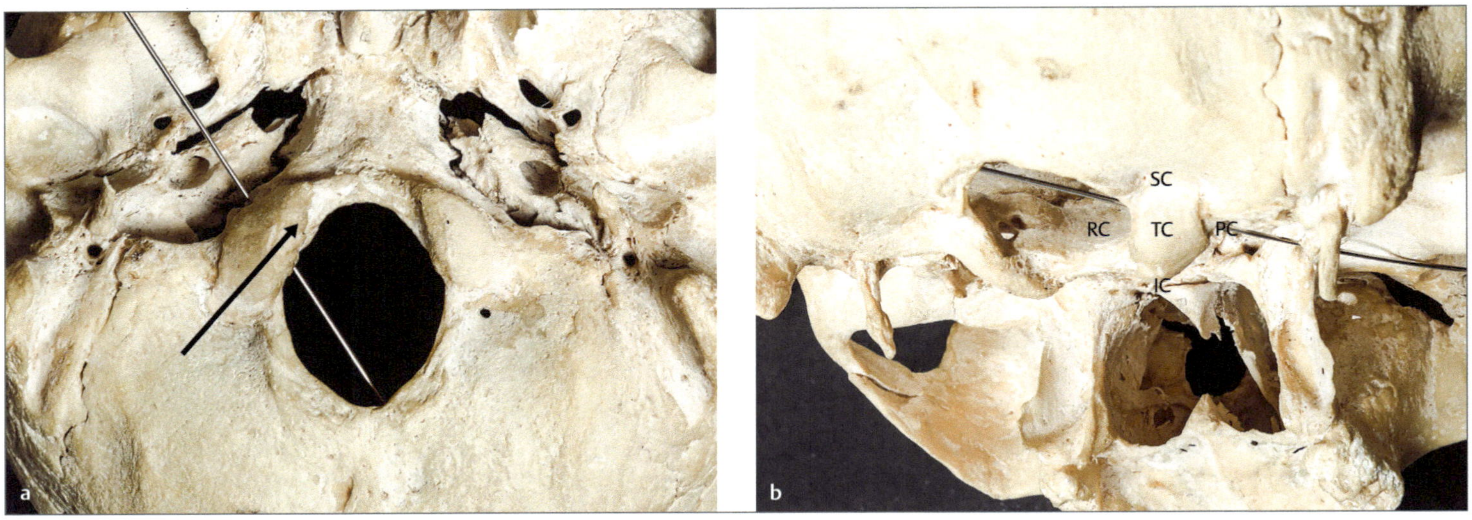

Fig. 6.52 (a, b) The XIIth nerve and the transcondylar approach. View of the foramen magnum from below **(a)** and surgeon's view **(b)**. The hypoglossal canal (wire) and the XIIth nerve exit at an angle of approximately 90° to the planned surgical trajectory. The XIIth nerve always represents an obstacle to the drilling and the approach, and all approaches have to work around it. This can be done either above or below the XIIth nerve, depending on the location and the size of the lesion.

As mentioned above, the far-lateral approach involves different degrees of skull base or lateral extension as shown in ▸Table 6.1.

Table 6.1 The concept of the different degrees of lateral extension

Degree of lateral extension	Name of approach	Resection of:	Surgical targets (examples)
	Supracondylar	• Posterolateral wall of the foramen magnum • Bone at the fossa condylaris • Drilling of the jugular tubercle may or may not be required	Anterolateral clivus
	Partially transcondylar	Plus • Posteromedial third or <50% of the occipital condyle or the atlanto-occipital joint	Midline
	Transcondylar	Plus • Complete or >50% removal of the occipital condyle or the atlanto-occipital joint. Requires occipitocervical instrumentation and fixation	Lesions at the base of the clivus in the midline
	Extreme lateral	Plus • Lateral mass of C1 • Transposition of the vertebral artery	Access to C2

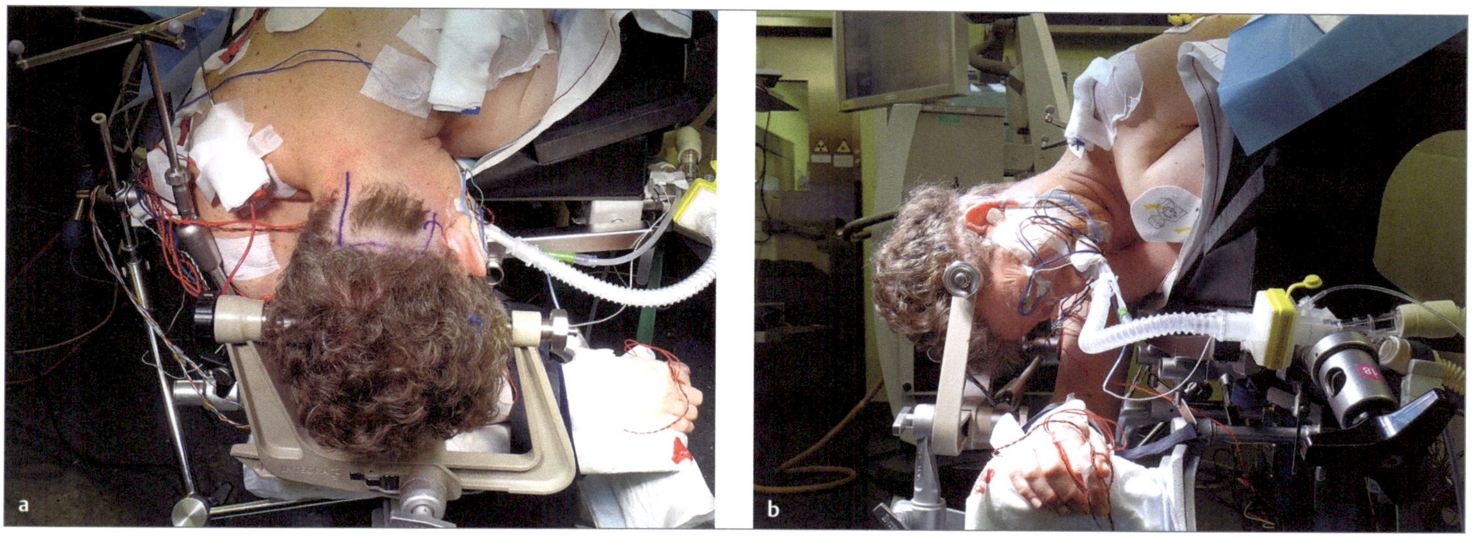

Fig. 6.53 (a, b) Positioning. The surgical corridor requires opening of the inferior paramedian suboccipital region and the craniocervical junction. The patient should be in the park bench position with the head turned 30° (15–45° according to the surgical target) to the contralateral side and maximally flexed (two fingers must fit between the chin and clavicle). Tilting the head toward the contralateral side further opens the region of the surgical corridor. The patient should be stabilized on the table to allow rotation and table tilting. A final check should be made to ensure that there is no venous congestion.

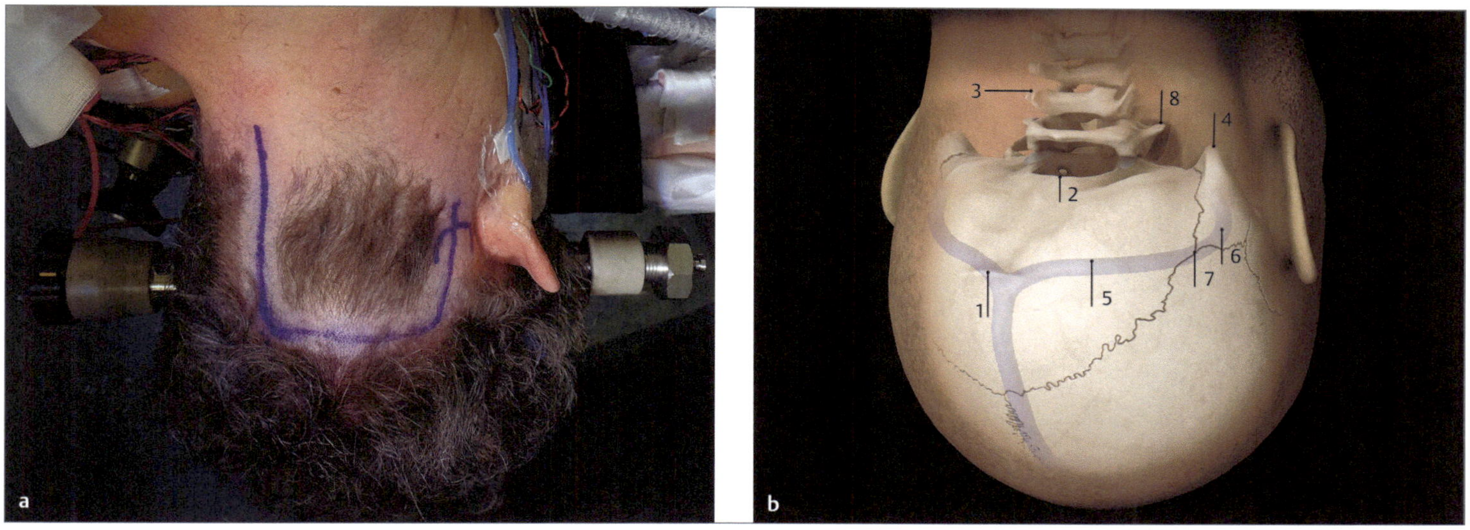

Fig. 6.54 (a, b) Anatomy overview. Important landmarks or structures are (1) inion, (2) foramen magnum, (3) spinous process of C2, (4) mastoid process, (5) transverse sinus, (6) sigmoid sinus, (7) asterion, and (8) transverse process of C1.

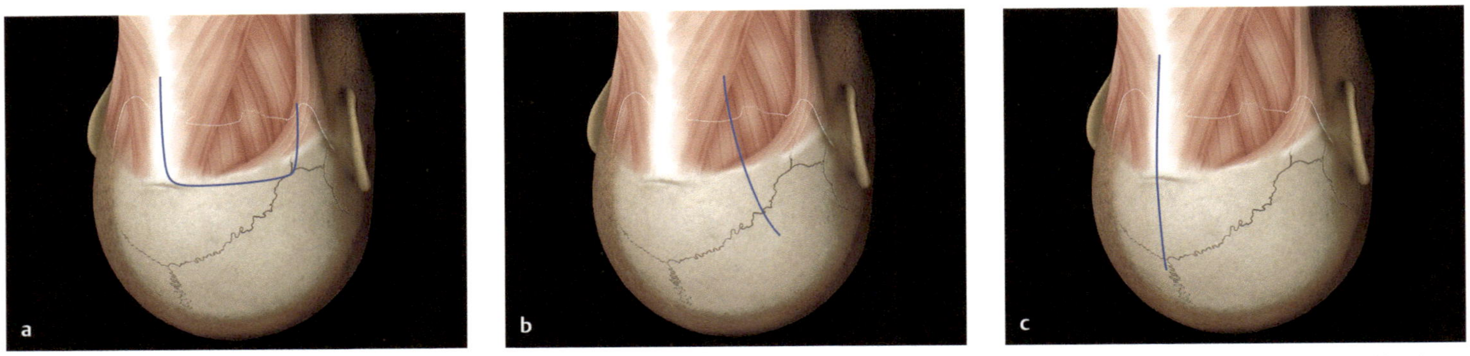

Fig. 6.55 (a–c) Skin incision. In contrast to midline craniotomies or retrosigmoid exposure, the region for the far-lateral approach is covered by the complex and multilayered nuchal muscles. To expose the region between the foramen magnum and the mastoid, three variants of skin incision may be used: **(a)** hockey stick incision (further illustrated), **(b)** incision centered straight or curved, and **(c)** a long midline suboccipital skin incision.

(a) Hockey stick skin incision: We prefer a hockey stick incision, because the nuchal muscles are composed of several layers with fibers crossing in different directions. They cannot be bluntly separated and for a straight or S-type incision a retractor has to be in place; this elevates the edges of the incision and increases the distance to the surgical field. The hockey stick incision uses the two muscle-free vertical lines, which are in the midline at the level of the mastoid. When the horizontal part of the incision is made just above the nuchal line, a combined muscle–skin flap can be elevated. The incision line starts just below the spinous process of C2, and follows the midline, curving in a horizontal direction above the inion and the superior nuchal line toward the region of the asterion. It then curves toward the mastoid process ending just below it.

(b) A linear or S-type skin incision: It is centered above the planned craniotomy, between the mastoid and the midline, ranging from 3 cm above the nuchal line to 3 cm below the tip of the mastoid. The muscles can then sometimes be separated layer by layer, either bluntly or sharply. Injury to the occipital artery and the greater occipital nerve may occur, especially when the incision is made more laterally. Placing it more medially will locate it above the nuchal muscles where the diameter is thickest. Therefore, incision may start at the superior edge more medially, and curve more laterally at the lower end. The advantage is a smaller incision, whereas the disadvantages are a much more difficult orientation, more muscle damage, and a deeper surgical situs when working through this muscle tunnel. The pressure of retraction must be checked to avoid muscle damage. Image guidance is always helpful when using this approach, especially when this straight and centered skin incision is used.

(c) Midline incision: Particularly when only minimal laterality is required, a larger but standard suboccipital midline incision may be sufficient. In the region of the foramen magnum and the suboccipital bone, the muscles are detached to the side of approach and a self-retaining retractor is placed. This is the least invasive variant; however, it should only be used with a supra- or retrocondylar approach for small anterolaterally situated lesions above the condyle where only a few degrees of laterality are required. The pressure of the retraction must be checked to avoid muscle damage.

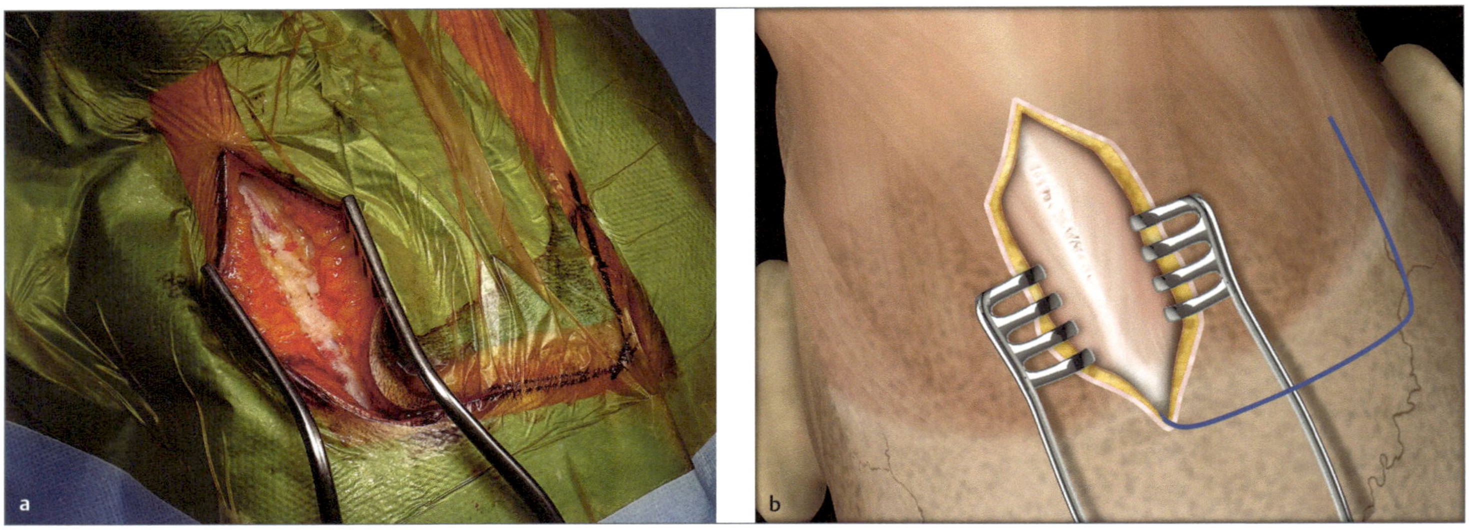

Fig. 6.56 (a, b) Hockey stick incision: midline incision along the ligamentum nuchae. We usually start with the midline incision. This makes it easier to stay in the muscle-free plane of the ligamentum nuchae along from the spinous process C2 to above the linea nuchae superior where the superficial layer of the nuchal muscles is attached.

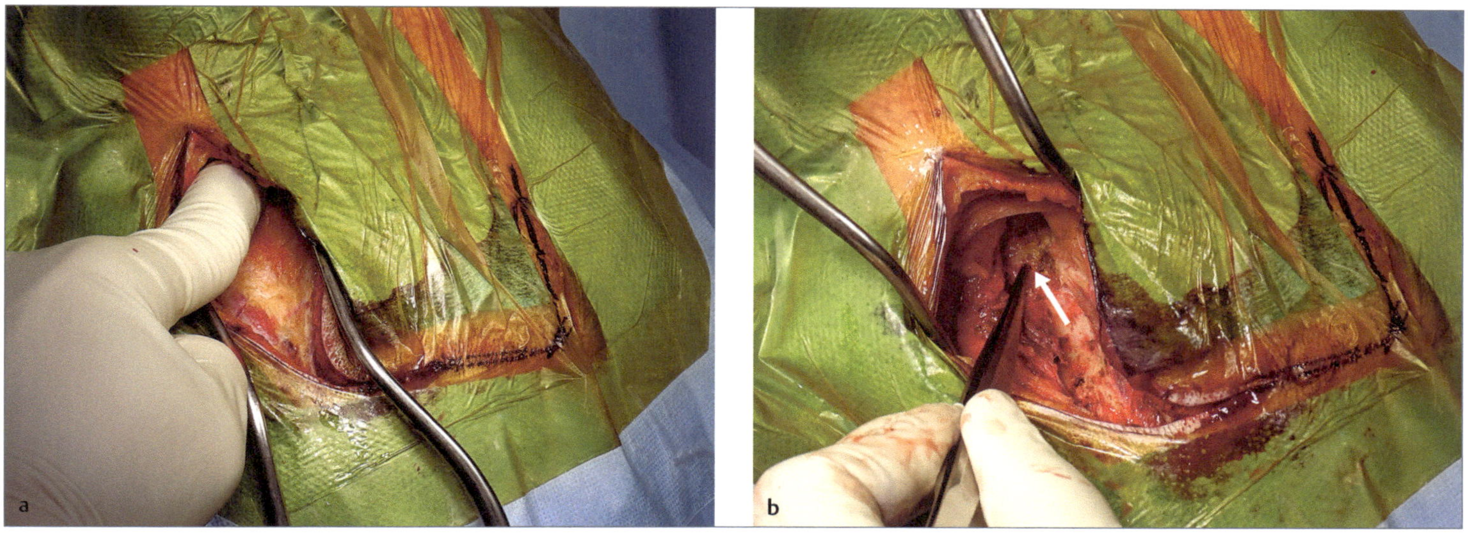

Fig. 6.57 (a, b) Exposure of C1 in the midline. The prominent spinous process of C2 serves as a landmark for the lower edge of the exposure and can be palpated at the lower edge of the incision. The arch of C1 is palpated superiorly to C2. The occipital bone and the arch of C1 (*arrow*) with the atlanto-occipital membrane is exposed in the midline.

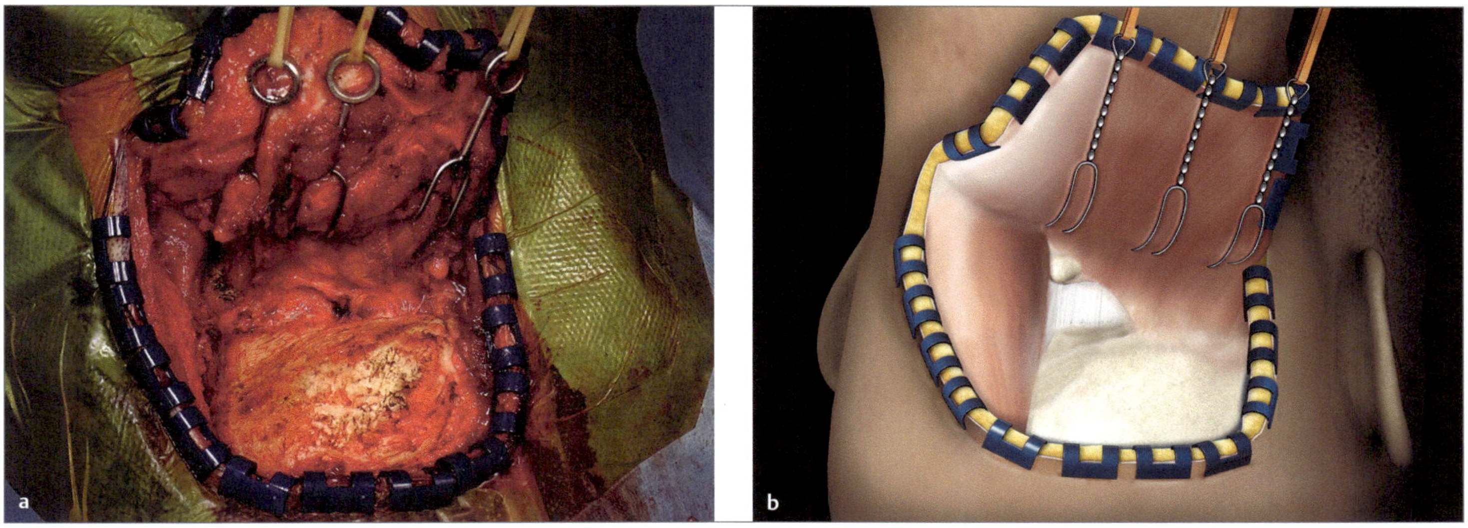

Fig. 6.58 (a, b) Elevation of the combined skin–muscle flap and exposure of the suboccipital region. The entire muscle package is sharply detached from the suboccipital region and the lineae nuchae and reflected inferiorly. Instead of detaching the muscles entirely from the nuchal line, a muscle cuff can be left for attachment of the muscles at closure. After detachment of the muscles and downward reflection of the musculocutaneous cuff, the lateral suboccipital region, the base of the mastoid process, the spinous process of C2, and the arch of C1 are exposed. The soft tissue covering the lateral arch of C1 is left untouched and further exposure of C1 is performed under the microscope.

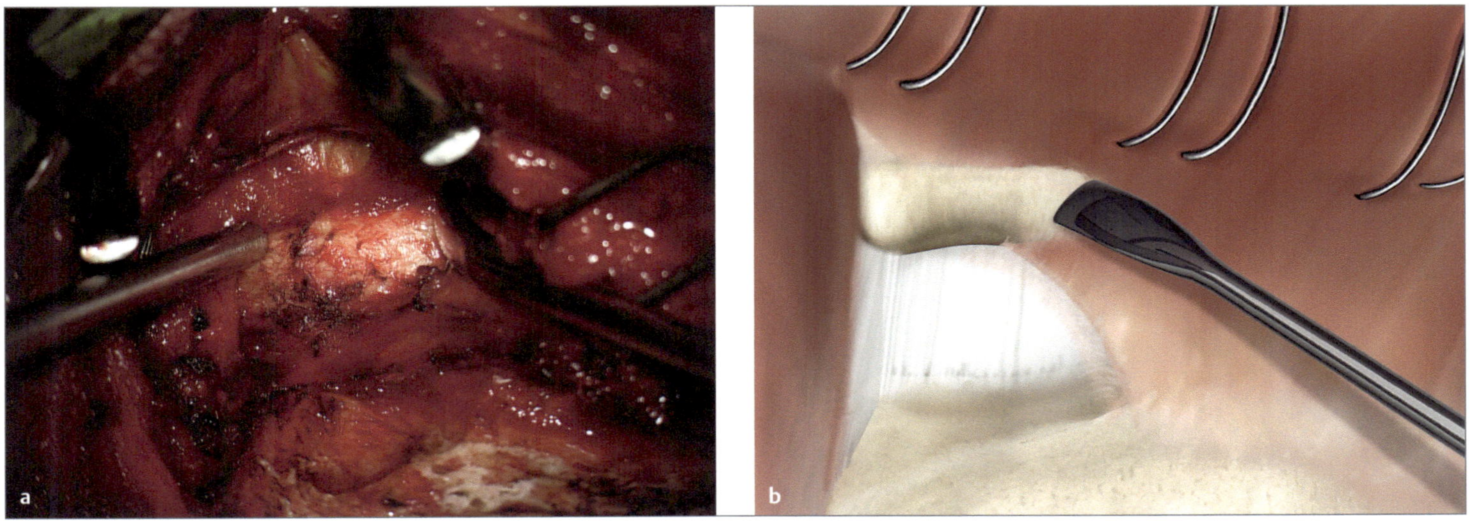

Fig. 6.59 (a, b) Dissection at C1. Using the surgical microscope, the soft tissue at the lateral C1 arch is detached subperiosteally from medial to lateral using a sharp rasp. The arch of C1 is followed from medial to lateral starting at the inferior side of the arch of C1. The sulcus arteriosus is located at the superior side of the C1 arch, which marks the medial edge of the vertebral artery (VA). Be aware that the VA may follow an aberrant course more medially (but almost always at the superior side of the arch). Therefore, dissection of the muscle and soft tissue between the foramen magnum and the arch of C1 is best performed under magnification using the microscope.

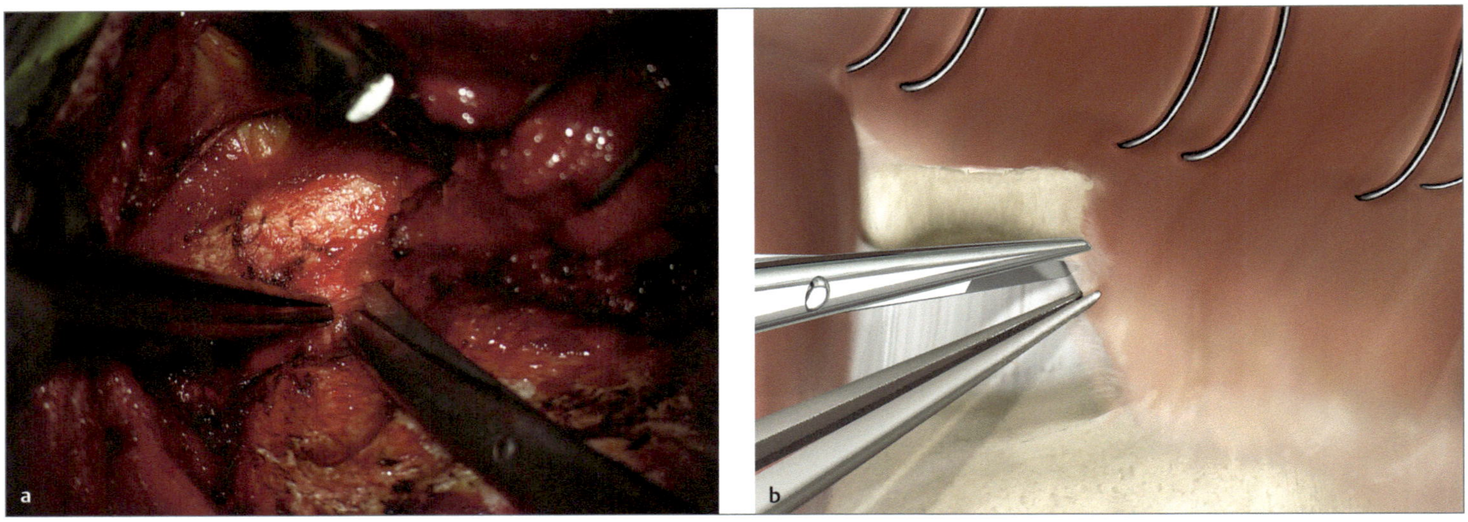

Fig. 6.60 (a, b) Dissecting the tissue from the C0-C1 interspace from medially to laterally. Using forceps and scissors, the visualized layer of tissue that attaches to the C0–C1 interspace can be dissected, separated, and incised millimeter by millimeter from medial to lateral. In many cases, the VA can be palpated or visualized. Usually, bleeding from the surrounding venous plexus of the VA indicates its vicinity. Care has to be taken not to tighten the tissue with fish hooks or the retractor. This stretches the wall of the VA and makes identification much more difficult. Therefore, the retractors should rather be loosened. A more medial VA course can be visualized before removing the arch of C1. If the course is more lateral, the artery is often encountered after removal of the arch of C1.

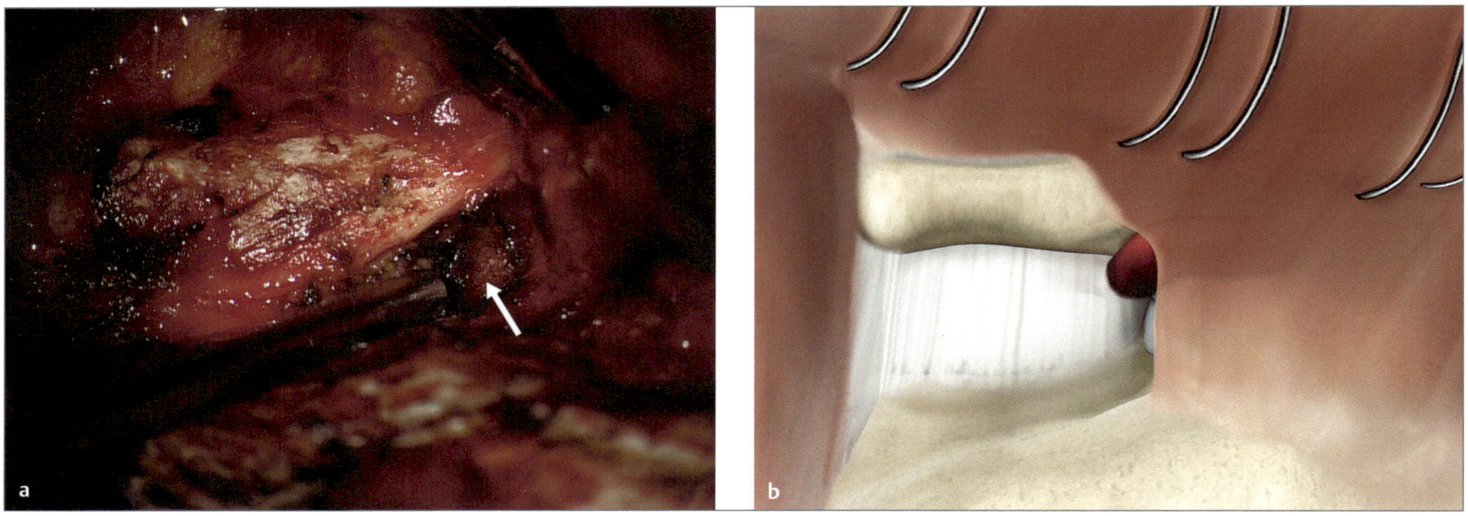

Fig. 6.61 (a, b) Visualization of the vertebral artery before removal of the left arch of C1. The VA runs from the foramen transversarium at C1 toward the lateral atlanto-occipital membrane and penetrates this membrane medial to the atlanto-occipital joint at the level of the C1 arch. The VA is usually located at the superior side in the arterial sulcus of the arch close to its connection to the lateral mass of C1. In some patients, the artery (*arrow*) can be easily identified before removal of the C1 arch. In others, it is hidden behind the lateral C1 arch.

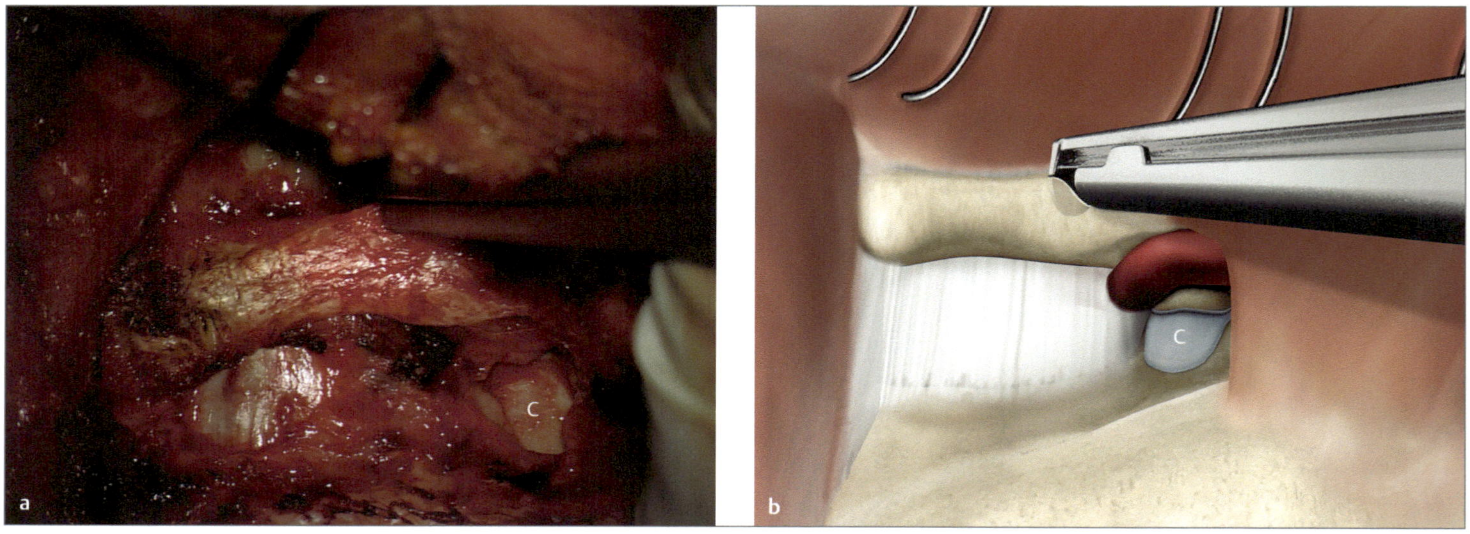

Fig. 6.62 (a, b) Removal of the C1 arch. After exposing the lateral C1 arch and making sure that the VA is identified or absent from the area of the planned hemilaminectomy, the bone is removed using a rongeur or the footplate of the craniotome. The lamina of C1 is removed to allow opening of the dura below the foramen magnum. C, occipital condyle.

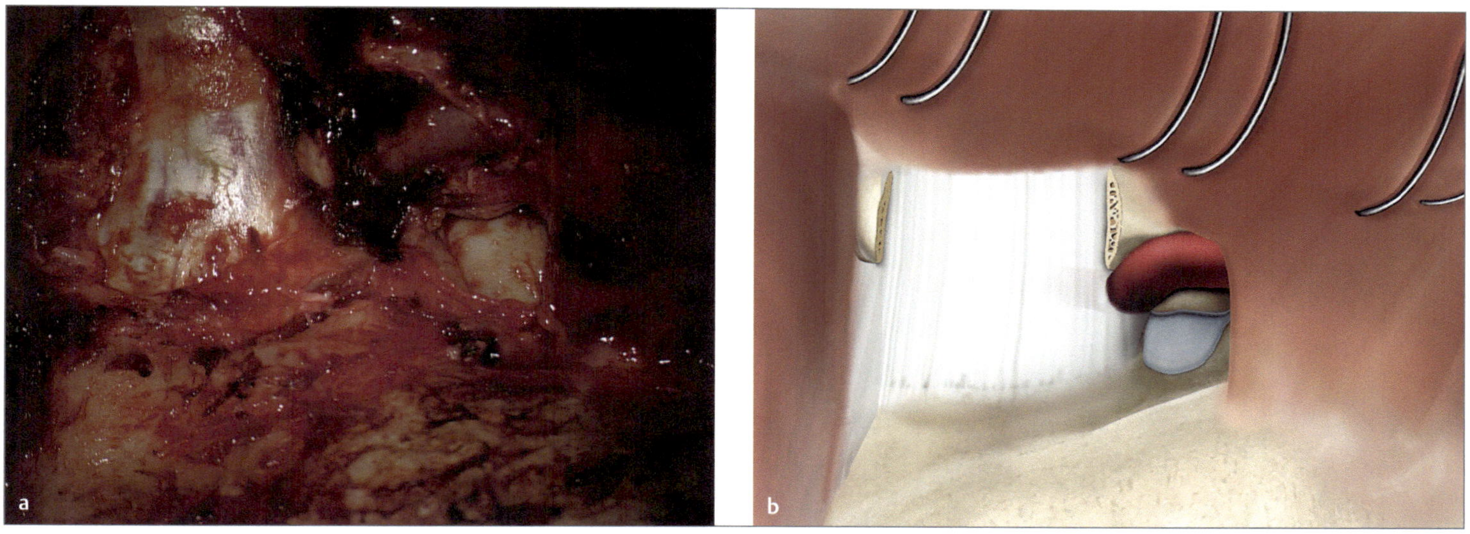

Fig. 6.63 (a, b) Visualization of the vertebral artery after removal of the left arch of C1. Although not required in most cases, the VA can often be visualized after removal of the hemilamina of C1. Bleeding from the venous plexus, which accompanies the VA, is controlled using Gelfoam powder, Gelfoam with fibrin glue or oxycellulose, or a similar hemostypticum.

Although often described in the literature as an important step in the far-lateral approach, there is no need to skeletonize the VA except when proximal extradural control is required.

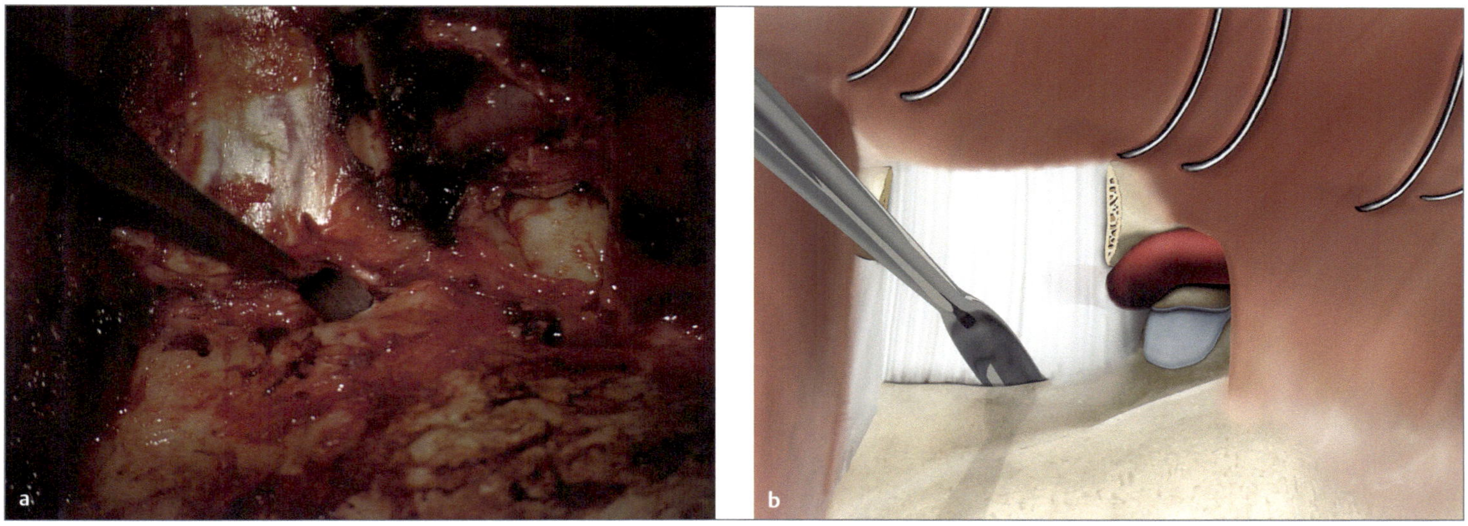

Fig. 6.64 (a, b) Detaching the endosteal dura layer from the bone at the foramen magnum. The outer, endosteal, layer of the dura is tightly attached to the foramen magnum. Before opening the foramen, the dura should be detached with a sharp rasp, subperiosteally around the foramen magnum.

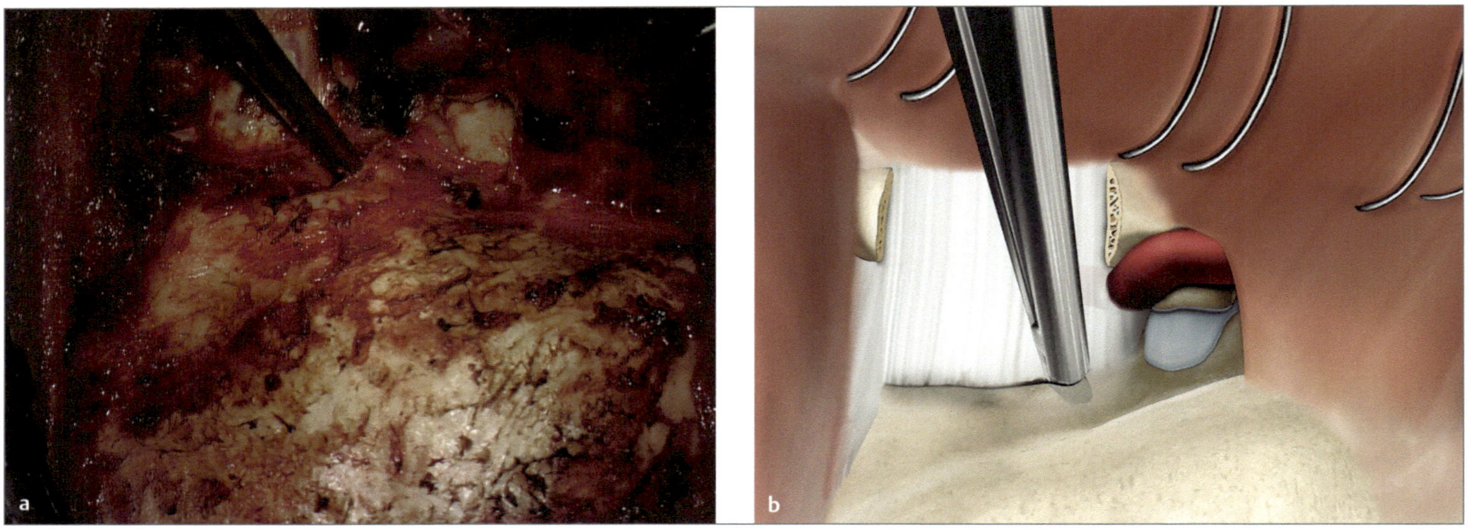

Fig. 6.65 (a, b) Preparing the foramen magnum for craniotomy. After detaching the endosteal layer from the bone at the foramen magnum, a Kerrison rongeur can be used to cross the lip of the foramen at the lateral and the medial side of the planned flap until the normal dura is reached. The craniotome can then be inserted into one of these grooves. Alternatively, a drill can be used to facilitate crossing the lip of the foramen magnum with the craniotome.

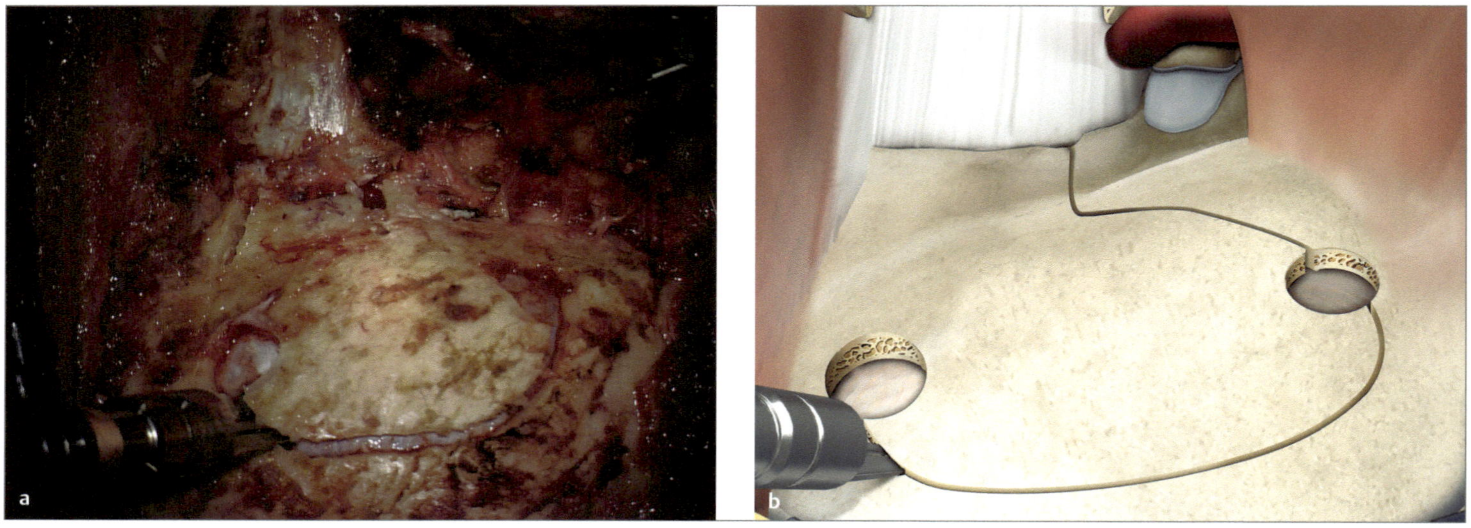

Fig. 6.66 (a, b) Craniotomy. In this example, two burr holes were made. The craniotomy can either start there or may start and end directly at the foramen magnum without the need for burr holes. The lateral edge of the craniotomy can best be found in a superolateral to an inferomedial direction when feeling the curvature of the infratentorial bone toward the base. Medially, there is usually no need to cross the midline. As usual, image guidance helps to determine the ideal line and the size of the craniotomy.

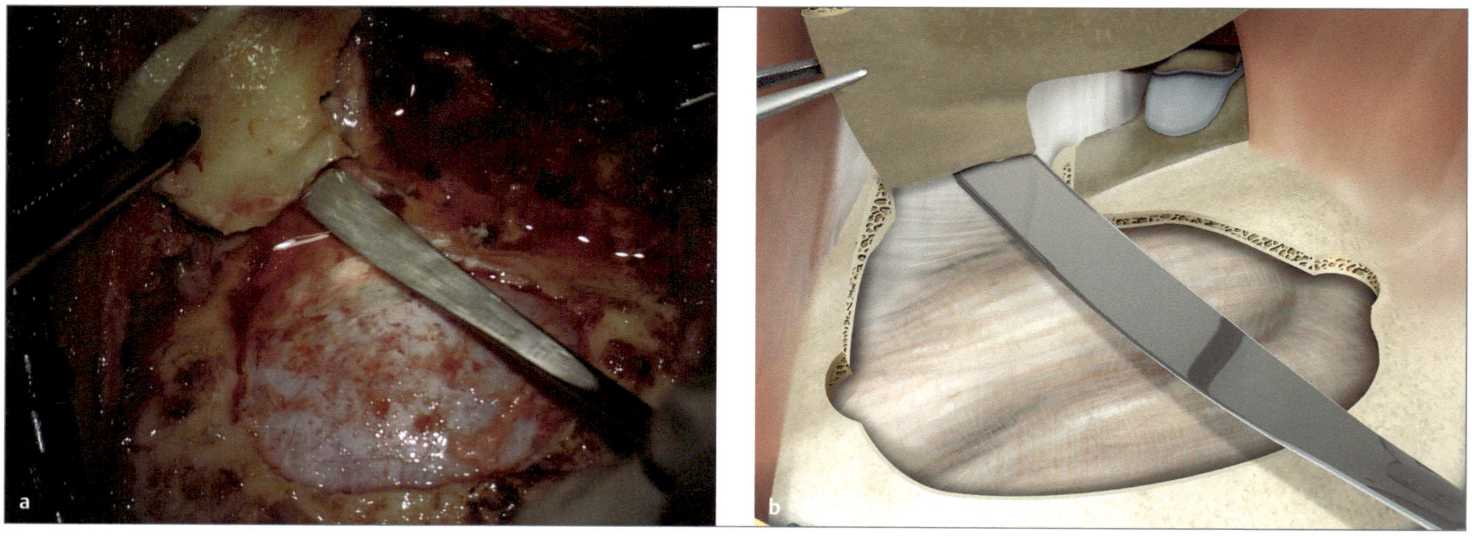

Fig. 6.67 (a, b) Lifting the bone flap. The bone flap usually adheres to the dura at the foramen magnum and needs to be sharply detached.

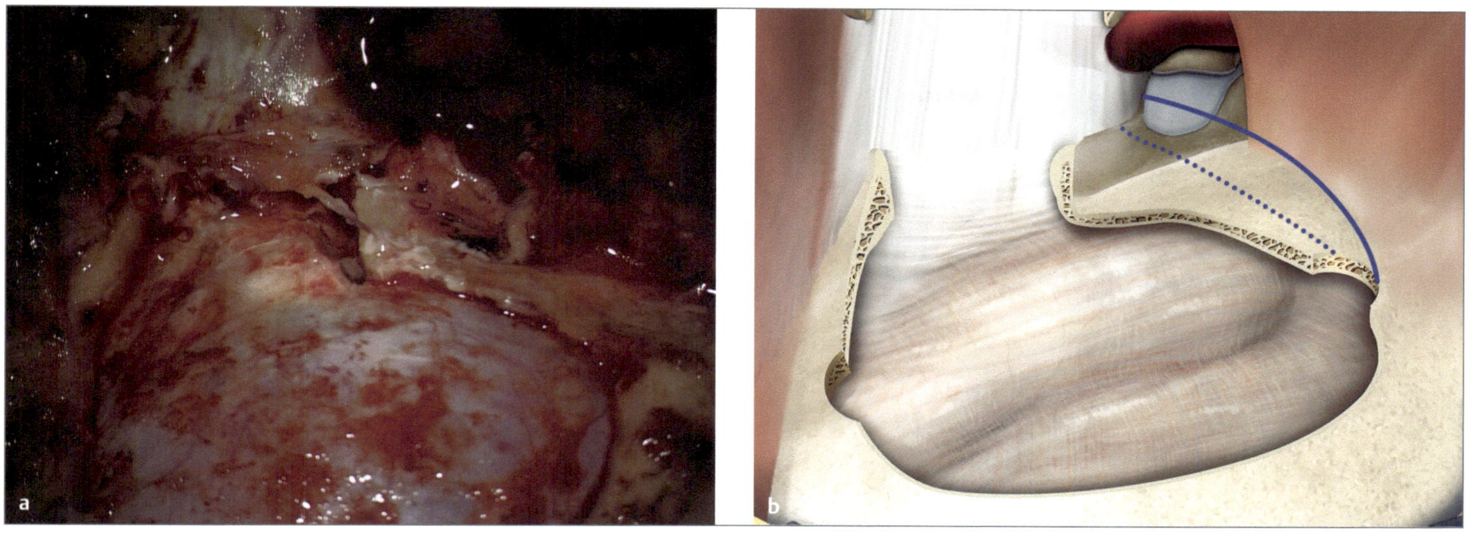

Fig. 6.68 (a, b) Drilling for the far "enough" lateral approach. After lifting the flap, the bony edge at the lateral foramen magnum can be seen as the obvious obstruction to reverting the opened dura laterally and to reaching the area anterolateral to the brainstem. The *dotted lines* indicate where further drilling is required—for the far "enough" lateral extension (*dotted line*), up to a partially transcondylar extension (*solid line*) resecting the superomedial aspect of the condylus.

How much bone needs to be removed at the lateral foramen magnum, the suboccipital bone, the condylar fossa, and the condyle depends on the lesion. Again, image guidance is very helpful. For the supracondylar approach, drilling only needs to complete bone removal flush to the lateral spinal canal without drilling the condyle (*dotted line*). Depending on the target, extra- or intradural drilling of a prominent tuberculum jugulare may also be necessary. In a partially transcondylar approach, the medial and/or superior occipital condyle is removed.

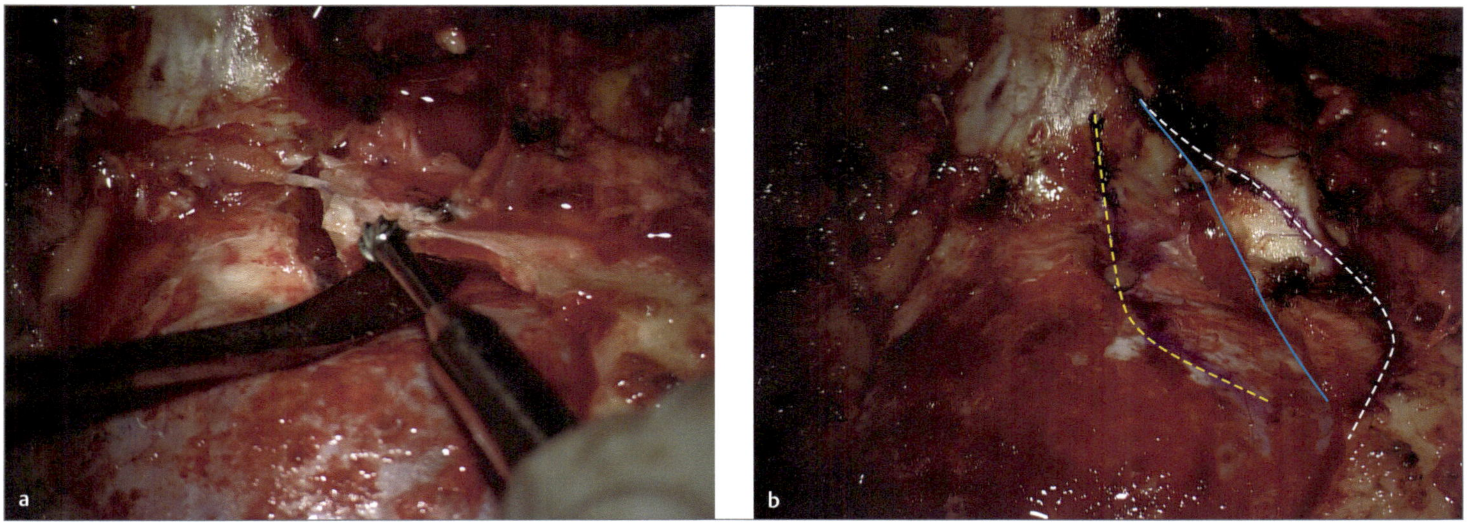

Fig. 6.69 (a, b) Bone removal for the retrocondylar and supracondylar approach. The dura is detached from the bone and drilling is performed using cutting and then diamond drills. The direction of drilling is toward the superior and median edge of the occipital condyle. ▸Fig. 6.71b shows the situs after completion of drilling for the far "enough" lateral approach. The *yellow dotted line* on the left shows the edge of the craniotomy before and the *blue line* after drilling. If a more lateral approach is needed, the medial and superior part of the condyle (transcondylar extension) and more bone at the occiput can be removed (*white dotted line*). For access to the anterior or anterolateral area of the foramen magnum and clivus, the dura can be opened slightly paramedian at the ipsilateral side. A prominent tuberculum jugulare can also be drilled intradurally, similarly to the intradural tailored drilling of the anterior clinoid process.

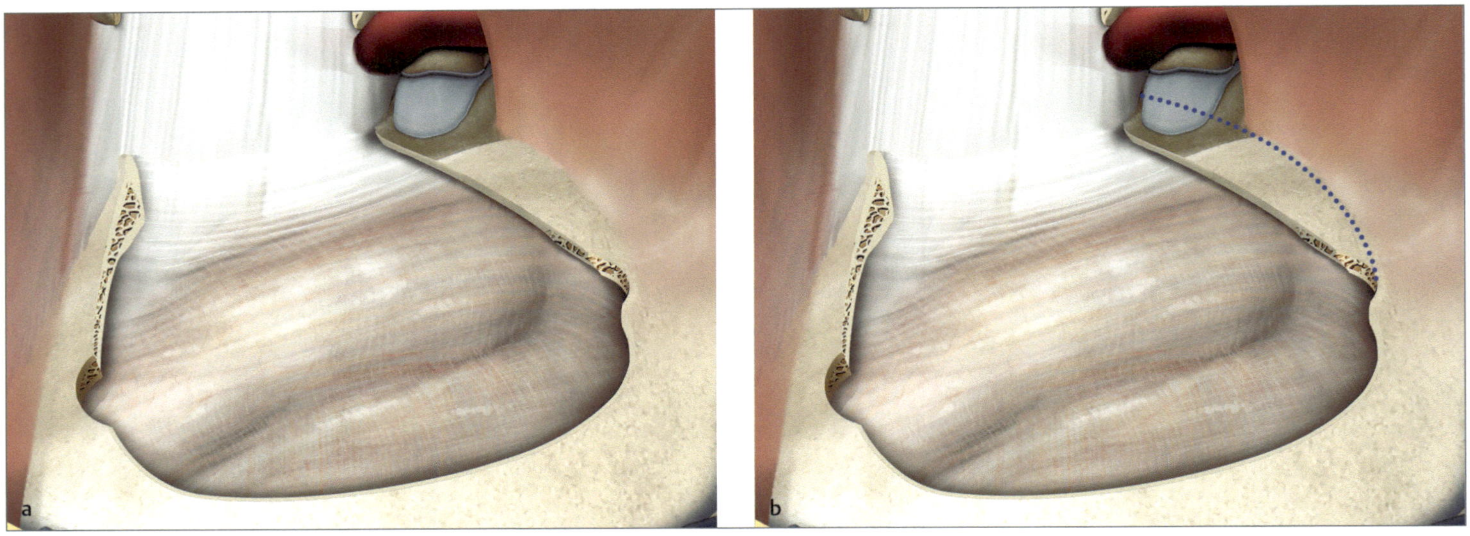

Fig. 6.70 (a, b) Bone removal for the retro- and supracondylar approach before and after drilling. These illustrations show schematically the extent of bone removal before **(a)** and after drilling **(b)** for the retro- and supracondylar approach. The *dotted line* illustrates the area of additional drilling for the partially transcondylar extension. If the surgeon is not sure whether the exposure is sufficient, opening the dura helps to decide whether the drilling and far-lateral extension need to be continued. Flipping the dura back and forth allows tailoring of the drilling.

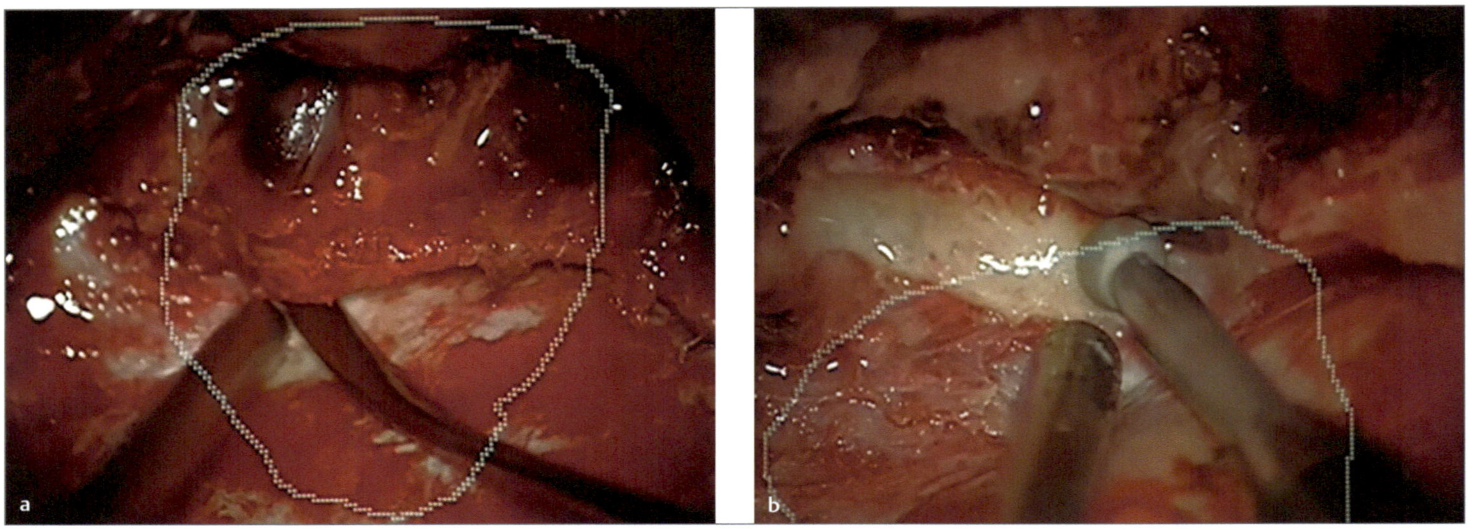

Fig. 6.71 (a, b) Tailored drilling using image guidance. Alternatively, image guidance, especially with microscope image injection of the contour of the target, can be used to tailor and minimize the drilling required, as demonstrated in these two images.

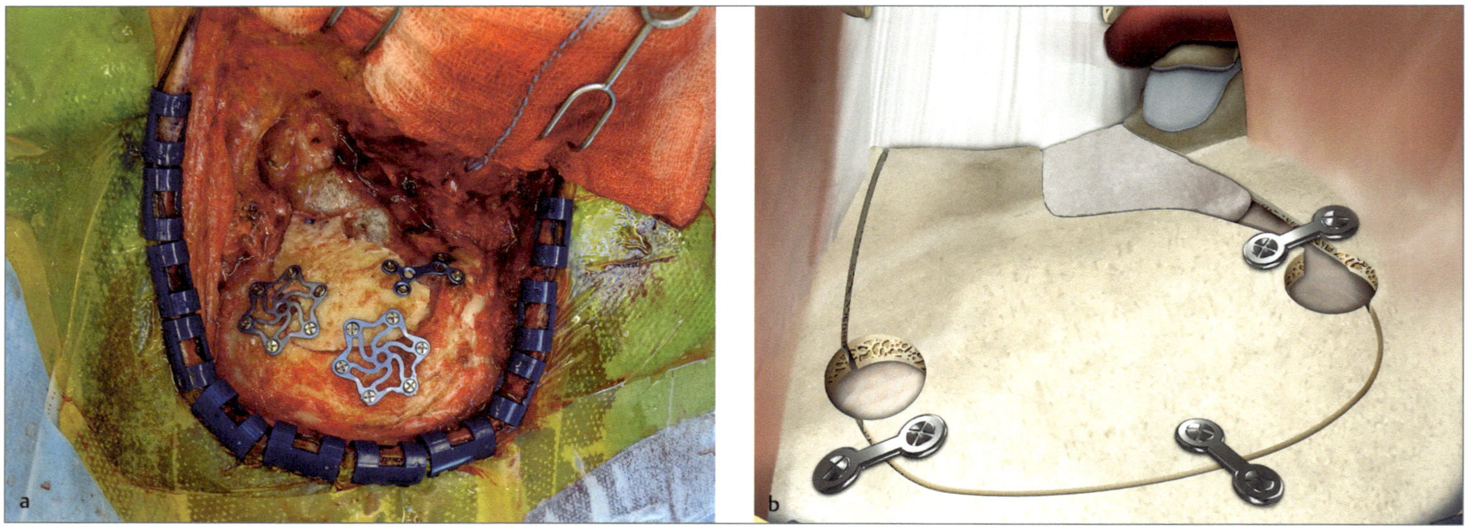

Fig. 6.72 (a, b) Dural suture, reinsertion of the bone flap, and wound closing. Watertight suturing of the dura is achieved by primary closure or using a patch such as lyophilized pericardium. We have found that a TachoSil sponge provides very good sealing and prevention of cerebrospinal fluid fistulas in critical places, such as the craniocervical junction, when covering the primary suture. The bone flap is reinserted using mini-plates or fixation caps.

The combined musculocutaneous flap is turned back. As mentioned at the beginning of the chapter, suturing the muscle and fascia back to a cuff that has been left below the linea nuchae during opening greatly facilitates tight muscle approximation. In the midline, the nuchal fascia is reattached to the contralateral side with slightly angled, single-stitched sutures that pull the tissue up. Then the galea is reattached and the skin is closed.

Checklist

- Mark the landmarks with a pencil to maintain correct orientation. Keep the orientation of the midline, the inion, the mastoid, and the spinous process of C2 after draping. Ideally, use image guidance.
- The hockey stick skin incision should be above the nuchal line where the nuchal muscles attach. Laterally and inferiorly, it should extend to the incisura mastoidea.
- Follow the midline in the muscle-free plane of the nuchal ligament.
- Feel the spinous process of C2. Continue incision and dissection in the midline and feel the arch of C1.
- Complete skin incision and lift the skin–muscle block.
- Dissect medially to laterally at the lamina of C1. Use sharp dissection and alternate between tension and relaxation of tissue to expose the arch of C1 and to identify an aberrant course of the vertebral artery.
- Detach the dura around the foramen magnum before craniotomy.
- Open the lip of the foramen magnum with the Kerrison rongeur to facilitate insertion of the craniotome.
- After craniotomy, detach the dura laterally and drill the bone.
- For better tailoring of the drilling, open the dura, check the line of intradural approach required to reach the target, and flip it back. Then continue drilling.

Further Readings

Nanda A, Vincent DA, Vannemreddy PS, Baskaya MK, Chanda A. Far-lateral approach to intradural lesions of the foramen magnum without resection of the occipital condyle. J Neurosurg 2002;96(2):302–309

Salas E, Sekhar LN, Ziyal IM, Caputy AJ, Wright DC. Variations of the extreme-lateral craniocervical approach: anatomical study and clinical analysis of 69 patients. J Neurosurg 1999;90(2, Suppl):206–219

Spektor S, Anderson GJ, McMenomey SO, Horgan MA, Kellogg JX, Delashaw JB Jr. Quantitative description of the far-lateral transcondylar transtubercular approach to the foramen magnum and clivus. J Neurosurg 2000;92(5):824–831

Seoane P, Kalb S, Clark JC, et al. Far-lateral approach without drilling the occipital condyle for vertebral artery-posterior inferior cerebellar artery aneurysms. Neurosurgery 2017;81(2):268–274

Lanzino G, Paolini S, Spetzler RF. Far-lateral approach to the craniocervical junction. Neurosurgery 2005;57(4, Suppl):367–371, discussion 367–371

Heros RC. Lateral suboccipital approach for vertebral and vertebrobasilar artery lesions. J Neurosurg 1986;64(4):559–562

Spetzler RF, Grahm TW. The far-lateral approach to the inferior clivus and the upper cervical region: technical note. Barrow Neurol Inst Q 1990;6:35–38

7 Transsphenoidal Approach

7.1 Microsurgical Endonasal Approach

Christian F. Freyschlag and Claudius Thomé

Introduction

Modern pituitary surgery using a transsphenoidal approach is relatively noninvasive, as it utilizes the nasal passages and regular sinus anatomy to reach the sella. Successful treatment requires the surgeon to navigate to the sella and visualize the lesion through a relatively narrow corridor with minimal damage to the surrounding tissues (sinonasal anatomy, nonadenomatous pituitary), while removing the tumor as completely as possible. Thus, a profound knowledge of the nasal anatomy and its variations is crucial.

Imaging

Imaging consists of MRI with a focus on sellar pathologies, including T1 sequences in three planes (axial, coronal, sagittal) with and without contrast enhancement. Additionally, dynamic contrast sequences should be obtained in cases of microadenomas. Individual anatomy has to be analyzed in every case, including size and location of the sphenoid sinus, its septations, the carotid arteries, and the attachment of the nasal septum to the anterior wall of the sphenoid sinus.

Particularly for less experienced transsphenoidal surgeons, intraoperative fluoroscopy and/or neuronavigation may be helpful and can prevent a too superiorly located approach toward the sphenoid plane and the risk of cerebrospinal fluid (CSF) leakage. CT and/or image guidance is especially helpful in cases of recurrence. ▶Fig. 7.1, ▶Fig. 7.2, ▶Fig. 7.3, ▶Fig. 7.4, ▶Fig. 7.5, ▶Fig. 7.6, ▶Fig. 7.7, ▶Fig. 7.8, ▶Fig. 7.9, ▶Fig. 7.10, ▶Fig. 7.11, ▶Fig. 7.12, and ▶Fig. 7.13).

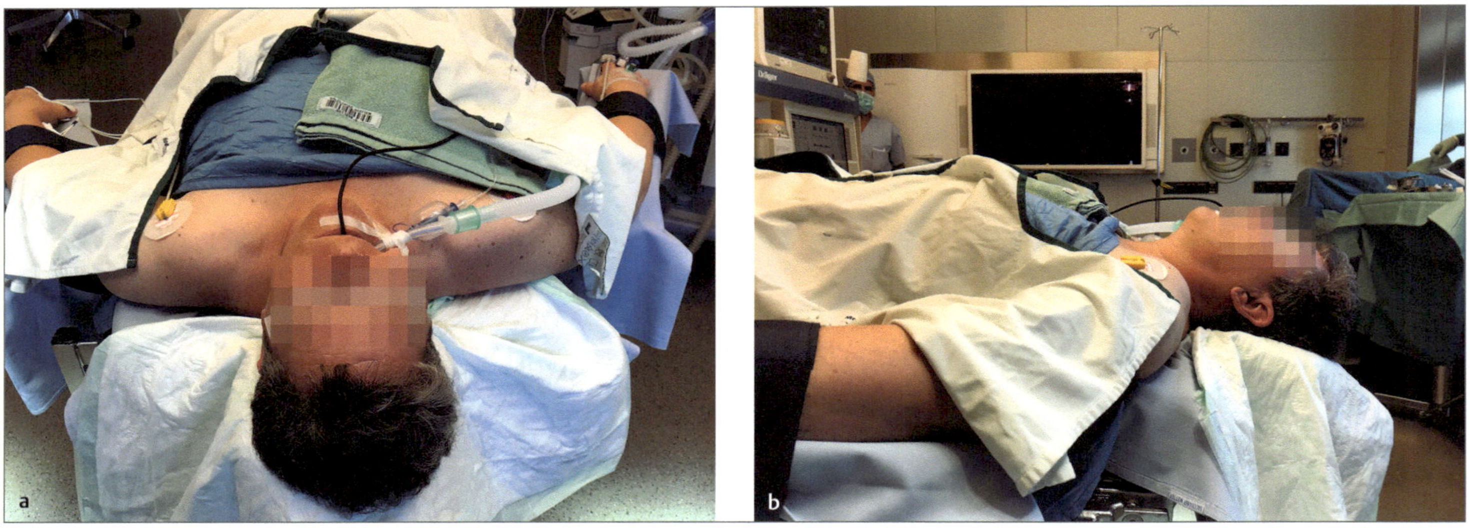

Fig. 7.1 (a, b) Positioning and draping. A patient undergoing microsurgical, endonasal transsphenoidal surgery is positioned strictly supine. It is recommended not to turn the head, which is placed in a horseshoe (or equivalent) and reclined slightly to achieve a vertical approach to the sella. The plane of the table is tilted to raise the level of the patient's head above her/his heart, in order to reduce venous bleeding. The surgeon's position is straight behind the patient, as for most cranial procedures.

In our department, draping (with a nontransparent drape) leaves only the nose uncovered. Different draping methods are possible, many of which leave the patient's face cleaned and at least partly uncovered (usual in ENT rhinosurgery, which allows intraoperative access to the eyes).

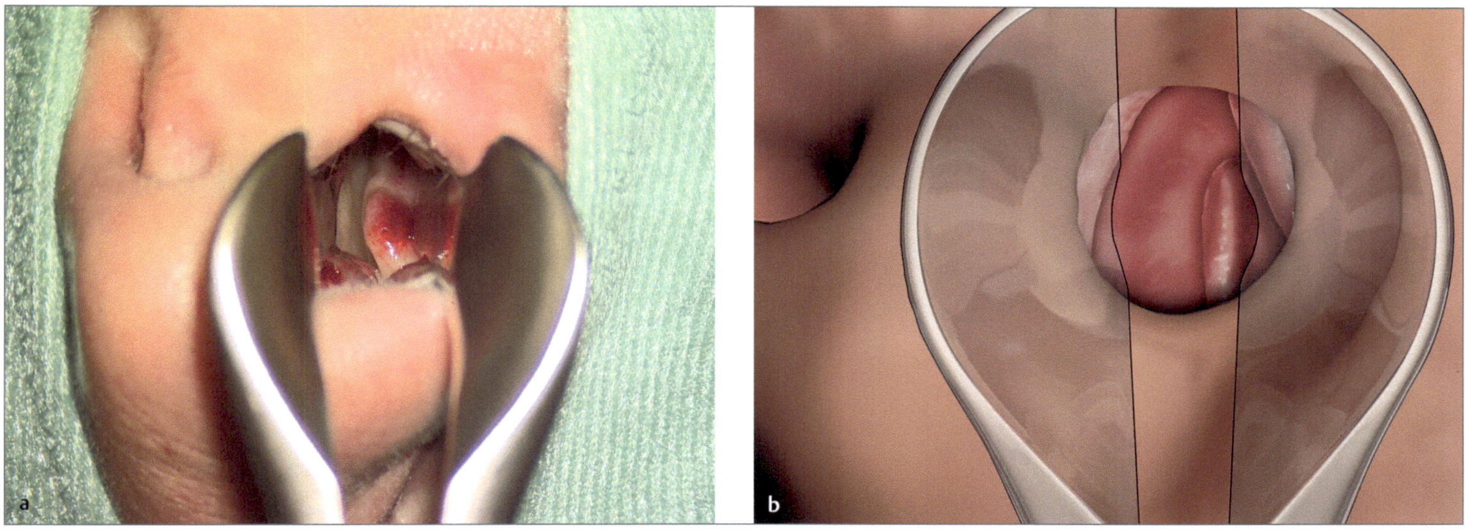

Fig. 7.2 (a, b) Nasal inspection and lateralization of the middle turbinate. View of the patient in the supine position; the surgeon stands behind the patient's head. Right-handed surgeons usually use the right nostril for the endonasal transsphenoidal approach. As anatomical variations within the nose might mean that the other nostril should be chosen, initial inspection of both nostrils is suggested.

After inspection of the nasal cavity, the middle turbinate is identified as the landmark and is lateralized in order to gain space within the nose. The speculum can be used to mobilize and push the turbinate laterally. In the endonasal approach, the anterior sphenoid wall is directly exposed without any incision into the septal mucosa. To make sure that the orientation is correct, fluoroscopy, image guidance, or orientation via nasal anatomy can be used. The choanae can be visualized as the most inferior structure and guide the surgeon's way more cranially to the anterior sphenoid wall and to the sphenoid ostium.

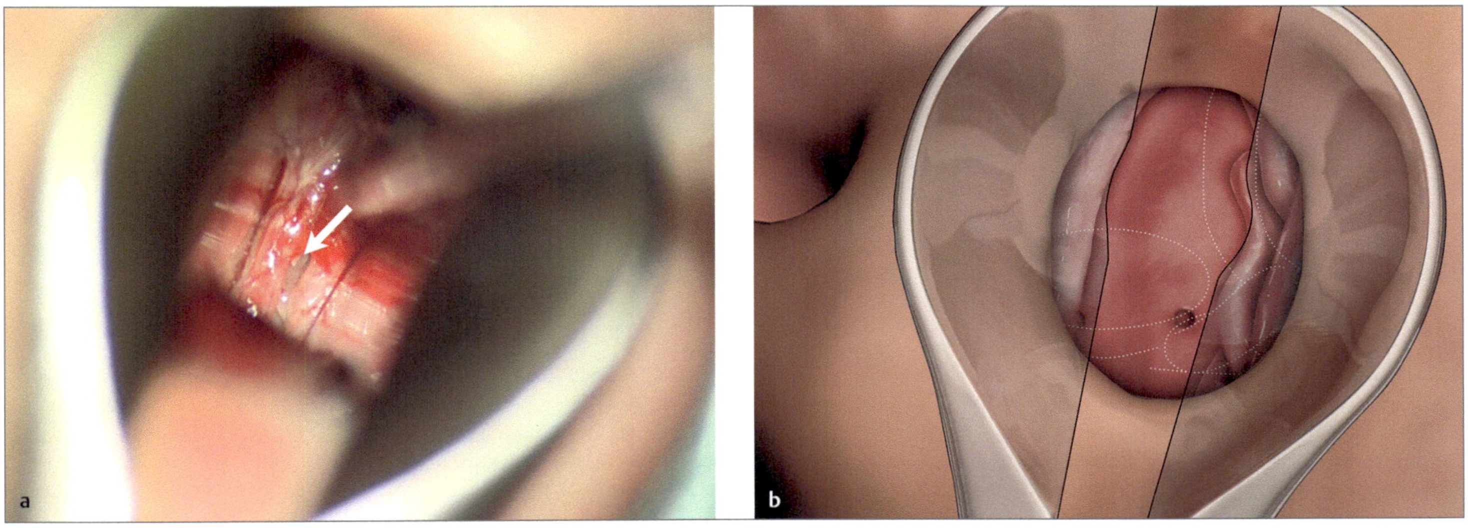

Fig. 7.3 (a, b) Identification of the sphenoid ostium. The orientation of the nasal speculum should not exceed a 20° angle to the bony palate. At the level of the middle turbinate, the sphenoid ostium (marked with an *arrow*) can be found and inspected. After definitive identification of the right sphenoid ostium, the mucosal dissection is carried on from the ostium in a caudal direction, including coagulation of the septal mucosal membrane and identification of the cartilage and vomer.

If CSF leakage was observed during surgery, a lumbar drain is placed at the level of L4/L5 immediately after surgery and kept in place for 3 to 5 days. A daily drainage of 120-mL CSF is recommended.

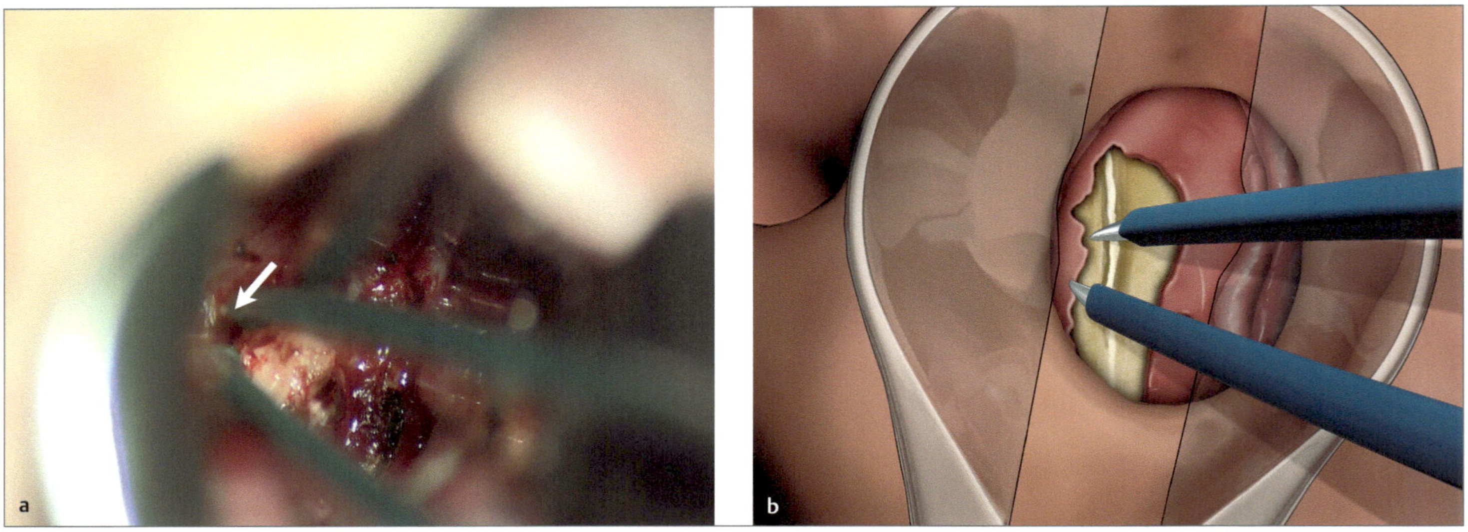

Fig. 7.4 (a, b) Mobilization of the nasal septum. As the septum is now mobilized from its mucosal layer, the speculum is used to crack the posterior bone of the nasal septum to the contralateral side. This reveals the vomer, shaped like a ship's keel. Further, the contralateral sphenoid ostium becomes visible.

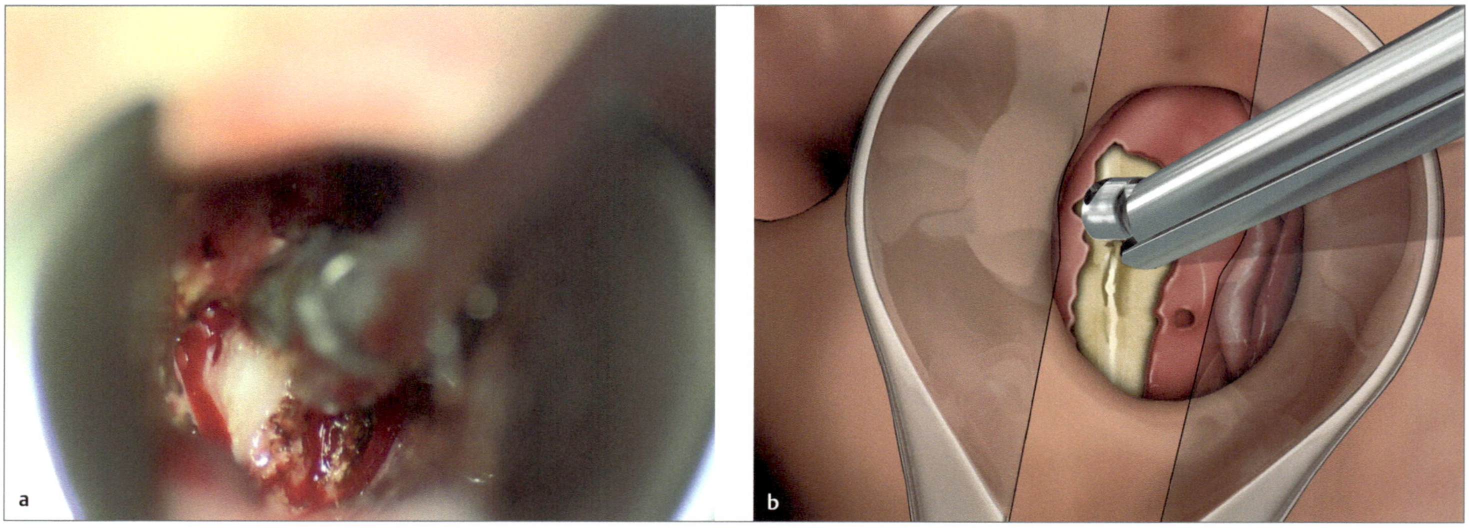

Fig. 7.5 (a, b) Partial removal of the vomer—opening the sphenoid sinus. After identification of the vomer and both sphenoid ostia, a Kerrison punch is used to combine the sphenoid ostia and remove the superior part of the vomer. Now the more lateral section of the anterior sphenoid wall is opened in a downward direction, using a Kerrison punch. After disconnection of the bony anterior sphenoid wall, the vomer is removed using Blakesley grasping forceps and kept for later reconstruction.

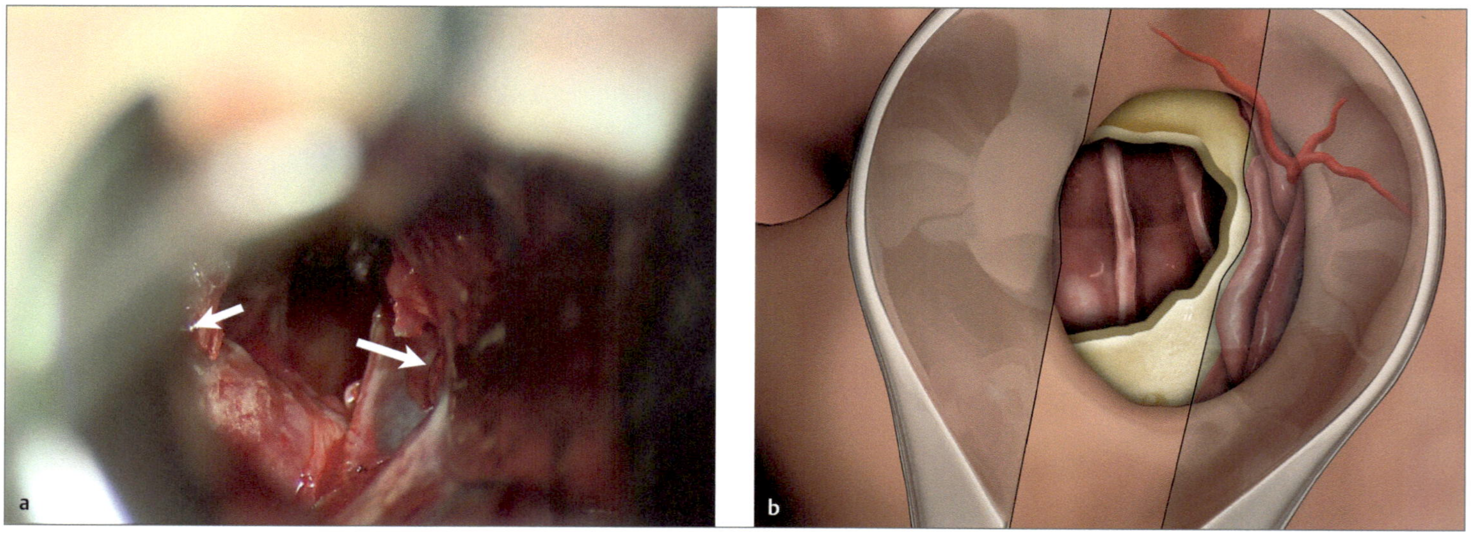

Fig. 7.6 (a, b) Lateral extension of the sphenoid opening. The approach has to be extended more laterally (*arrows*) by further resection of the anterior sphenoid wall, using different punches. Extending the approach laterally often leads to bleeding from sphenopalatine artery branches, which can be easily controlled by bipolar coagulation.

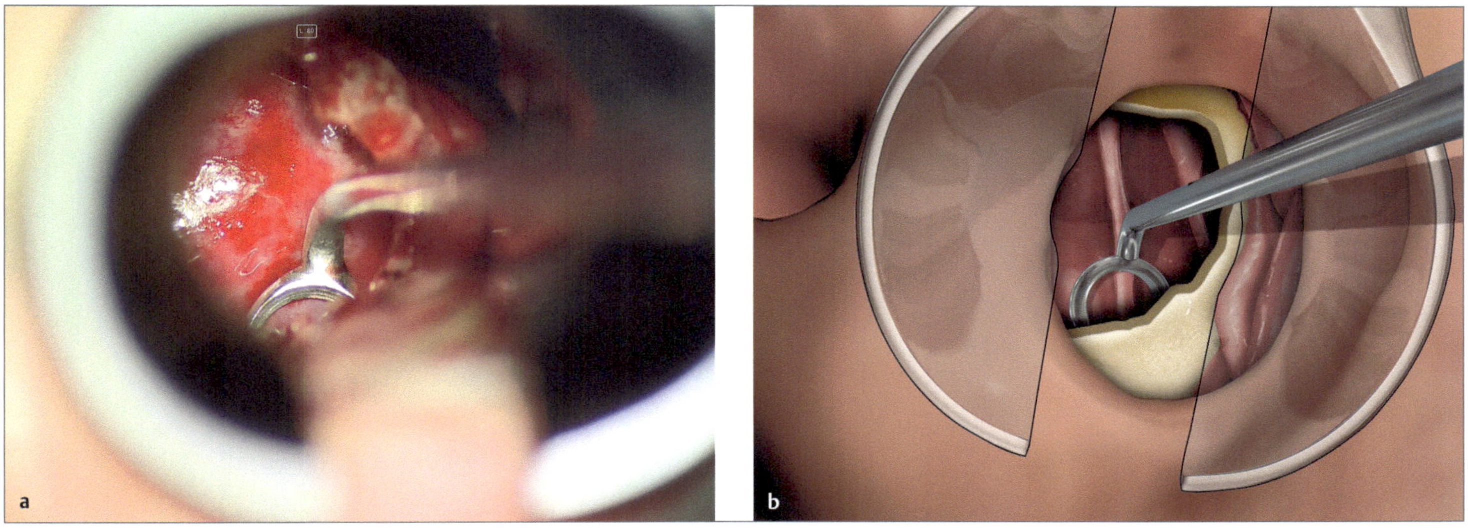

Fig. 7.7 (a, b) Superior extension of the sphenoid opening. Using standard curettes, the lateral and superior extension of the approach can be verified and extended, if necessary. This palpation secures a sufficient exposure cranially and allows identification of the tuberculum sellae in lesions with suprasellar extension.

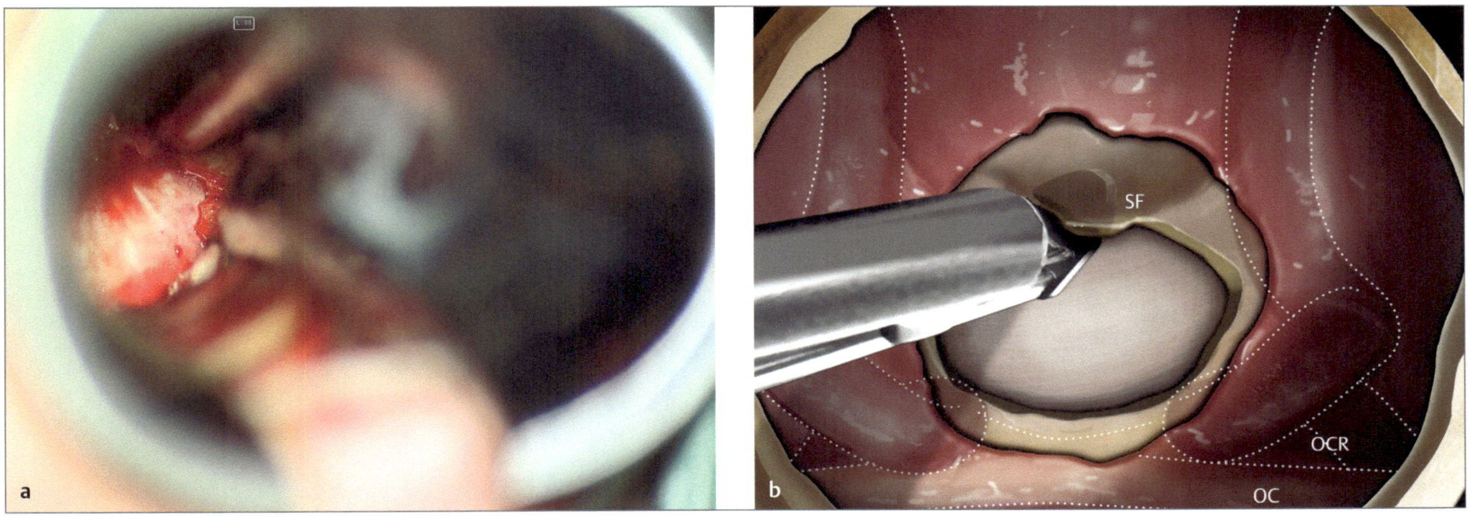

Fig. 7.8 (a, b) Removal of the sellar floor. After removal of the sphenoid mucosa, the complete floor of the sella is visualized and the bony floor can be resected with punches. Note that the opening should be tailored to the size of the adenoma. The lateral opening of the sellar floor should extend to the cavernous sinus, which can be identified by both its blueish color and often a dural ridge. The carotid artery is located just laterally. Cranially, it is recommended to leave a small bony rim to cover the dural reflection to avoid CSF leakage.

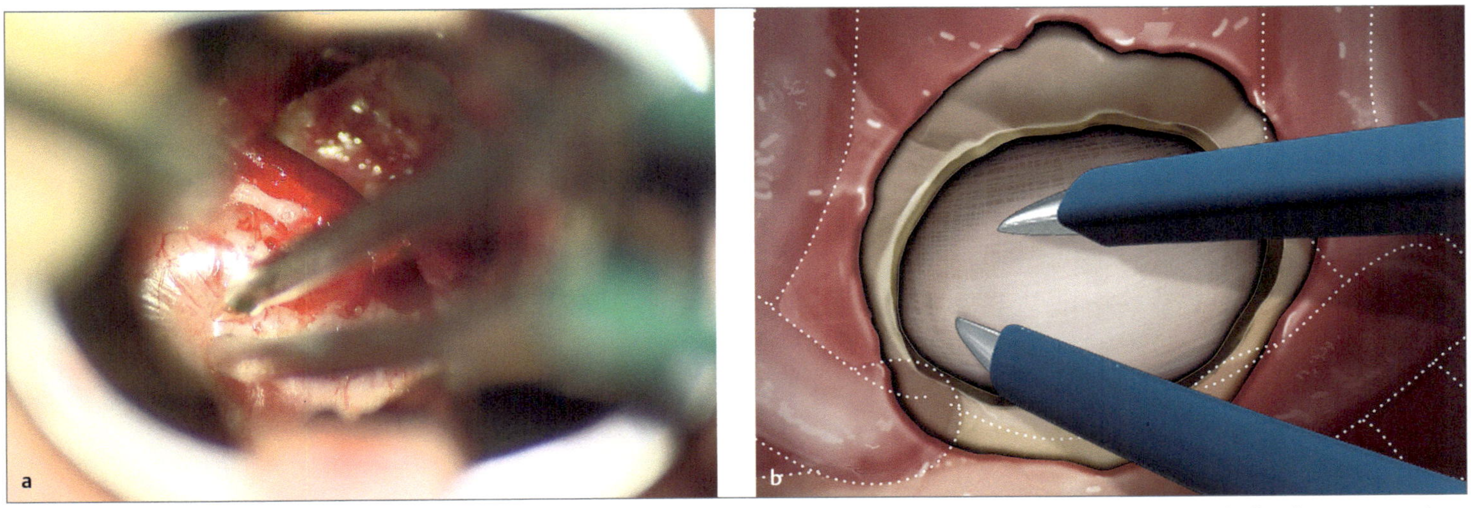

Fig. 7.9 (a, b) Opening the endosteum (dura) and removal of the adenoma. Following bipolar coagulation, the endosteum/sellar dura is opened in a cruciate fashion. Care is taken not to incise too cranially, as this may open the dural duplication anterior to the pituitary gland (CSF leakage!). Usually, the adenoma prolapses through the incision as a sign of elevated intrasellar pressure. Pulsation of the brain will push the grayish adenoma tissue toward the opening. Blunt curettes are used to dissect the tumor and anterograde movement of the instruments toward sellar structures is applied, instead of pulling in the direction of the surgeon. It is recommended to start the dissection of the adenoma inferiorly and then proceed laterally. In infiltrative tumors, the noninfiltrated side is dissected first, as opening of the cavernous sinus causes venous bleeding. To reach the more cranial portions of adenomas, various maneuvers have been applied (compression of jugular veins or saline injections to the subarachnoid space). In our experience, gentle manipulation of the adenoma and diligent dissection in tissue planes is sufficient. Sometimes, a pseudocapsule can be helpful.

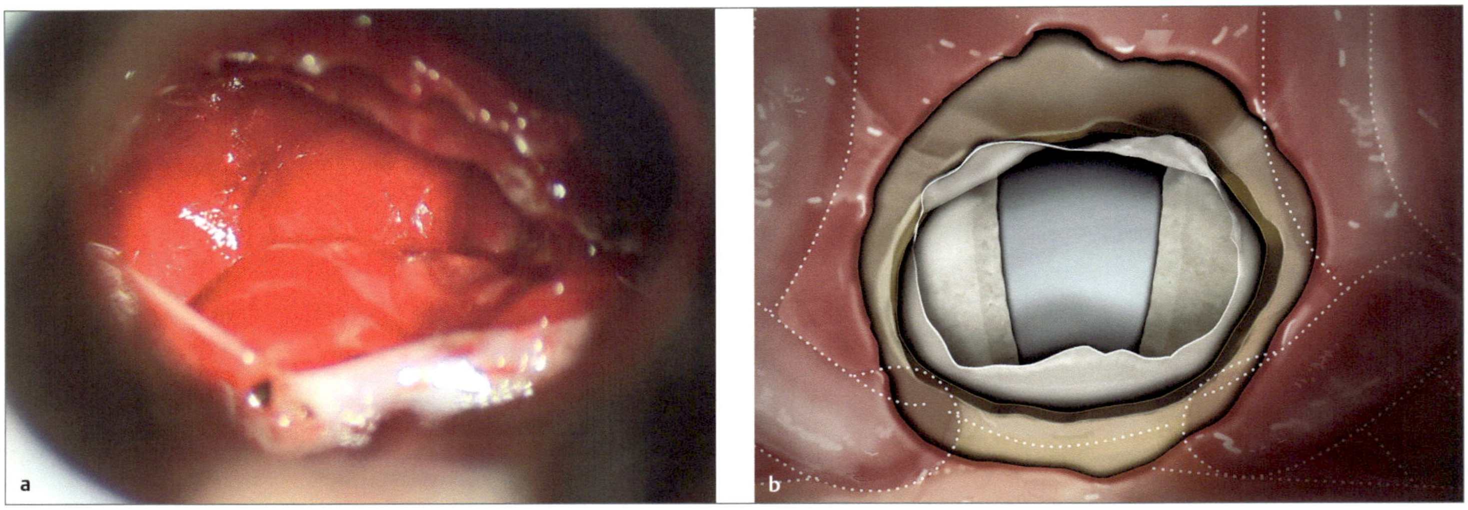

Fig. 7.10 (a, b) Hemostasis. Hemostasis can be achieved through bipolar coagulation if needed. Blood oozing from the cavernous sinus is easily stopped with small pieces of Gelfoam, placed laterally on each side of the sella. Temporary compression with cottonoids and/or elevation of the head may be required.

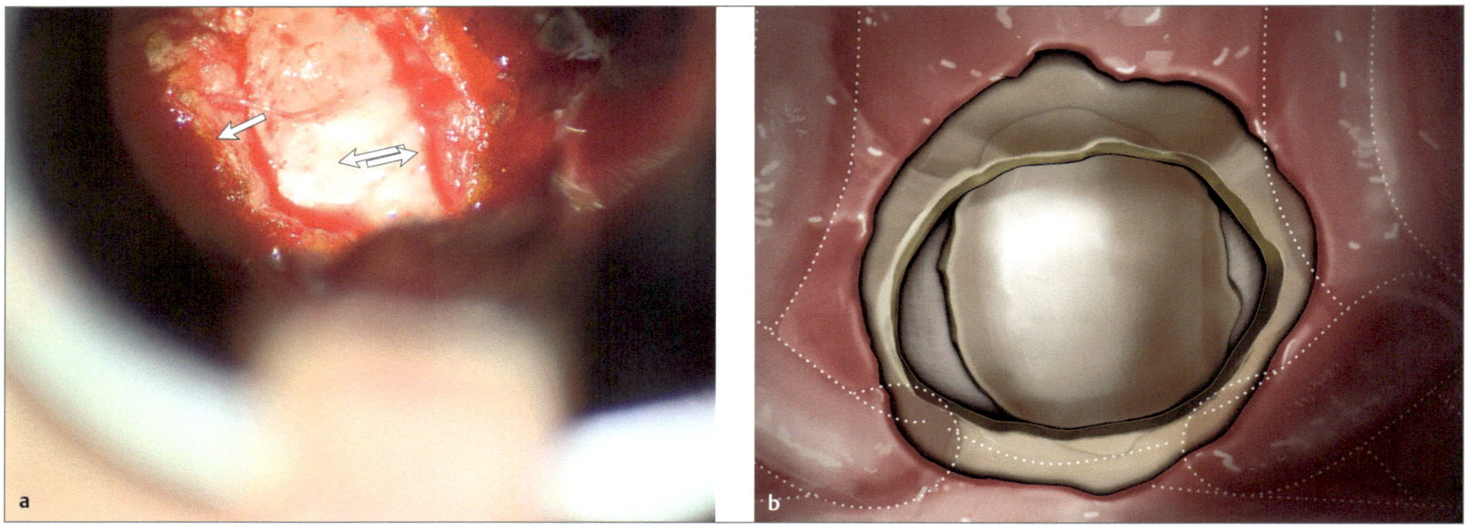

Fig. 7.11 (a, b) Reconstruction of the sellar floor—closure. Methods of reconstruction and closure of the sellar floor are still a matter of debate and range from no specific closure (in the absence of CSF leakage intraoperatively) to routine use of subcutaneous fat from the abdomen or fascia lata. As the latter adds to the overall risk of morbidity of the procedure, we use Gelfoam and fibrin sealant-coated collagen fleece (*arrow*), which is stuck to the diaphragm to prevent CSF leakage. For closure of the dura and the sellar floor, the coated collagen fleece and autologous bone (*double arrow*), harvested during opening, is applied. Most importantly, the piece of bone is interlocked with the bone of the sellar floor to achieve a robust buttress and keep the applied materials in place.

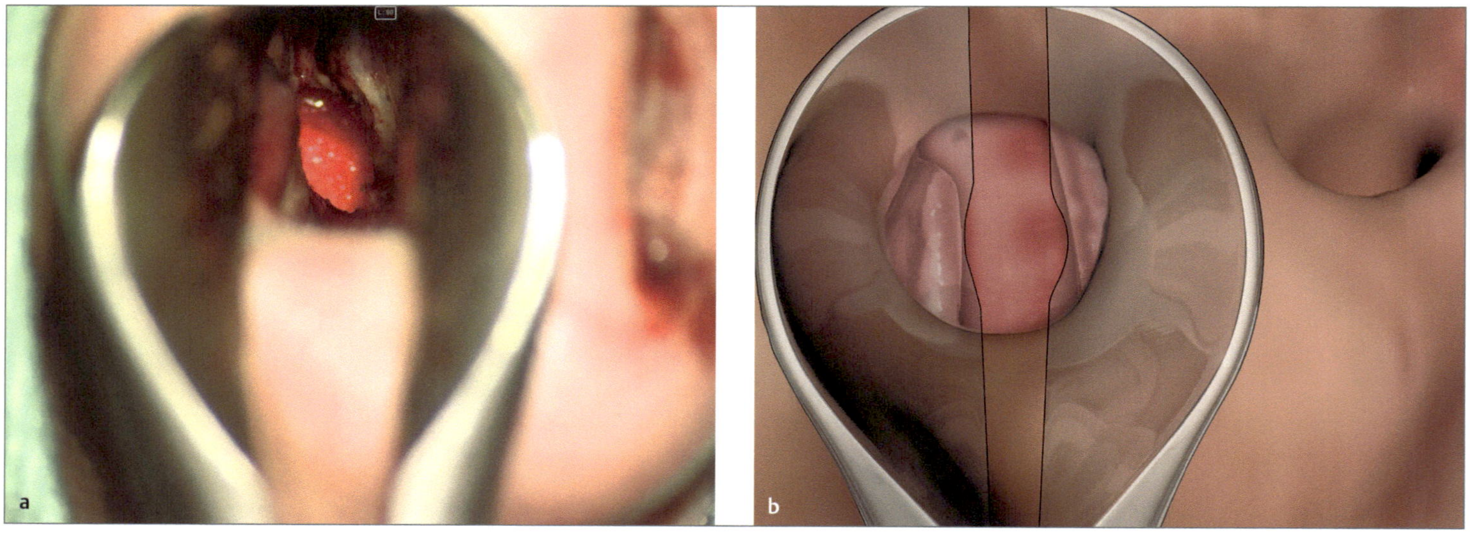

Fig. 7.12 (a, b) Repositioning of the nasal septum and the middle turbinate. After removal of the speculum, the septum is repositioned medially and inspected meticulously. Iatrogenic damage to the septum may occur, although it is very rare, and needs to be readapted with absorbable sutures. Finally, the middle turbinate is repositioned in order to prevent an artificial recess with accumulation of blood and mucosal exudate.

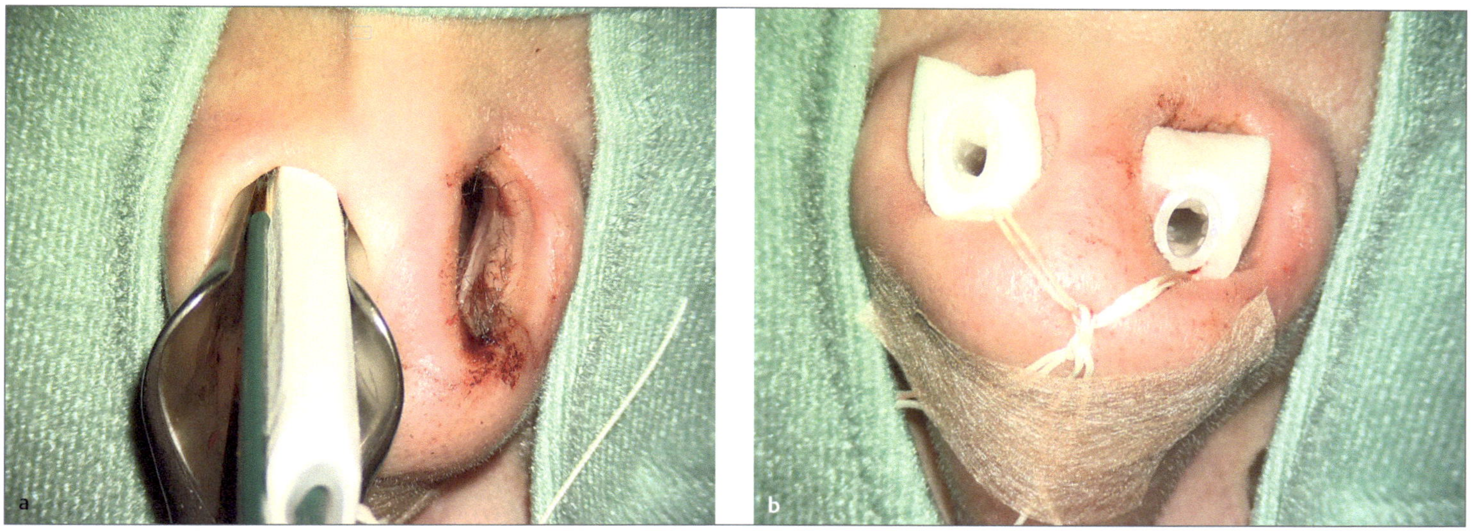

Fig. 7.13 (a, b) **Placement of tamponades—finish line.** Finally, two tubed tamponades can be used for gentle nasal packing to prevent blood oozing from the nasal mucosa. These are placed using the speculum and remain for approximately 24 hours.

Checklist

- Use fluoroscopy or image guidance in anatomical variants and recurrent tumor surgery.
- Inspect both nostrils to identify anatomical variations and pathological obstructions.
- To find the sphenoid ostium, work your way up from the choana to the anterior wall of the sphenoid sinus.
- Aim to remove the anterior sphenoid wall (or a sphenoid septum) in one piece—and retain harvested bone for closure.
- Make sure your sphenoid opening does not extend too far cranially—use curettes to check cranial (and lateral) extension.
- Perform hemostasis before opening the dura.
- Cavernous sinus bleeding can easily be controlled using Gelfoam and head elevation.
- Reconstruction of the sellar floor should be done meticulously to prevent CSF leakage.
- Repositioning of the middle turbinate and the nasal septum is mandatory.
- In case of intraoperative CSF leakage, use lumbar CSF drainage for 3 to 5 days.

7.2 Endoscopic Approach

Henry Schroeder and Jörg Baldauf

In all patients undergoing endoscopic endonasal surgery, CT scans with bone window and MR imaging (when no contraindication exists) are obtained. Fluoroscopy is never used and neuronavigation is not routine. Navigation is usually not required for standard approaches to the sella and anterior skull base when the sinuses are well pneumatized. We use navigation in conchal types of sphenoid sinus, in kissing carotids, in extended transclival–transpterygoid approaches, and recurrent cases when the landmarks are not easy to see (▶ Fig. 7.14, ▶ Fig. 7.15, ▶ Fig. 7.16, ▶ Fig. 7.17, ▶ Fig. 7.18, ▶ Fig. 7.19, ▶ Fig. 7.20, ▶ Fig. 7.21, ▶ Fig. 7.22, ▶ Fig. 7.23, ▶ Fig. 7.24, ▶ Fig. 7.25, ▶ Fig. 7.26, ▶ Fig. 7.27, ▶ Fig. 7.28, ▶ Fig. 7.29, ▶ Fig. 7.30, ▶ Fig. 7.31, ▶ Fig. 7.32, ▶ Fig. 7.33, ▶ Fig. 7.34, ▶ Fig. 7.35, ▶ Fig. 7.36, ▶ Fig. 7.37, ▶ Fig. 7.38, ▶ Fig. 7.39, ▶ Fig. 7.40, and ▶ Fig. 7.41).

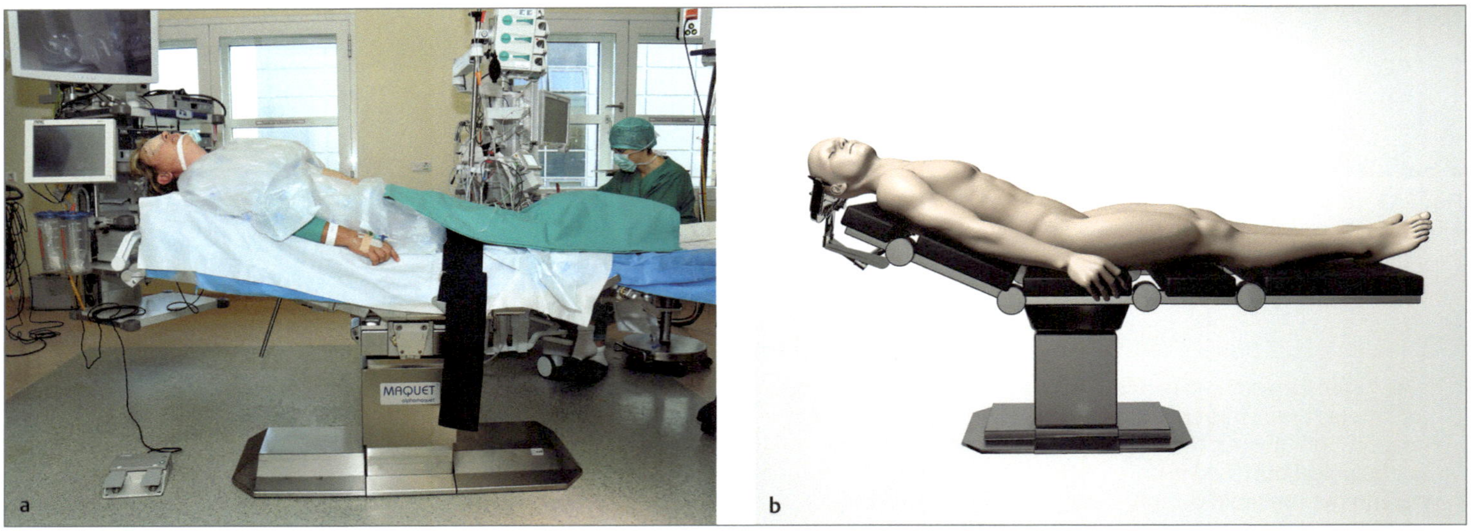

Fig. 7.14 (a, b) Positioning. The position of the patient is supine with the back elevated up to 30° to reduce the venous pressure within the cavernous sinus. The arms are placed by the patient's sides. Note that the anesthesiologist sits at the left-hand side at the foot of the operating table. As well as the preparation of the nose and nasal cavity with iodine solution, the periumbilical region is disinfected in case a fat graft is needed. Before draping, cottonoids soaked in epinephrine 1:1,000 are placed within both nasal cavities to assure good decongestion of the mucosa.

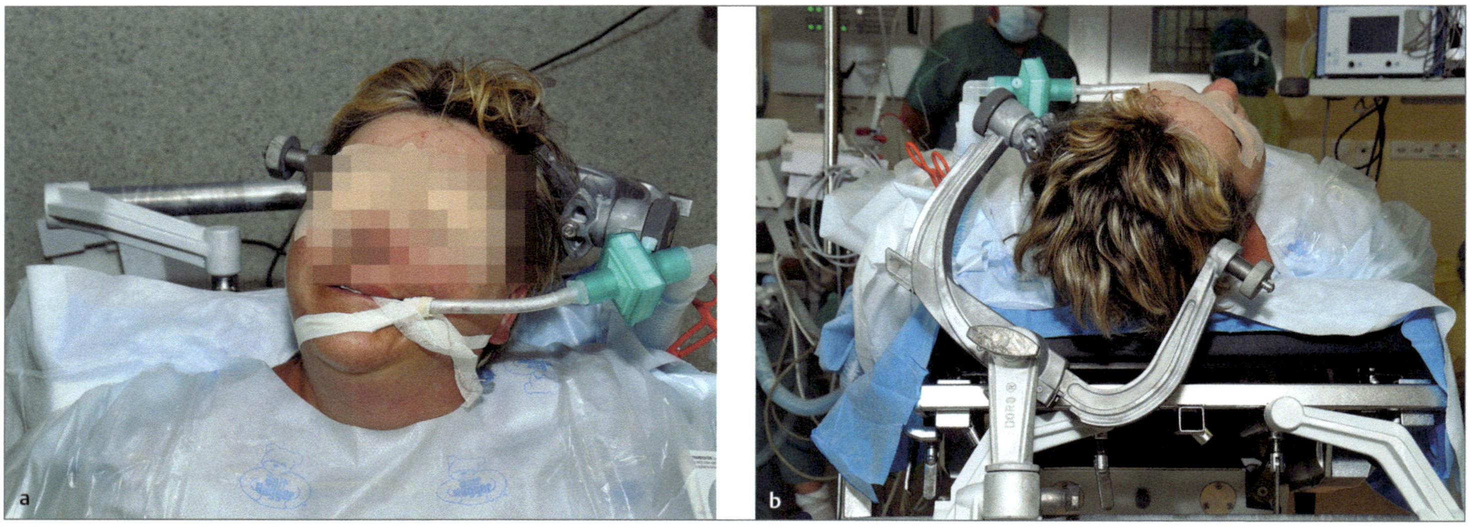

Fig. 7.15 (a, b) Head positioning. The neck is gently tilted to the left and the head, fixed in a Mayfield clamp, is slightly extended, and turned toward the surgeon.

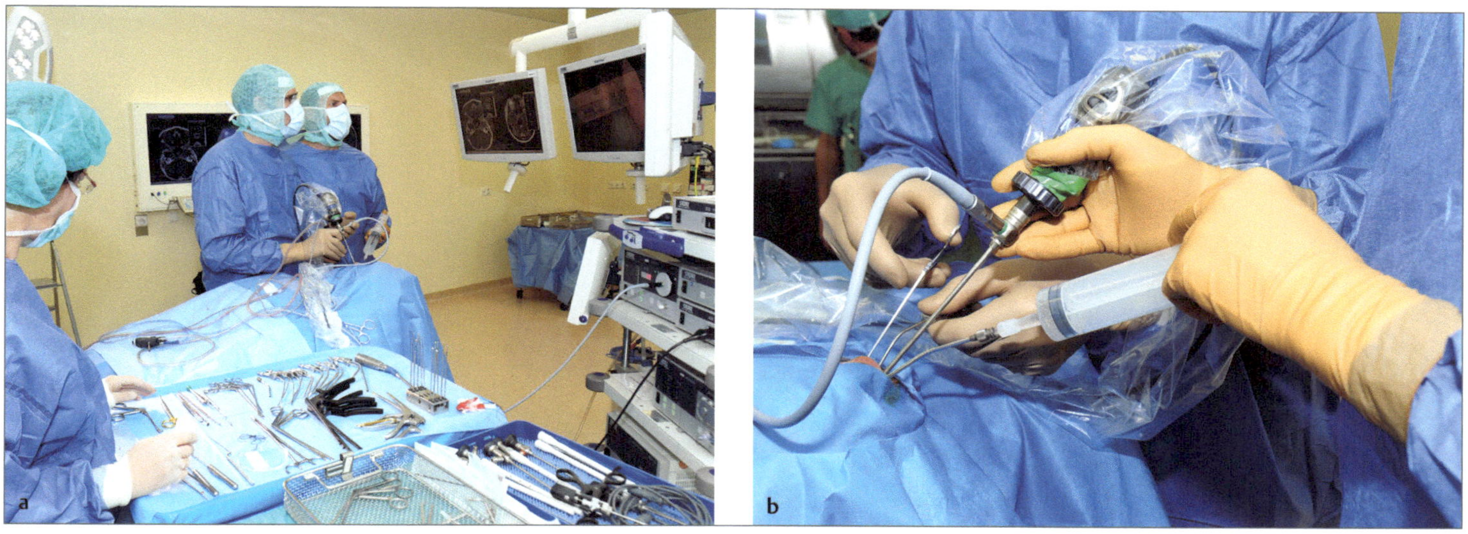

Fig. 7.16 (a, b) **Operating theater setup.** **(a)** The patient is draped and the videoendoscopic equipment needed during surgery is positioned at the level of the patient's head, including monitors for each surgeon. The two surgeons stand on the right side of the patient. The scrub nurse stands on the opposite side to allow easy changing of the surgical instruments. **(b)** It is a two-surgeon, three- or four-handed operation. This technique enables one surgeon to work bimanually in the depth, while the other surgeon moves the endoscope. This offers flexible mobility of the endoscope with respect to the operating field.

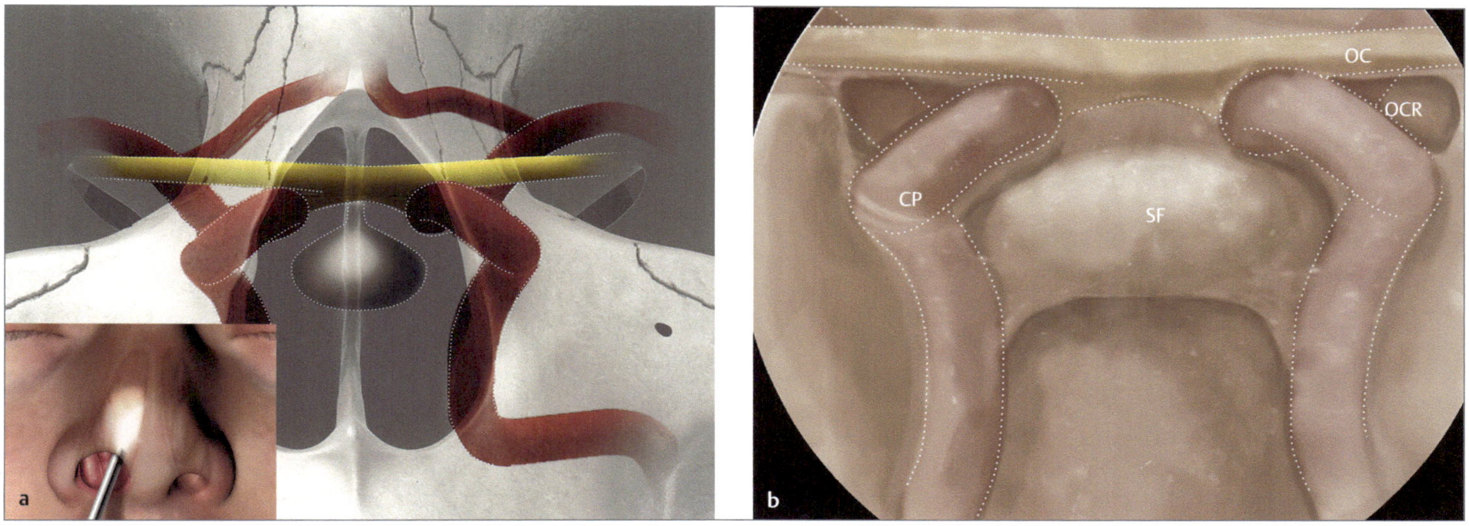

Fig. 7.17 (a, b) **Anatomical overview.** Schematic drawing of the endoscope inserted through the right nostril. The inferior, middle, and superior turbinates and nasal septum are hidden below the surface of the skin (inlay in **b**). The same projection is shown in **(a)** for the optic nerve and the anterior part of the circle of Willis with respect to the pituitary gland. **(b)** The projection of the anatomy at the level of the sphenoid sinus (explained in greater detail in ▸Fig. 7.31). CP, carotid prominence; OC, optic canal with optic nerve; OCR, lateral opticocarotid recess; SF, sellar floor.

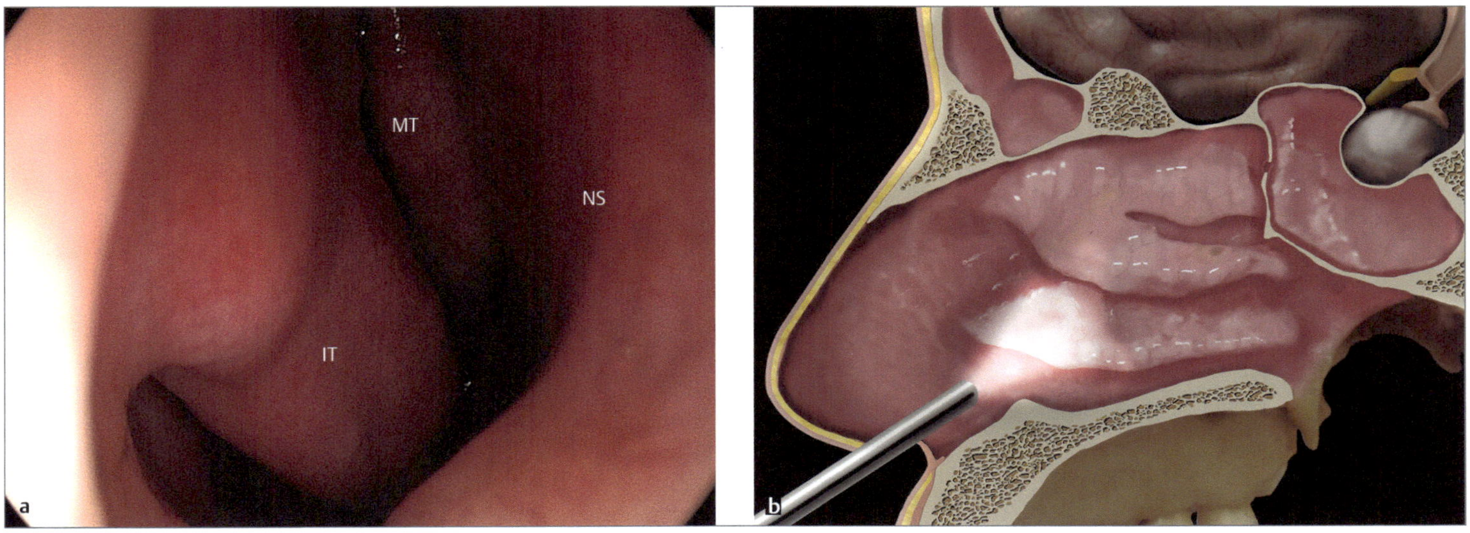

Fig. 7.18 (a, b) **The nasal phase: inferior and middle turbinate inspection.** Initial approach through the right nostril. Inspection of the inferior (IT) and middle turbinate (MT) and nasal septum (NS).

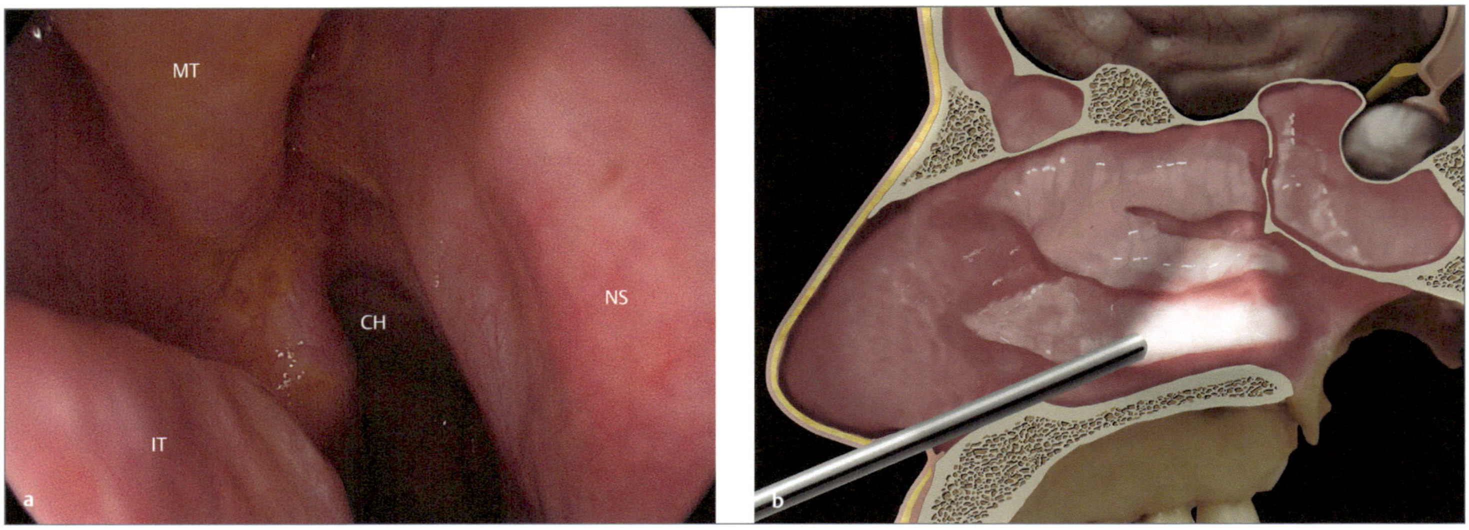

Fig. 7.19 (a, b) Nasal phase: posteroinferior inspection. Inspection of the posteroinferior part of the nasal cavity. Identification of the choana (CH), middle turbinate (MT), inferior turbinate (IT), and nasal septum (NS).

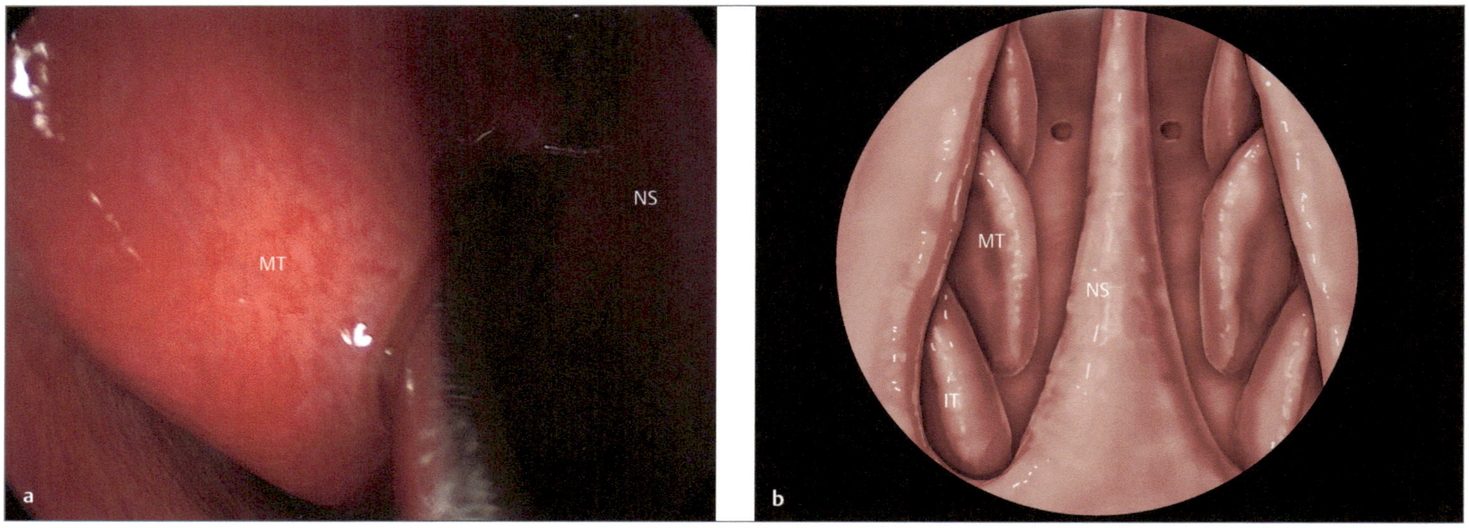

Fig. 7.20 (a, b) Creating working space at the level of the inferior and middle turbinates. The middle turbinate and lower turbinate are pushed laterally using a dissector to create working space. A cottonoid can be placed between the inferior and middle turbinate and the nasal septum to protect the mucosa.

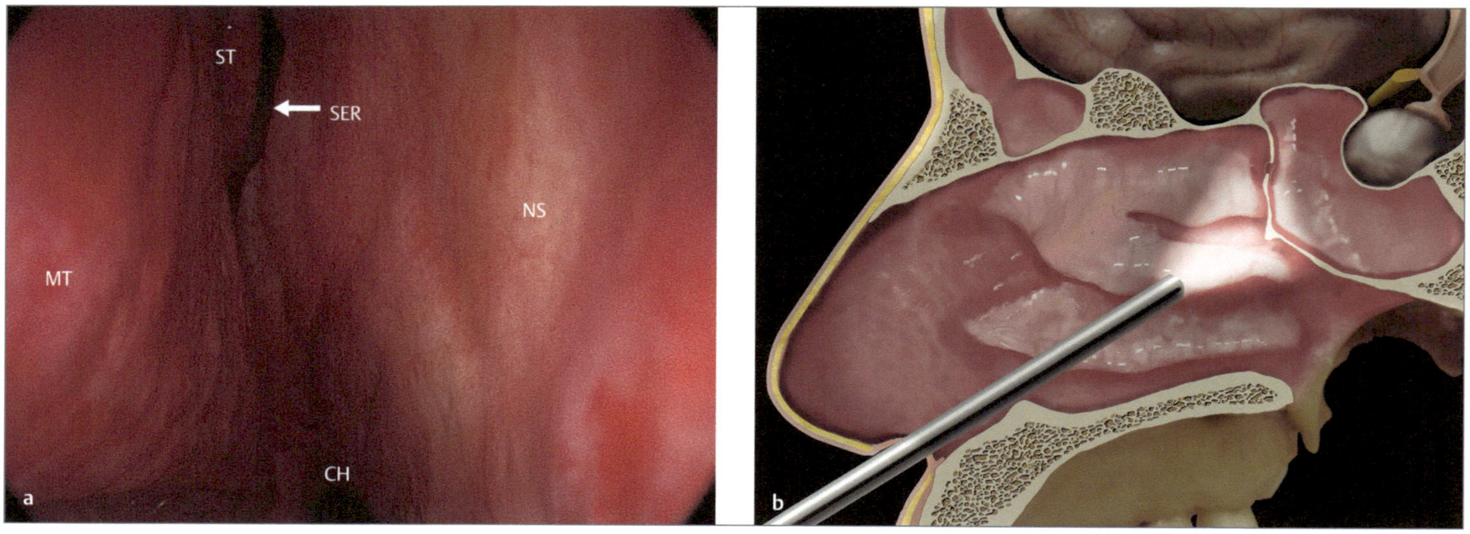

Fig. 7.21 (a, b) Nasal phase: visualization of the superior nasal cavity. Visualization of the superior turbinate (ST) and sphenoethmoid recess (SER). The upper margin of the choana is visible.

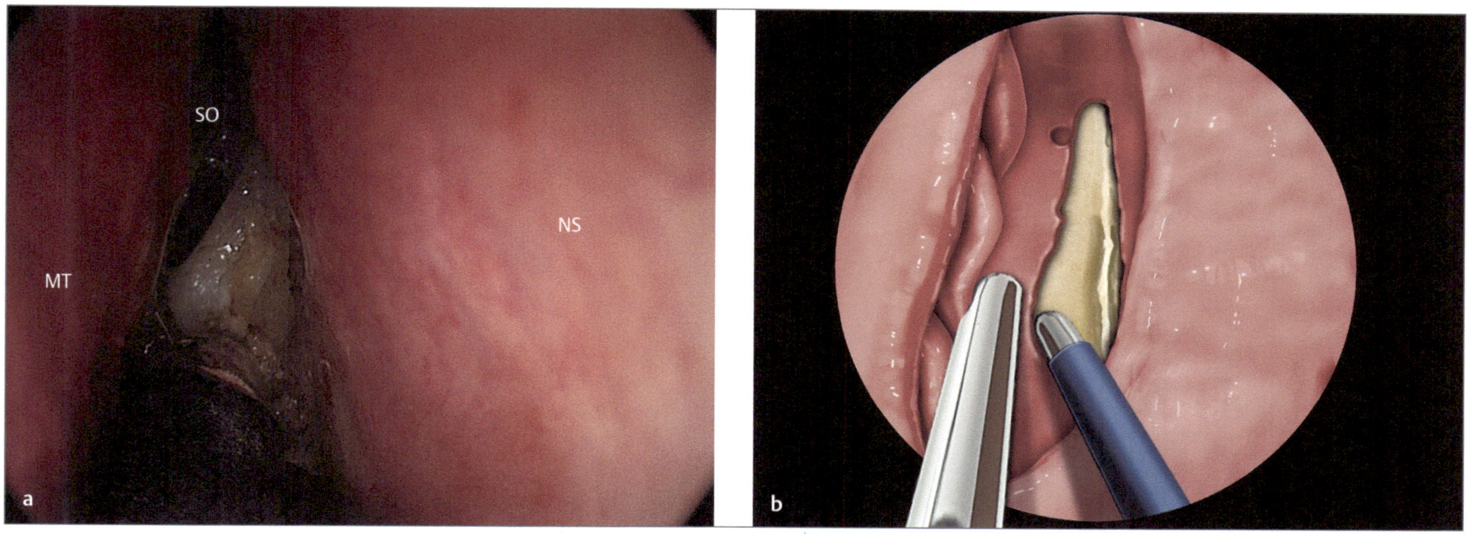

Fig. 7.22 (a, b) Identification of the site of the sphenoid ostium. Approximately 1.5 cm above the choana, the sphenoid ostium can sometimes be identified. However, it might be completely covered by mucosa. This point is the landmark to gain access to the sphenoid cavity. Blunt perforation opens the sphenoid sinus. The mucosa in front of the sphenoid sinus is coagulated from the choana up to the sphenoid ostium (1 cm) with a monopolar suction-coagulation device, as well as the dorsal part of the nasal septum. Once this step has been finished, the whole procedure is repeated on the left side.

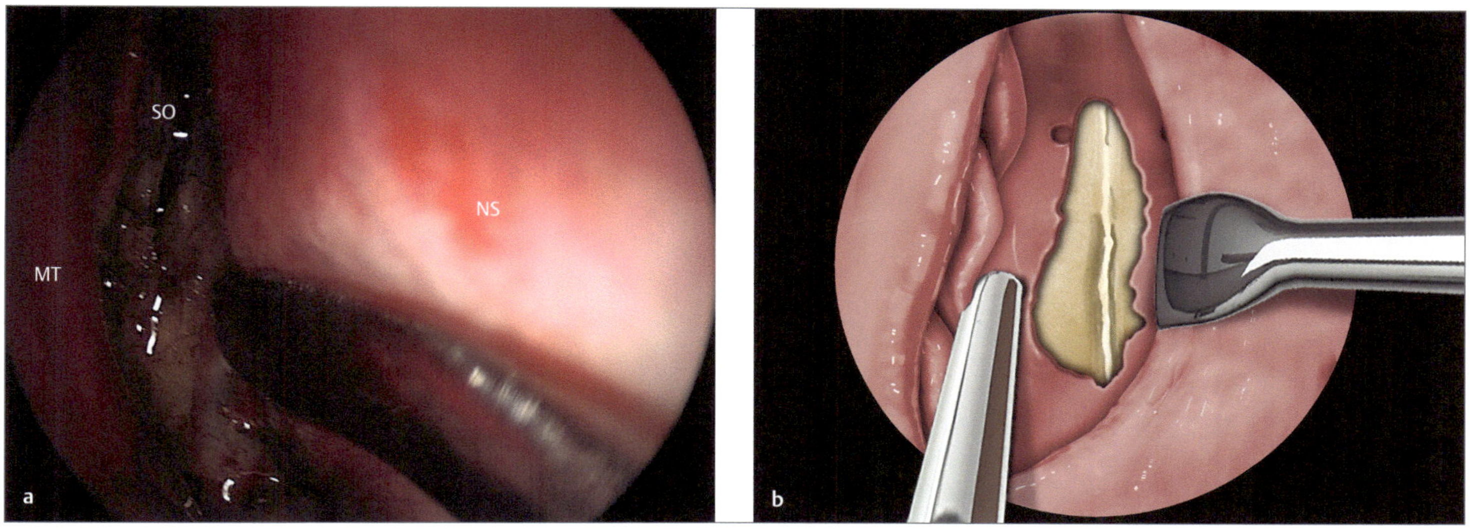

Fig. 7.23 (a, b) Exposing the anterior wall of the sphenoid sinus and dislocating the nasal septum. After the anterior wall of the sphenoid sinus has been exposed on both sides, the nasal septum is dislocated from the right side to the left with a blunt dissector.

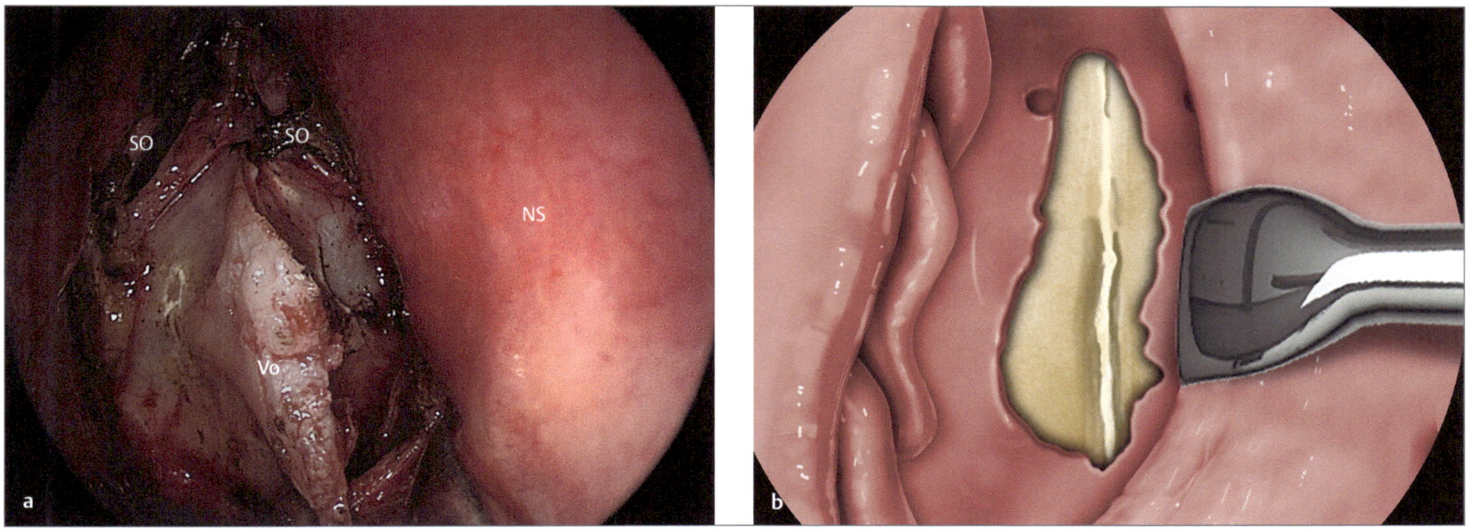

Fig. 7.24 (a, b) Visualization of the vomer as the midline landmark. The vomer (Vo) comes into view. In contrast to the nasal septum and the sphenoid septum, the vomer is a reliable landmark for the midline in both endoscopic and microscopic surgery.

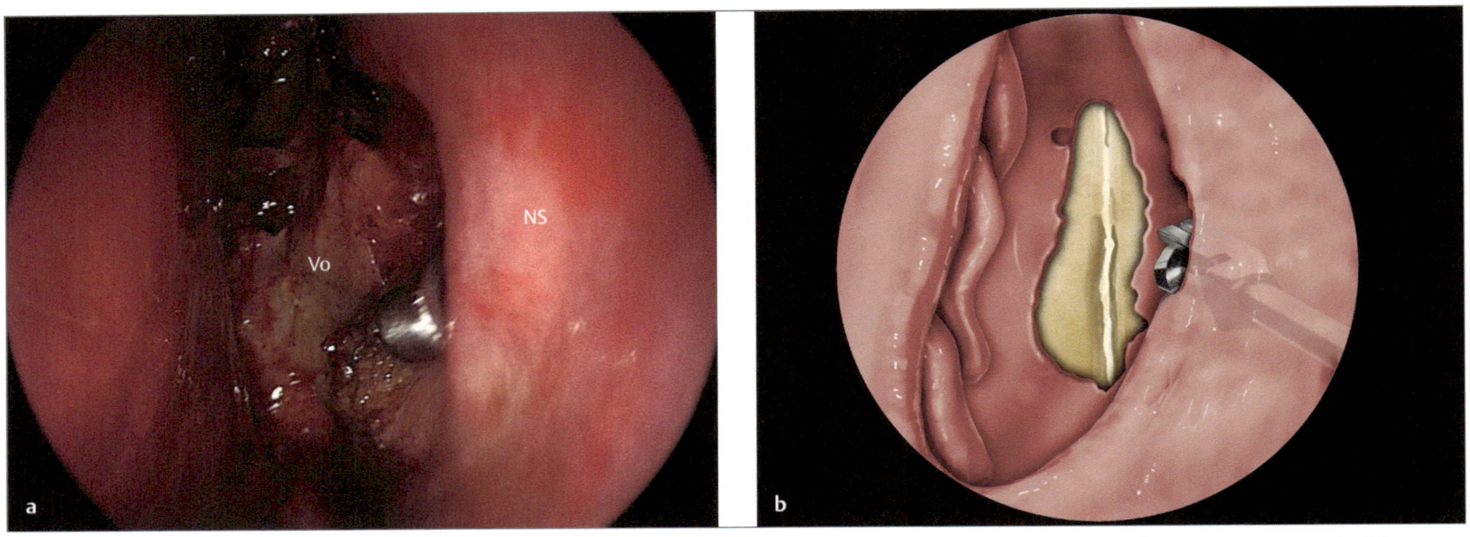

Fig. 7.25 (a, b) **Resection of the posterior third of the nasal septum.** Then, less than one third of the posterior nasal septum is resected with a retrograde cutting punch to create working space.

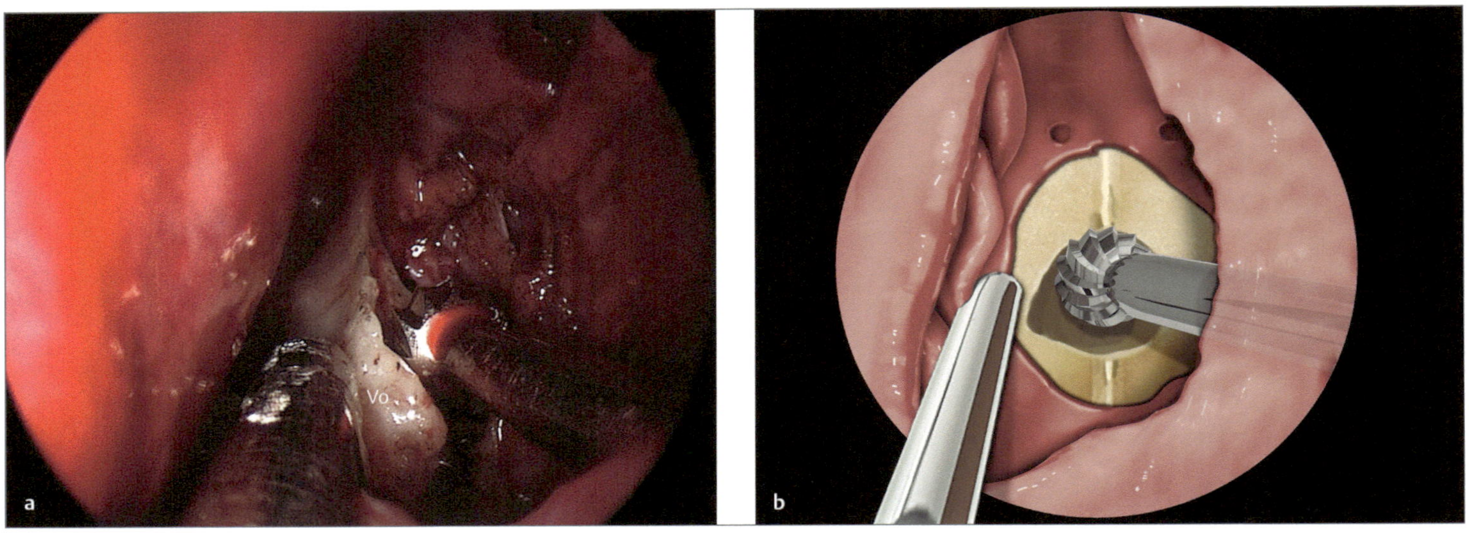

Fig. 7.26 (a, b) **The sphenoid phase.** In the sphenoid phase, both nostrils are used for bimanual manipulation. The vomer and rostrum of the sphenoid sinus is removed with the aid of a high-speed drill. The drill is held in one hand and a suction device is held in the other hand to remove bone dust and fumes. The assisting surgeon holds the endoscope and irrigates the area simultaneously to prevent heating of the drill and generation of bone dust.

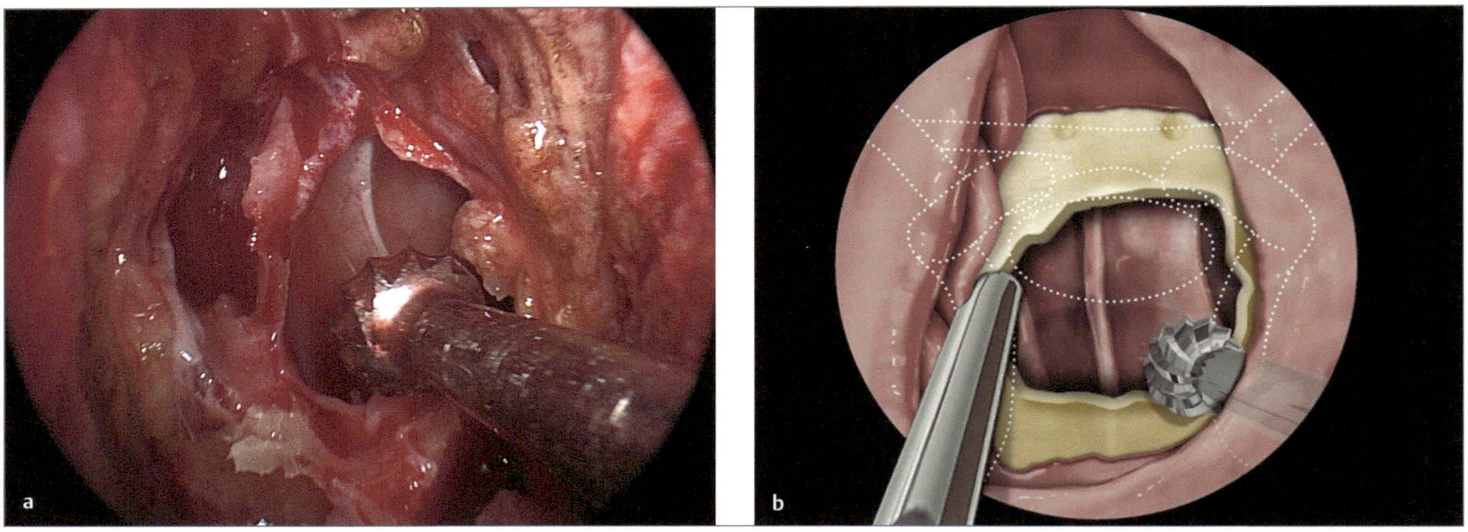

Fig. 7.27 (a, b) **Further opening of the sphenoid sinus using the drill.** The sphenoid sinus is opened wide in all directions to create sufficient space for the bimanual dissection. A high-speed drill is usually used for this. The extent of the sphenoid sinus opening depends on the lesion and the aim of the surgery. The mucosa and the sphenoid septum come into view.

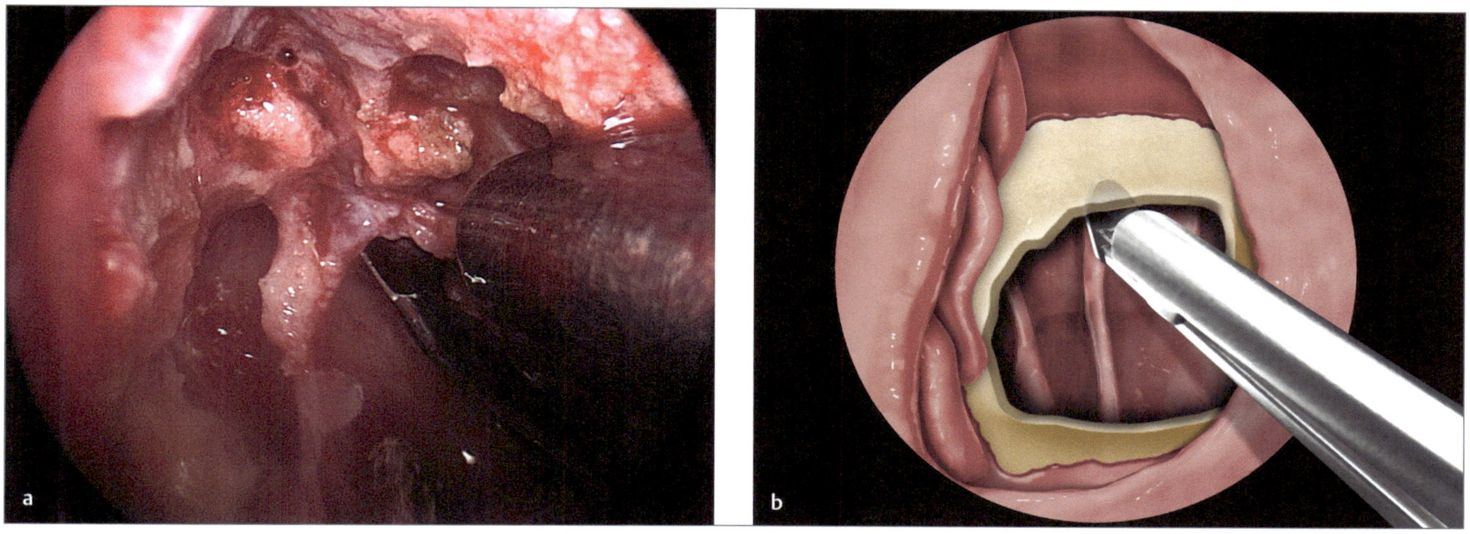

Fig. 7.28 (a, b) Further opening of the sphenoid sinus using the rongeur. Kerrison rongeurs are used to enlarge the sphenoidotomy in all directions until it reaches the size required for the surgery.

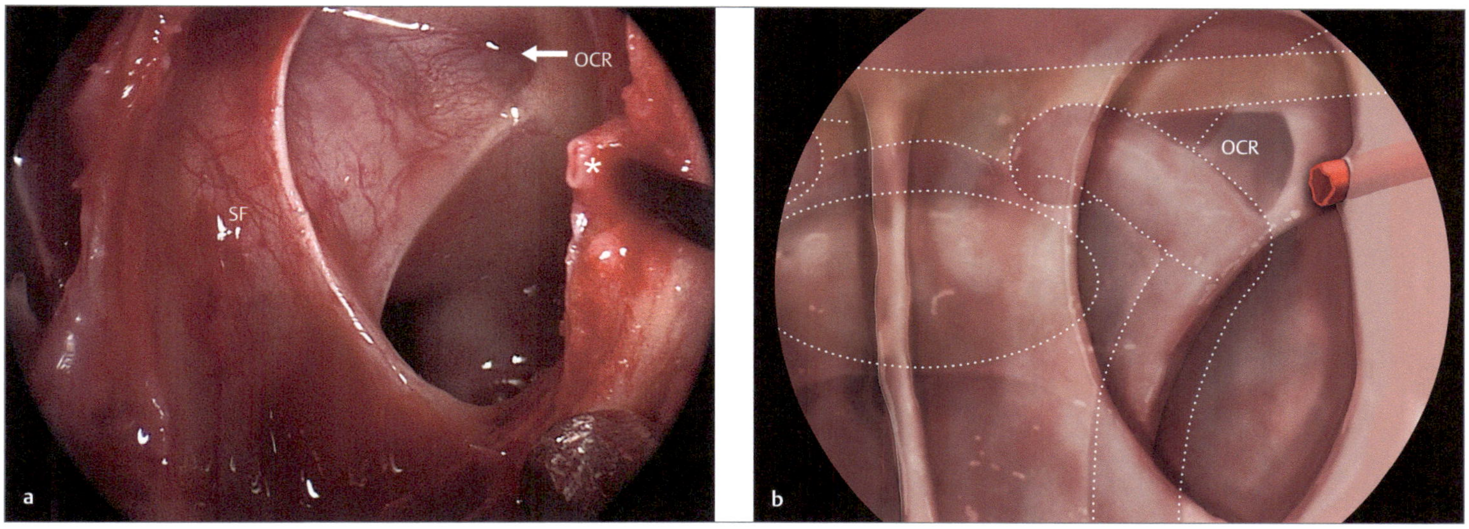

Fig. 7.29 (a, b) Sphenopalatine artery and its branches. At the lateral border of the opening of the sphenoid sinus, the posterior nasal arteries (one or more branches of the sphenopalatine artery, asterisk) are identified. OCR, = opticocarotid recess; SF, sellar floor.

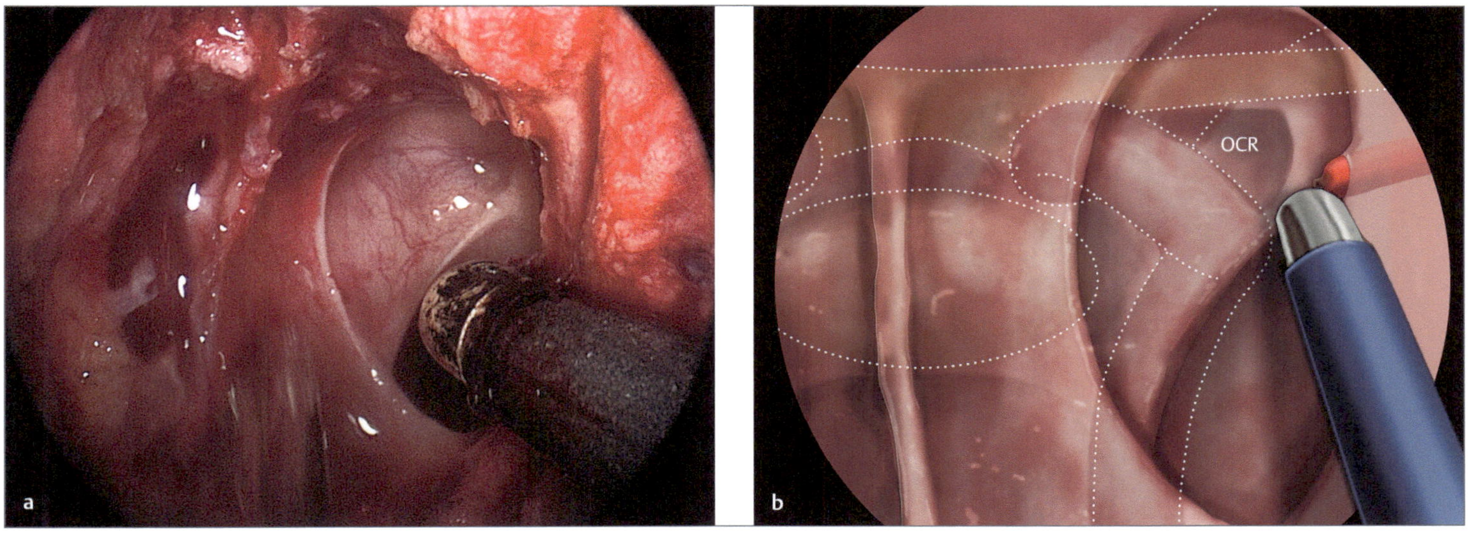

Fig. 7.30 (a, b) Coagulation of the posterior nasal artery branch. Coagulation of the posterior nasal artery with the monopolar suction-coagulation device is performed. It is of the utmost importance to coagulate the artery thoroughly to avoid nasal hemorrhage after surgery.

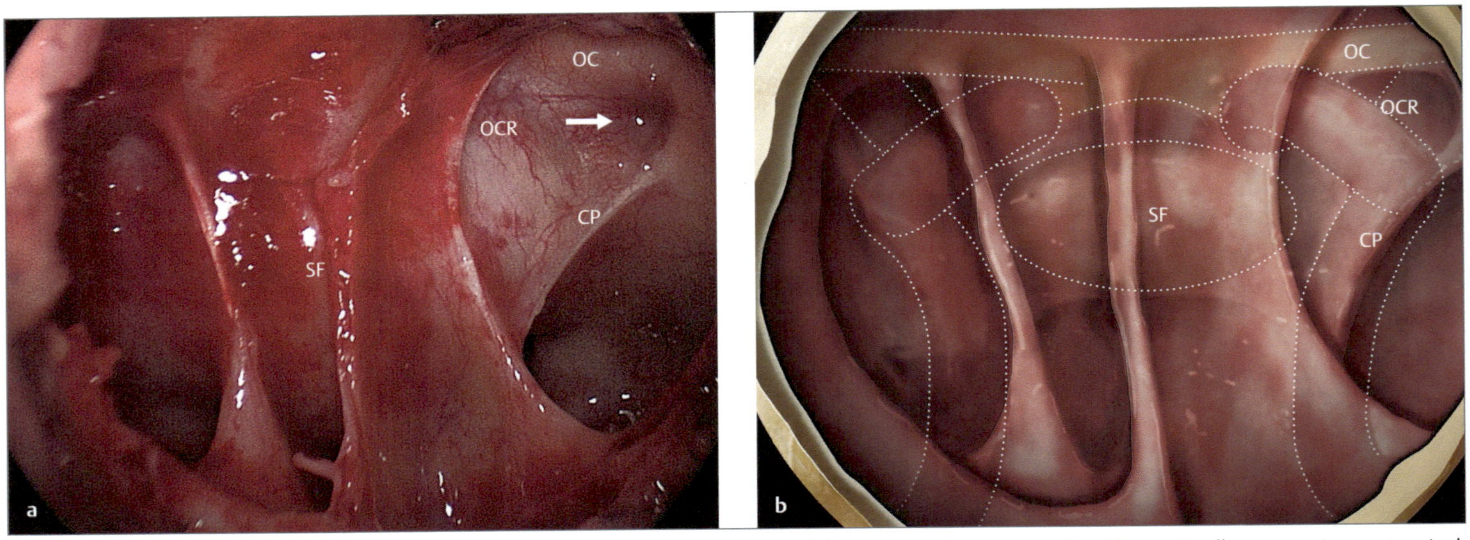

Fig. 7.31 (a, b) Intrasphenoidal bony anatomy. The anatomy of the intrasphenoidal bony septa is very variable. The septa allow a precise anatomical orientation, especially the relation to the carotid arteries. When the sphenoid sinus is well pneumatized, the important anatomical landmarks can be identified, such as the optic canals (OC), carotid protuberances (CP) of the clinoidal, cavernous, and clival carotid artery, clivus, and lateral opticocarotid recesses (OCR). Neuronavigation helps the surgeon to stay oriented when the sphenoid sinus is not well pneumatized.

The septa are drilled flat with the high-speed drill or are removed using rongeurs and punches. The space created must be sufficient to allow an optimal dissection within the sphenoid cavity and to avoid collisions of the instruments during surgical maneuvers.

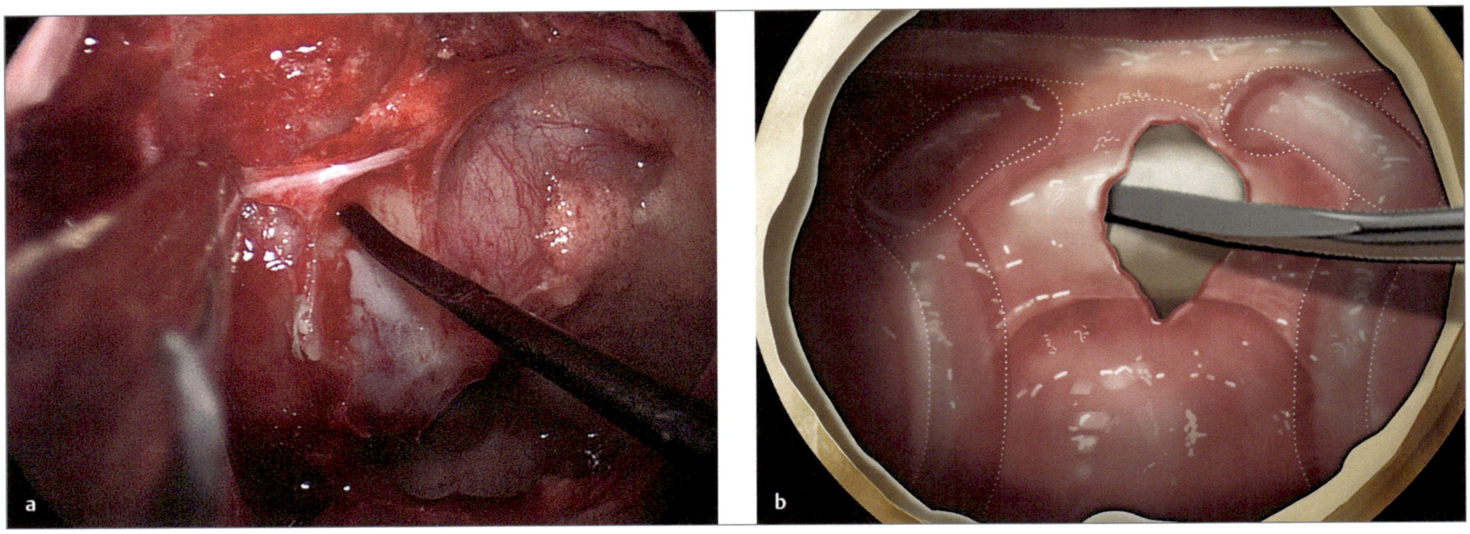

Fig. 7.32 (a, b) Removal of the mucosa. The mucosa is removed only from the sellar floor to reduce the degree of crusting and discharge. It is peeled off with the dissector and sometimes cut with scissors.

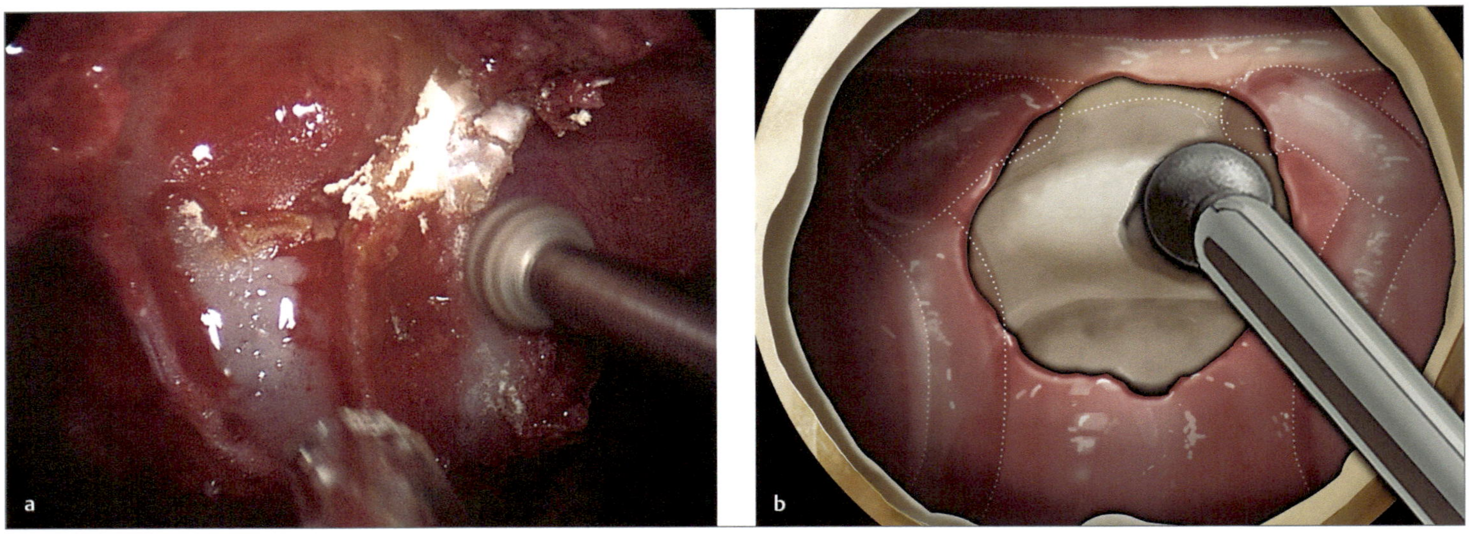

Fig. 7.33 (a, b) Opening of the sellar floor using the drill. The sellar floor is drilled with a diamond high-speed drill to expose the dura of the sella.

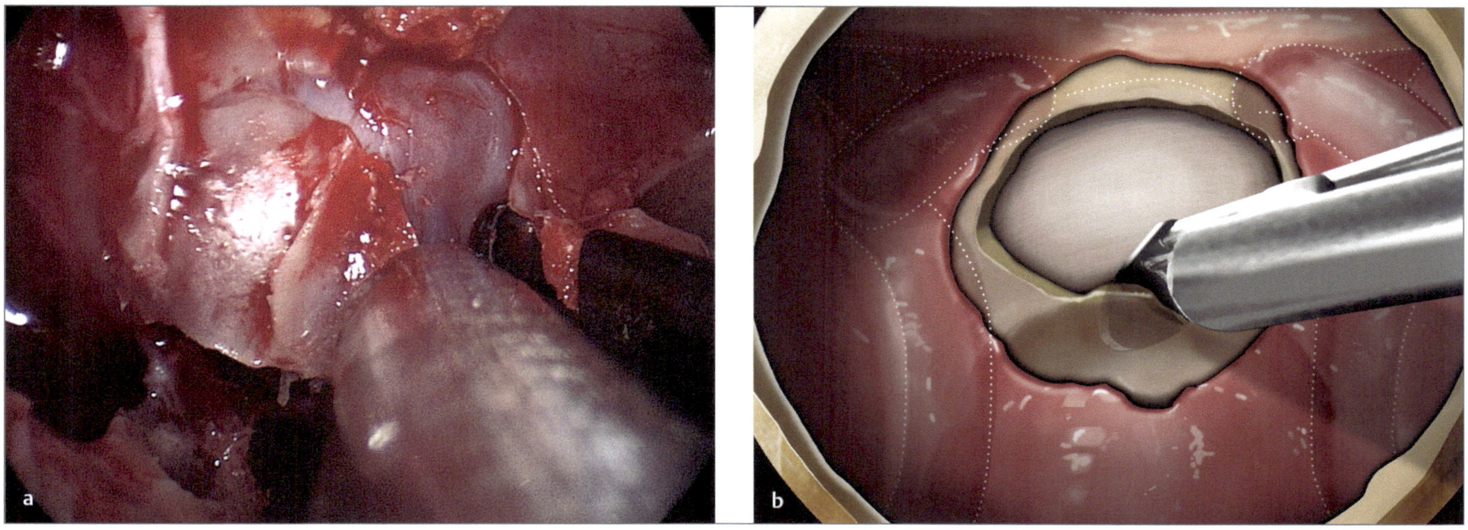

Fig. 7.34 (a, b) Enlargement of the opening using the rongeur. Sellar bone removal is extended laterally with a Kerrison rongeur until sufficient access to the lesion is obtained. When performing surgery for large adenomas, the opening should expose both the cavernous sinus and the superior intercavernous sinus. Venous bleeding from the sinus may occur. The latter can easily be controlled with application of FloSeal hemostatic sealant (Baxter Healthcare Corporation, Hayward, California, United States).

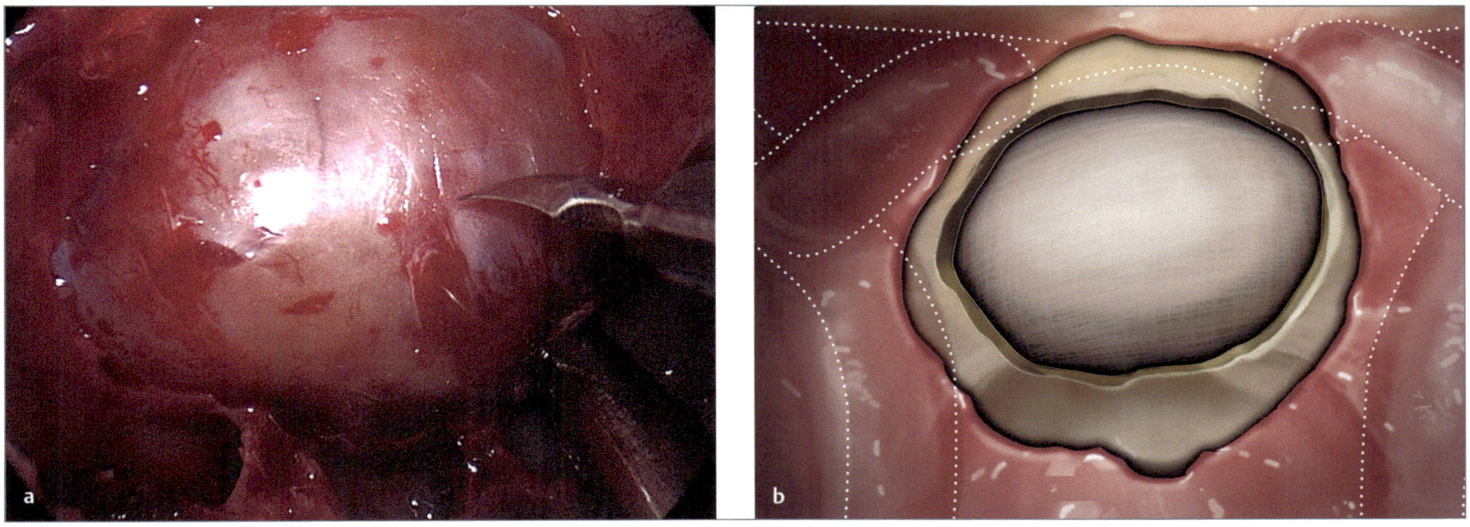

Fig. 7.35 (a, b) The sellar dura mater. The sellar dura is now exposed. A sharp incision of the dura mater is made in the midline with a knife.

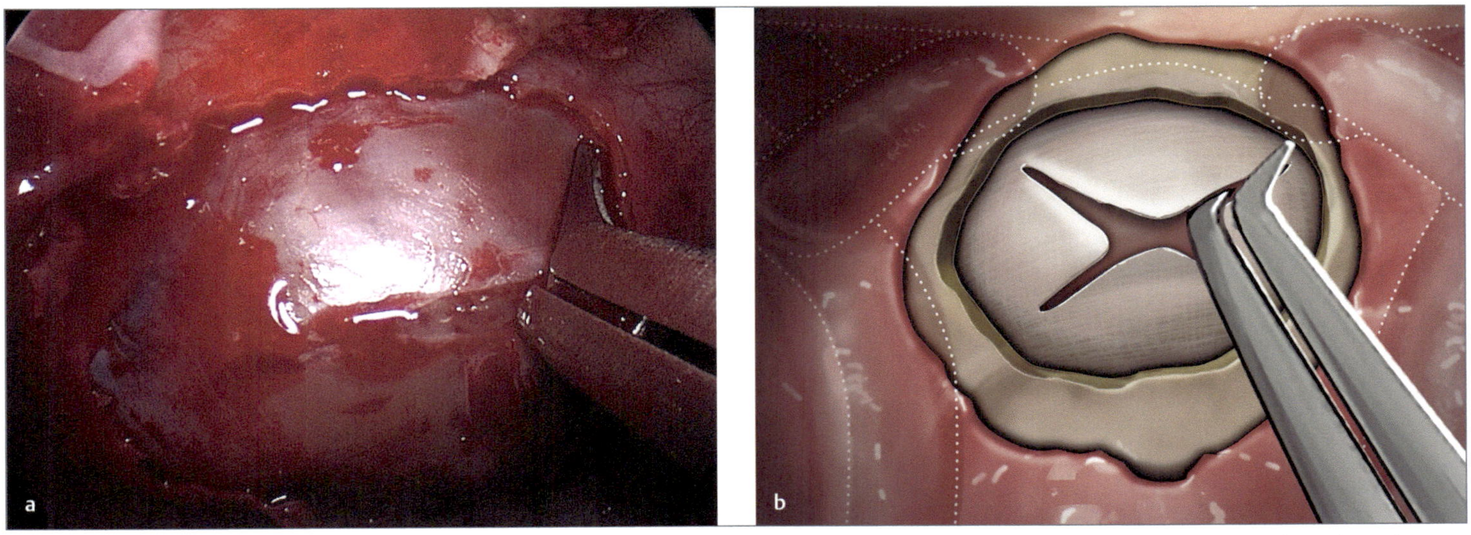

Fig. 7.36 (a, b) Opening of the sellar dura. Angled scissors are used to create a wide dural opening. The opening can be cross- or door-shaped.

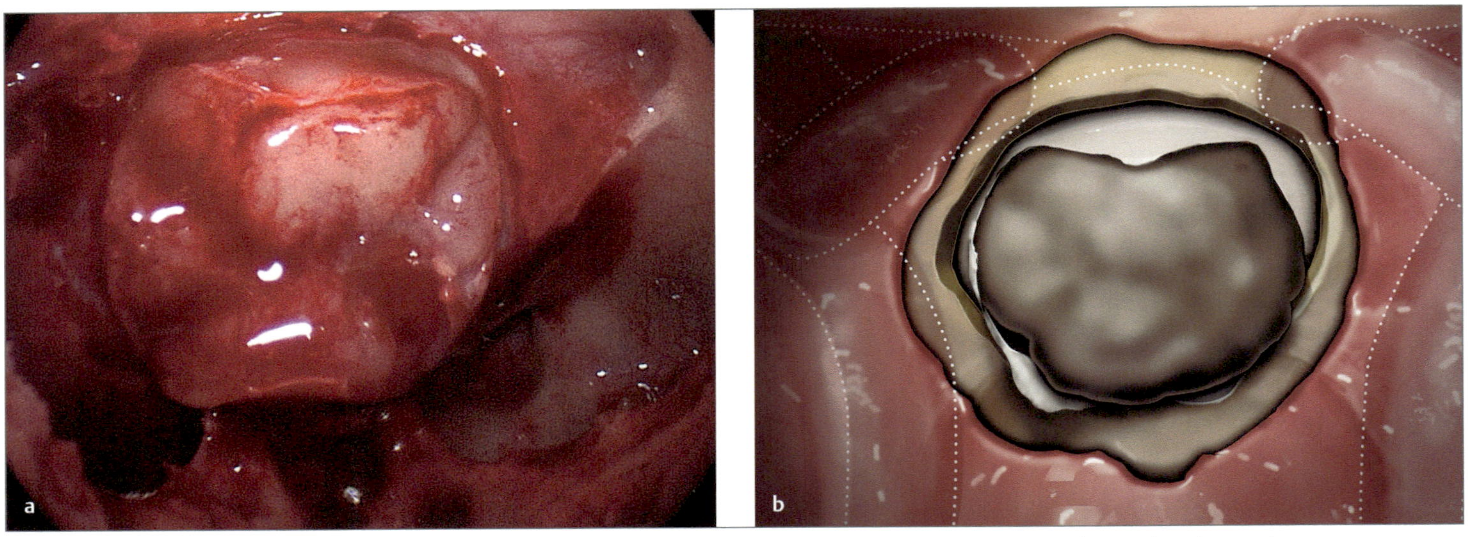

Fig. 7.37 (a, b) **Tumor removal.** After the dural opening has been made, access to the lesion (e.g., pituitary adenoma) is obtained.

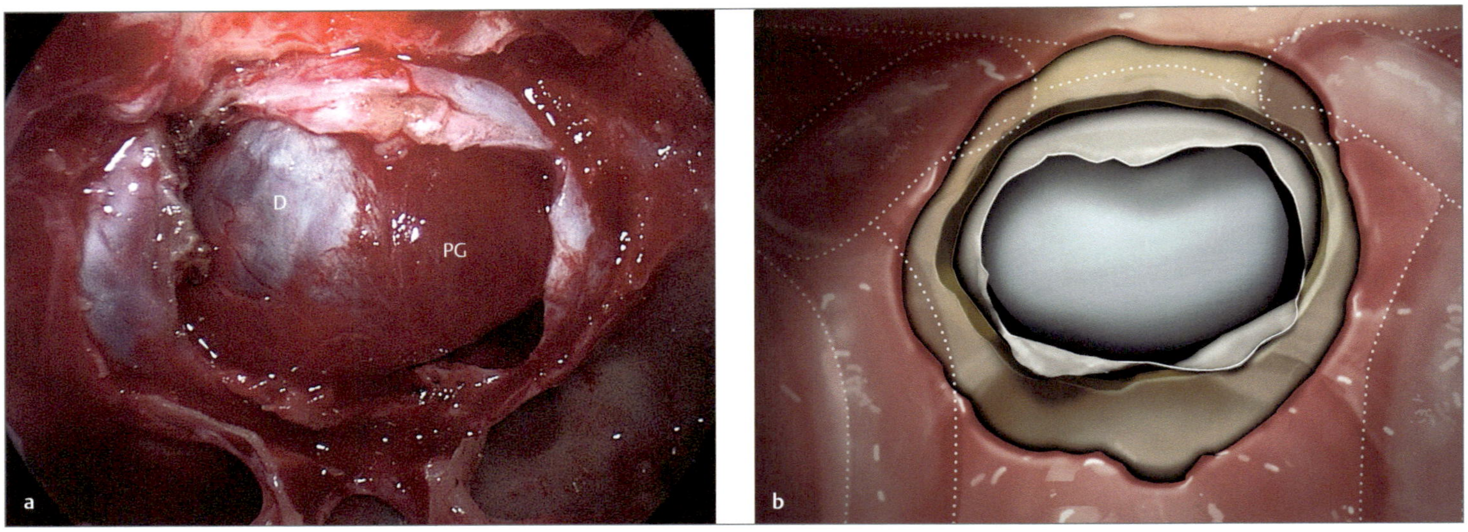

Fig. 7.38 (a, b) **Closure.** After surgery for small adenomas when no cerebrospinal fluid (CSF) leak was observed during the surgery and the Valsalva maneuver did not lead to CSF flow, a piece of Gelfoam is placed in the resection cavity or on the gland. In the case of larger lesions, when the thin diaphragm is coming down to the sellar floor level or beyond, a sellar floor reconstruction is performed even when no CSF flow was observed. On the diaphragm (D), a thin layer of normal pituitary gland (PG) is seen.

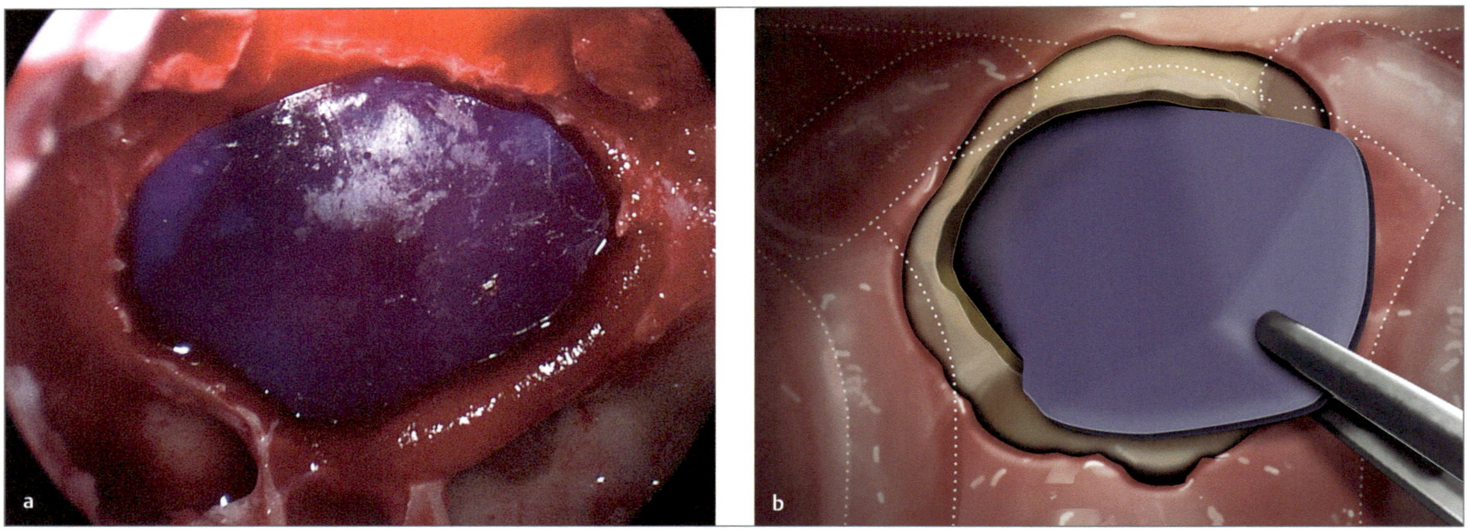

Fig. 7.39 (a, b) **Placing a PDS plate for the reconstruction of the bony sellar floor.** For larger CSF leaks, we place a fat graft into the sellar space. For small leaks, dura collagen substitutes are used. After resection of a large adenoma with no CSF leak, we simply place Gelfoam in the resection cavity. To avoid dislocation of the material, we place a PDS plate (poly-p-dioxane) trimmed to an appropriate size into the margin of the bony sella opening overlapping the dural defect. The plate is anchored epidurally to the bony borders.

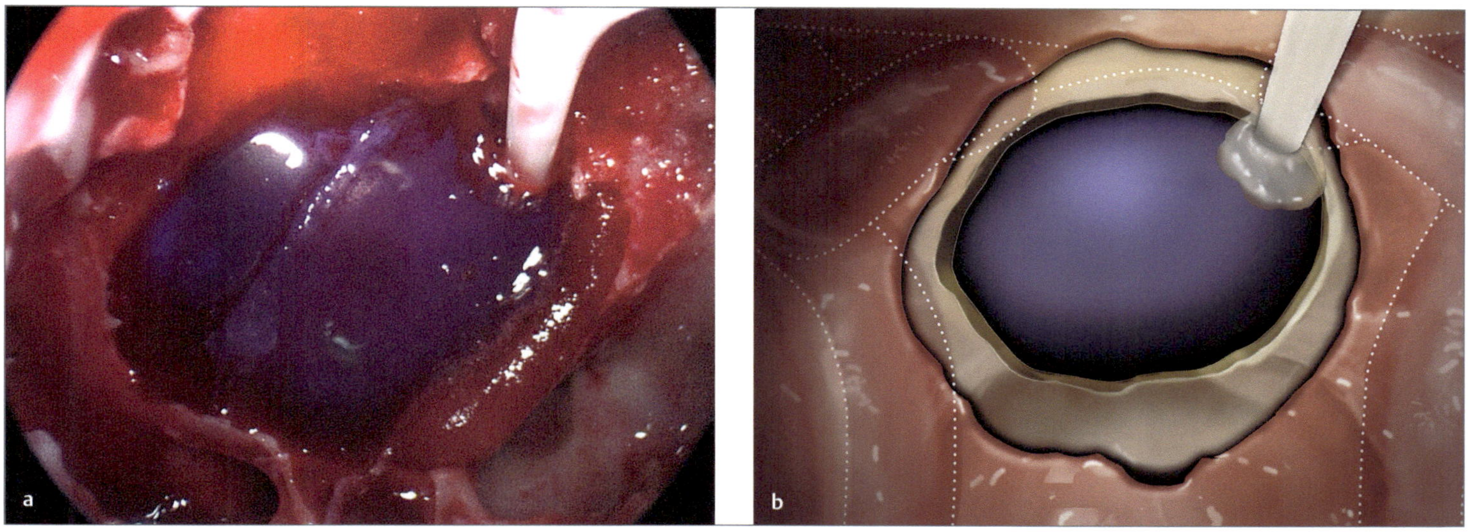

Fig. 7.40 (a, b) Sealing with fibrin glue. Fibrin glue is used only when a CSF leak is obvious.

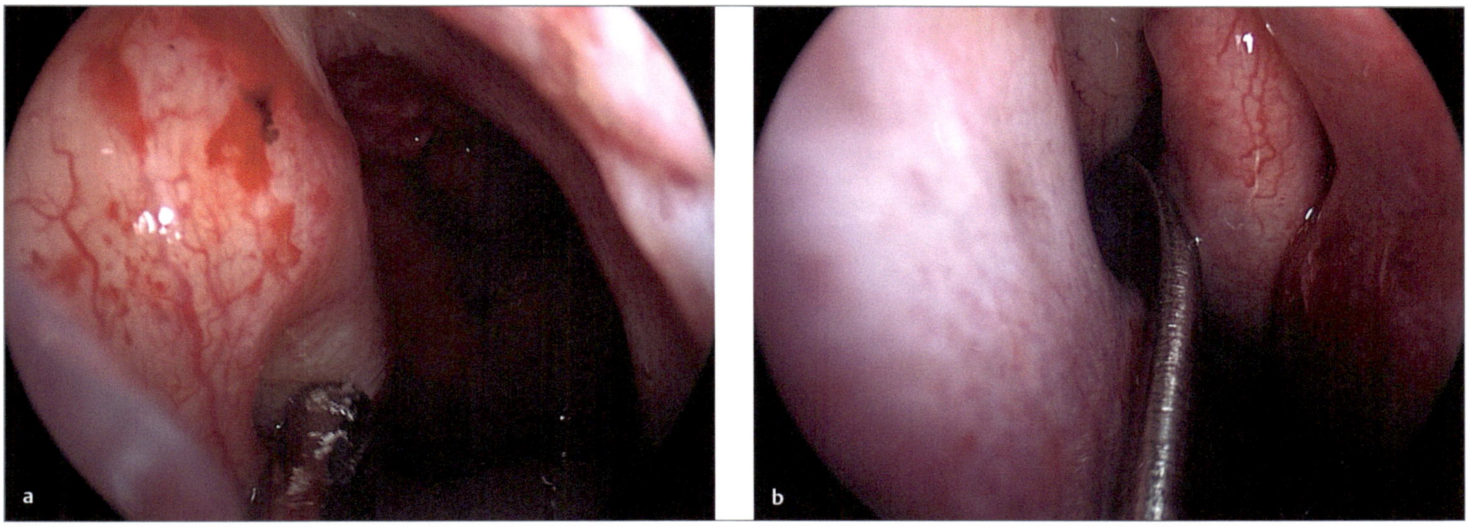

Fig. 7.41 (a, b) Nasal cleaning. The nasopharynx is cleaned to remove blood and bony fragments **(a)**. Finally, the middle turbinates are repositioned medially **(b)**.

Checklist

- Look at CT and MR images to become familiar with the individual's nasal anatomy. Cave: septal deviation, size of sphenoid sinus, position of intrasphenoid septi, intercarotid distance.
- Decongestion of mucosa is a most important step to allow a good view throughout the surgery.
- Identify all turbinates and sphenoid ostia.
- Ensure careful coagulation of the posterior nasal arteries to avoid postoperative nasal hemorrhage.
- Wide opening of the sphenoid sinus is necessary to allow unobstructed bimanual dissection.
- Identify optic canals and carotid protuberances.
- Ensure wide opening of the sellar floor.
- Adequate sellar floor reconstruction is required to avoid CSF leakage.
- No tamponade of the nasal cavity.

8 Decompressive Hemicraniectomy

Jürgen Beck

See ▸Fig. 8.1, ▸Fig. 8.2, ▸Fig. 8.3, ▸Fig. 8.4, ▸Fig. 8.5, ▸Fig. 8.6, ▸Fig. 8.7, ▸Fig. 8.8, ▸Fig. 8.9, ▸Fig. 8.10, ▸Fig. 8.11, and ▸Fig. 8.12.

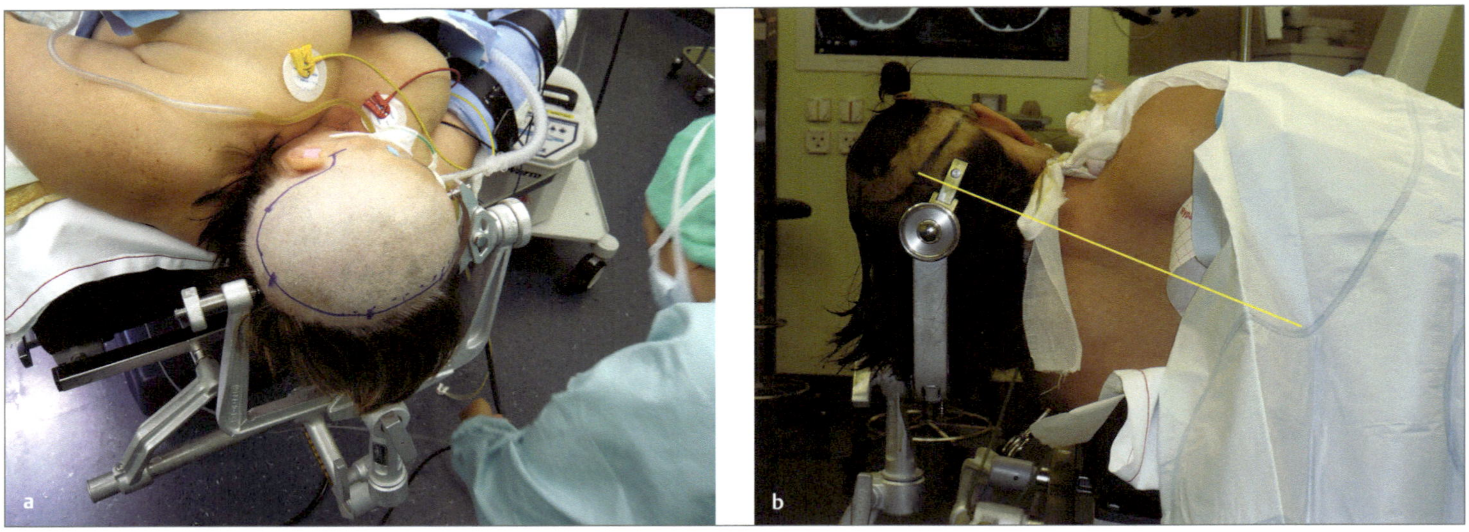

Fig. 8.1 (a,b) Positioning. The head is placed horizontally. The body position is either supine, supine 30°, or lateral. The body and head are elevated approximately 15° to reduce intracranial pressure (ICP) and to facilitate venous return. Care is taken not to angle the head in relation to the body (see *straight yellow line* in **b**). In trauma patients, check the cervical spine (C-spine) before positioning. If it is not possible to clear the C-spine, a lateral body position with the neck collar in place is preferred. A horizontal orientation for the Mayfield head holder gives the surgeon more space. Pins, placed at a distance from the skin incision, facilitate skin closure. A Leyla bar on the occipital site enables placement of skin/fish hooks for retraction of the myocutaneous flap.

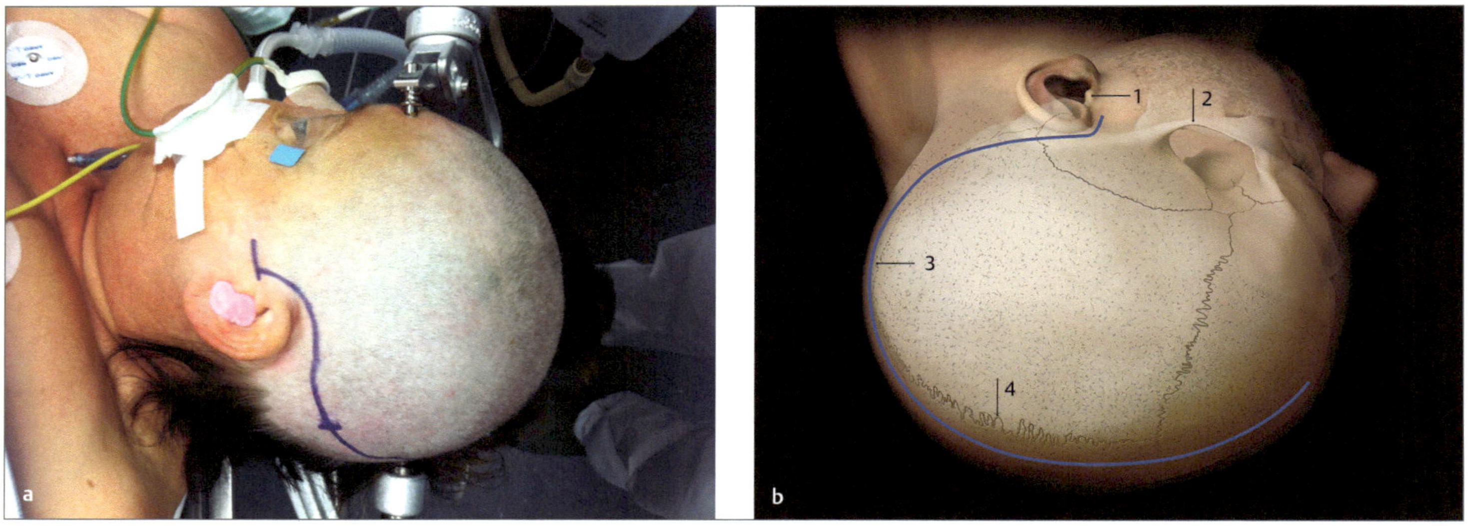

Fig. 8.2 (a,b) Anatomy overview. Landmarks are (1) the tragus for the lower limit of skin incision, (2) zygomatic process of the frontal bone for the anterior cranial base, (3) opisthocranion as the most posterior part of the skull for the posterior inferior limit of skin incision, and (4) the midline. A landmark for the transverse sinus and the torcular is the line drawn from the epicanthus lateralis to the point where the ear (helix) connects to the scalp. The extension of this line approximates the position of the transverse sinus and the torcular/inion.

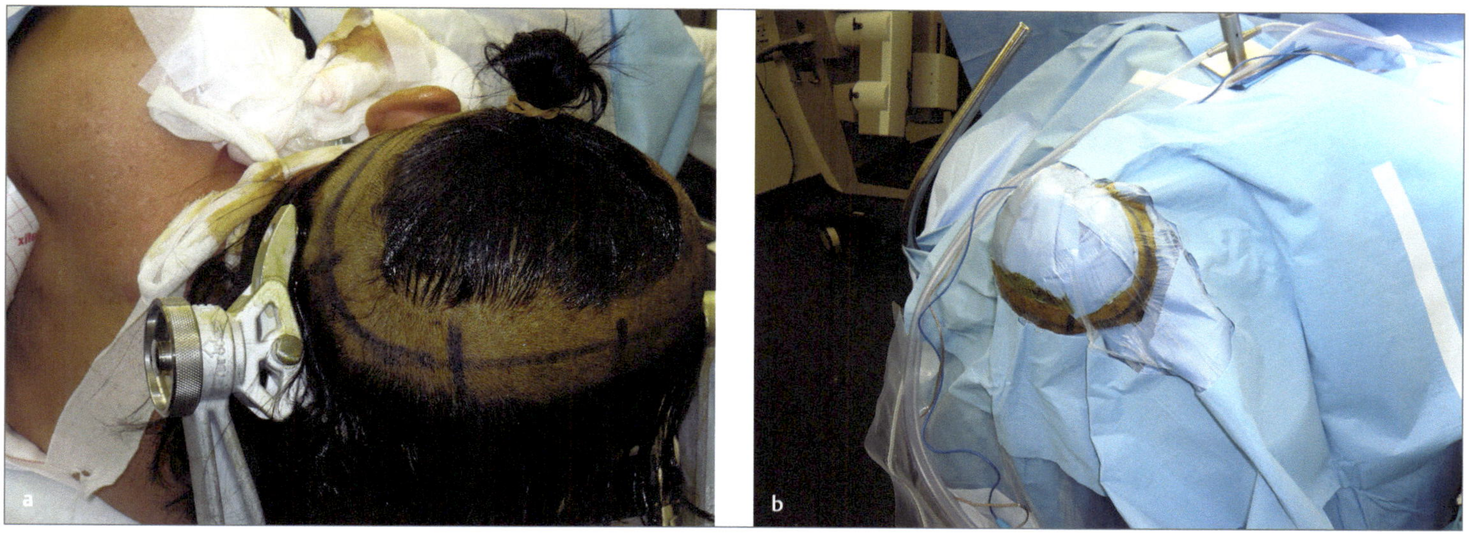

Fig. 8.3 (a,b) Shaving and draping. Simply shave a strip (as broad as the width of the clipper) or the hemicranium.

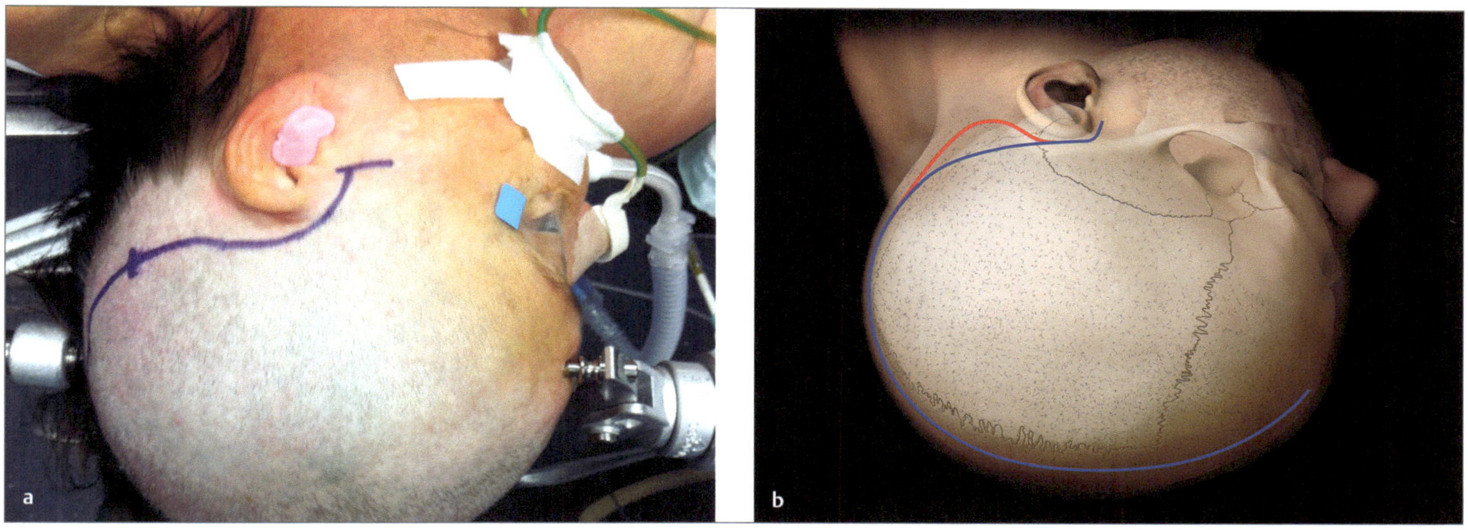

Fig. 8.4 (a,b) Skin incision. The question-mark-like skin incision follows the four landmarks mentioned above. Because a common mistake is to perform a craniectomy that is too small to allow extension of the brain without shearing at the bone edges, the skin incision should be large enough to perform a temporal decompression and follow more or less the transverse and sagittal sinus. Avoiding a sharp angle behind the ear leads to less scalp necrosis and better wound healing.

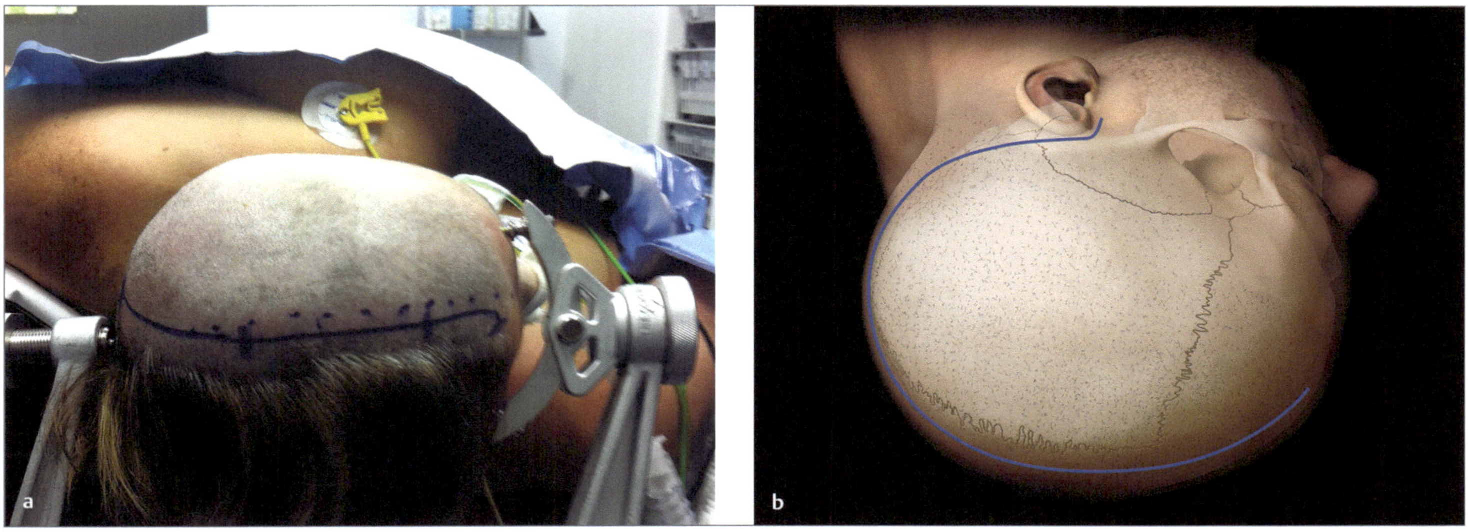

Fig. 8.5 (a,b) Contralateral midline crossing. The cross-midline skin incision is used to facilitate reinsertion of the bone flap. The craniectomy should extend close (~1.5 cm) to the midline. The skin incision should be made outside the craniectomy line. It simplifies the surgical procedure of reinsertion of the bone flap, because it allows to cut the skin down through the scar straight to the level of the bone. By contrast, if the scar lies over the craniectomy, i.e., over brain tissue, it takes much longer to find and dissect the desired layer, and complications are more likely. Therefore, the cross-midline skin incision is recommended to facilitate reinsertion of the bone flap.

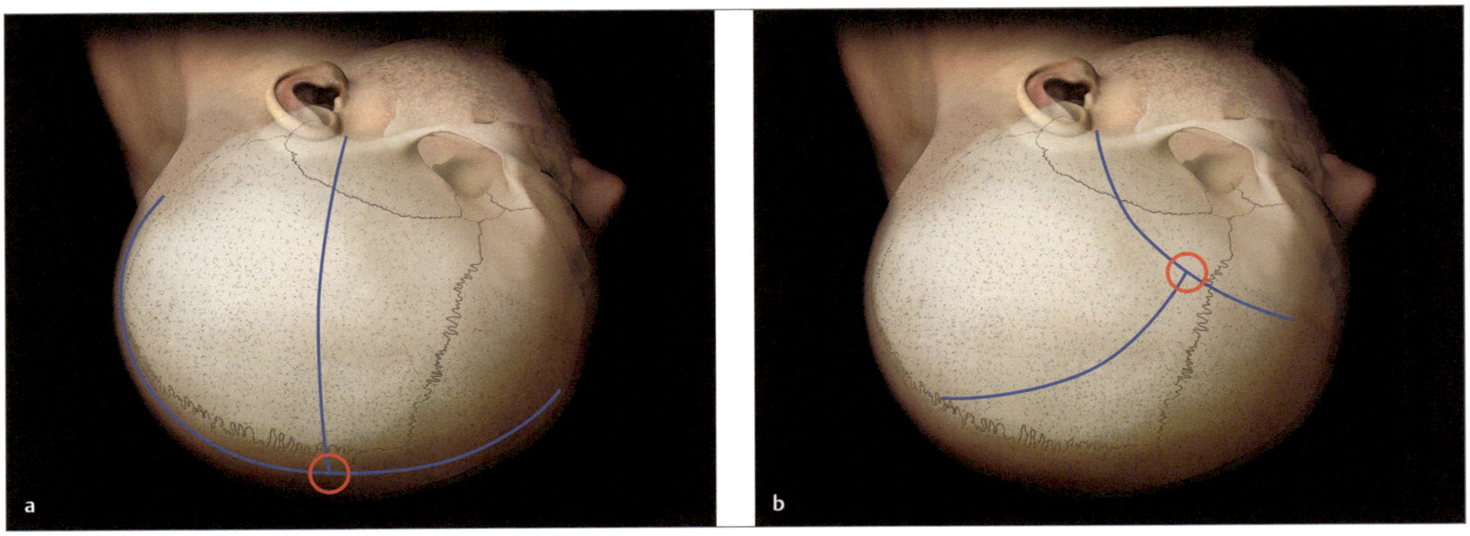

Fig. 8.6 (a,b) **Alternative skin incision.** A T-shaped skin incision is an alternative to a hockey stick **(a)**. However, it may somewhat increase wound healing complications compared to the question mark incision because it requires cutting two 90° angles. Sometimes a decompressive hemicraniectomy has to be performed secondarily after a smaller craniotomy, for example, after aneurysm clipping or the removal of a subdural hematoma **(b)**. In these cases, a skin incision already exists and can be extended. Then, a more or less T-shaped skin incision can be performed allowing exposure of the hemicranium while still enabling good wound healing **(b)**. This approach faces the same problem of two 90° cuts. Coagulation in this area (circle) should be avoided and the skin suture at these edges should be tightened only gently to maintain blood supply.

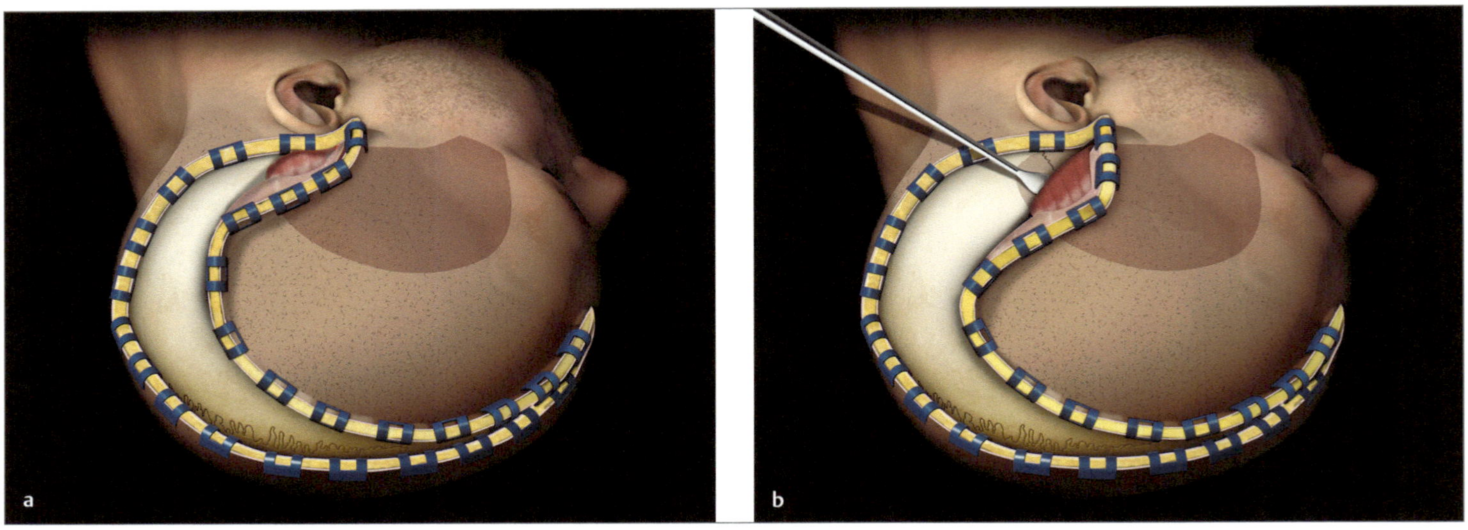

Fig. 8.7 (a,b) **Myocutaneous flap and muscle handling.** The skin is incised down to the level of the bone. Skin clips are placed to control bleeding. The main trunk of the superficial temporal artery (see Chapter 5.2.2) and the parietal branch should be saved. The skin flap is elevated from frontal and parietal toward the temporal muscle which is still fixed to the bone and the galea. Upon reaching the edge of the muscle, it is sharply incised and detached from the temporal bone, but left completely attached to the skin and galea flap.

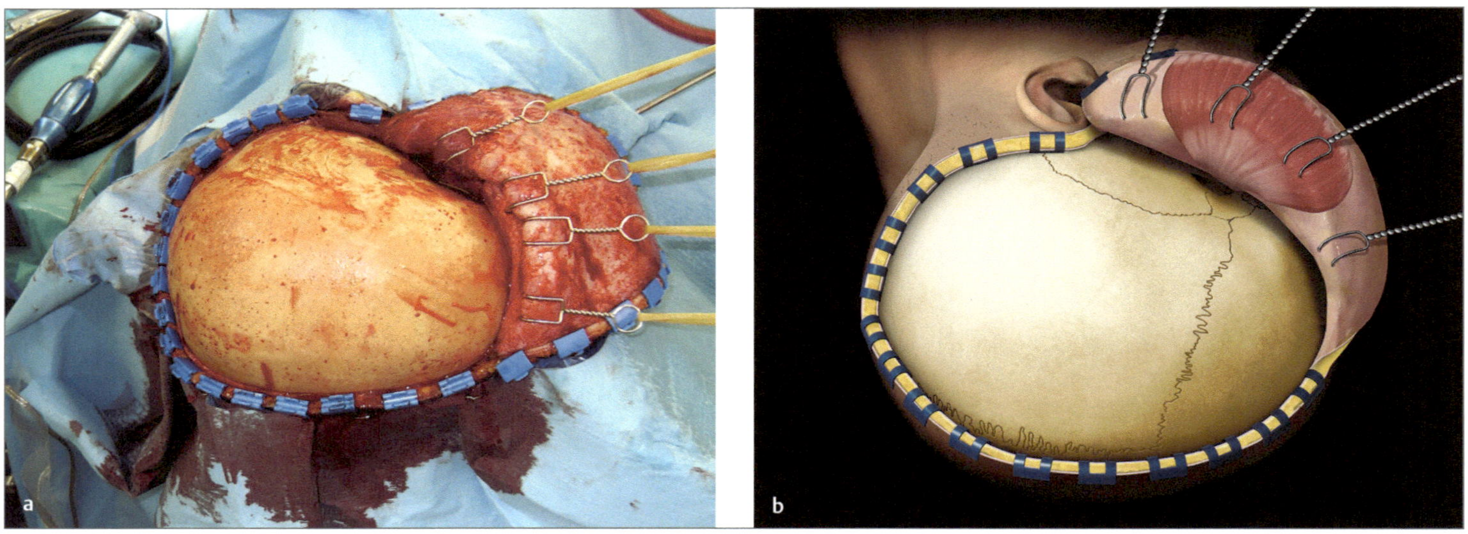

Fig. 8.8 (a,b) **Exposure of the hemicranium.** Then the single myocutaneous flap is developed toward the frontal and temporal base. Fish hooks are used to retract the flap.

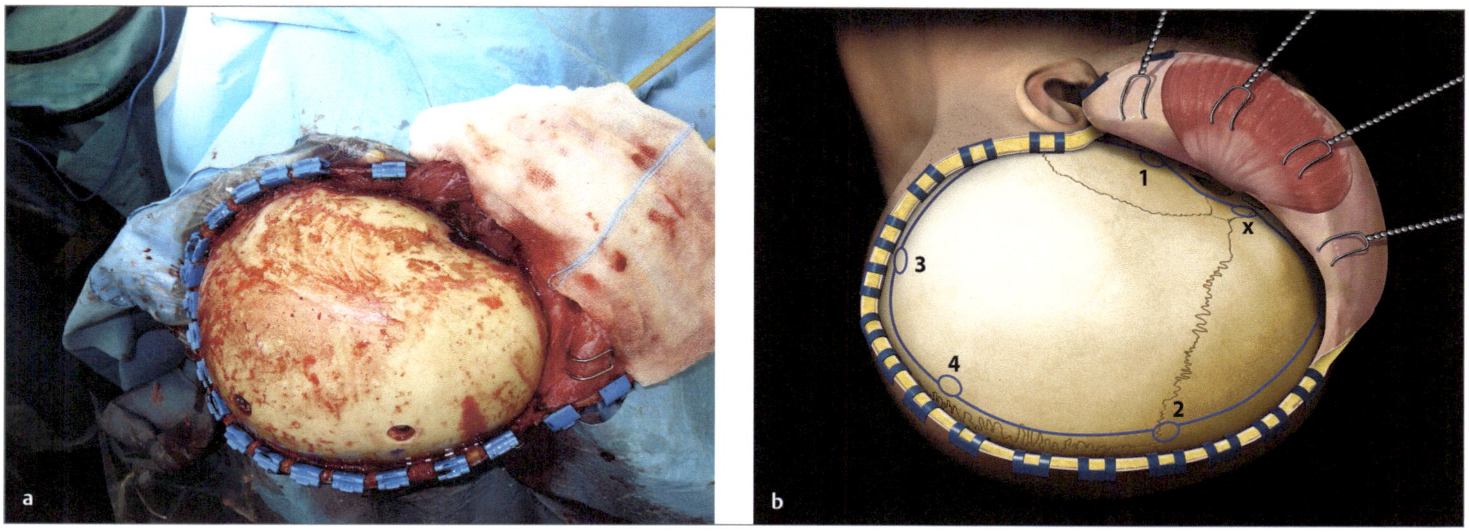

Fig. 8.9 (a,b) Burr holes and craniotomy. Placing the burr holes should not follow any dogma. The goal is to saw the bone flap quickly and easily without damaging the dura or the sinuses. One practical routine is the following four-burr hole technique: (1) one at the temporal base, root of zygoma, (2) one at the bregma, approximately 1.5–2 cm from the midline (use the width of the burr: one width from midline), (3) one just behind the lambdoid suture, (4) one between the bregma and the lambdoid hole, next to the midline (one burr-width away from the midline).

There is a reason for the location of every burr hole: (1) to mark the level of the skull base at the middle fossa—remember to decompress osteoclastic down to the level of the middle fossa and not to leave any form of balcony that is sufficient for the temporal bone to serve as a support for herniation into the temporal notch: (2) safe mark for midline and cosmesis—the burr hole is usually way behind the hairline: (3) makes sure that the bone flap is wide enough: (4) enables straightforward sawing down along the superior sagittal sinus (SSS) without running into the SSS (just make a line between burr holes 2 and 4).

Cave: remember the basal temporal bone is sometimes very pneumatized with a high risk of rhinoliquorrea after decompressive craniectomy. Seal air cells (e.g., with bone wax, muscle, or glue).

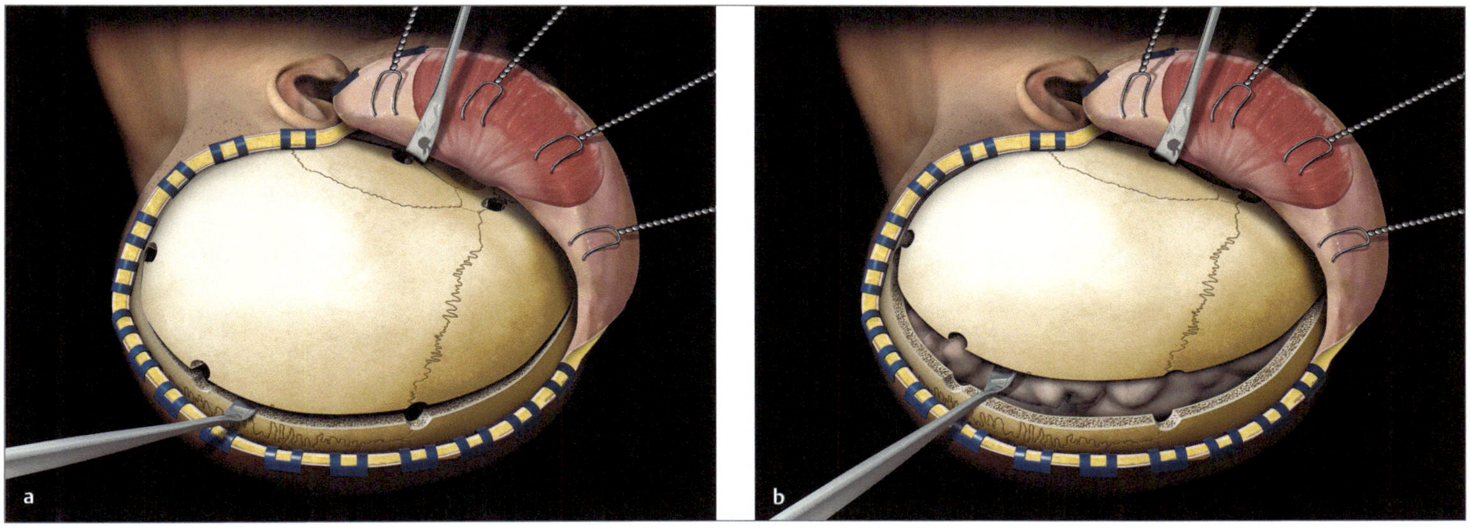

Fig. 8.10 (a,b) Lifting the bone flap. It is usually difficult to lift the bone flap. It is tightly fixed by the dura and lifting one edge to allow better access to the inner table to detach the dura often pushes the other side into the brain. Sometimes several elevators have to be used to prevent this. One or more additional burr holes (x) may help in detaching the dura.

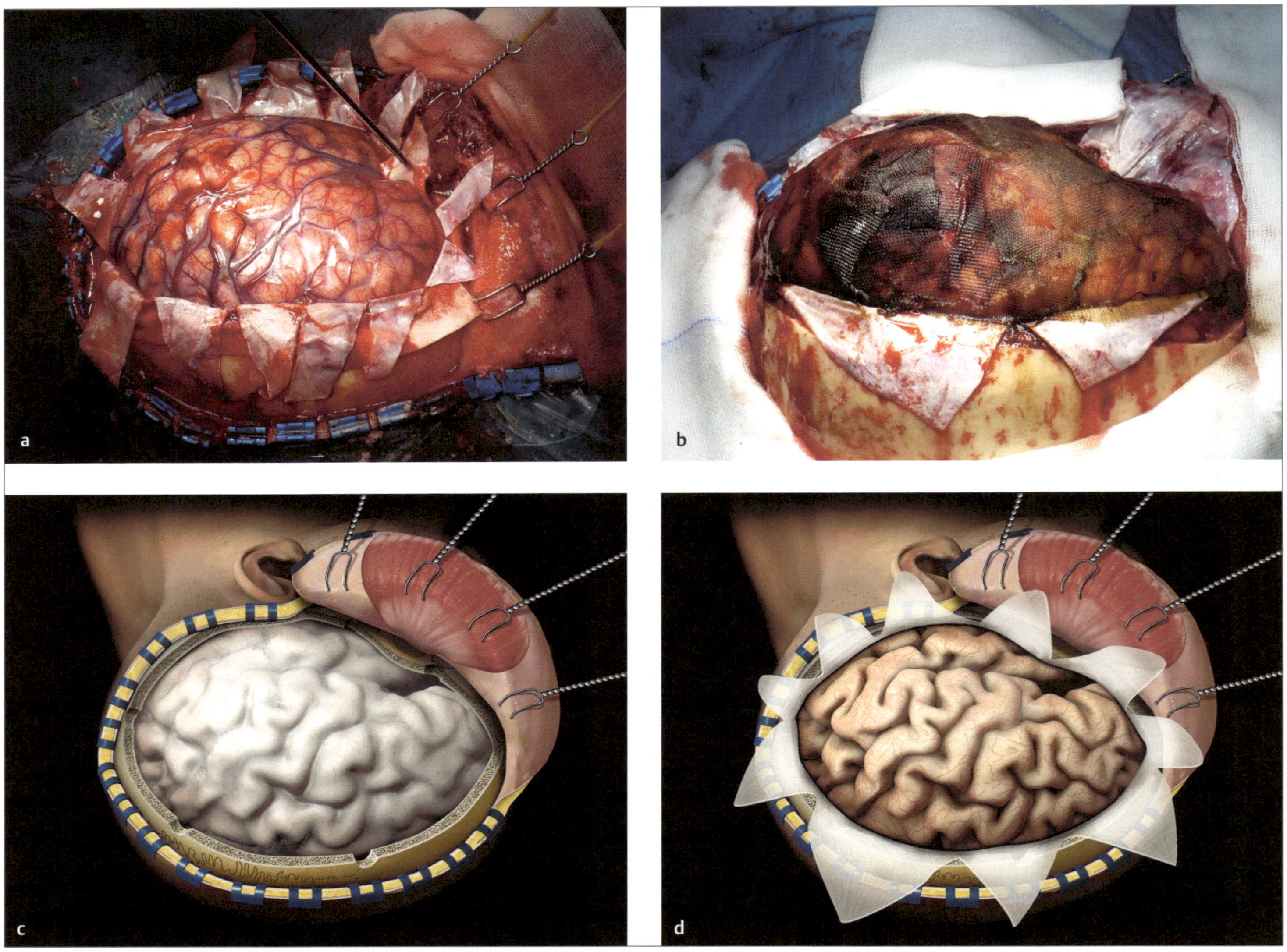

Fig. 8.11 (a–d) Dural opening. Open the dura in a C-shaped fashion around the sylvian fissure and then release the dura in stellate fashion up to the bony edges (stellate: because of the bridging veins; be careful not to cut these veins that run, often attached to the dura, close to the sinuses).

Cover brain with Tabotamb or any other (reasonably priced and rapidly available) material. The goal is to promote the formation of a neo-dura that covers the brain and provides a readily available plane for dissection at the time of reinsertion of the bone. There is no need to add any form of dura plastic.[1]

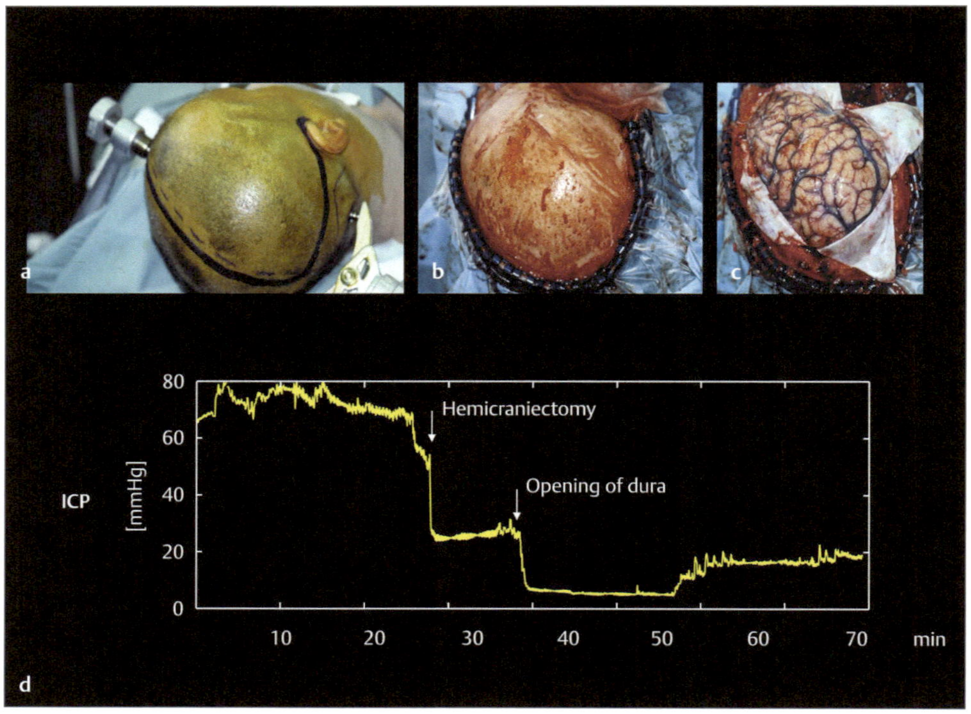

Fig. 8.12 (a–d) Decompressive hemicraniectomy to treat increased ICP. Decompressive craniectomy in a patient with an ICP probe. **(a)** The cross midline skin incision, **(b)** the one-layer myocutaneous flap, and **(c)** the dural opening. **(d)** After lifting of the bone flap (hemicraniectomy) ICP drops from around 70 to 25 mm Hg and only after large opening of the dura, the ICP decreases further to around 8 mm Hg.

Skin Closure

Before closure, think about an ICP monitor. An intraparenchymatous ICP probe can facilitate the management of the patient on the ICU.

After covering the brain loosely with dura mater (do not use sutures) and placing a subgaleal drain without active suction, the myocutaneous skin flap is turned back. The galea is sutured subcutaneously, before applying skin staples or running skin suture, or the skin–galea is sutured with large stitches.

In the case of a T-shaped skin incision: do not apply tension to the edges where the T-shaped incision approximates, because this is the most vulnerable site (to avoid necrosis of the skin).

Measures in Case of Massive Bleeding

Cover sinus with Gelfoam (-/+ glue) or suture dura/sinus against the bone. Cave: never push any material into the sinus; the goal is to cover the sinus and not to plug it.

Checklist

- Cross-midline skin incision.
- Question mark skin flap.
- Myocutaneous flap.
- Four burr holes (temporobasal, bregma, lambda, between bregma and lambda) for orientation.
- Saw the bone along the sinus last.
- Control sinus bleeding by covering the sinus (immediately: finger, cottonoids; permanent: Gelfoam, Gelfoam with fibrin glue).
- Open dura wide, stellate fashion (90°) to the sinus.
- Think about pressure monitoring (eases management during stay in ICU).
- Cover brain with dura and scar-forming dural substitute (Surgicel, Audio-mesh, Gelfoam).
- Place drain subgaleal (passive, cave suction).
- Suture subcutaneously and then suture skin.

Reference

[1] Güresir E, Vatter H, Schuss P, et al. Rapid closure technique in decompressive craniectomy. J Neurosurg 2011;114(4):954–960

9 Approaches to the Orbita

9.1 Frontolateral Approach to the Orbit

Torstein R. Meling

A frontolateral craniotomy can be combined with a superior orbitotomy to give wide superior and lateral exposure of the orbital contents for microsurgical removal of orbital tumors. It is particularly suitable for large orbital neoplasms, tumors in the orbital apex, optic canal lesions, lesions with intracranial extensions, and medial orbital tumors (see ▶ Fig. 9.1, ▶ Fig. 9.2, ▶ Fig. 9.3, ▶ Fig. 9.4, ▶ Fig. 9.5, ▶ Fig. 9.6, ▶ Fig. 9.7, ▶ Fig. 9.8, ▶ Fig. 9.9, ▶ Fig. 9.10, ▶ Fig. 9.11, ▶ Fig. 9.12, ▶ Fig. 9.13, and ▶ Fig. 9.14).

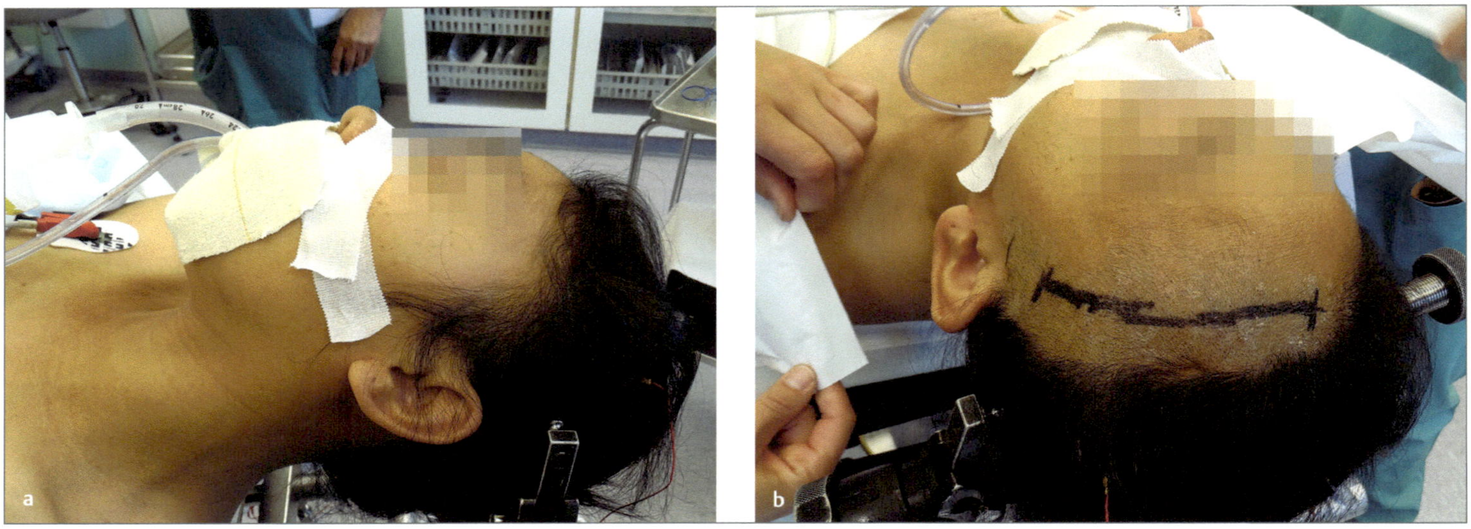

Fig. 9.1 (a, b) Positioning. The patient is placed in the supine position with the body slightly elevated. The head is fixed in a three-pin headrest and elevated above the level of the heart. The head is rotated 15–20° to the contralateral side and tilted laterally to increase the surgeon's working space. The head is then retroflexed 15° so that gravity causes the frontal lobe to fall away from the anterior cranial fossa and allow for retractor-free intracranial dissection.

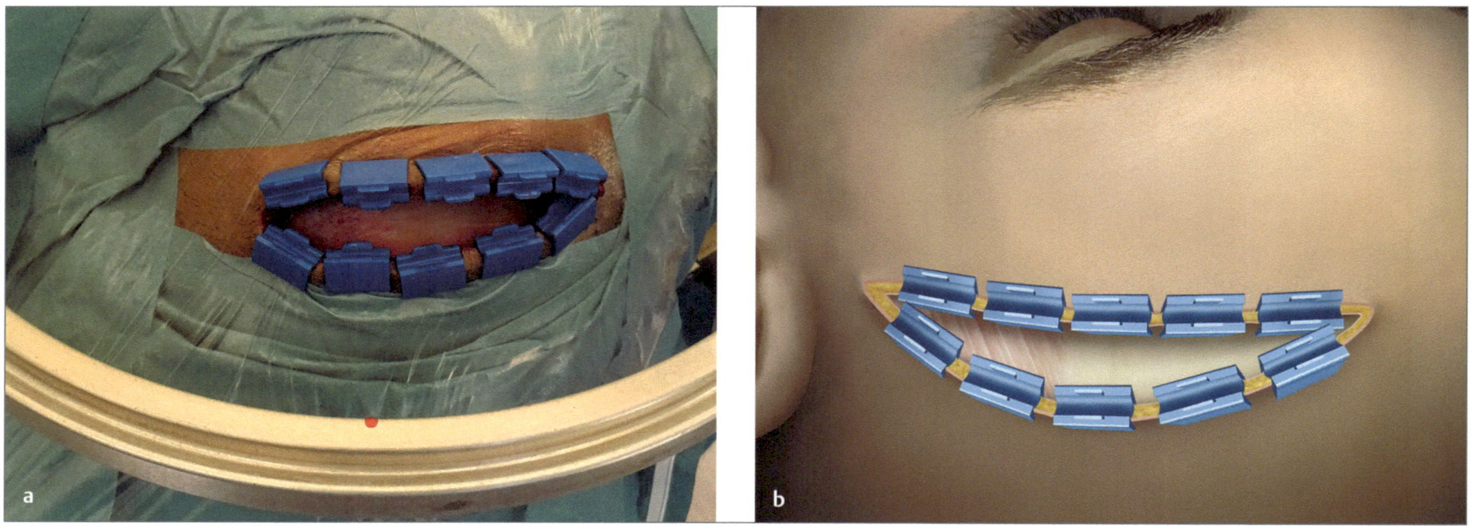

Fig. 9.2 (a, b) Skin incision. The skin is minimally shaved and infiltrated using 1% Xylocaine with 1:200,000 adrenaline. Using a No. 20 knife blade, a slightly curved frontotemporal skin incision is made behind the hairline. The incision stops 2 cm from the midline and 3 cm above the zygoma. Hemostatic clips are placed on the margins of the incision.

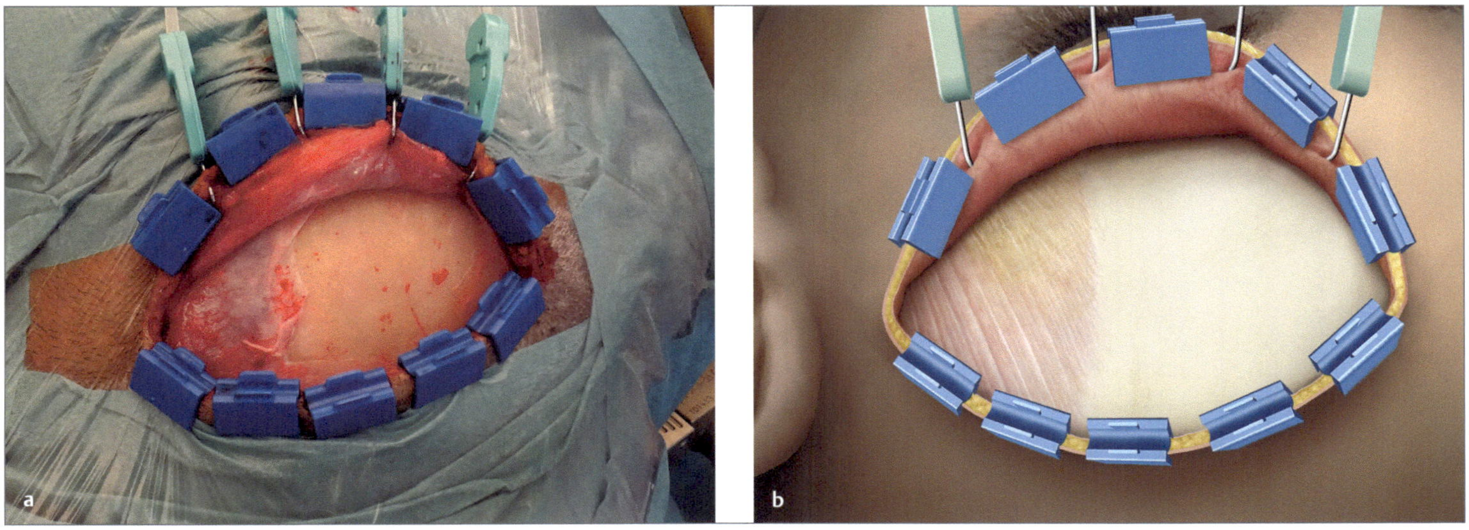

Fig. 9.3 (a, b) Skin flap. The skin flap is retracted anteriorly using three or four small fishhooks with elastic bands. The temporal muscle is left in place. To avoid injury to the supraorbital nerve, the superior orbital margin should not be exposed.

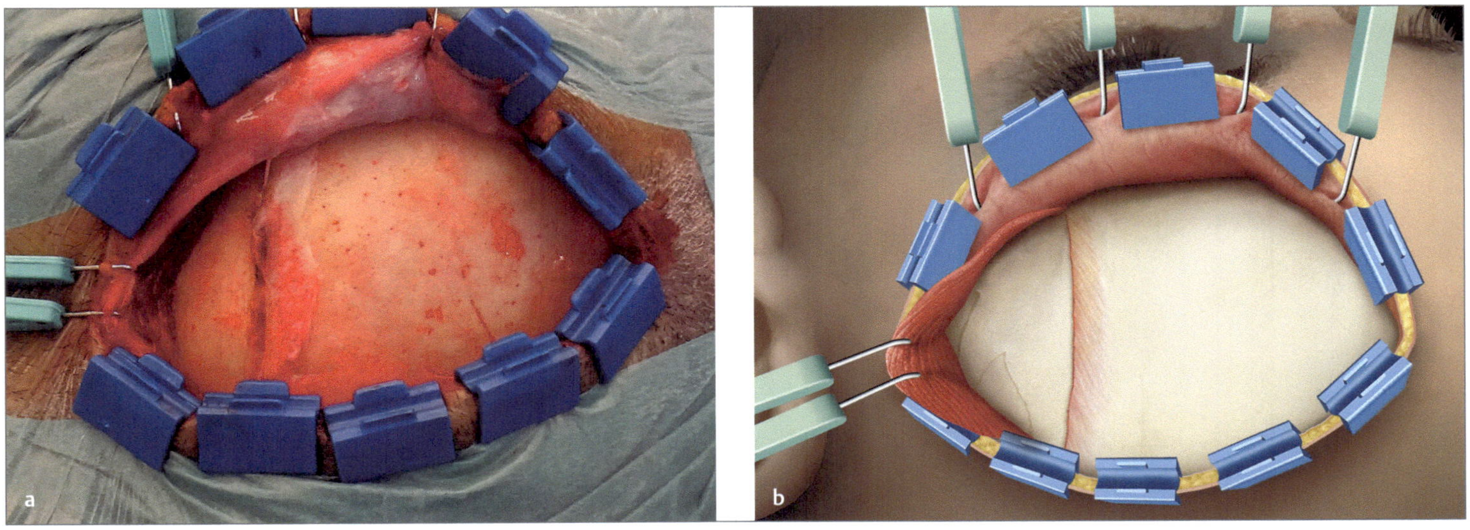

Fig. 9.4 (a, b) Detachment of the temporal muscle. Superiorly, the temporal muscle is detached along the muscle insertion. The temporalis muscle is also detached from its insertion at the zygomatic process of the frontal bone and the temporal fossa and retracted inferiorly toward the zygomatic arch with one or two fishhooks. It is lifted up rather than retracted by force.

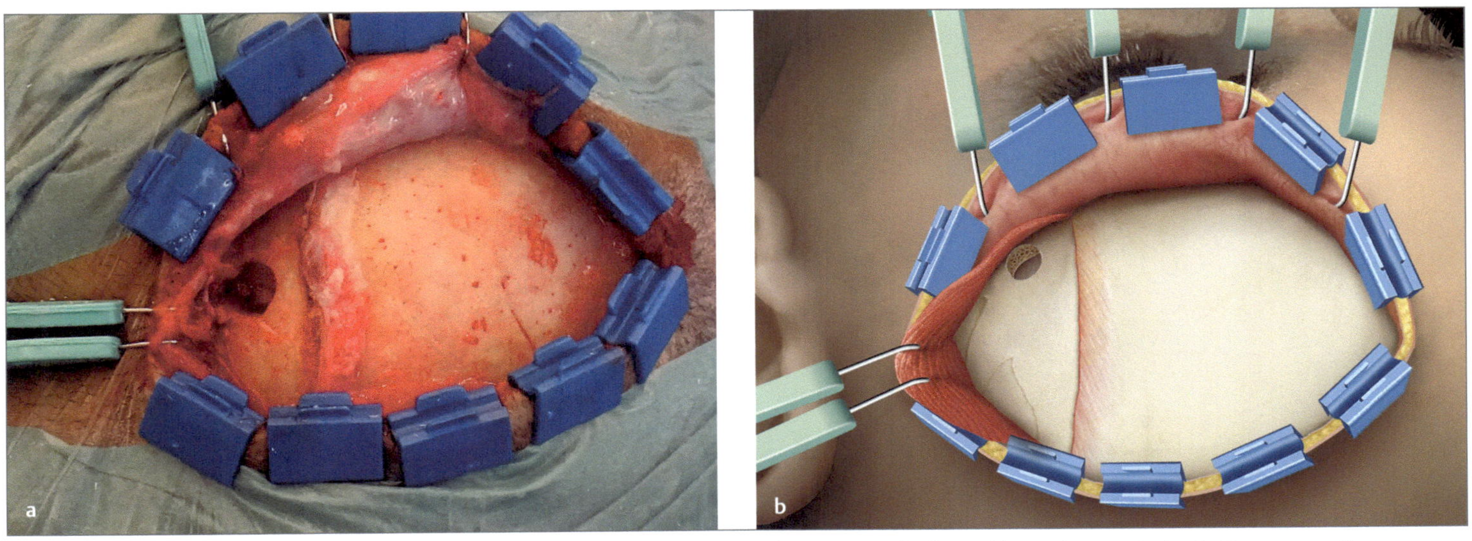

Fig. 9.5 (a, b) Burr hole. Using a 2-mm, sharp burr, a small burr hole (3–5 mm) is made in the frontal bone, just posterior to the zygomatic process and caudal to the superior temporal line, so as to be covered by the temporalis muscle when this is later reattached.

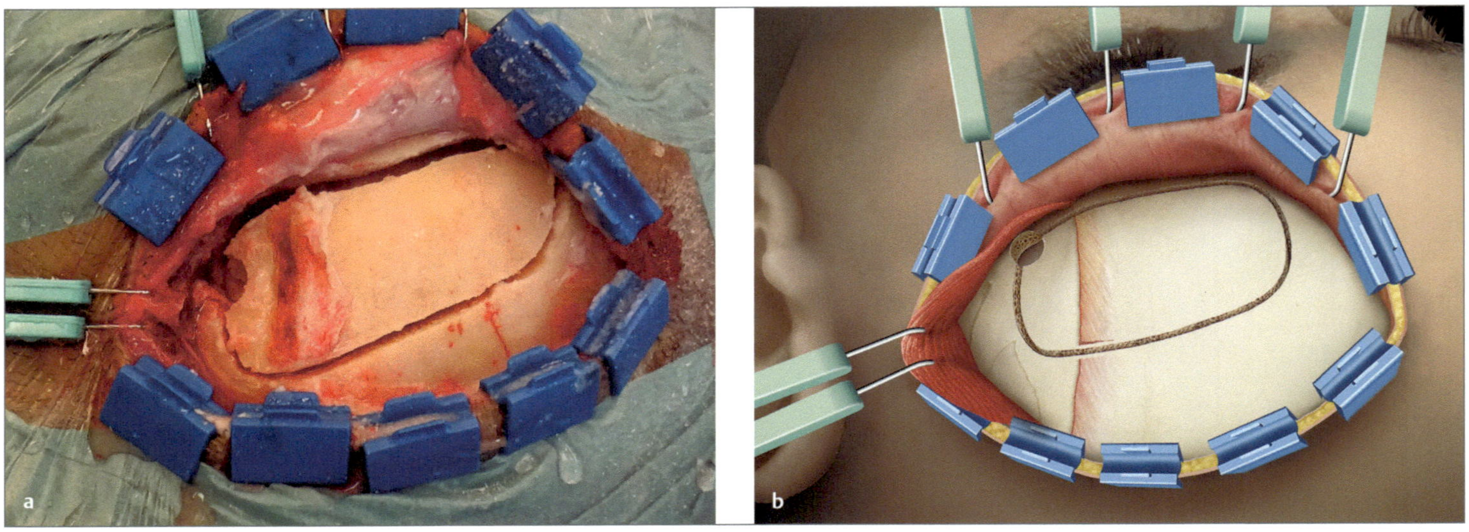

Fig. 9.6 (a, b) Bone flap. Using a high-speed electric craniotome, a lateral frontotemporal craniotomy is performed. A straight anterior cut is made as close to the superior orbital rim as possible in a lateral-to-medial direction, avoiding the lateral border of the frontal paranasal sinus as measured on preoperative MR scans. Next, a C-shaped line is cut from the burr hole to the medial border of the previously made frontobasal line. The size of the bone flap depends on whether the intraorbital lesion is medial or lateral to the levator muscle, with the medial location requiring a wider exposure. As the most common intraorbital corridor is between the levator and lateral rectus muscles, the almost superelliptic bone flap is usually 5 cm wide (coronal plane) and 2.5 cm deep (sagittal plane).

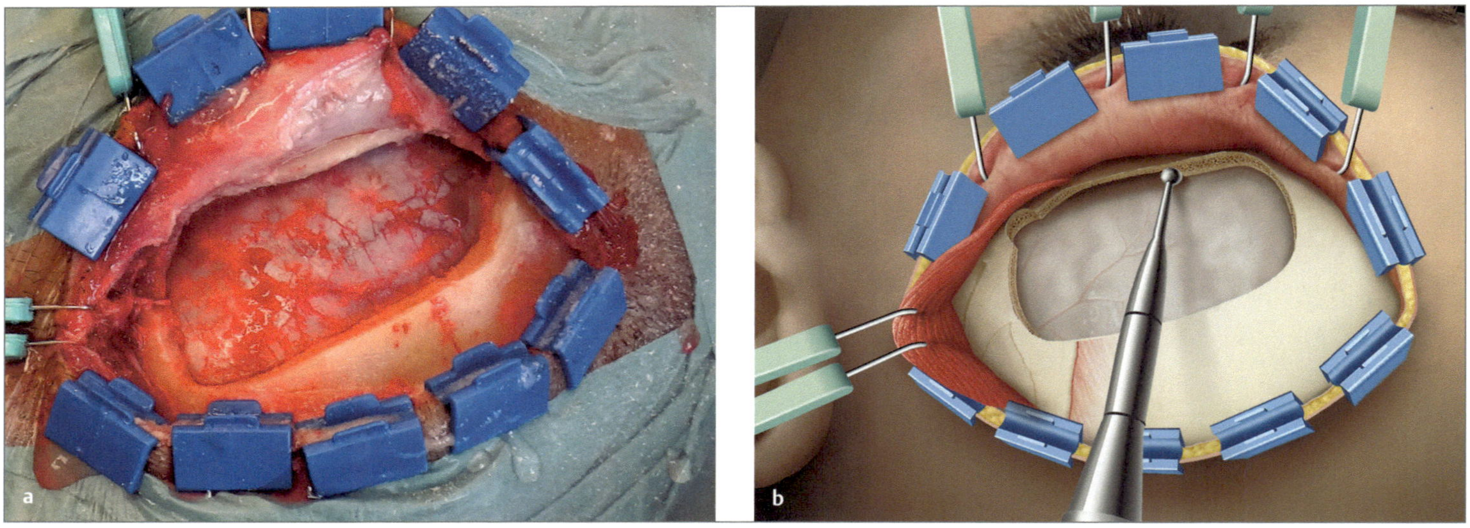

Fig. 9.7 (a, b) Additional bone drilling. The inner edge of the orbital bar is drilled away expanding the view along the skull base.

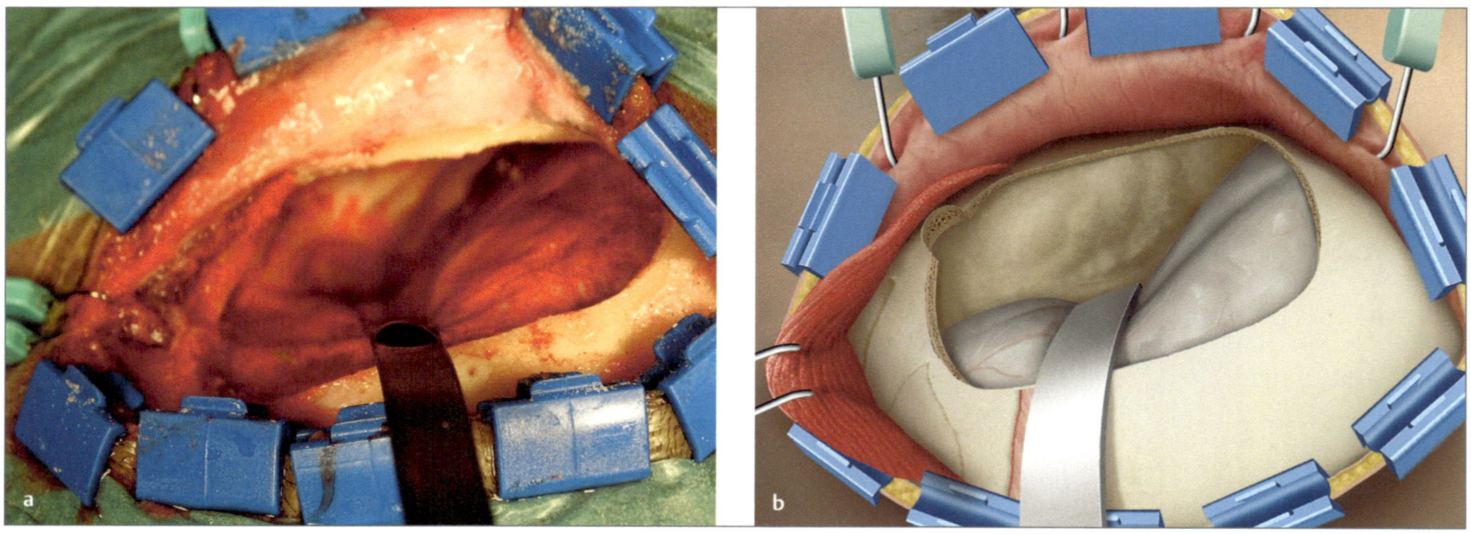

Fig. 9.8 (a, b) Extradural dissection. The dura is lifted off the inner table of the frontal bone and the orbital roof. Care is taken not to come too far medially, so as not to injure the ipsilateral olfactory nerve in the olfactory groove. No lumbar drain is inserted, as head elevation and good neuroanesthesia are sufficient for brain relaxation. Lesions confined entirely to the orbit can be removed without opening the dura, whereas intradural exposure is required for those lesions involving the intracranial segment of the optic nerve.

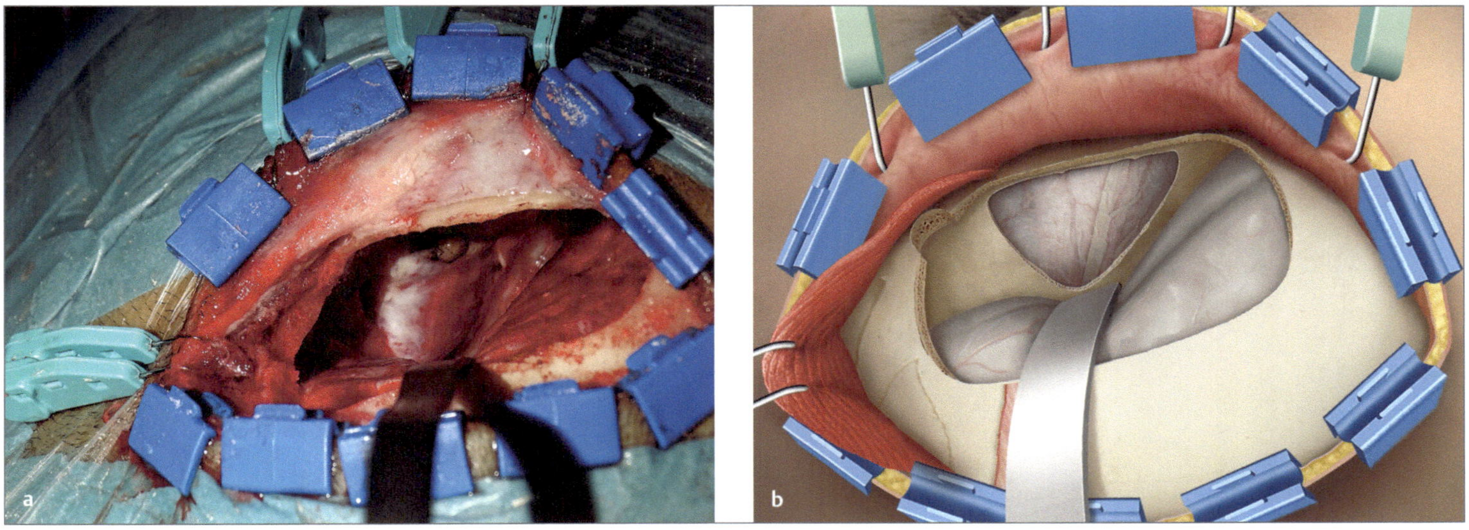

Fig. 9.9 (a, b) Superior orbitotomy, visualization of the periorbita, and underlying anatomy of the orbit. Using a Misonix electric 1-mm bone scalpel, straight cuts are made in the superior orbital roof, creating a trapezoid bone flap. The bone flap can be supplemented by a craniectomy over the optic canal if the most posterior parts of the orbit and the intracanalicular segment of the optic nerve need to be exposed. Care should be taken not to injure the underlying periorbita and the trochlear and frontal nerves in the midline and the lacrimal nerve laterally. The periorbita is frequently thinned by the raised intraorbital pressure caused by the lesion and is often very difficult to preserve.

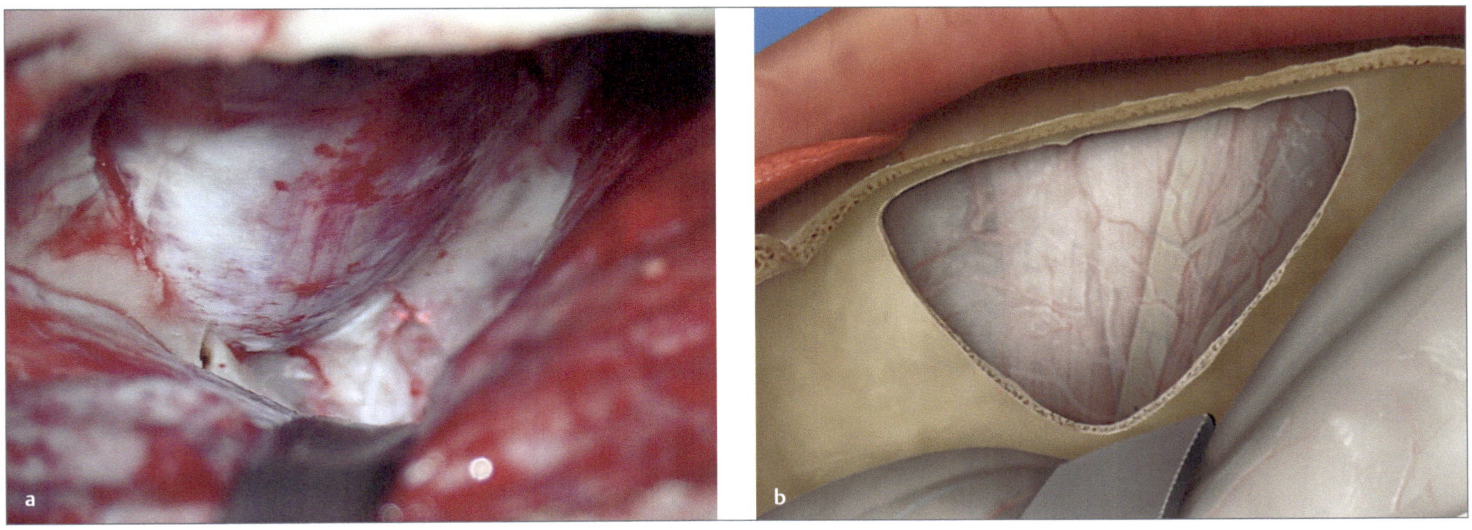

Fig. 9.10 (a, b) Periorbital dissection. The periorbita is incised using a diamond knife or microscissors. A V-shaped incision is made and the periorbita flap is retracted anteriorly. This exposes the trochlear nerve and the supraorbital and supratrochlear branches of the frontal nerve, all of which run immediately beneath and can often be seen through the periorbita. The trochlear nerve passes medially above the levator muscle to reach the superior oblique muscle. The frontal nerve is a branch of the ophthalmic nerve (V1) and passes through the superior orbital fissure to course superiorly on the levator muscle. It divides into a supratrochlear nerve, which passes above the trochlea of the superior oblique muscle, and the supraorbital nerve, which passes through the supraorbital foramen or notch in the supraorbital margin. The lacrimal nerve passes above the lateral rectus muscle to innervate the lacrimal gland and convey sensation to the area around the lateral part of the supraorbital margin.

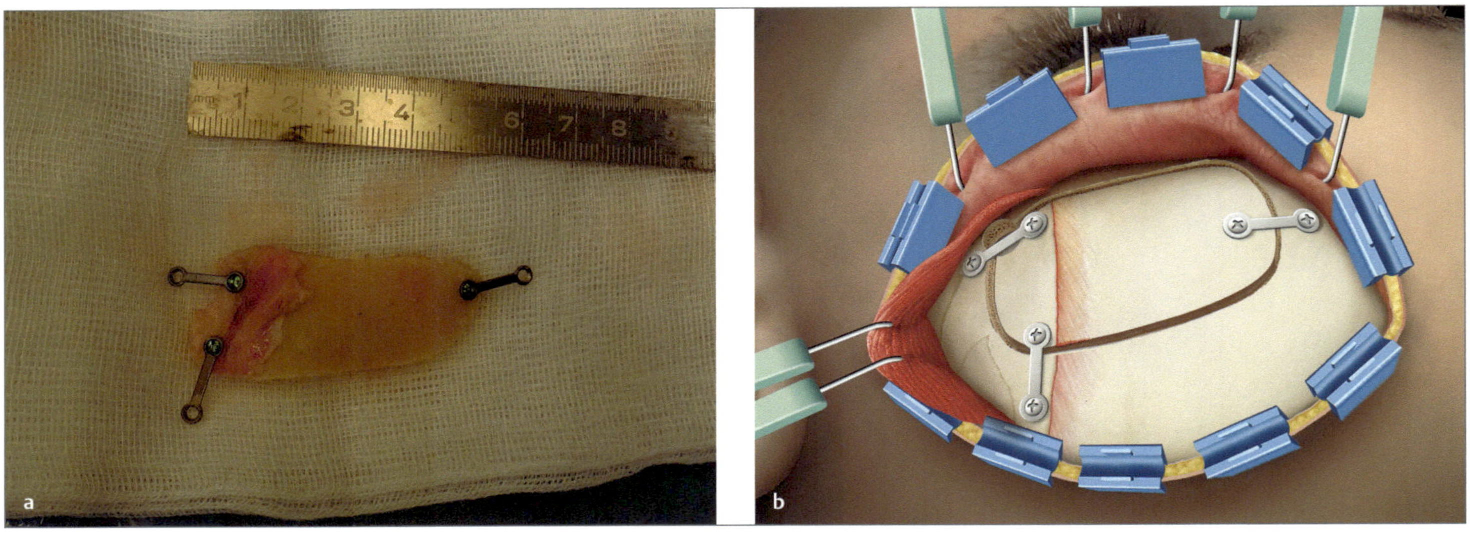

Fig. 9.11 (a, b) Closure. After the resection, any bleeding is controlled by applying FloSeal hemostatic matrix rather than bipolar diathermy. A small piece of Tachosil is placed over the intraorbital fat to reconstruct the periorbita. To avoid a pulsating exophthalmos, the orbital bone flap is replaced and fixed with 1-mm titanium mini-plates.

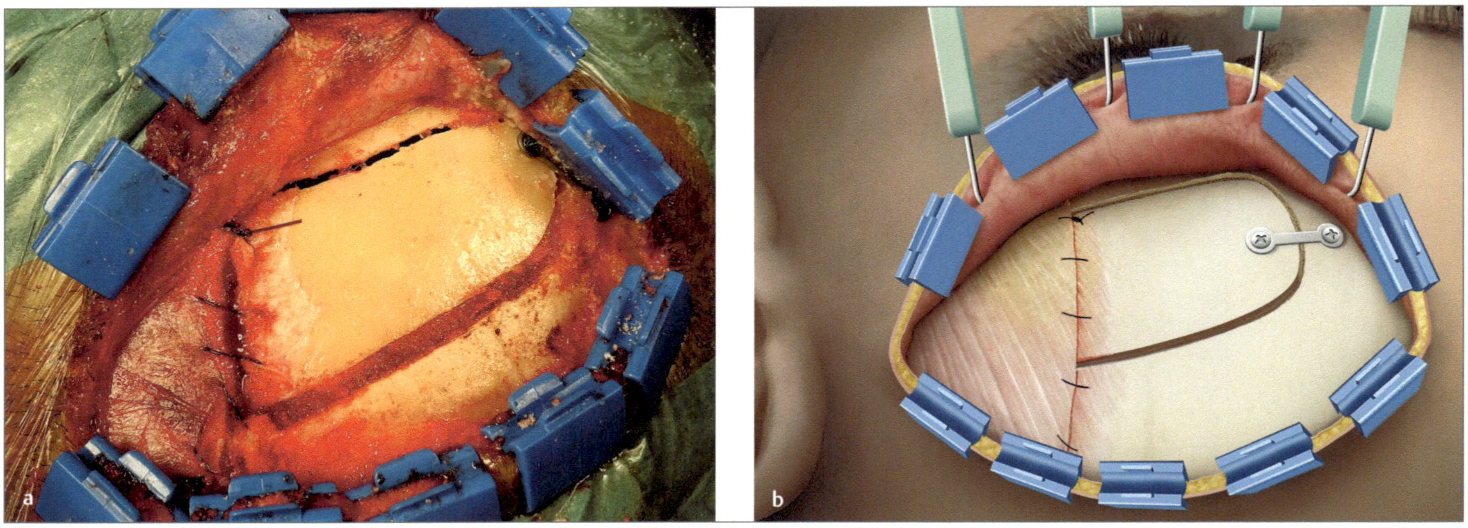

Fig. 9.12 (a, b) Bone closure. The craniotomy bone flap is replaced and secured using 1-mm titanium mini-plates. Care is taken to ensure that the bone flap is level with the surrounding cranium. The muscle is reattached to the cuff.

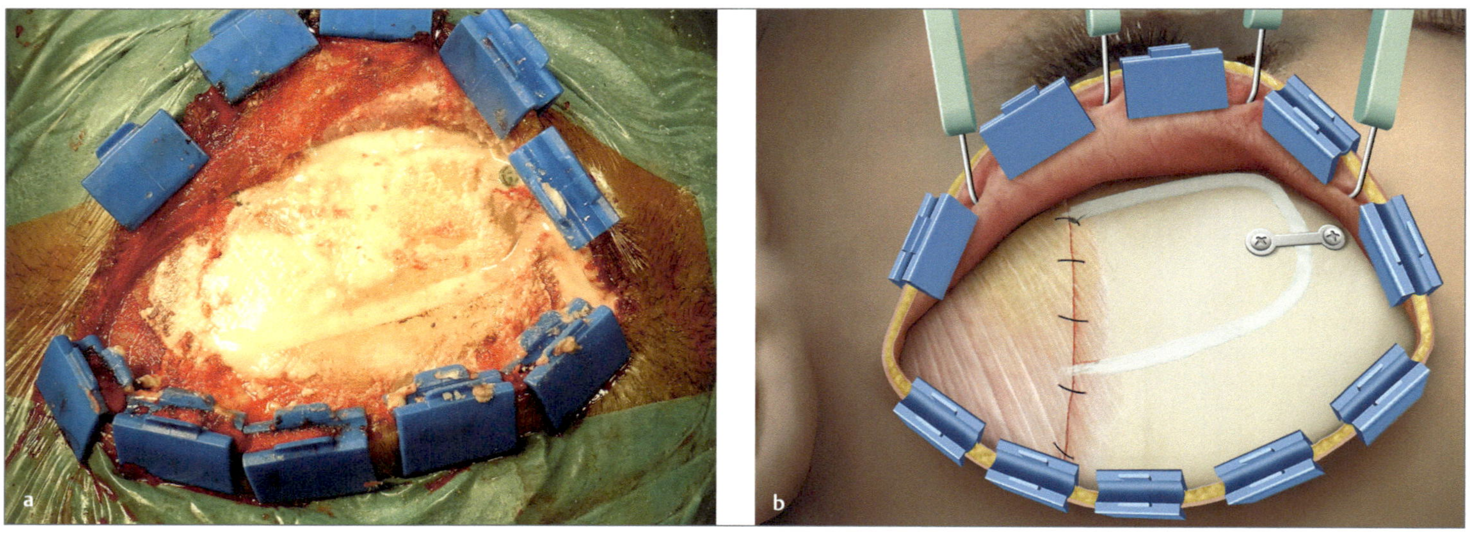

Fig. 9.13 (a, b) Bone closure. Any irregularities or larger gaps can be filled using BoneSource hydroxyapatite cement.

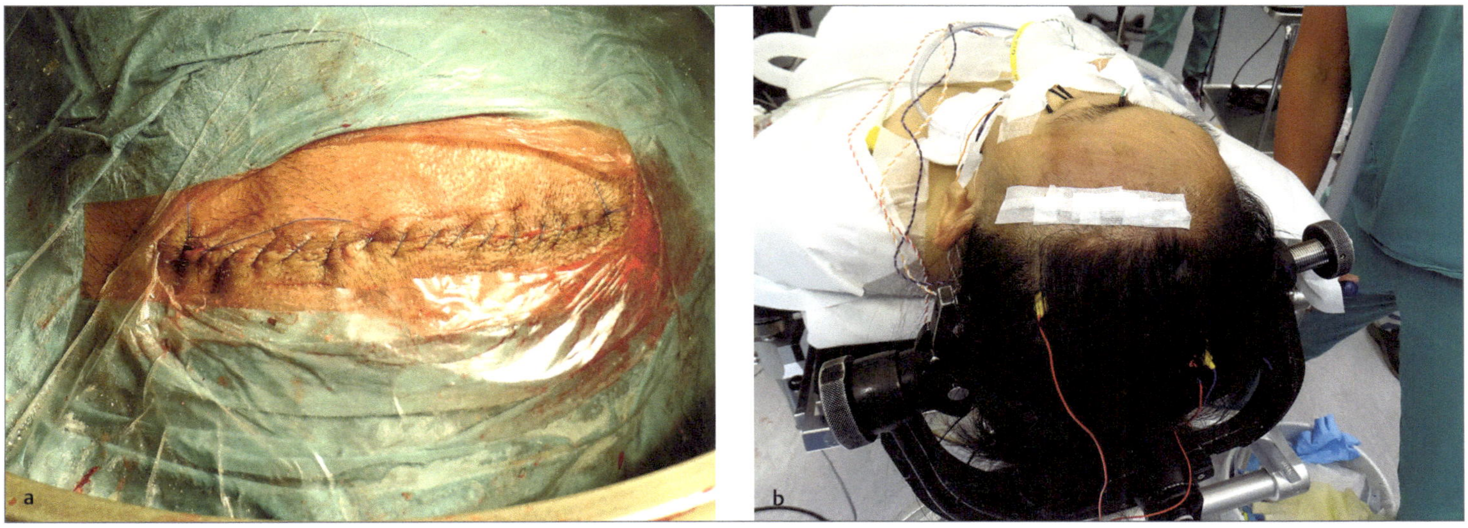

Fig. 9.14 (a, b) Skin closure. The pericranium is closed with a running Monocryl 3–0 suture. The skin is closed using skin sutures. The wound is dressed using 3M Steri-Strips.

Checklist

- Look at CT and MR images to familiarize yourself with the frontal sinus anatomy. Cave: very lateral extensions.
- Before skin incision, make sure the head is retroflexed enough to allow the frontal lobe to fall away from the anterior cranial fossa and enable retractor-free intracranial dissection.
- Make the skin incision > 1 cm behind the hairline and ensure that it is sufficiently large.
- When performing the interfascial dissection, stay directly on the superficial layer of the deep temporal fascia *at all times* to avoid injury to the temporal branch of the facial nerve.
- Detach the temporalis muscle from its anterior insertion and retract it inferiorly toward the zygomatic arch.
- Use neuronavigation to identify the lateral border of the frontal sinus.
- Make a small burr hole posterior to the zygomatic process of the frontal bone and caudal to the superior temporal line to improve cosmesis.
- Make the first cut straight and run it as close to the superior orbital rim as possible in a lateral-to-medial direction. Cave: very medial cuts can injure the supraorbital nerve if not properly detached from its canal/groove.
- Make the last cut C-shaped, starting from the burr hole and running to the medial border of the first cut.
- Drill the tabula interna of the orbital bar to expand the field of view while leaving the tabula externa intact for cosmesis.
- When lifting the dura off the frontal bone and the orbital roof, be careful not to go too far medially, so as not to injure the ipsilateral olfactory nerve in the olfactory groove.
- Use a Misonix electric 1-mm bone scalpel or a pediatric craniotome to make the cuts in the superior orbital roof so as to avoid losing too much bone.
- After opening the periorbita, identify the trochlear nerve and the supraorbital and supratrochlear branches of the frontal nerve as landmarks.
- For the intraorbital part of surgery, retract the rectus muscles gently using PDS 5–0 traction sutures.
- Gently dissect the intraorbital fat lobules using cotton swaps as blunt dissectors to avoid rupture of the lobules.
- Avoid bipolar electrocoagulation or, if unavoidable, use at a very low power setting. Try to stop bleeding with FloSeal hemostatic matrix rather than bipolar diathermy.
- To avoid a pulsating exophthalmus, fix the orbital bone flap with Lorentz 1-mm titanium mini-plates or PDS sutures.
- Ensure that the bone flap is level with the surrounding cranium so as to avoid any irregularities and use hydroxyapatite cement to fill any larger gaps.

9.2 Lateral Orbitotomy

Torstein R. Meling

Kronlein's original lateral orbitotomy technique, which was first described in the late 1800s, has undergone many modifications, especially with respect to the skin incision. The lateral approach is useful for tumors located in the lateral, superior, or inferior compartment in the orbit (see ▶ Fig. 9.15, ▶ Fig. 9.16, ▶ Fig. 9.17, ▶ Fig. 9.18, ▶ Fig. 9.19, ▶ Fig. 9.20, ▶ Fig. 9.21, ▶ Fig. 9.22, ▶ Fig. 9.23, and ▶ Fig. 9.24).

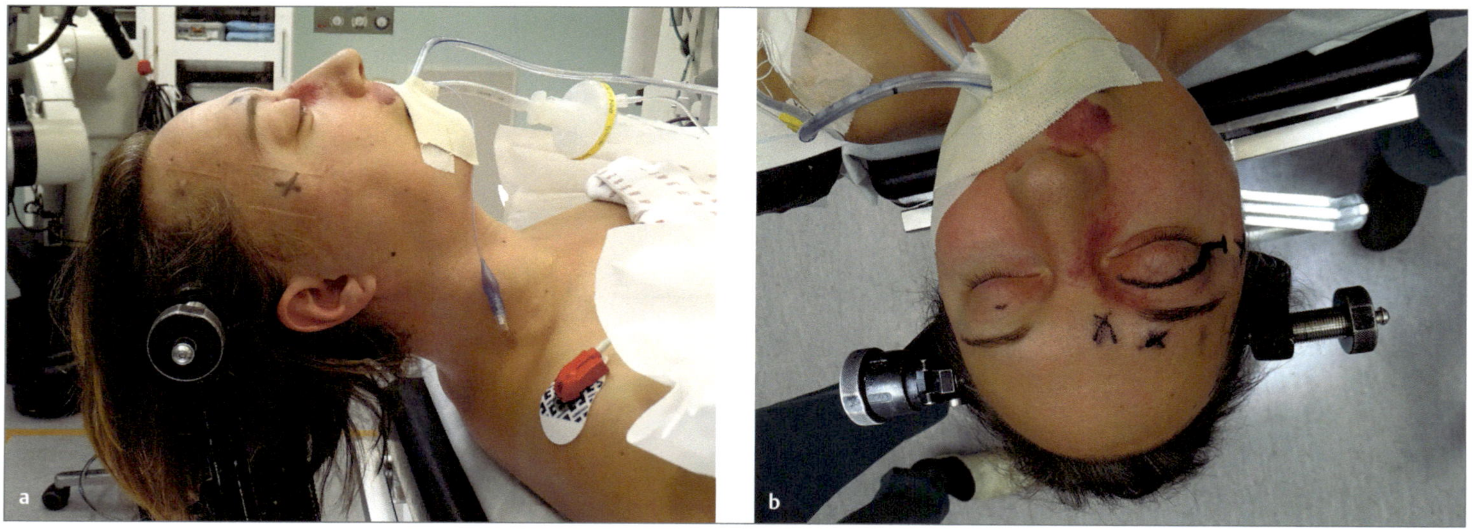

Fig. 9.15 (a, b) Positioning. The patient is in the supine position with the body slightly elevated. The head is fixed in a three-pin headrest and elevated above the level of the heart. The head is rotated 10–15° to the contralateral side and the neck is slightly extended and tilted laterally.

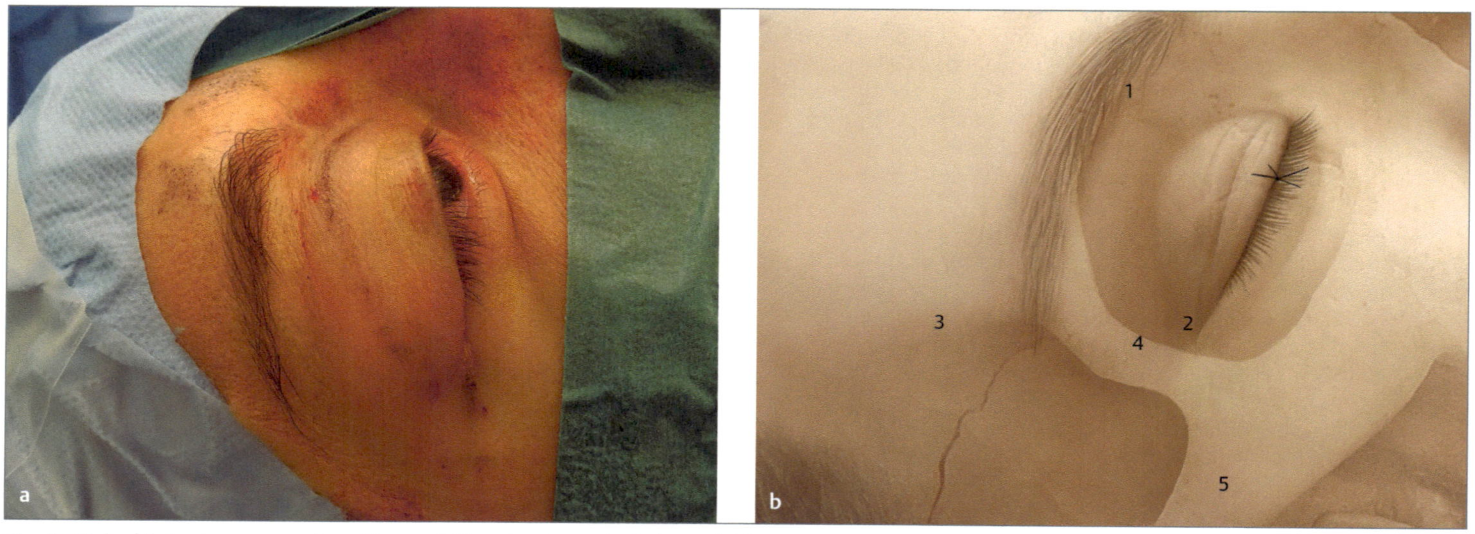

Fig. 9.16 (a, b) Anatomy overview. The eyelid incision is particularly useful for gaining access to the superior and lateral orbital space. The skin incisions are made perpendicular to the skin surface, with one important exception: if an eyebrow incision is used, the cut is made at a 45° angle following the angulation of the hair follicles for cosmetic reasons.

Important anatomical landmarks are: (1) supraorbital foramen/notch, (2) lateral canthus, (3) frontotemporale = palpable zygomatic process of the frontal bone, (4) lateral orbital rim, (5) anterior superior edge of the zygomatic arch.

Skin incisions of the eyelids and periorbital area should follow the relaxed skin tension lines. For reasons of cosmesis, the incision line should be marked with a fine-tipped surgical pen prior to any injection of local anesthetics. A 2.5- to 3.5-cm incision of the upper eyelid is marked on the mid-eyelid crease. The medial limit of the skin incision is just lateral to a vertical plane running through the supraorbital notch. The lateral limit is usually at a horizontal plane running through the lateral canthus.

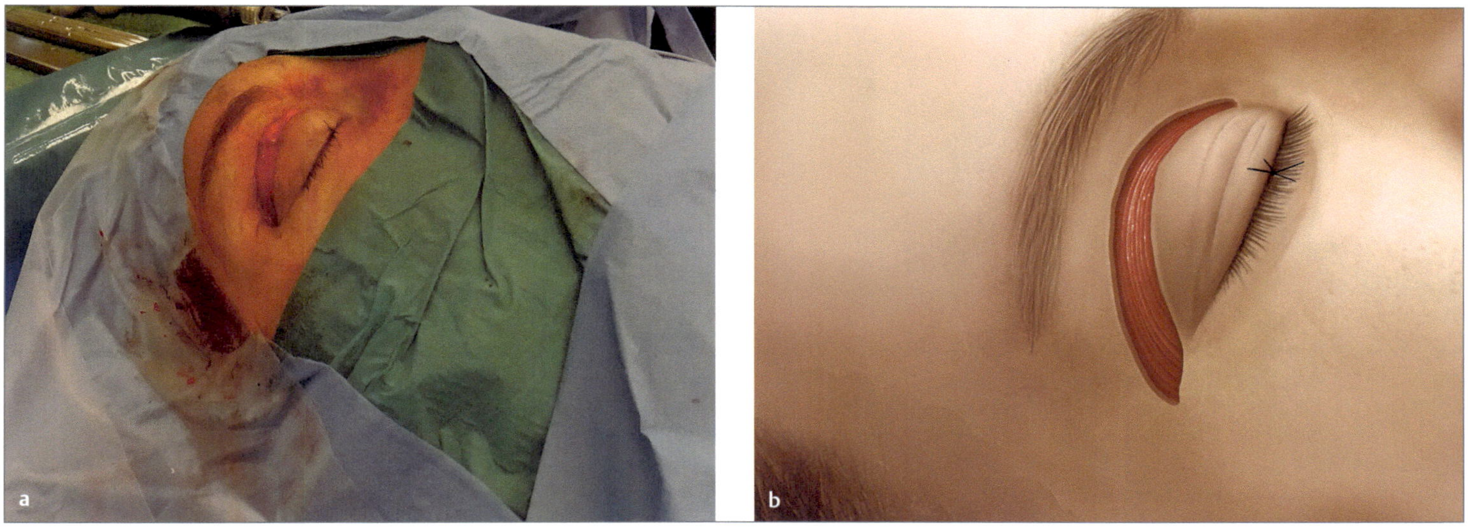

Fig. 9.17 (a, b) Eyelid crease incision. Initially, a temporary tarsorrhaphy is performed to protect the cornea. The skin is infiltrated using Xylocaine 1% with 1:200,000 epinephrine. The skin incision is made under the microscope with a No. 15 blade knife. The entire length of the incision should be completed in one sweep from medial to lateral. Care should be taken to cut only the skin, so as not to injure the underlying structures.

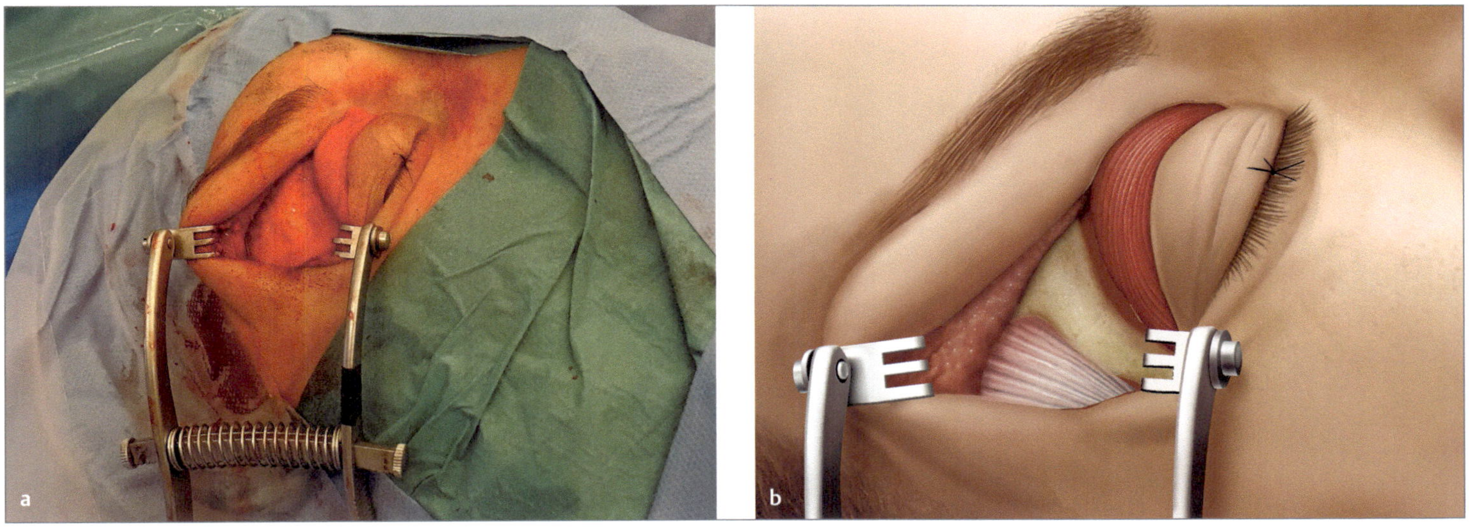

Fig. 9.18 (a, b) Subcutaneous dissection. The skin flap is retracted using a low-profile, curved, self-retaining retractor.

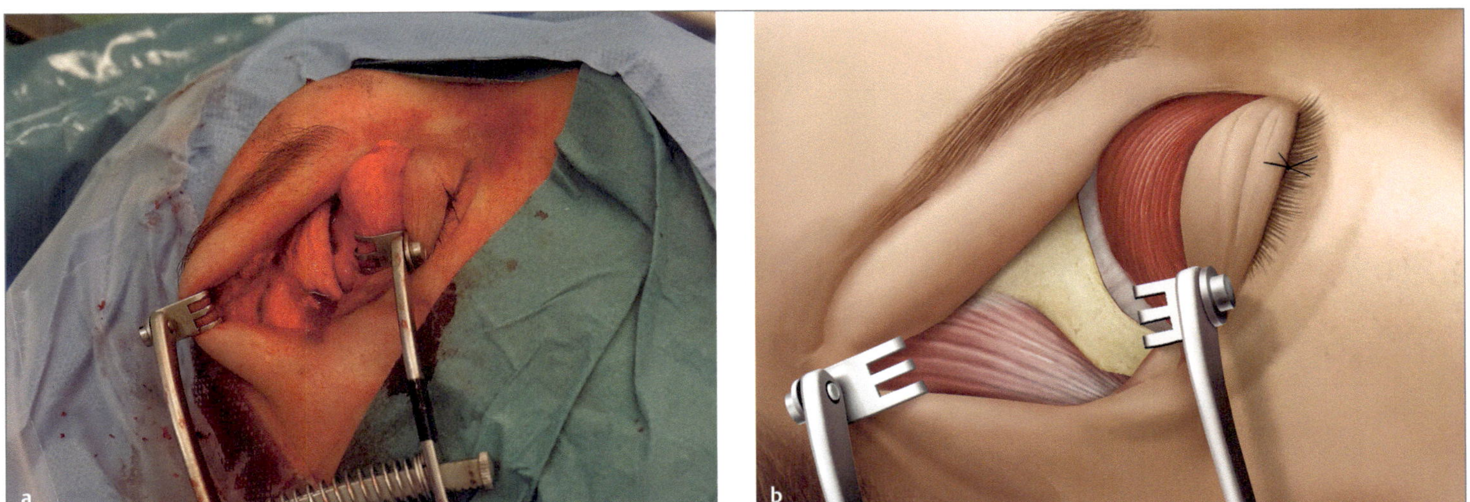

Fig. 9.19 (a, b) Subcutaneous dissection. The orbicularis oculi muscle is traversed by blunt dissection using curved scissors with blunt tips to reach the periosteum of the superior and lateral orbital rim. The periorbita is dissected and mobilized.

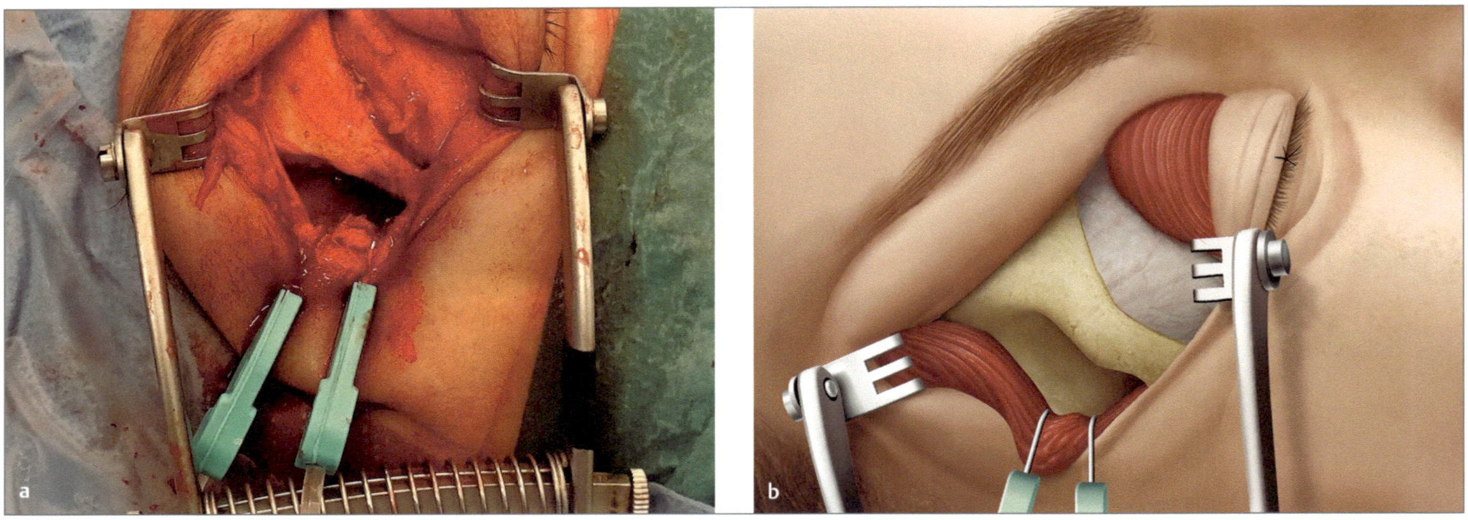

Fig. 9.20 (a, b) Intraorbital dissection. The periosteum is incised sharply with a knife or using a monopolar with a Colorado needle tip. Subperiosteal dissection is performed to expose the lateral orbital rim and wall externally in the frontotemporozygomatic region. The temporalis aponeurosis is detached from its insertion along the zygomatic process of the frontal bone and frontal process of the zygomatic bone anteriorly. This allows for elevation of the temporal muscle from the lateral orbital wall and retraction of the muscle posteriorly using one or two small fishhooks with elastic bands. The subperiosteal dissection is carried medially to expose the lateral orbital wall internally. It is important to stay subperiosteal so as not to injure the periorbita and bulbus oculi. The depth of this dissection depends on the location of the lesion, but should usually extend beyond the equator of the orbit to prevent injury to the soft tissues during the orbitotomy and to expose the anterior two-thirds of the lateral orbital wall.

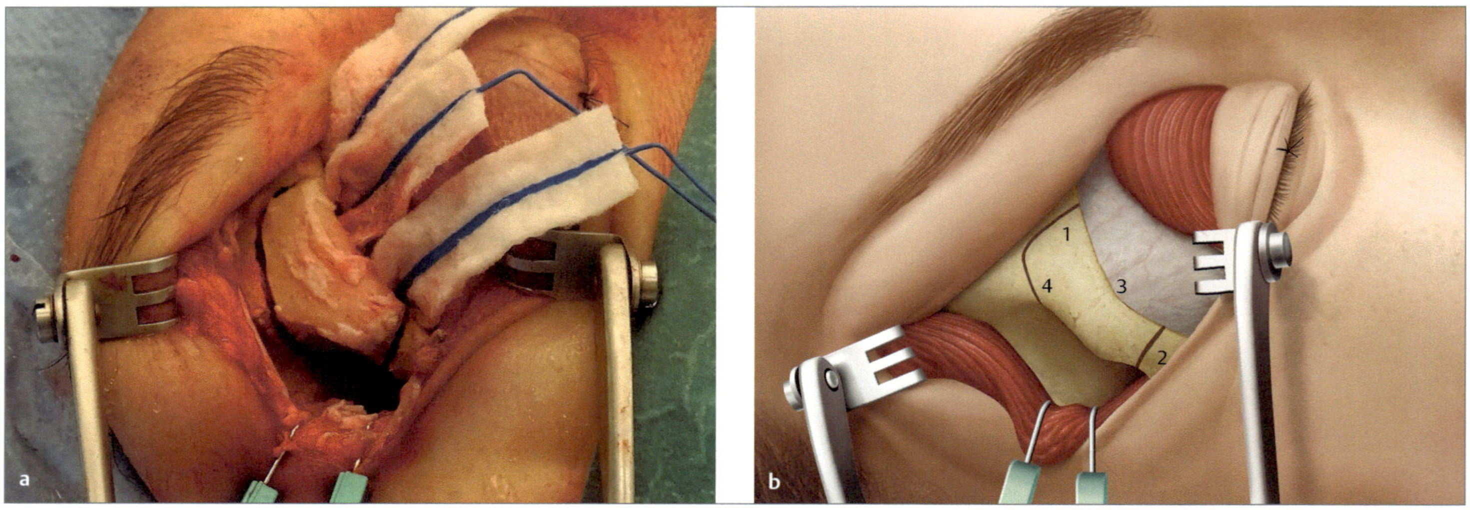

Fig. 9.21 (a, b) Lateral orbitotomy. Using an electric 1-mm bone scalpel, four straight cuts are made in the orbital wall. These comprise two horizontal cuts in the lateral orbital ring, one superiorly in the superior orbital rim of the frontal bone (2), and one inferiorly in the frontal process of the zygomatic bone (2). The cuts usually extend posterior to the equator of the orbit. Next, two vertical cuts are made: one internally in the orbit pointing posterolaterally (3) and one externally through the greater sphenoid wing in the temporal region pointing anteromedially (4). Care should be taken to avoid thermal damage to the surrounding tissue.

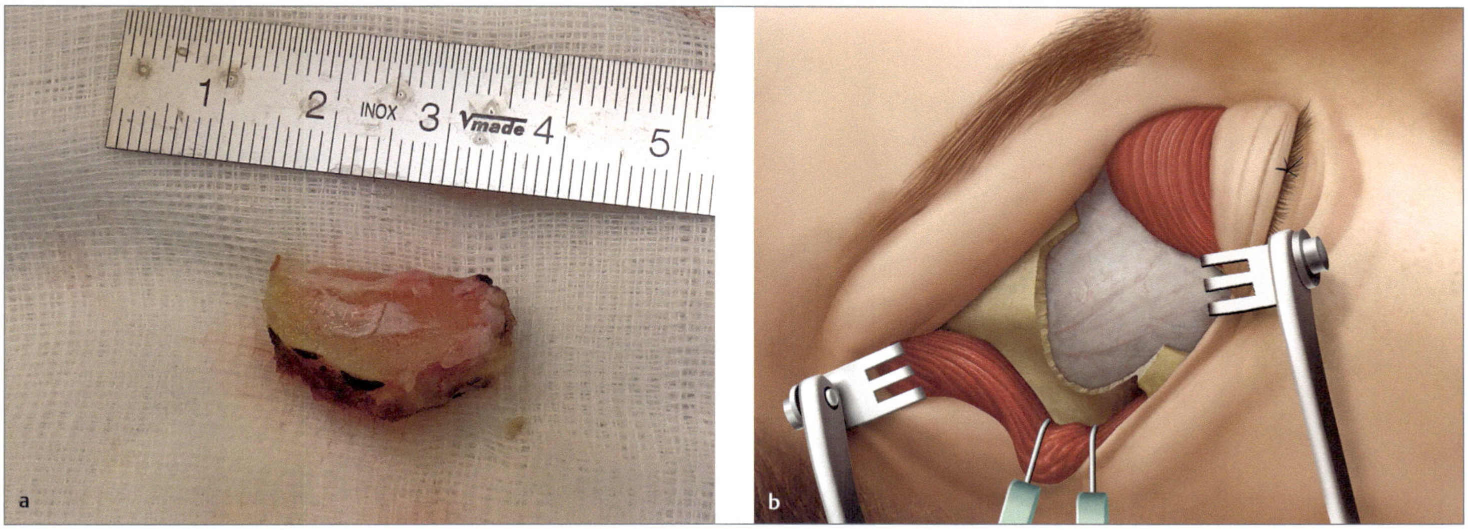

Fig. 9.22 (a, b) Lateral orbitotomy. The two vertical cuts should meet, resulting in a single bone flap 1.5–2.0 cm high and 2.5–3.0 cm wide. Additional bone can be drilled out using the bone scalpel or a high-speed drill to extend the orbitotomy in a posterior direction if needed. The periorbita is incised using a diamond knife or microscissors. The periorbita is often thinned by the raised intraorbital pressure caused by the lesion and the lateral rectus muscle, which is situated immediately beneath, can often be seen through the periorbita.

Opening the periorbita exposes the lateral rectus muscle, the lacrimal artery and nerve, and the lacrimal gland. A PDS 5–0 traction suture can be used to retract the muscle superiorly or inferiorly. Dissection proceeds by gently manipulating the intraorbital fat lobules using cotton swabs as blunt dissectors and exposes the structures lateral to and above and below the optic nerve, as well as the insertion of the lateral rectus and inferior oblique muscles on the globe.

The intraorbital tumors are resected using standard microsurgical techniques. Sharp dissection is preferred as blunt dissection can injure the fine intraorbital nerves, especially in the posterior intraconal area. Bipolar electrocoagulation with a very low power setting is often useful to shrink large intraorbital cavernomas to facilitate en bloc resection, whereas large neurinomas and meningiomas are resected in a piecemeal fashion.

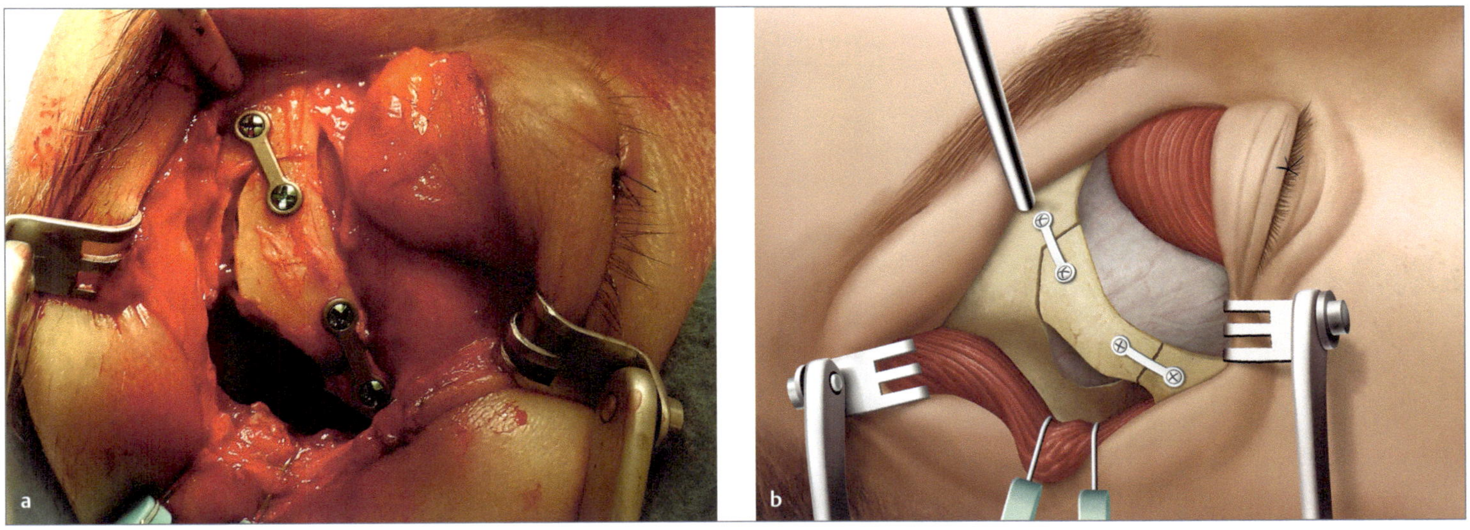

Fig. 9.23 (a, b) Closure. After the resection, any bleeding is controlled by applying hemostatic matrix rather than bipolar diathermy. A small piece of TachoSil is placed over the intraorbital fat to reconstruct the periorbita. The lateral orbital rim and wall, which has been elevated in a single piece, is replaced after removing the intraorbital lesion and fixed with 1-mm titanium mini-plates.

Care is taken to ensure that the bone flap is flush with the surrounding cranium to avoid any irregularities that will be noticeable by the patient on palpation. Irregularities or gaps can be filled using hydroxyapatite cement.

Closure is performed under the microscope to assure the best possible result. The wound is closed in three layers. The temporal muscle is reattached to the posterior margin of the zygomatic process of the frontal bone to ensure a good cosmetic outcome, using a 3–0 suture. The subcutaneous layer is closed with a running suture of the same material.

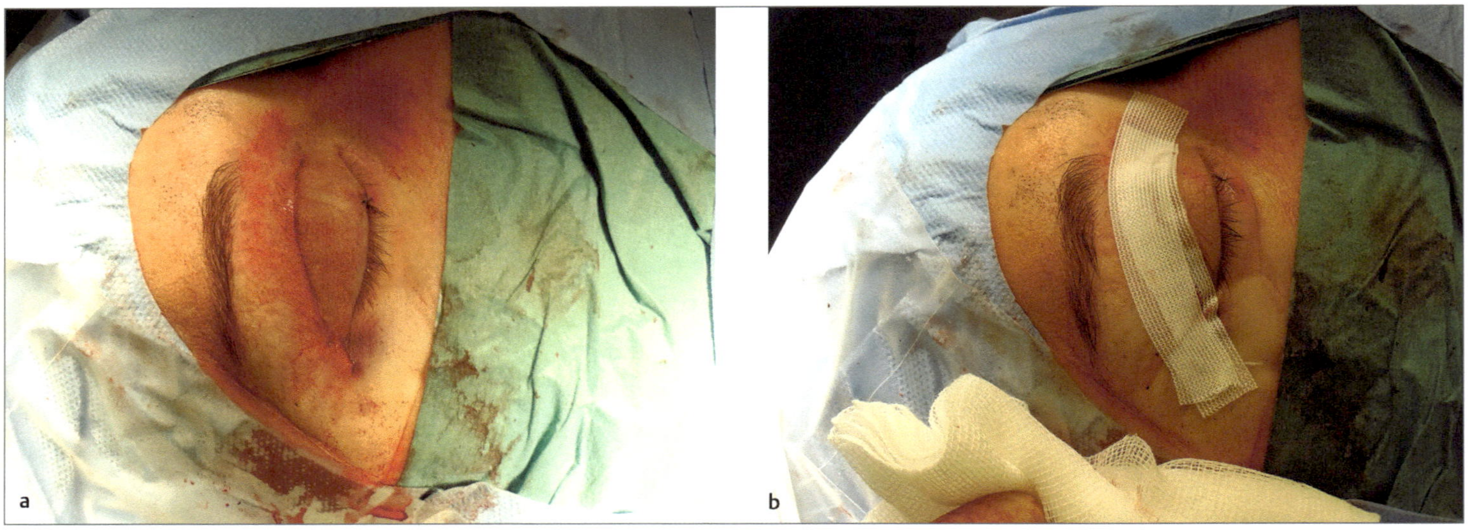

Fig. 9.24 (a, b) Closure. The skin is closed using intracutaneous Vicryl Rapid 4–0. The wound is dressed using Steri-Strip.

Checklist

- Look at CT or MR images to familiarize yourself with the frontal sinus anatomy. Cave: very lateral extensions.
- Before skin incision, make sure the patient's head is elevated enough to avoid venous congestion.
- Make a temporary tarsorrhaphy to protect the cornea.
- The skin incisions should follow the relaxed skin tension lines for optimal cosmesis.
- Mark the skin incision with a fine-tipped permanent marker pen before injecting local anesthetics.
- Make the skin incision perpendicular to the skin surface when an eyelid incision is used, or at a 45° angle when an eyebrow incision is used.
- Traverse the orbicularis oculi muscle by blunt dissection.
- Incise the periosteum sharply and stay directly on the bone when exposing the lateral orbital wall internally and externally, so as not to injure the periorbita and bulbus oculi.
- Use an electric 1-mm bone scalpel or a pediatric craniotome for the bone cuts so as to reduce bone loss.
- Fix the orbital bone flap with Lorentz 1-mm titanium mini-plates.
- Take care to level the bone flap so that it is flush with the surrounding cranium to avoid any irregularities, and use BoneSource hydroxyapatite cement to fill any larger gaps.
- Close the wound under the microscope to assure optimal cosmetic results.

Index

Note: Page numbers set in **bold** or *italic* indicate headings or figures, respectively.